SURGICAL INFECTIONS

SURGICAL INFECTIONS

Edited by

DONALD E. FRY, MD

Adjunct Professor of Surgery
Northwestern University Feinberg School of Medicine
Chicago, Illinois
Emeritus Professor of Surgery
University of New Mexico School of Medicine
Albuquerque, New Mexico
USA

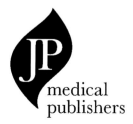

JP
medical
publishers

London • St Louis • Panama City • New Delhi

Published by JP Medical Ltd, 83 Victoria Street, London, SW1H 0HW, UK
Tel: +44 (0)20 3170 8910   Fax: +44 (0)20 3008 6180
Email: info@jpmedpub.com   Web: www.jpmedpub.com

ISBN: 978-1-907816-26-0

British Library Cataloguing in Publication Data
A catalogue record for this book is available from the British Library

Library of Congress Cataloging in Publication Data
A catalog record for this book is available from the Library of Congress

JP Medical Ltd is a subsidiary of Jaypee Brothers Medical Publishers (P) Ltd, New Delhi, India.

Publisher:	Geoff Greenwood
Development Editor	Gavin Smith
Design:	Designers Collective Ltd

Indexed, typeset printed and bound in India.

Preface

The management of infection has a long history and continues to be a major challenge for surgeons in all specialties, for whom infectious disease had its earliest major relevance in the management of battlefield casualties. Ambroise Paré identified that the topical treatment of traumatic wounds influenced the outcome. His substitution of a turpentine-based topical treatment, as opposed to the boiled oil and cauterization method, was a beginning for antisepsis at the injury site. In the 17th century, Leewenhoek first observed bacteria and became the 'Father of Microbiology'. Bacteria were not viewed as being of pathologic significance at that time. In the 18th century, the Scottish surgeon John Hunter observed the value of open management and delay closure of battlefield wounds, an observation that should be remembered today.

The 19th century saw significant progress in understanding and managing infections of the surgical patient. The Hungarian Semmelweis, working at the Vienna General Hospital, identified the role of obstetricians in potentially introducing a toxin or poison into birthing women with the pre-partum pelvic examination. He studied the benefits of hand-washing with sodium hypochlorite solution and demonstrated a reduction in the rate of what was called 'child bed fever'. Of course, the germ theory of disease was not yet formulated and an infectious agent (*Streptococcus pyogenes* as it turned out) was not suspected. Despite clinical evidence of benefit, the work of Semmelweis was not accepted at the time.

It was Louis Pasteur who developed the germ theory of disease, which largely originated in his work on the bacterial contamination of French wine and his studies of silkworm infections. He proposed microbes as infectious pathogens in man but unfortunately a stroke prevented him from claiming the scientific achievement of proving his theory. Nevertheless, his contributions subsequently led to the development of the rabies and anthrax vaccines. Perhaps his ultimate contribution was the Pasteur Institute, which prospers to this day, with original research into infection and the host response. Elie Metchnikoff was one of the first appointees at the Pasteur Institute, and is generally credited with being the father of immunology. Metchnikoff earned the Nobel Prize in 1908 for the discovery of phagocytic cells.

Robert Koch, a German physician, developed the scientific evidence to prove the germ theory and the internationally recognized Koch postulates. His early research with anthrax in the 1870s was conducted in a home laboratory using a microscope given to him by his wife. He discovered *Mycobacterium tuberculosis* in 1882, for which he received the Nobel Prize in 1905.

With the dawn of the 20th century came the hope that specific treatments could be developed to treat specific infections. Paul Ehrlich discovered salvarsan as a treatment for syphilis. With this first treatment for an established bacterial infection, Ehrlich's work led to the concept of the 'magic bullet' that would be microbe specific and eradicate infection. This was conceptually different from the Pasteur and Metchnikoff idea of host enhancement through vaccines.

The discovery of penicillin and the development of sulfa compounds in the late 1920 and 1930s resulted in specific chemotherapy (Ehrlich's term) becoming the mainstay for the treatment of infection. Thus, after World War II, antibiotics were widely deployed for the treatment of infection, with different antibiotics used against different organisms. Microbial resistance patterns developed for specific pathogens and this required the development of newer drugs, or the re-engineering of older ones.

The treatment of clinical infections largely became the purview of internal medicine practitioners. It was William Altemeier who pioneered interest in the treatment and prevention of infectious problems that were unique to the surgical patient. In the 1950s, Altemeier and others began to look at antibiotics as a potential avenue not only to treat infection, but to prevent infections in the patient undergoing invasive procedures. However, early clinical trials failed to show any clinical benefit. The shortcomings of these early trials were due to very heterogeneous patient populations, but more importantly to the fact that the antibiotics were not initiated until the postoperative period. Ashley Miles at the Lister Institute in London became the father of preventive antibiotics in surgery, by conducting basic experimental studies in 1957 with John Burke from Boston, which demonstrated that the antibiotics needed to be given before the insult to achieve benefit. In 1969 Hiram Polk provided the critically stratified, prospective, randomized clinical trial to provide proof of concept. Thus, the use of antibiotics and the evolution of preventive strategies became commonplace in surgical care. The work of all of these international investigators led to the establishment of the Surgical Infection Society of North America, The Musculoskeletal Infection Society, The Surgical Infection Society of Europe, and the Japan Society for Surgical Infection.

The management of the infectious disease problems covered in this book form an integral part of surgeons' clinical duties. First, there is the patient who presents with a community-acquired infection. These infections commonly include soft tissue infections following traumatic injury (chapter 5) or intra-abdominal infections after perforation of a viscus (chapter 6). They may include brain abscess (chapter 22), empyema from pneumonia (chapter 15), or osteomyelitis (chapter 19). In community-acquired infection, treatments require combinations of surgical management of the primary focus of infection, antimicrobial therapy for the offending micro-organisms, and supportive care to manage physiologic perturbations created by the infectious event.

Second, surgical site infection (SSI) continues to be a complication of care that has defied control (chapter 4). SSI rates have dramatically improved since the times of Ambroise Paré and Joseph Lister. However, the design of surgical interventions has become more innovative with transplantation procedures, extensive surgical oncology efforts, and the general deployment of prosthetic materials to replace effete tissues. The surgical host has clearly become more susceptible, with increasing age at the time of intervention, more advanced diseases at the time of operation, and immunosuppression either associated with therapeutic interventions (e.g. corticosteroids) or loss of homestasis (e.g. trauma, shock, resuscitation). While progress has been made in the prevention of SSI, newer methods and strategies are needed.

Third, nosocomial infections of the surgical patient at anatomic sites remote from the operation have continued to complicate surgical care. The surgical intensive care unit (ICU) has provided dramatic support for critically ill patients, but has become a reservoir of increasingly resistant pathogens. Support technology has yielded endotracheal tubes (chapter 8), intravenous infusion sites and arterial lines (chapter 10), drainage catheters (chapter 9), and many other invasive devices that serve an important support function but which have become portals for microbial access to the host. Not only has our invasive support technology created the opportunity for infection, but systemic antibiotic treatment has changed the ecology of the host to one where resistant bacteria are the rule and not the exception. Thus, meticillin-resistant *Staphylococcus aureus*, extended-spectrum β-lactamase Gram-negative bacteria, and *Clostridium difficile* have become common problems of hospital-acquired infection for surgical patients.

The prevention and management of surgical infection has become a part of the management for every patient that has a surgical procedure, and justifies books that, like this one, attempt to address all of these contemporary issues. The role of infection and surgery is a dynamic one that is constantly changing. Who would have believed 40 years ago that peptic ulcer disease was an infection of the gastric mucosa with *Helicobacter pylori*? Over the last 40 years, community-acquired staphylococcal infections have been transformed from being penicillin-sensitive to being meticillin-resistant. Bacterial infections in the ICU are now commonly pan-resistant to virtually all available antibiotics. Fungal infections are all too common in severely ill surgical patients but were barely identified 40 years ago. The future of head and neck cancer is likely to be more commonly associated with human papilloma virus infection and not tobacco-associated. Finally, contagious disease has now been associated with misfolded neuroproteins (new-variant Creutzfeldt–Jakob disease) rather than nucleotide-bearing pathogens such as bacteria, fungi, or viruses. Indeed, the germ theory of disease may be returning to theory status.

Reflections on changes in infectious diseases within a surgical setting over the last 40 years can only beg the question: 'What will happen in the next 10 or so years as we go forward?' How will a text on surgical infections change over the next decade? Many of the following may occur, with some being more likely than others:

- Bacterial resistance will continue and the need for additional antibiotics will continue. *Staphylococcus aureus* will become progressively more resistant and additional mechanisms of resistance will likely be seen among Gram-negative pathogens.
- Will a post-antibiotic era of preventing and treating infections emerge? It can be anticipated that there may be increased investigation to develop vaccines and passive immunity with antitoxins and immunoglobulins. In surgery, topical agents to prevent or treat infections that modulate microbial virulence such as phosphates or siderophores will be developed.
- Immune enhancement of the host has been explored in the past with levamasole and muramyl dipeptide. Will non-specific enhancement of the host before major operations be desirable, and what will be the consequences for the enhanced host if a systemic inflammatory response emerges?
- Hospital-acquired infections with unusual pathogens are likely to increase as support technology maintains the patient through critical illness in the intensive care unit. It is likely that more fungal infections will be identified and that viruses may emerge as a new group of pathogens for postoperative surgical patients.
- What will be the influence of new diagnostic methods upon the recognition and treatment of surgically-associated infections? Amplification of microbial DNA has already become a common method in the diagnosis of *Clostridium difficile* infection. Some studies have found increased sensitivity to the detection of blood-borne DNA where conventional cultures have not identified pathogens. Will enhanced molecular detection be overly sensitive in the detection of microbes that have long since been extinguished but have left residual genetic material within the host?
- Will other infectious proteins similar to prions be uncovered to explain other neurodegenerative diseases, and will infectious protein be yet another source for nosocomial transmission in patient care?

It is certain that prevention and management of infection in the surgical patient will remain a challenge. We trust that the many contributions to *Surgical Infections* will have a useful role as we all move forward from this point in time.

Donald E. Fry

Contents

Contributors

Shawn M. Allen, MD
Resident in Otolaryngology
Department of Otolaryngology –
Head and Neck Surgery
University of Tennessee
Memphis, Tennessee
USA

Dennis F. Bandyk, MD
Professor of Vascular Surgery
Sulpizio Cardiovascular Center
University of California San Diego School of Medicine
La Jolla, California
USA

Philip S. Barie, MD, MBA
Professor of Surgery and Public Health
Department of Surgery
Weill Cornell Medical College
New York, New York
USA

Rebecca E. Barnett, MBBS, MRCS
Research Fellow
Hiram C. Polk Jr. Department of Surgery
University of Louisville
Louisville, Kentucky
USA

Adrian T. Billeter, MD, PhD
Ferguson Fellow
Hiram C. Polk Jr. MD Department of Surgery
University of Louisville School of Medicine
Louisville, Kentucky
USA

Culley C. Carson, MD
Rhodes Distinguished Professor
Division of Urology
The University of North Carolina
School of Medicine
Chapel Hill, North Carolina
USA

Shannon L. Castle, MD
Pediatric Surgery Research Fellow
Children's Hospital Los Angeles
Los Angeles, California
USA

Mitchell Challis, MD
University of Tennessee Health Science Center
Department of Otolaryngology
Memphis, Tennessee
USA

William G. Cheadle, MD
Professor of Surgery; Associate Chief of Staff for Research
and Development
Veterans Affairs Medical Center – Louisville
Department of Surgery, University of Louisville
Louisville, Kentucky
USA

Jeffrey A. Claridge, MD
Director, Trauma and Critical Care,
Metro Health Medical Center
Associate Professor of Surgery
Department of Surgery
Case Western Reserve University
Cleveland, Ohio
USA

Edwin A. Deitch, MD, FACS, FRCS Ed (Hons)
Professor of Surgery
Department of Surgery
New Jersey Medical School
University of Medicine and Dentistry of New Jersey
Newark, New Jersey
USA

Charles A. Dietl, MD
Associate Professor of Surgery
Department of Surgery
Division of Cardiothoracic Surgery
University of New Mexico Health Sciences Center
Albuquerque, New Mexico
USA

Constance Faro, MD
Department of Obstetrics and Gynecology
The Woman's Hospital of Texas
Houston, Texas
USA

Jonathan Faro, MD, PhD
Assistant Professor of Obstetrics and Gynecology
Department of Obstetrics, Gynecology and
Reproductive Sciences
University of Texas Health Science Center at Houston
Houston, Texas
USA

Sebastian Faro, MD, PhD
John T. Armstrong Professor and Vice Chairman
Chief, Obstetrics and Gynecology, Lyndon B. Johnson
General Hospital
Department of Obstetrics, Gynecology and Reproductive
Sciences
University of Texas Health Science Center at Houston
Houston, Texas
USA

Jordan E. Fishman, MD, MPH
General Surgery House Officer
Department of Surgery
New Jersey Medical School
University of Medicine and Dentistry of New Jersey
Newark, New Jersey
USA

Henri R. Ford, MD, MHA
Vice President and Surgeon in Chief
Children's Hospital Los Angeles
Professor and Vice Chair of Surgery
Vice Dean of Medical Education
Keck School of Medicine
University of Southern California
Los Angeles, California
USA

Donald E. Fry, MD
Adjunct Professor of Surgery
Northwestern University Feinberg School of Medicine
Chicago, Illinois
Emeritus Professor of Surgery
University of New Mexico School of Medicine
Albuquerque, New Mexico
USA

Susan Galandiuk, MD
Professor, Department of Surgery
Program Director, Section of Colon and Rectal Surgery
Director, Price Institute of Surgical Research, University of
Louisville
Department of Surgery
University of Louisville School of Medicine
Louisville, Kentucky
USA

James J. Gallagher, MD
Assistant Attending Surgeon
Assistant Professor of Surgery
William Randolph Hearst Burn Center
Weill Cornell Medical College – New York Presbyterian Hospital
New York, New York
USA

Saadi Ghatan, MD
Vice Chairman, Department of Neurological Surgery
Continuum Healthcare
New York, New York
USA

Joseph F. Golob, MD
Assistant Professor of Surgery
Department of Surgery
Case Western Reserve University
Cleveland, Ohio
USA

David N. Herndon, MD
Professor of Surgery
Jesse H. Jones Distinguished Chair in Burn Surgery
University of Texas Medical Branch – Galveston
Chief of Staff and Director of Research
Shriners Hospital for Children – Galveston
Galveston, Texas
USA

Kelley D. Hodgkiss-Harlow, MD
Clinical Assistant Professor of Vascular Surgery
Section of Vascular Surgery
Kaiser Permanente
San Diego, California
USA

Ziad Kanaan, MD, PhD
Resident in Medicine
Department of Internal Medicine
Wayne State University
Detroit, Michigan
USA

Raj Kurpad, MD
Resident, UNC Division of Urology
The University of North Carolina
School of Medicine
Chapel Hill, North Carolina
USA

Gal Levy, MD
Surgical House Officer
Department of Surgery
New Jersey Medical School
University of Medicine and Dentistry of New Jersey
Newark, New Jersey
USA

John C. Marshall, MD, FRCSC
Professor of Surgery
Department of Surgery
St Michael's Hospital
University of Toronto
Toronto, Ontario
Canada

John E. Mazuski, MD, PhD
Professor of Surgery
Section of Acute and Critical Care Surgery
Department of Surgery
Washington University School of Medicine
Saint Louis, Missouri
USA

Katrina Blackburn Mitchell, MD
General Surgery Resident
Weill Cornell Medical College – New York Presbyterian Hospital
New York, New York
USA

Lena M. Napolitano MD, FACS, FCCP, FCCM
Professor of Surgery
Division Chief, Acute Care Surgery (Trauma, Burn,
Critical Care, Emergency Surgery)
Associate Chair of Surgery
Department of Surgery
Director, Trauma and Surgical Critical Care
University of Michigan Health System
Department of Surgery
University of Michigan
Ann Arbor, Michigan
USA

Michael J. Patzakis, MD
Professor of Orthopedic Surgery
Chairman, Department of Orthopaedic Surgery
Vincent and Julia Meyer Chair in Orthopaedic Surgery
Department of Orthopaedic Surgery
LAC + USC Medical Center
Keck School of Medicine
University of Southern California
Los Angeles, California
USA

Mathew C. Raynor, MD
Assistant Professor
Division of Urology
The University of North Carolina
School of Medicine
Chapel Hill, North Carolina
USA

Jianan Ren MD, FACS
Professor of Surgery, Vice-Director
Research Institute of General Surgery
Jinling Hospital, Nanjing University
Nanjing, Jiangsu
China

Noe A. Rodriguez, MD
General Surgery Resident
Department of Surgery
University of Texas Health Science Center – San Antonio
San Antonio, Texas
USA

William P. Schecter, MD
Professor of Clinical Surgery Emeritus
Department of Surgery
University of California, San Francisco
San Francisco General Hospital
San Francisco, California
USA

Jess D. Schwartz, MD
Assistant Professor of Surgery
University of New Mexico
Department of Surgery
Division of Thoracic and Cardiovascular Surgery
Albuquerque, New Mexico
USA

Joseph S. Solomkin, MD
Professor of Surgery (Emeritus)
Department of Surgery
University of Cincinnati College of Medicine
Cincinnati, Ohio
USA

Ian Udell, MD
Resident, UNC Division of Urology
The University of North Carolina
School of Medicine
Chapel Hill, North Carolina
USA

Francisco O. M. Vieira, MD
Assistant Professor of Otolaryngology –
Head and Neck Surgery
Department of Otolaryngology – Head and Neck Surgery
University of Tennessee
Director of Otolaryngology – Head and Neck Surgery
Regional Medical Center at Memphis
Memphis, Tennessee
USA

Jorge A. Wernly, MD
Professor of Surgery
Department of Surgery
University of New Mexico
Albuquerque, New Mexico
USA

H. Richard Winn, MD
Professor of Neurosurgery
Director of Neurosurgery
Lenox Hill Hospital
New York, New York
Professor of Neurosurgery
Hofstra University School of Medicine
Hempstead, New York
USA

Charalampos G. Zalavras, MD, PhD, FACS
Professor of Orthopedic Surgery
Department of Orthopaedic Surgery
LAC + USC Medical Center
Keck School of Medicine
University of Southern California
Los Angeles, California
USA

Dedication

To Hiram C. Polk, Jr, M.D.

In recognition of his lifetime contribution to surgical education and research in the science of surgical infection

Chapter 1 Microbiology of surgical pathogens

Donald E. Fry

The number of pathogens responsible for infections in the surgical patient increases with each passing year. Microorganisms that were previously thought to have little pathologic significance emerge as having clinical relevance. Many accepted pathogens develop new virulence characteristics that create new clinical challenges. Bacterial pathogens, in particular, respond to environmental threats from new antibiotic therapy and evolve mechanisms of resistance that give them a new role in clinical infection. Fungi and viruses have become pathogens of concern in selected patients, in addition to the ever-expanding number of bacterial species.

It is the unique structure and function of each microbial species that results in the pathogenic expression of the organism. As the generation time of microbes may be measured in minutes when ideal growth conditions are present, mutant species that are better adapted for survival rapidly become dominant in the microenvironment. Newly acquired genetic material or mutation yields new virulence characteristics and new mechanisms for resistance to antimicrobial treatment. To understand virulence and the direction of new treatments, it is essential to understand the basics of microbiology of surgical pathogens.

▇ BACTERIA

Bacterial cells share many of the same structural features of mammalian cells. They have a cell membrane composed of a lipoprotein bilayer which is similar to human cells. DNA is the molecular template for orchestrating the synthesis of new proteins. Translational processes occur with cytoplasmic ribosomes that are quite similar in all animal and plant species.

There are important features of the bacterial cell that set it apart from other cell types. Bacteria have a rigid cell wall external to the plasma membrane, which serves in protecting the cell from mechanical injury but also gives unique features in the interaction with other bacteria and with phagocytes of the potentially infected host (Silhavy et al. 2010). Bacteria do not have a nuclear membrane to partition their genetic material from the cytoplasm, although the genetic material is centrally located within the cell. The genome is single-stranded DNA which is anchored in a single location to the plasma membrane. This mesosomal attachment of the DNA demarcates the cleavage point for cellular division of the mature mother cell into two daughter cells.

The cell wall–plasma membrane complex is a very important feature of each bacterial species in dictating the virulence of that species, but also in determining the sensitivities of specific bacterial cells to antibiotic therapy. The relationship of the cell wall and the plasma membrane are different between Gram-positive and Gram-negative bacteria (**Figure 1.1**).

Gram-positive bacteria have a cell wall that may be 20–50 times thicker than that of Gram-negative bacteria. Although of different thickness, the cell wall comprises a cross-linked peptidoglycan matrix that is similar in Gram-positive and -negative bacteria. The larger thickness and volume of peptidoglycan give the positive blue coloration on

the Gram stain, whereas the scant amount of the peptidoglycan matrix is responsible for the negative Gram stain of Gram-negative bacteria. The cell wall serves an important role in providing protection for Gram-positive and -negative species against adverse osmotic conditions by the prevention of cell lysis. The peptidoglycan may play a role in the virulence of Gram-positive organisms (Myhre and Aasen 2006).

Gram-positive bacteria have only a single plasma membrane that lines the internal surface of the cell wall. The cell wall and the plasma membrane adhere closely to each other; there is no periplasmic space between the cell wall and around the plasma membrane of Gram-positive bacteria. By contrast, Gram-negative bacteria have both an outer and an inner plasma membrane with the cell wall "sandwiched" in between. The outer membrane provides the unique virulence factors (e.g., endotoxin) that are not present in Gram-positive species. Furthermore, a periplasmic space exists between the internal surface of the cell wall and the inner plasma membrane. This space serves as a repository for β-lactamase accumulation and Gram-negative resistance.

The special membrane configuration of the Gram-negative bacteria has significance relative to the diffusion of macromolecules, ions, and various nutrients into the cell. The cell wall of peptidoglycan is very permeable to most macromolecules especially in Gram negatives where it is so thin. The permeability of solutes into the cell of Gram-negative bacteria is dictated by the parallel plasma membranes.

In Gram-negative bacteria, penetration of the outer cell wall–plasma membrane complex requires the presence of pores for solute transport into the cell. These pores are lined with specialized proteins, known as porins, which have permissive and exclusive qualities with respect to the passage of specific macromolecules and solutes

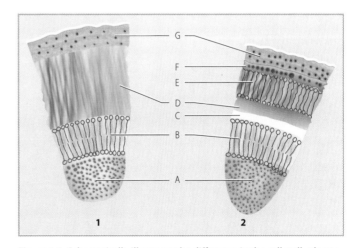

Figure 1.1 Schematically illustrates the difference in the cell wall–plasma membrane relationships of Gram-positive (1) and Gram-negative (2) bacteria. (A) Cytoplasm; (B) plasma membrane; (C) periplasmic space; (D) cell wall; (E) outer plasma membrane (only in Gram negatives); (F) location of endotoxin (only in Gram negatives); (G) bacterial capsule.

(Zeth and Thein 2010). The proteins that line the porin channel are hydrophilic passages through the ordinarily hydrophobic lipid bilayer of the Gram-negative plasma membrane complex (**Figure 1.2**). Porins may have unique electrical charge and allosteric properties that permit passage of certain water-soluble compounds while excluding others. Mutations that affect these porin molecules may confer changes to the way in which molecules enter the cell, so they will be excluded (e.g., antibiotics). The growth and division of the bacterial cell can be significantly altered by the macromolecules and solutes that can navigate the porin channel. Antibiotic access through porin channels may affect resistance or sensitivity.

The outer membrane of the Gram-negative bacterial cell presents unique antigens to the external environment. One particularly unique antigen is the lipopolysaccharide endotoxin (Brandenburg et al. 2010). Endotoxin has particular significance as a virulence factor, but also as an important recognition antigen for the host response.

Many bacteria have a capsule that is external to the cell wall and completely surrounds the microorganism (Roberts 1996). The capsule has a different composition for different bacterial species. The capsule may protect the microorganism from certain noxious environmental threats by retarding passage of selected molecules. Most importantly, the capsule provides protection from antibody or opsonic adherence and prevents phagocytosis by neutrophils from the infected host. In addition, the capsular material may have virulence factors that facilitate tissue invasion.

The bacterial cell may have a large number of external appendages with various biological functions. Flagella occur as single or multiple structures on the cell surface, and commonly are eccentrically located at one end of the cell, or may be found across the entire bacterial surface (Sowa and Berry 2008). Flagella are important in locomotion, but also have specific antigens that are recognized by the host through toll-like receptors. Sex pili are found on Gram-negative bacteria and assume importance in the exchange of extrachromosomal genetic material (e.g., plasmids), which are of significance in the transfer of acquired antibiotic resistance and perhaps other virulence factors. Fimbriae and the smaller fibrillae are external filaments that primarily facilitate adherence to other cells and surfaces. Fimbriae and fibrillae may be found on Gram-positive and -negative bacteria, and are important virulence factors in that the protein receptors on these structures mediate binding to epithelial cells of the host as the first phase of invasive infection. Likewise, these proteins are targets for immunoglobulin IgA antibodies which neutralize adherence to host surface cells.

The major components of the bacterial cell cytoplasm are ribosomes and metabolic enzymes. The ribosomes are temperature-sensitive structures and are of critical significance for the synthesis of proteins by the process of translation. Bacterial cells do not have mitochondria, but rather have the machinery of oxidative phosphorylation on the internal surface of the plasma membrane. The analogy of the internal oxidative phosphorylation apparatus of bacteria to the internal location of the electron transport particles within the mitochondria of mammalian cells provides inferential evidence of the bacterial origin of mitochondria.

■ FUNGI

Fungal cells have morphologic characteristics that are more analogous to mammalian cells than bacterial cells. Fungal cells may grow as individual yeast forms or divide and maintain continuous cell-to-cell contact as filamentous growth. The filamentous growth can be viewed as a primitive effort at tissue formation. Despite the numerous similarities of the fungal cell to mammalian cells, the presence of the cell wall still makes these microorganisms plants.

Similar to mammalian cells, fungal cells have a nuclear membrane that segregates the chromosomal material from the cytoplasm. The DNA genetic material is organized as chromosomal strands rather than the circular DNA of bacteria. Fungal cells have mitochondria within the cytoplasm for oxidative phosphorylation. Ribosomes and metabolic enzymes make up most of the cytoplasm.

The rigid cell wall of fungi provides osmotic regulation and protection similar to bacteria. However, the fungal cell wall has a different composition from bacteria. The fungal cell wall is a polysaccharide rather than the peptidoglycan of bacteria. For most species the polysaccharide is N-acetylglucosamine polymers, commonly known as chitin. An external capsule may be found on the surface of the cell wall and may contain virulence factors.

Fungi have a dimorphic character (**Figure 1.3**). They commonly occur as molds in nature, but are transformed into yeast forms when present in a suitable host with favorable temperature conditions (Nemecek et al. 2006). *Candida* spp. are a yeast that forms hyphae when

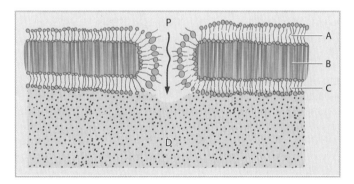

Figure 1.2 Schematically illustrates the porin channels through the cell wall-plasma membrane complex of Gram-negative bacteria. (A) Outer plasma membrane; (B) cell wall; (C) inner plasma membrane; (P) porin channel with negatively charged molecules lining the passage into (D) the cytoplasm of the bacterial cell.

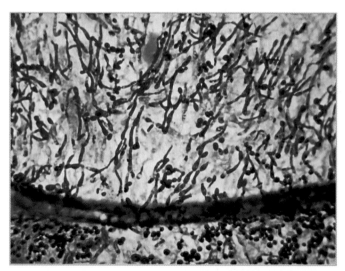

Figure 1.3 This photomicrograph demonstrates the yeast and hyphae phases of Candida albicans in a case of endocarditis. (From the Public Health Image Library, Centers for Disease Control, Atlanta, Georgia. Courtesy of Sherry Brinkman.)

present as an invasive pathogen in tissues (Sudbery 2011). Fungi of clinical significance to surgeons are discussed further in Chapter 13.

Fungi have fewer recognized virulence factors than bacteria and they are less competitive for nutrients within the microenvironment. However, the generalized use of antibiotics results in a reduction in the density and composition of bacterial colonization on epithelial surfaces, which enhances fungal colonization of the surgical host during hospitalization. The immunosuppressive drugs used in transplant recipients and the generalized immunosuppression of sustained illness or severe injury then results in increased frequency of fungal infections in the surgical patient. Given a favorable environment and an impaired host, surface adhesins facilitate binding to epithelial surfaces, and secreted aspartyl proteinases and phospholipases contribute to tissue invasion (Calderone and Fonzi 2001).

■ VIRUSES

Viruses are generally viewed as the most primitive form of infectious pathogens. Viruses not only are infectious in animal cells, but also infect plants (e.g., tobacco mosaic virus) and bacteria (e.g., bacteriophages). Viruses are extremely small, a feature that makes them not filterable by methods customarily used to entrap bacteria. Viral particles are in the range of 10–50 nm in diameter, whereas bacterial cells are 1–3 μm and fungi 4 μm. These sizes compare with the human red cell which is 6–8 μm in diameter.

The primitive viral particle is best exemplified by the fact that viruses are obligate intracellular parasites. They have no intrinsic mechanisms for cellular energy production. Without ribosomes, they cannot independently synthesize protein, so metabolic activity and replication can occur only when the virus utilizes the bioenergy and protein synthesis resources of the infected host cell.

The complete viral particle requires basically only two structural elements but may have as many as three. All viruses have nuclear material that is either DNA or RNA. DNA viruses have double strands, but RNA viruses may be either single or double stranded. One or more nucleoproteins may be associated with the viral genome. The viral genome is contained within a shell known as the capsid, which is a symmetrical structure that may be helical in configuration or icosahedral. The capsid is made up of capsomere subunits that are viral proteins. All DNA viruses are icosahedrons whereas RNA capsids may be icosahedron or helical. The capsid function is prevention of degradation of the nuclear contents as the viral particle passes from one infected cell to another. The capsid may have surface protein receptors that mediate the binding of a specific viral particle (e.g., hepatitis virus) to a specific target cell (e.g., hepatocyte).

Only the nuclear genetic material and the capsid are necessary for a complete viral particle (virion) capable of causing infection. However, some viral particles will have a third component that is an envelope around the perimeter of the nucleocapsid complex (**Figures 1.4** and **1.5**). The envelope contains both lipid and carbohydrate components, which are derived from the plasma membrane of the previously infected host cell at the time of release of the particle. The plasma membrane from the host cell in the envelope may be modified by viral glycoproteins to facilitate adherence to new host cellular targets. As the viral genome contains only the enzyme capacity to synthesize proteins, only the protein "spikes" that protrude through this envelope are of actual viral origin. The spikes are important for viral adherence to target cells. Viruses with envelopes are vulnerable to lipid solvents and non-ionic detergents where naked viruses are not.

Infection of the host cell may depend on whether the virus has an envelope or not, and whether the virus is a DNA or an RNA particle.

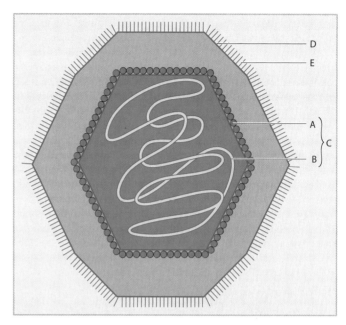

Figure 1.4 Schematically illustrates a viral particle with the envelope component. (A) The capsid shell made of capsomeres; (B) the DNA or RNA nuclear material; (C) the nucleocapsid unit; (D) the viral envelope; (E) spikes of viral protein.

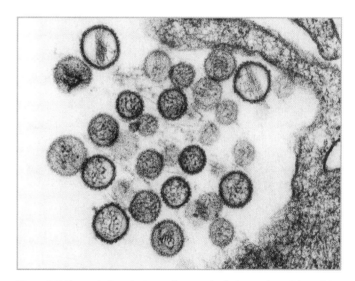

Figure 1.5 Transmission electron micrograph of a hantavirus virion with an outer envelope. (From the Public Health Image Library, Centers for Disease Control, Atlanta, Georgia. Courtesy of Brian WJ Mahy, Luanne H Elliott.)

Infection of the host cell begins with penetration through the plasma membrane into the cytoplasm. For the viral particle with an envelope, the envelope fuses with the host cell plasma membrane, which results in release of the nucleocapsid into the cytoplasm. The nucleocapsid is then degraded and the nuclear material is released. Naked viruses (those without an envelope) bind directly to the target cell surface and, by the process of endocytosis, are incorporated into a vacuole within the infected cell. Both the membrane of the vacuole and the capsid are subsequently degraded with release of the viral genome.

The pattern of infection, after release of the viral genetic material into the host cytoplasm, differs between DNA and RNA viruses. For DNA viruses, the viral genome migrates into the host cell nucleus where incorporation into the host cell chromosomal complement occurs. Transcription from the viral DNA template then becomes the means for synthesis of viral proteins and new viruses. The RNA genome may be "sense stranded" in that it becomes a direct template for the translational phase of protein synthesis in the host cell cytoplasm. The RNA genome may be "negative sense stranded" and requires synthesis of a RNA copy that is readable for translation of proteins. A notable exception to this pattern of RNA infection is the retrovirus group, as is best illustrated by human immunodeficiency virus (HIV). With retroviruses, the RNA nuclear material becomes the template for the synthesis of a complementary DNA in the cytoplasm of the host by the enzyme reverse transcriptase, and this complementary DNA then enters the nucleus of the infected cell and proceeds with viral protein transcription. Viruses of interest to surgeons are discussed in Chapter 14. New viruses of clinical significance continue to be identified and viruses of surgical significance will continue to increase.

VIRULENCE FACTORS IN MICROORGANISMS

Virulence represents the biologic potential for a given microorganism to cause infections. Although some microorganisms are viewed as having different intrinsic potential to cause infection, the emergence of clinical infection is not solely dependent on microbial virulence. It is rather determined by the microbial inoculum, the environment of infection, and the integrity of the host. Nevertheless, virulence is an important issue and it is assuming greater importance as newer treatment regimens attempt to neutralize specific virulence factors.

Virulence factors are essentially grouped into three categories. First, the microorganisms may have structural components that are shed into the local environment or released with microbial cell lysis. Second, the microorganisms may synthesize and secrete toxins, enzymes, or other biological products that injure host tissues or facilitate bacterial growth and proliferation. Finally, an important virulence factor is the development of resistance to antimicrobial chemotherapy.

Structural components

Structural components of the bacterial cell that promote virulence include specific capsular polysaccharides that are external to the cell wall (Comstock and Kasper 2006). One of the most notable of these capsular elements is the M protein coat of *Streptococcus pyogenes*. The M protein provides significant protection to the microorganism by retardation of phagocytosis by host leukocytes. The M-protein coat also appears to facilitate binding of the streptococcal pathogen to epithelial cell surfaces. The capsules of *Streptococcus pneumoniae, Neisseria meningitides,* and *Hemophilus influenzae* are also well known to resist phagocytosis. Although these organisms are efficiently cleared from the blood without opsonization by the spleen, the capsule makes them inefficiently cleared by other elements of the reticuloendothelial system (e.g., Kupffer cells). Accordingly, these microorganisms have assumed a special pathogenic role in the postsplenectomy sepsis syndrome. Isolation of these capsular polysaccharides has been used for the development of vaccines against these encapsulated bacterial strains.

The capsular polysaccharide of *Bacteroides fragilis* has been extensively studied and appears to similarly retard phagocytosis. Purification and injection of the capsular material into the peritoneal cavity of experimental animals cause abscesses without the presence of live bacteria. Thus, it would appear that the capsule of *B. fragilis* may actually exert some of its pathologic potential by being leuko-

toxic. "Shedding" of the capsule of *B. fragilis* into the environment of infection may then actually provide protection of the aerobic partner in polymicrobial infections of the peritoneal cavity or diabetic foot.

Gram-positive bacteria have unique adhesion proteins of the cell wall that mediate the binding to the extracellular matrix of the infected host tissues. These adhesion proteins are collectively referred to as **mi**crobial **s**urface **c**omponents **r**ecognizing **a**dhesive **m**atrix **m**olecules, or MSCRAMMs (Patti et al. 1994). Several unique MSCRAMMs are associated with increased microbial virulence, especially in *Staphylococcus aureus*. These surface molecules are of interest in the development of vaccines and specific immunotherapy for staphylococcal infections.

The most notable of any structural element that has virulence potential is endotoxin, the lipopolysaccharide of Gram-negative bacteria. Endotoxin is almost uniformly found in all aerobic, enteric, Gram-negative bacteria. It is a component of the outer membrane and appears to shed into the microenvironment by actively dividing bacteria; it is certainly released in large quantities with the lysis of Gram-negative bacterial cells.

Although each bacterial strain has a genetically different endotoxin, Gram-negative endotoxins customarily have the lipid A component that is associated with many of the virulent features of these bacteria. Selected endotoxins such as the endotoxin from *B. fragilis* do not have the lipid A component, and accordingly the virulence of this pathogen is mediated by mechanisms other than endotoxin.

The biologic effects of endotoxin are numerous. It is a potent activator of the complement cascade through the alternative, or properidin, pathway. The release of potent cleavage products by complement activation stimulates mast cells to release inflammatory proteins and likewise activates neutrophils and macrophages. Endotoxin is identified to directly activate neutrophils without the requirement of an intermediary macrophage cytokine. This activated state occurs through the formation of an endotoxin complex to lipopolysaccharide-binding protein, which in turn binds to the CD-14 receptor site on the neutrophil. Neutrophil activation leads to the synthesis and production of reactive oxygen intermediates, which serve an important role in intracellular killing of ingested bacteria, but may have destructive effects on tissues and the microcirculation.

Endotoxin is a potent direct stimulus to macrophages and provokes the release of biologically active cytokines. Endotoxin-stimulated macrophages produce tumor necrosis factor (TMF). Endotoxin is particularly noted for causing fever either through the release of Interleukin-1 (IL-1) from macrophages or even from direct hypothalamic stimulation without a cytokine mediator. In addition to IL-1, IL-6, IL-8, and many other important chemical signals, all of which are redundant signals that mediate various components of the acute-phase response, fever, and other sequelae of inflammation, are produced by stimulated macrophages. Furthermore, the role of endotoxin as an agonist signal to stimulate the neuroinflammatory response and the modulation of the numerous pro- and counterinflammatory responses remain to be fully elucidated.

Endotoxin activates both the intrinsic and the extrinsic pathways of the coagulation cascade. Similarly it provokes platelet aggregation and the release of vasoactive compounds (e.g., thromboxane A_2) from this source. These combined effects of endotoxin on coagulation proteins and platelets result in its clinical association with disseminated intravascular coagulation.

Secreted toxins

Secreted products by the bacterial cell result in the expression of virulence. Secretable expanded repertoire adhesion molecules are identified from *S. aureus* that are the soluble analogues of the MSCRAMMs in the facilitation of binding to host tissues (Chavakis et al. 2005). Other secreted products include the exotoxins, which are most notably produced by *Clostridium* spp. and have hemolytic, neurotoxic, cytotoxic, and enteropathogenic effects.

Hemolytic secretory products are synthesized by other groups of pathogenic bacteria besides the *Clostridium* spp. Potent hemolysins are produced by strains of both group A streptococci and *S. aureus*. The production of these hemolysins is best exemplified when the microorganisms are cultured on blood agar plates. The hemolytic character of streptococci has long been used to classify these bacteria and has been associated with those strains that have the greatest pathogenic potential.

In addition to expressing toxicity to red blood cells, white blood cell toxicity is another virulence factor that can be secreted by selected pathogenic bacteria. Leukocidins have been traditionally recognized as secretory products of *S. pyogenes* and *S. aureus*. In studies designed to elucidate the pathologic adjuvant effects of hemoglobin, Pruett et al. (1984) identified a product from the metabolism in hemoglobin by *Escherichia coli* that appears to be toxic to leukocytes. This feature of certain Gram-negative bacteria may play a significant role in the suppurative character of selected Gram-negative infections, particularly those within the peritoneal cavity. Panton–Valentine leukocidin (PVL) is a unique exotoxin produced by community-associated meticillin-resistant *S. aureus* (CA-MRSA). PVL consists of two proteins that create plasma membrane damage in host cells and is a contributor to the virulence of CA-MRSA (Boyle-Vavra and Daum 2007).

Coagulase activity is another virulence factor that provokes activation of the coagulation cascade. This secretory activity has been associated with pathogenic *S. aureus* and has been generally identified as a marker for bacterial virulence. The activation of fibrinogen to fibrin by this enzyme results in the precipitation of fibrin about the staphylococcal microorganisms and provides a measure of protection against phagocytosis. This enzyme results in thrombosis of the microcirculation in staphylococcal infections and contributes to the local ischemia and pyogenic character of these infections. Although coagulase production has been customarily identified with *S. aureus*, it can also be identified with *E. coli*, *Serratia* spp., and *Pseudomonas aeruginosa*.

An important host defense mechanism for the eradication of bacteria is the production of reactive oxygen intermediates by phagocytic cells in the process of intracellular killing of phagocytosed microorganisms. A significant virulence factor is the ability of bacteria to produce enzymes that neutralize the effects of these toxic oxygen intermediates. *B. fragilis* can produce superoxide dismutase, which converts superoxide ion to hydrogen peroxide and attenuates the cytotoxic effects of this phagocytic cell product. *E. coli* may produce catalase, which then completes the neutralization process by the conversion of hydrogen peroxide to water. Thus, the combined effects of these two bacterial strains, which are commonly identified in polymicrobial infections within the abdominal cavity, can totally neutralize a major phagocytic cell mechanism for the eradication of bacteria.

The production of enzymes that degrade the extracellular matrix of host tissues and facilitate bacterial proliferation is also an important virulence factor. Collagenase production degrades the fundamental collagen structure that constitutes the "skeleton" of many tissues. Collagenase is produced by *S. pyogenes*, *S aureus*, and selected strains of *P. aeruginosa*. Hyaluronidase and heparinase similarly have the biologic function of degradation of the intercellular matrix. Hyaluronidase and heparinase are produced by *S. pyogenes*, *S. aureus*, and by selected strains of *Clostridium* spp. Siderophores are chelating proteins secreted by selected bacteria that provide a competitive advantage in capturing ferric iron (Fe^{3+}) from the microenvironment (Krewulak and Vogel 2008). Ferric iron is essential for metabolic processes and cellular division, and siderophore proteins facilitate solubility and capture. Siderophore-producing bacterial cells have a competitive advantage for virulence compared with non-producing bacteria in the microenvironment and are considered more virulent. Examples of siderophores include enterobactin from *E. coli*, bacillibactin from *Bacillus* spp., and pyoverdine from *P. aeruginosa*.

A particularly interesting virulence factor that is of considerable recent interest is the production of biofilm (Cogan et al. 2011). This secreted polysaccharide is produced when selected bacteria establish contact with natural or foreign body surfaces. The biofilm facilitates microbial adherence to surfaces, but retards cellular and humoral elements of host defense from contacting the pathogen. It will also interfere with antimicrobial contact with the microbe. Biofilms are receiving more attention because they are being recognized as being more prevalent in many clinical infections. The rigid character of this extracellular polysaccharide in selected circumstances (e.g., vascular graft infections) may also pose special problems in attempts to culture the putative pathogens. Thus, sonication of suspected foreign bodies and tissue implants may be necessary to disrupt the rigid configuration of this polysaccharide, to permit effective cultures to be performed.

Superantigens are secreted protein toxins that bind to the major histocompatibility class II and T-cell receptors to provoke a massive proinflammatory response in the host (Alout and Müller-Alouf 2003). The toxic shock syndromes associated with staphylococcal and streptococcal infections are the most common clinical scenarios. A broad array of superantigens has been identified (Fraser and Proft 2008) and more than one unique toxin may be produced by a given clinical isolate. Fortunately, genetic encoding for these superantigens is identified only in a minority of staphylococcal and streptococcal strains. Targeting superantigens for newer treatment strategies is being pursued.

◼ Antimicrobial resistance

Resistance to antibiotic treatment has emerged as the major virulence factor for the surgical patient. Pathogens with only ordinary virulence characteristics can become extraordinarily difficult to manage in clinical infections because of the development of resistance. It has been the adaptation of resistance more than the development of new virulence characteristics that has significantly yielded suboptimal results in the prevention and management of clinical infection. Selected bacterial species (e.g., *S. aureus*) have been uncanny in the development of resistance in very short periods of evolutionary time. This emergence of resistance to specific antibiotics has meant that the search for new agents will be an endless one.

As microorganisms are identified as being sensitive or resistant to a given antibiotic, it is important to understand what resistance means. Antibiotic sensitivity is described as being bacteriostatic or bactericidal for a specific microbial density (microbes/ml) and at a specific concentration of the drug. An antibiotic is deemed to be bactericidal if it actually kills the microbe, and it is bacteriostatic if the organism remains viable but has growth inhibited by the drug. There may also be subtherapeutic effects of the drug that neither kill nor inhibit microbial replication but may change the phenotype of the bacterium.

Antibiotics generally work by binding to a target receptor. The target receptor is usually an enzyme that is instrumental in a critical process for synthesis or metabolism of the organism. For a given bacterial cell, binding of the antibiotic molecule must occur to a critical threshold of receptor sites before bactericidal or bacteriostatic effects are seen.

If the drug is present in an inadequate concentration to bind the necessary threshold of target sites, a resistant phenotype is observed. If the organism is present in very high or very low concentrations, then the number of target sites will be great or small, and the effect of a given drug is influenced by the total number of target sites that are bound to achieve antimicrobial effect. Determinations of resistance and sensitivity are generally indexed to a microbial concentration of 10^5 organisms/ml for definition of cidal or static effects at achievable drug concentrations. The "breakpoint" is the concentration of drug at which 90% inhibition is observed against the reference 10^5/ml concentration of bacteria. The *inoculum effect* is the identification of microbial resistance at high concentrations of the bacteria when the organism is sensitive at the reference 10^5/ml. Although not often discussed, the inoculum effect explains in part why treatment with appropriate antibiotics may yield suboptimum results if microbial density at the site of infection is very high (e.g., abscesses).

Another consideration in antibiotic use is the *post-antibiotic effect*. The antibiotic may be irreversibly bound to the target receptor or it may dissociate when environmental drug concentration drops below a critical level. If the drug is irreversibly bound, the effects of the drug are sustained after drug elimination from the microenvironment. Thus, antibiotics such as the aminoglycosides bind irreversibly to the ribosomal target site and have sustained effects even though the drug has been cleared. This is the basis for once-daily treatment of selected infections with this group of antibiotics. Other drugs such as the cephalosporins in the treatment of Gram-negative infections generally require maintenance of the critical drug concentration to have sustained effects, because clearance of the drug leads to dissociation of the molecules from the target site and loss of antimicrobial effect.

It must be emphasized that antibiotic sensitivity is determined in the clinical laboratory under ideal environmental conditions. For aerobic pathogens, ideal growth conditions are chosen with appropriate oxygenation, optimum pH, and no protein present in the environment. Unfortunately, the microenvironment of infection is not ideal (Fry et al. 1982). The microenvironment may have predominantly anaerobic conditions that adversely affect those drugs (e.g., aminoglycosides) that require oxygen for effectiveness (Verklin and Mandell 1977). The pH of pus and inflammation is acidic rather than neutral and this too may affect the affinity of the drug at the target site. Furthermore, the microenvironment of inflammation and suppuration is rich in fibrin and protein, which is likely to affect highly protein-bound antibiotics. These observations about the microenvironment, when combined with the discussion about the inoculum effect, indicate that in vitro microbial activity may not linearly translate into clinical effectiveness, especially in pyogenic infections. Microbial sensitivity as portrayed by the microbiological laboratory must be validated by clinical trials.

Genetics of resistance

Bacteria may be resistant to specific antibiotics because the organism may not have a susceptible target site for that drug (Young and Mayer 1979), e.g., conventional penicillin has never had activity against enteric Gram-negative bacteria. The development of resistance by formerly sensitive bacteria means that a structural or functional change in the target site within the microorganism has mediated the susceptibility change. The receptor site has changed, the target metabolic enzyme has been bypassed by an alternative, or efflux pumps are excluding the drug from the cell. These structural or functional changes are mediated by either acquired genetic material (e.g., plasmids) or chromosomal mutation. The fact that resistance can develop during a course of antibiotic therapy clearly indicates that random chromosomal mutation is not the only mechanism that is responsible for this rapid phenotypic

change. Once a genetic change has occurred, the single mutated and phenotypically changed microorganism then becomes the predominant strain within a given environment because sustained antibiotic pressure within that environment "selects out" the resistant form.

Mutation is a relatively rare event among bacteria. During a single generation of a bacterial cell, a mutation is estimated to have a probability of 10^{-7}–10^{-8}. Many mutations that occur have no particular significance to the microorganism. Others may actually make the microorganism less resilient and result in the less suitably adapted mutant becoming extinct. An occasional mutation may lead to changes that confer a state of less vulnerability to antibiotic activity.

Extrachromosomal acquisition of additional genetic material in the form of plasmids is probably the most important mechanism for acquired resistance. Plasmids are circular pieces of genetic material that can be acquired by bacterial cells and result in acute structural or functional changes that mediate acute changes in bacterial resistance. Plasmids doubtlessly had their origin from liberated chromosomal material after the death and lysis of bacterial cells. Much of this liberated genetic material is degraded. However, those plasmids that could serve functional value for the recipient bacterial cell which can internalize this external DNA result in phenotypic changes.

The internalization of external genetic material can occur by several mechanisms. Transformation is the process where external genetic material is directly acquired from the surrounding environment by the bacterial cell. Plasmids may gain passive entrance into other bacterial cells via the pores, which have been previously described. This external genetic material remains in an extrachromosomal location within the cytoplasm of the recipient cell, where transcriptional processes may then lead to genetic expression. Replication of the plasmid likewise occurs from the cytoplasmic compartment, totally independent of the bacterial cells' normal chromosomal complement.

Transduction is the process where the extrachromosomal genetic material is transported into the bacterial cell by a bacteriophage. Bacteriophages may have free plasmids within their primitive structure from previously infected bacterial cells. Bacterial genetic material may actually have been incorporated into the genome of the viral particle itself. Thus, viral DNA that is inserted into the genome of the infected bacterial cell may carry other bacterial DNA material with it, which results in the incorporation of plasmid DNA into the chromosomal complement of the bacteriophage-infected cell.

Conjugation refers to the process where bacteria may exchange plasmids by direct cell-to-cell transfer (Llosa et al. 2002). Many species of bacteria have sex pili that serve as direct conduits for the passage of cytoplasmic components from one bacterial cell to another. The process of conjugation can permit the transfer of plasmids and antibiotic resistance among bacterial cells within a given environment. Plasmids can be exchanged from one species of bacteria to another. Conjugation is most commonly appreciated among the Gram-negative *Enterobacteriaceae*.

Mechanisms of resistance

Antibiotics within the major subgroups share common mechanisms of activity and likewise share common patterns of resistance. Resistance that develops to one drug within a group may actually confer resistance to the entire group. Thus, it becomes appropriate to discuss resistance by antibiotic group.

β-Lactams

As discussed earlier, the β-lactam group of antibiotics has the principal action of inhibition of cell wall synthesis. Inhibition of cell wall synthesis results in lysis of actively dividing cells because of loss of osmotic control (Tomasz 1979). Inhibition of cell wall synthesis may also acti‑vate autolysins that actually mediate death of the organism (Tomasz et al. 1970). The activity of β‑lactam antibiotics does require binding to target sites that are on the inner aspect of the plasma membrane.

The most important mechanism for resistance in β‑lactam antibiot‑ics is β‑lactamase. β‑Lactamases represent a broad array of enzymes that are produced by virtually every known bacterial organism. These enzymes cleave the amide bond of the lactam ring by hydrolysis and thus neutralize the drug effect on the cell wall target. Since the initial isolation of an enzyme that hydrolyzed penicillin (Abraham and Chain 1940), literally hundreds of these types of β‑lactamases have been isolated.

This β‑lactamase activity appears to be ubiquitous among all bacte‑rial species and found even among some yeast isolates. β‑Lactamases are coded as part of the normal chromosomal genetic information and have been identified from bacteria recovered from times before the use of antibiotics. Naturally occurring β–lactamases may play a role in the cleavage of chemical intermediates in the polymerization of peptidoglycans as part of normal cell wall biosynthesis.

However, the development of acquired bacterial β‑lactamases from plasmids has become a more clinically important source of β‑lactamase production and resistance. The threat of acquired resis‑tance by this mechanism can be so great and acquired so efficiently that resistance may occur even during the course of treatment.

The activity of each β‑lactamase enzyme appears to be unique, with each enzyme having substrate specificity. As there are nearly 1000 dif‑ferent β‑lactamases that have been identified, efforts have been made to categorize these enzymes by functional or molecular criteria (Bush and Jacoby 2010). These enzymes are commonly viewed as being on a continuum, with some being principally penicillinases, cephalospo‑rinases, or even carbapenemases (**Table 1.1**). Unique enzymes are identified in Gram‑positive, Gram‑negative, and anaerobic bacteria.

The mechanisms whereby β‑lactamases mediate resistance are actually twofold. First, the enzyme may simply be synthesized by the organism, released into the environmental milieu, and then it hydro‑lyzes the lactam ring of the antibiotic. However, strains of *Pseudomo‑nas* spp. have been isolated that appear to have developed β‑lactam resistance, but the new β‑lactamase does not hydrolyze the drug.

This non‑hydrolytic activity of β‑lactamase appears to be secondary to the enzyme binding to the antibiotic by a tight and non‑reversible bond. The subsequent antibiotic–enzyme complex may effectively neutralize drug activity by interfering with binding to the protein‑bind‑ing site on the plasma membrane. This mechanism may actually be activated by de‑repression of genes within the normal chromosomal genome. The rapidity of this de‑repression and induction of enzyme production may be important in the emergence of resistance during therapy. β‑Lactamase induction by this mechanism has been associ‑ated with cross‑resistance to other drugs within the group.

Although β‑lactamases have been the major focus of investigation into acquired resistance for β‑lactam antibiotics, non‑β‑lactamase mechanisms may mediate resistance. Movement of the antibiotic through the cell wall may be impeded by acquired or mutational phenotypic changes. Changes in the penicillin‑binding proteins them‑selves may alter the affinity of the drug. Either reduced binding or en‑hanced ability of the bacterial cell to synthesize new penicillin‑binding sites will result in attenuation of the drug effect on the organism.

Aminoglycosides

Aminoglycoside antibiotics are actively transported into the bacterial cell where binding to cytoplasmic ribosomes results in inhibition of protein synthesis. The transport process is energy dependent and requires an electrochemical gradient of protons. The active transport process results in concentrations that are much greater within the cell than in the external environment. The absence of a transport mecha‑nism excludes aminoglycosides from human cells, except proximal renal tubule and cochlear cells. An additional undefined mechanism of aminoglycoside activity has been suspected, because inhibition of protein synthesis alone may not account for the potent bactericidal effect of the aminoglycosides (Hancock 1981). The aminocyclitol antibiotics (e.g., spectinomycin) have chemical and mechanism simi‑larities to aminoglycosides (Holloway 1982), although the ribosomal target appears to be different.

Resistance to the aminoglycosides (and presumably the aminocy‑clitols) may be mediated by several mechanisms (Jana and Deb 2006). First, drug transport into the bacterial cell may be impaired or efflux pumps exclude the drug from the bacterial cell. Another mechanism of

Table 1.1 Identifies the functional group and the molecular class of the commonly identified β‑lactamase enzymes.

Functional group	Molecular class	Genetics	Comments
1. Cephalosporinases	C	Mostly chromosomal Some plasmid	Most active on cephalosporins, cephamycins, aztreonam. Resistant to clavulanate. Large amounts affect carbapenems
2. Serine β‑lactamases			
2a	A	Mostly chromosomal	Responsible for Gram‑positive resistance to benzyl penicillin; Inhibited by clavulanate
2b	A	Plasmids	Hydrolyze cephalothin and cephaloridine; inhibited by clavulanate; 2b(e) subset are extended‑spectrum β‑lactamases that hydrolyze cefotaxime, ceftazidime, and aztreonam; subgroup 2b(r) are resistant to clavulanate; subgroup 2b(er) are extended spectrum enzymes and are resistant to clavulanate
2c	A	Plasmids	Rapid hydrolysis of carbenicillin and ticarcillin; easily inhibited by clavulanate; 2c(c) subgroup hydrolyzes cefepime
2d	D	Plasmids	Rapid hydrolysis of cloxacillin, oxacillin, and carbenicillin; inhibited by clavulanate; subgroup 2d(e) hydrolyzes oxyimino‑β‑lactams; subgroup 2d(f) hydrolyzes carbapenems
2e	A	Plasmids	Hydrolyze extended‑spectrum cephalosporins; inhibited by clavulanate
2f	A	Chromosomal or plasmid	Hydrolyze carbapenems
3. Metallo‑β‑lactamases	B	Chromosomal or plasmid	Hydrolyze carbapenems but not aztreonam. Not inhibited by clavulanate
4. Unknown	Not Classed	Unknown	Penicillinases not inhibited by clavulanate

resistance is alteration of the molecular target on ribosomal proteins. Drug transport is normal but the host cell ribosomes are not bound by the drug. Enzymatic conjugation or degradation of the aminoglycoside can occur after the drug is internalized into the bacterial cell. Every known aminoglycoside is vulnerable to enzymatic neutralization by any one of several known enzymes. Plasmid exchange allows this resistance to then be transmitted to other organisms. No inhibitors of these anti-aminoglycoside enzymes have yet been identified.

Tetracyclines

Tetracyclines are actively transported across the plasma membrane of bacterial cells. Adequate intracellular concentrations result in threshold binding to the 30-S ribosome and blocks protein synthesis by the bacterial cell. Tetracycline binding to ribosomes is reversible and concentration dependent. As many as 46 different determinants have been identified that account for tetracycline resistance (Nelson and Levy 2011). Most are plasmid mediated and include: Reduced drug penetration of the bacterial cell, efflux pump systems, ribosomal protection proteins that dislodge the antibiotic from the ribosomes, and clinical inactivation of the antibiotic by specific enzyme systems.

Trimethoprim–sulfamethoxazole

These two separate antibiotics have a very similar mechanism of antibacterial action in that both drugs inhibit different enzyme systems involved in the biosynthesis of tetrahydrofolate by the bacterial cell. The sulfonamides competitively inhibit the enzyme dihydropteroate synthetase, which is essential for the chemical reaction of aminohydroxy-tetrahydropteridine and p-aminobenzoic acid. Sulfamethoxazole is the most commonly used sulfonamide at the present time. Trimethoprim has its focus of activity at a subsequent step in tetrahydrofolate synthesis by the inhibition of dihydrofolate reductase. The sequential inhibition of sulfonamide and trimethoprim has resulted in the two agents being used together to impede folate synthesis among susceptible organisms.

Naturally occurring resistance to sulfonamides and trimethoprim occurs by the inability of either drug to penetrate the cytomatrix of the bacterial cell. Acquired resistance occurs from plasmid-mediated alternative enzyme pathways that permit folate metabolism to proceed by bypassing both dihydropteroate synthetase and dihydrofolate reductase. This results in resistance to both sulfonamide and trimethoprim. Other resistance mechanisms include increased endogenous synthesis of p-aminobenzoic acid to overcome competitive inhibition, enzymatic degradation of the sulfonamide, mutational changes to both sulfonamide and trimethoprim target sites, and efflux pumps (Masters et al. 2003).

Erythromycin

Erythromycin is transported into the cell where it has reversible binding to the 50-S ribosome, blocks transpeptidation or translocation, and subsequently inhibits protein synthesis. Plasmid-mediated resistance results in changes in the binding sites on the ribosomes. This mechanism has its greatest significance among Gram-positive organisms. Chromosomal mutation may result in decreased cell wall penetration in Gram-negative bacteria, loss of ribosomal binding sites similar to that seen with plasmid acquisition, and synthesis of an esterase enzyme that hydrolyzes erythromycin. Efflux pumps have recently been implicated in Gram-positive resistance (Varaldo et al. 2009).

Clindamycin

The lincosamide antibiotics have a similar action to erythromycin with reversible binding to the 50-S ribosome. Resistance occurs in a similar fashion to erythromycin, and resistance to one drug may carry resistance to both. CA-MRSA will be identified that is sensitive to clindamycin but resistant to erythromycin. These organisms will develop inducible resistance if treated with clindamycin, and the D-test should be used to avoid this adverse event in treatment (Woods 2009).

Vancomycin

Vancomycin is a bactericidal drug that interferes with glycopeptide polymerization, or transglycosylation, after monomeric units of the peptidoglycan are synthesized in the cell cytoplasm. Cell lysis ensues when actively replicating bacteria have an incomplete cell wall. Vancomycin does affect the growth of protoplasts, reflecting a level of bacterial action that is not just the inhibition of cell wall synthesis.

Vancomycin resistance is increasing as the minimum inhibitory concentration for MRSA is increasing, and intermediate and frankly resistant staphylococci are being identified (Linden 2008). Emerging resistance likely relates to impaired penetration of the cell wall or mutation, which reduces and precludes binding of drug to the target site.

Metronidazole

Resistance to metronidazole among anaerobic bacteria remains uncommon (Löfmark et al. 2010). The drug activity is characterized by penetration of the bacterial cell, followed by reduction of the drug, binding to DNA and other macromolecular structures being the result. Cell penetration of the drug into resistant strains is slower, and reduction of the compound after penetration is dramatically slower. These changes are probably chromosomal mutation.

Quinolones

The quinolones have anti-bacterial action by inhibition of DNA synthesis and inhibition of DNA gyrase enzymes, which are important in the supercoiling of bacterial DNA. Resistance is mediated by mutation in the gene for DNA gyrase, which appears to reduce affinity of the drug target, or chromosomal changes in porin proteins, which excludes access of the quinolones from the intracellular compartment (Drlica et al. 2009). Although plasmid replication is potentially inhibited by the DNA gyrase, this acquired mechanism for resistance has assumed greater significance with the identification of several plasmids that mediated quinolone resistance.

Other antibiotics

Many other antibiotics are being employed in patient care and are summarized relative to mechanisms of action and mechanisms of resistance in **Table 1.2**. The pressure of evolving resistance among *S. aureus* and Gram-negative bacteria has resulted in new drug development but also in the revival of older drugs (e.g., rifampicin). It should be apparent that new drug development must continue or that treatment of clinical infections will need to pursue alternative treatment models for the future.

Table 1.2 Details less frequently used antibiotics, their mechanisms of action, and the mechanisms of resistance that have been identified.

Antibiotic	Mechanisms of action	Resistance mechanisms
Linezolid (Nannini et al 2010)	Binds reversibly to ribosomal receptors and inhibits protein synthesis	Mutational changes in ribosomal target sites; *cfr* gene encoding a ribosomal RNA methyltransferase
Daptomycin (Nannini et al 2010)	Inserts into and damages bacterial plasma membrane	Cell wall and membrane changes adversely affecting drug binding to target sites
Lipoglycopeptides (dalbavancin, telavancin, oritavancin) (Zhanel et al 2010)	Impair cell wall synthesis, bacterial plasma membrane effects	Changes in peptidoglycan synthesis target sites
Teicoplanin (Jung et al 2009)	Inhibits final stage of peptidoglycan synthesis	Alternative pathways for peptidoglycan synthesis; reducing binding affinity for target sites
Polymixins (polymixin B, colistin) (Falagas et al 2010)	Binding to lipopolysaccharides and disruption of outer plasma membrane	Modification of outer membrane structure
Tigecycline (Peterson 2008)	Strongly and reversibly bound to ribosomal targets to inhibit protein synthesis	Anecdotally reported; mechanism undefined
Rifampicin (Tupin et al 2010)	Inhibition of RNA polymerase	Target site mutation
Fosfomycin (Karageorgopoulos et al 2012)	Inhibits peptidoglycan synthesis	Decreased drug uptake; target site modification; drug inactivation

■ REFERENCES

Abraham EP, Chain E. An enzyme from bacteria able to destroy penicillin(letter). *Nature* 1940;**146**:837.

Alouf JE, Müller-Alouf H. Staphylococcal and streptococcal superantigens. molecular, biological and clinical aspects. *Int J Med Microbiol* 2003;**292**:429–40.

Boyle-Vavra S, Daum RS. Community-acquired methicillin-resistant *Staphylococcus aureus*. the role of Panton–Valentine leukocidin. *Lab Invest* 2007;**87**:3–9.

Brandenburg K, Schromm AB, Gutsmann T. Endotoxins. relationship between structure, function, and activity. *Subcell Biochem* 2010;**53**:53–67.

Bush K, Jacoby GA. Updated functional classification of β-lactamases. *Antimicrob Agents Chemother* 2010;**54**:969–76.

Calderone RA, Fonzi WA. Virulence factors of *Candida albicans. Trends Microbiol* 2001;**9**:327–35.

Chavakis T, Wiechman K, Preissner KT, Hermann M. *Staphylococcus aureus* interaction with the endothelium. the role of bacterial "secretable expanded repertoire adhesion molecules" (SERAM) in disturbing host defense systems. *Throm Haemost* 2005;**94**:278–85.

Cogan NG, Gunn JS, Wozniak DJ. Biofilms and infectious diseases. biology to mathematics and back again. *FEMS Microbiol Lett* 2011;**322**:1–7.

Comstock LE, Kasper DL. Bacterial glycans. key mediators of diverse host immune responses. *Cell* 2006;**126**:847–50.

Drlica K, Hiasa H, Kerns R, et al. Quinolones. action and resistance updated. *Curr Top Med Chem* 2009;**9**:981–98.

Falagas ME, Rafailides PI, Matthaiou DK. Resistance to polymixins. mechanisms, frequency, and treatment options. *Drug Resist Update* 2010;**13**:132–8.

Fraser JD, Proft T. The superantigens and superantigen-like proteins. *Immunol Rev* 2008;**225**:226–43.

Fry DE, Garrison RN, Rink RD, et al. An experimental model of intraabdominal abscess in the rat. *Adv Shock Res* 1982;**7**:7–11.

Hancock REW. Aminoglycoside uptake and mode of action. with special reference to streptomycin and gentamicin. II. Effects of aminoglycoside on cells. *J Antimicrob Chemother* 1981;**8**:429.

Holloway WJ. Spectinomycin. *Med Clin N Am* 1982;**66**:169.

Jana S, Deb JK. Molecular understanding of aminoglycoside action and resistance. *Appl Microbiol Biotechnol* 2006;**70**:140–50.

Jung HM, Jeya M, Kim SY, et al. Biosynthesis, biotechnological production, and application of teicoplanin. current state and perspectives. *Appl Microbiol Biotechnol* 2009;**84**:417–28.

Karageorgopoulos DE, Wang R, Xu-hong Y, Falagas ME. Fosfomycin. revaluation of the published evidence on the emergence of antimicrobial resistance in Gram-negative pathogens. *J Antimicrob Chemother* 2012;**67**:255–68.

Krewulak KD, Vogel HJ. Structural biology of bacterial iron uptake. *Biochim Biophys Acta* 2008;**1778**:781–1804.

Linden PK. Vancomycin resistance. are there better glycopeptides coming? *Expert Rev Anti Infect Ther* 2008;**6**:917–28.

Llosa M, Gomis-Rüth FX, Coll M, de la Cruz FdF. Bacterial conjugation. a two-step mechanism for DNA transport. *Mol Microbiol* 2002;**45**:1–8.

Löfmark S, Edlund C, Nord CE. Metronidazole is still the drug of choice for treatment of anaerobic infections. *Clin Infect Dis* 2010;**50**(suppl 1):S16–23.

Masters PA, O'Bryan TA, Zurlo J, et al. Trimethoprim-sulfamethoxazole revisited. *Arch Intern Med* 2003;**163**:402–10.

Myhre AE, Aasen AO, Thiemermann C, Wang JE. Peptidoglycan-an endotoxin in its own right? *Shock* 2006;**25**:227–35.

Nannini E, Murray BE, Arias CA. Resistance or decreased susceptibility of glycopeptides, daptomycin, and linezolid in methicillin-resistant *Staphylococcus aureus. Curr Opin Pharmacol* 2010;**10**:516–21.

Nelson ML, Levy SB. The history of the tetracyclines. *Ann N Y Acad Sci* **1241**:17–32.

Nemecek JC, Wüthrich M, Klein BS 2006;Global control of dimorphism and virulence in fungi. *Science* 2011;**312**:583–8.

Patti JM, Allen BL, McGavin MJ, et al. MSCRAMM-mediated adhesive of microorganisms to host tissues. *Annu Rev Microbiol* 1994;**48**:585–617.

Peterson LR. A review of tigecycline-the first glycylglycine. *Int J Antimicrob Agents* 2008;**32**(suppl 4):S215–22.

Pruett TL, Rotstein OD, Fiegel VD, et al. Mechanism of the adjuvant effect of hemoglobin in experimental peritonitis. VIII. A leukotoxin is produced by *Escherichia coli* metabolism in hemoglobin. *Surgery* 1984;**96**:375–83.

Roberts IS. The biochemistry and genetics of capsular polysaccharide production in bacteria. *Annu Rev Microbiol* 1996;**50**:285–315.

Silhavy TJ, Kahne D, Walker S. The bacterial cell envelope. *Cold Spring Harb Perspect Biol* 2010;**2**:a000414.

Sowa Y, Berry RM. Bacterial flagellar motor. *Q Rev Biophys* 2008;**41**:103–32.

Sudbery PE. Growth of *Candida albicans* hyphae. *Nat Rev Microbiol* 2011;**9**:737–48.

Tomasz A. The mechanism of the irreversible antimicrobial effects of penicillins. how the beta-lactam antibiotics kill and lyse bacteria. *Annu Rev Microbiol* 1979;**33**:113–37.

Tomasz A, Albino A, Zanatle E. Multiple antibiotic resistance in a bacterium with suppressed autolytic system. *Nature* 1970;**227**:138–40.

Tupin A, Gualtieri M, Roquet-Banères F, et al. Resistance to rifampicin. at the crossroads between ecological, genomic, and medical concerns. *Int J Antimicrob Agents* 2010;**35**:519–23.

Varaldo PE, Montanari MP, Giovanetti E. Genetic elements responsible for erythromycin resistance in streptococci. *Antimicrob Agents Chemother* 2009;**53**:343–53.

Verklin RM, Mandell GL. Alterations of effectiveness of antibiotics by anaerobiosis. *J Lab Clin Med* 1977;**89**:65–71.

Woods CR. Macrolide-inducible resistance to clindamycin and the D-test. *Pediatr Infect Dis J* 2009;**28**:1115–18.

Young FE, Mayer L. Genetic determinants of microbial resistance to antibiotics. *Rev Infect Dis* 1979;**1**:55–63.

Zeth K, Thein M. Porins in prokaryotes and eukaryotes. common themes and variations. *Biochem J* 2010;**431**:13–22.

Zhanel GC, Calic D, Schweizer F, et al. New lipoglycopeptides. a comparative review of dalbavancin, oritavancin, and telavancin. *Drugs* 2010;**70**:859–86.

Chapter 2 Antimicrobial agents

Lena M. Napolitano

The initial management of all surgical infections should include the initiation of early empiric antimicrobial therapy to cover all potential possible pathogens, because early and appropriate empiric antibiotic therapy improves patient outcomes (**Box 2.1**) (Kollef et al. 1999, Kumar et al. 2006, Napolitano 2010). The choice of early empiric antimicrobial therapy is guided by the specific site of infection, the common pathogens associated with that infection, and local and regional antibiograms. The goal of antimicrobial therapy is to achieve antibiotic concentrations at the site of the infection that exceed the minimum inhibitory concentration (MIC) of the microbial pathogens present. In surgical infections, antimicrobial agents are used together with adequate source control of the initial infection. This chapter reviews antimicrobial agents that are currently available and in development.

Box 2.1 Appropriate antimicrobial therapy of surgical infections

- Early diagnosis of surgical infection
- Early initiation of appropriate empiric broad-spectrum antimicrobial therapy
- Adequate source control
- Pathogen identification and appropriate de-escalation of antimicrobial therapy

---

ANTIMICROBIALS – SPECTRUM OF ACTION

The range of bacteria or other microorganisms that are affected by a certain antibiotic is expressed as its spectrum of action. Antibiotics effective against a wide range of Gram-positive and Gram-negative bacteria are said to be *broad spectrum* or *expanded spectrum*. If antibiotics are effective mainly against Gram-positive or -negative bacteria, they are *narrow spectrum*. If effective only against a single organism, they are referred to as *limited spectrum*. Empiric antibiotic therapy should be broad spectrum to cover all possible pathogens, but should always be followed by directed narrow-spectrum therapy once the organism's identify and sensitivity to antibiotics have been established – this is the process of "de-escalation" of antibiotics. Antimicrobials should be selected based on the likely bacterial pathogens that are responsible for the infectious disease, categorized as Gram-positive, Gram-negative, or anaerobes (**Table 2.1**).

Antibiotic effect

Antibiotics may have a *bactericidal* (killing) effect or a *bacteriostatic* (inhibitory) effect on a range of microbes. Bactericidal drugs may be desirable in infections characterized by poor regional host defenses, such as endocarditis and meningitis. But in most surgical infections, particularly complicated intra-abdominal infections or complicated skin and skin structure infections, there are few data to suggest that bactericidal antibiotics are associated with better outcomes than bacteriostatic antibiotics. Clinical efficacy of antimicrobials in large clinical trials should be considered rather than whether the specific antimicrobial is bactericidal or bacteriostatic.

Mechanisms of action of antibiotics

Antibacterial drugs prevent bacterial growth by disrupting the function of a wide variety of molecular targets located within bacteria and at the cell surface (**Figure 2.1**). The penicillins, cephalosporins, and carbapenems all target cell wall synthesis by inhibiting transpeptidases required for peptidoglycan formation and the crosslinking of structures in the cell wall. Metronidazole interacts with DNA and inhibits nucleotide synthesis, leading to cell death. The fluoroquinolones block DNA synthesis by inhibiting DNA gyrase, which is responsible for folding and supercoiling of the replicating DNA. The sulfonamides and trimethoprim–sulfamethoxazole (TMP-SMX) inhibit the metabolism of bacteria by inhibiting enzymes of folic acid synthesis. The peptide antibiotics (e.g., vancomycin) form complexes with the peptidoglycans

Table 2.1 Spectrum of activity of specific antimicrobials for specific pathogens.

Antibiotic	Gram negative	Gram positive	Resistant Gram negative	Resistant Gram positive	Anaerobe	Pseudomonas spp.
β-Lactam/β-lactamase inhibitor	+	+	#	0	+	#
First-generation cephalosporins	0	+	0	0	0	0
Second-generation cephalosporins	#	#	0	0	0	0
Third-generation cephalosporins	+	+	#	0	0	#
Fourth-generation cephalosporins	+	+	#	0	0	#
Fifth-generation cephalosporins	0	+	0	+	0	0
Tigecycline	+	+	+	+	+	0
Glycopeptides	0	+	0	+	0	0
Carbapenems	+	+	#	0	+	#
Quinolones	+	+	0	0	#	#

0 = no activity; + = activity; # = activity, but varies by product within class.

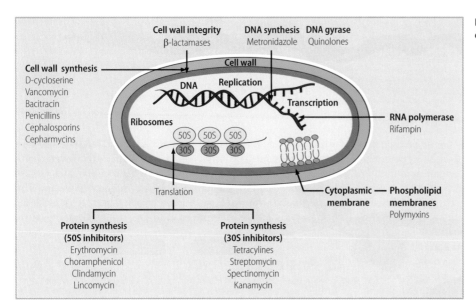

Figure 2.1 Antimicrobial mechanisms of action of various antibiotics.

that prevent binding to the transpeptidases responsible for crosslinking cell membrane structures into a rigid matrix.

A large number of antibiotics, including the aminoglycosides, macrolides, oxazolidinones, streptogramins, lincosamides, and tetracyclines/glycylcyclines, interact with bacterial ribosomes to inhibit protein synthesis (**Tables 2.2** and **2.3**).

■ Antimicrobial resistance mechanisms

Bacteria employ one or more of five basic mechanisms for developing resistance to antibiotics (**Figure 2.2**), as follows.

Antibiotic modification

The bacteria avoid the antibiotic's deleterious effects by inactivation of the antibiotic, such as enzymatic degradation of the antibiotic itself, as seen in β-lactamase-producing bacteria that destroy the β-lactam ring of penicillins and cephalosporins.

Alterations of the targets of antibiotic agents

Bacteria can also evade antibiotic action through the alteration of the compound's target, e.g., *Streptococcus pneumoniae* may express

Table 2.2 Mechanisms of action of selected antibiotics.

Antibiotic	Mechanism
Inhibitors of cell wall synthesis	
Penicillin	Inhibits transpeptidase enzymes. Activates lytic enzymes of cell wall. The affected bacterium will eventually lyse because the unsupported cell wall cannot withstand its growth
Carbenicillin	Inhibits transpeptidation enzymes. Activates lytic enzymes of cell wall
Vancomycin	Inhibits transpeptidation in crosslinking peptidoglycans. Interferes with bacterial cells at many levels, disrupting cell wall synthesis, interfering with RNA, and damaging the plasma membrane
Inhibitors of nucleic acid synthesis	
Ciprofloxacin	Inhibits DNA gyrase; interferes with DNA replication
Rifampin	Blocks RNA synthesis by binding to and inhibiting RNA polymerase
Inhibitors of protein synthesis	
Tetracyclines	Binds to the 30-S subunit and blocks the addition of amino acids, producing incomplete and probably nonfunctional proteins
Linezolid	Binds rRNA to prevent translation initiation and thus protein synthesis
Erythromycin	Binds the 50-S subunit and blocks translocation of the new protein on the ribosome, thus effectively halting synthesis
Chloramphenicol	Blocks formation of new peptide bonds during protein synthesis by binding to the 50-S subunit of the ribosome
Streptomycin	Binds the 30-S ribosomal subunit of the tuberculosis bacterium and prevents the ribosome from forming the complex necessary to initiate protein translation
Fusidic acid	Blocks translocation
Metabolic inhibitors	
Sulfonamides	Competitively inhibits dihydropteroate synthase, an enzyme that converts p-aminobenzoic acid into folic acid. These drugs can also be incorporated into a compound that resembles dihydrofolate and which in turn can inhibit another enzyme in the pathway, dihydrofolate reductase
Trimethoprim	Inhibits dihydrofolate reductase, blocking tetrahydrofolate synthesis

Table 2.3 Classes of antibiotics and their properties.

Chemical class	Examples	Biological source	Spectrum (effective against)	Mode of action
β-Lactams (penicillins and cephalosporins)	Benzylpenicillin, cephalothin	*Penicillium notatum* and *Cephalosporium* spp.	Gram-positive bacteria	Inhibits steps in cell wall (peptidoglycan) synthesis and murein assembly
Semisynthetic β-lactams	Ampicillin, amoxicillin		Gram-positive and -negative bacteria	Inhibits steps in cell wall (peptidoglycan) synthesis and murein assembly
Clavulanic acid	Augmentin is clavulanic acid plus amoxicillin	*Streptomyces clavuligerus*	Gram-positive and -negative bacteria	Inhibitor of bacterial β-lactamases
Monobactams	Aztreonam	*Chromobacterium violaceum*	Gram-positive and -negative bacteria	Inhibits steps in cell wall (peptidoglycan) synthesis and murein assembly
Carbapenems	Imipenem, meropenem, doripenem, ertapenem	*Streptomyces cattleya*	Gram-positive and -negative bacteria	Inhibits steps in cell wall (peptidoglycan) synthesis and murein assembly
Aminoglycosides	Streptomycin	*Streptomyces griseus*	Gram-positive and -negative bacteria	Inhibits translation (protein synthesis)
	Gentamicin	*Micromonospora* spp.	Gram-positive and -negative bacteria, especially Pseudomonas spp.	Inhibits translation (protein synthesis)
Glycopeptides	Vancomycin	*Amycolatopsis orientalis*, *Nocardia orientalis* (former designation)	Gram-positive bacteria, especially Staphylococcus aureus	Inhibits steps in murein (peptidoglycan) biosynthesis and assembly
Lincomycins	Clindamycin	*Streptomyces lincolnensis*	Gram-positive and -negative bacteria, especially anaerobic Bacteroides spp.	Inhibits translation (protein synthesis)
Macrolides	Erythromycin, azithromycin	*Streptomyces erythreus*	Gram-positive bacteria, Gram-negative bacteria not enterics, Neisseria, Legionella, Mycoplasma spp.	Inhibit translation (protein synthesis)
Polypeptides	Polymyxin	*Bacillus polymyxa*	Gram-negative bacteria	Damages cytoplasmic membranes
	Bacitracin	*Bacillus subtilis*	Gram-positive bacteria	Inhibits steps in murein (peptidoglycan) biosynthesis and assembly
Rifamycins	Rifampicin	*Streptomyces mediterranei*	Gram-positive and -negative bacteria, Mycobacterium tuberculosis	Inhibits transcription (bacterial RNA polymerase)
Tetracyclines	Tetracycline	*Streptomyces* spp.	Gram-positive and -negative bacteria, rickettsiae	Inhibit translation (protein synthesis)
Semisynthetic tetracycline	Doxycycline		Gram-positive and -negative bacteria, rickettsiae, Ehrlichia, Borrelia spp.	Inhibit translation (protein synthesis)
Glycylcycline	Tigecycline		Gram-positive and -negative bacteria. No activity against *Pseudomonas* spp. or *Proteus* spp.	Inhibit translation (protein synthesis)
Chloramphenicol	Chloramphenicol	*Streptomyces venezuelae*	Gram-positive and -negative bacteria	Inhibits translation (protein synthesis)
Fluoroquinolones	Ciprofloxacin, levofloxacin	Synthetic	Gram-negative and some Gram-positive bacteria (Bacillus anthracis)	Inhibits DNA replication

modified penicillin-binding proteins (PBPs) which renders them resistant to penicillins.

Active efflux of antibiotic

Bacteria can actively pump out and expel the antibiotic from the cell with the production of efflux pumps. Efflux pumps can be drug specific, as is the case in tetracycline-resistant Gram-negative bacteria, or may expel a wide variety of antibiotics from multiple classes, such as those seen in some strains of *Escherichia coli*, *Staphylococcus aureus*, *Streptococcus pneumoniae*, and *Pseudomonas aeruginosa*. An example would be the energy-dependent efflux of tetracyclines widely seen in *Enterobacteriaceae*. Tetracycline resistance results from acquisition of genetically mobile tetracycline resistance genes, which encode efflux pump proteins that expel tetracyclines from the cell or code for proteins that protect the ribosomes.

Prevention of antibiotic entry into the cell

Bacteria may induce changes in cell wall permeability that reduce antibiotic entry into the bacteria. These alterations can arise from point mutations in bacterial DNA or through the exchange of DNA fragments via the processes of transformation (i.e., "naked" DNA transfer), bacteriophage-mediated transduction, or plasmid-mediated

Figure 2.2 Antimicrobial resistance mechanisms.

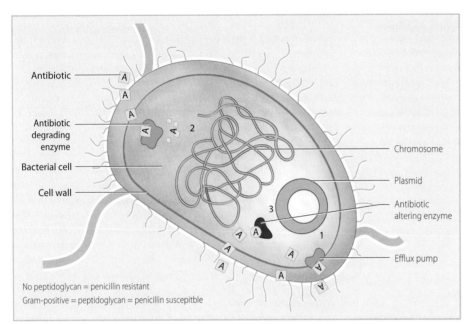

Antibiotic

Antibiotic degrading enzyme

Bacterial cell

Cell wall

Chromosome

Plasmid

Antibiotic altering enzyme

Efflux pump

No peptidoglycan = penicillin resistant
Gram-positive = peptidoglycan = penicillin suscepitble

conjugation. Production of enzymes that degrade or otherwise alter antibiotics and synthesis of antibiotic-insensitive targets are the primary mechanisms for resistance to trimethoprim and the sulfonamides, aminoglycosides, and quinolones. Reduced permeability is implicated in resistance to β-lactam antibiotics, aminoglycosides, and quinolones. In Gram-negative bacteria, porins are transmembrane proteins that allow for the diffusion of antibiotics through their highly impermeable outer membrane. Modification of the porins can bring about antibiotic resistance, as is the case of *Pseudomonas aeruginosa* resistance to imipenem.

Bypassing drug's action

The bacteria can bypass the deleterious effect of the drug without changing the original sensitive target. Examples are the alternative PBPs produced by meticillin-resistant *Staphylococcus aureus* (MRSA) in addition to the normal PBPs, and some sulfonamide-resistant bacteria that use environmental folic acid such as mammalian cells, and in this way bypass the sulfonamide inhibition of folic acid synthesis.

■ Pharmacokinetics and pharmacodynamics of antimicrobial agents

The goal of antimicrobial therapy is to select an appropriate antibiotic to eradicate microorganisms at the site of the infection, and correct dosing must be used to achieve the maximal effect and avoid toxicity. Pharmacokinetics refers to the disposition of drugs in the body and includes absorption, bioavailability, distribution, protein binding, metabolism, and elimination. Pharmacodynamics relates to the interaction between the drug concentration at the site of action over time and the desired antimicrobial effect. Both of these concepts are important to optimize antimicrobial use in surgical patients, particularly in critically ill patients. Impairment of renal or hepatic function may require alteration of the drug dosage or the dosing interval, and knowledge about which antimicrobials require dosing adjustment is mandatory.

■ SPECIFIC ANTIMICROBIALS

■ β-Lactam antibiotics

β-Lactam antibiotics are among the most commonly prescribed drugs, and are grouped together based on a shared structural feature, the β-lactam ring. β-Lactam antibiotics include the following:

- Penicillins
- Cephalosporins
- Cephamycins
- Monobactams
- Carbapenems
- β-Lactam/β-lactamase inhibitor combinations.

β-Lactam antibiotics are generally bactericidal. The mechanism of bacterial cell killing is an indirect consequence of the inhibition of bacterial cell wall synthesis.

■ Penicillins

Penicillin, derived from the penicillium mold, is one of the earliest discovered antibiotics (Zaffiri et al. 2012). Originally noticed by a French medical student, Ernest Duchesne, in 1896, penicillin was rediscovered by bacteriologist Sir Alexander Fleming working at St Mary's Hospital in London in 1928. But it was not until the 1940s that the use of penicillin began when Howard Florey and Ernst Chain developed a useful form of the antibiotic. Fleming, Florey, and Chain were awarded the 1945 Nobel Prize in Physiology or Medicine for the discovery of penicillin.

Penicillins are β-lactam antibiotics that bind to PBPs and transpeptidases on the bacterial cell surface, and inhibit cell wall synthesis and crosslinking of the peptidoglycan chains. Penicillins are excreted unchanged in urine via both glomerular filtration and tubular secretion. Ampicillin and nafcillin are also excreted in bile.

Natural penicillins include benzylpenicillin or penicillin G (administered parenterally) and phenoxymethylpenicillin or penicillin V (administered orally) and are active against streptococci, peptostreptococci, oral anaerobes, *Bacilllus anthracis*, actinomycoses, *Corynebacterium*, *Listeria*, *Neisseria*, and *Treponema* spp. Natural penicillins are commonly used for oral infections. Anti-staphylococcal penicillins include meticillin, nafcillin, oxacillin, cloxacillin, and dicloxacillin, and resist penicillinase degradation. Nafcillin is the preferred parenteral drug for the treatment of meticillin-sensitive *S. aureus* (MSSA) infections, including bacteremia.

Aminopenicillins (ampicillin, ampicillin/sulbactam, amoxicillin, amoxicillin/clavulanate) have extended the antimicrobial spectrum for Gram-negative organisms, and sulbactam and clavulanate increase activity against β-lactamase-producing organisms. These agents are used as first-line therapy for acute otitis media and sinusitis; however, they should not be used in the empiric treatment of intra-abdominal infections. The recent guidelines by the Surgical Infection Society and the Infectious Diseases Society of America (SIS/IDSA) state: "Ampicillin–sulbactam is not recommended for use in the treatment of complicated intra-abdominal infections because of high rates of resistance to this agent among community-acquired *E. coli*" (Solomkin et al. 2010a, 2010b).

Anti-pseudomonal penicillins (piperacillin, ticarcillin, piperacillin/tazobactam, ticarcillin/clavulanate) have increased activity for *Pseudomonas* spp. and other Gram-negative isolates, and decreased activity against Gram-positive organisms. In particular, piperacillin/tazobactam is commonly used for the treatment of surgical infections.

A recent study documented that avoidable metronidazole use occurred in 23.4% of all days of therapy, and that piperacillin/tazobactam was the most commonly administered drug with avoidable metronidazole use (Huttner et al. 2012). Clearly, additional education is necessary for clinicians about the adequacy of anaerobic coverage with piperacillin/tazobactam and that metronidazole is not necessary. Penicillins are associated with a hypersensitivity reaction in 5% of patients; anaphylaxis occurs only in 1 in 10 000 patients but has a 10% mortality rate.

■ Cephalosporins

Cephalosporins are β-lactam antibiotics that act on the bacterial cell wall, similar to penicillins. Cephalosporins demonstrate concentration-independent bactericidal activity, with maximal killing at four to five times the MIC of the organism. A clinically significant post-antibiotic effect is not observed with cephalosporins. Given these pharmacodynamic properties, it is imperative that optimal dosing regimens continuously maintain drug concentrations above the MIC of the pathogens. Bacterial resistance to cephalosporins is via β-lactamases. Cephalosporins are divided into five generations based on antimicrobial spectrum (**Table 2.4**).

Table 2.4 Cephalosporin antibiotics.

Spectrum of activity		Infectious diseases
First-generation cephalosporins		
Cephalothin Cefazolin Cephapirin Cephadrine Cephalexin Cefadroxil	**Gram positive** Activity against penicillinase-producing, meticillin-susceptible staphylococci and streptococci (although they are not the drugs of choice for such infections). No activity against meticillin-resistant staphylococci or enterococci. **Gram negative** Activity against *Proteus mirabilis*, some *Escherichia coli* strains, and *Klebsiella pneumoniae*, but no activity against *Pseudomonas*, *Acinetobacter*, *Enterobacter*, indole-positive *Proteus*, or *Serratia* spp.	
Second-generation cephalosporins		
Cefuroxime Cefamandole Cefoxitin Cefotetan Cefaclor	**Gram positive** Less than first-generation **Gram negative** Greater than first generation: Hemophilus influenzae, Enterobacter aerogenes, and some Neisseria and Proteus spp., E. coli, and K. pneumoniae described above	
Third-generation cephalosporins		
Cefotaxime Ceftriaxone Ceftazidime Cefoperazone Cefixime	**Gram positive** Some (especially those with anti-pseudomonal activity) have decreased activity against Gram-positive organisms **Gram negative** Further increased activity against Gram-negative organisms. Increasing ESBLs are reducing the clinical utility of this class of antibiotics. They are also able to penetrate the CNS, making them useful against meningitis caused by pneumococci, meningococci, *H. influenzae*, and susceptible *E. coli*, *Klebsiella* spp., and penicillin-resistant *Neisseria gonorrhoeae*. Since 2007, third-generation cephalosporins (ceftriaxone or cefixime) have been the only recommended treatment for gonorrhea in the USA	
Fourth-generation cephalosporin		
Cefipime	**Gram positive** They are extended-spectrum agents with similar activity against Gram-positive organisms as first-generation cephalosporins **Gram negative** Fourth-generation cephalosporins are zwitterions that can penetrate the outer membrane of Gram-negative bacteria. They have greater resistance to β-lactamases than third-generation cephalosporins; used for *Pseudomonas aeruginosa* infections. Can cross the blood–brain barrier and are effective in meningitis	Pneumonia, febrile neutropenia, urinary tract infection, skin infection, complicated intra-abdominal infection
Cephalosporin with expanded Gram-positive activity including MRSA		
Ceftaroline	**Gram positive** Broad expanded Gram-positive activity, including MRSA and vancomycin-resistant *S. aureus* **Gram negative** Activity against common respiratory pathogens and *Enterobacteriaceae* isolates	FDA approved for treatment of complicated skin and skin structure infections; community-acquired pneumonia

CNS, central nervous system; ESBLs, extended-spectrum b-lactamases; FDA, Food and Drug Administration.

Cephalosporins are one of the most widely prescribed class of antimicrobials due to their broad spectrum of activity and safety profile. The earlier generation cephalosporins are commonly used for community-acquired infections, whereas the later generation agents (with their better spectrum of activity against Gram-negative bacteria) make them more useful for nosocomial, hospital-acquired, or complicated community-acquired infections.

Hypersensitivity reactions to cephalosporins are manifested by rashes, eosinophilia, fever (1–3%), and interstitial nephritis. Given the structural similarity of cephalosporins and penicillins, an estimated 10% of patients with penicillin allergies will also be hypersensitive to cephalosporins. Cephalosporins should be avoided in patients with immediate allergic reactions to penicillins (e.g., anaphylaxis, bronchospasm, hypotension). Cephalosporins may be tried with caution in patients with delayed or mild reactions to penicillin. Among individuals with true immediate-type allergy to penicillin, desensitization to cephalosporins is usually an option in cases where no alternate antimicrobials are available (Lagacé-Wiens and Rubinstein 2012).

First-generation cephalosporins are most commonly used for surgical site infection prophylaxis where skin pathogens are the common causative pathogens. *Second-generation cephalosporins* fall into two groups, including the "true" second-generation cephalosporins (cefuroxime, cefamandole) and the cephamycins (cefoxitin, cefotetan). The cephamycins are active against most anaerobes found in the mouth and colon (e.g., *Bacteroides* spp., including *B. fragilis*). The "true" second-generation agents are useful for community-acquired infections of the respiratory tract (*Hemophilus influenzae, Moraxella catarrhalis, Streptococcus pneumoniae*) and uncomplicated urinary tract infections (*Escherichia coli*). The cephamycin group is useful for mixed aerobic/anaerobic infections of the skin and soft tissues, intra-abdominal, and gynecological infections, and surgical site infection prophylaxis in abdominal surgery. In a recent, randomized, double-blind trial of antimicrobial prophylaxis in elective colorectal surgery, ertapenem was found to be more effective than cefotetan (17.1% skin structure infection [SSI] rate in ertapenem group vs. 26.2% in cefotetan group (absolute difference –9.1; 95% confidence interval [CI] –14.4 to –3.7) (Itani et al. 2006).

Third-generation cephalosporins have increased activity against the *Enterobacteriaceae* associated with hospital-acquired infections. Some agents are also active against *Pseudomonas aeruginosa*. However, nosocomial Gram-negative isolates have a tendency to acquire antimicrobial resistance during cephalosporin therapy, and caution is required in prescribing these agents, particularly in critically ill patients. Ceftriaxone is a notable agent in this group because of its long half-life requiring less frequent dosing, adequate drug concentrations in the cerebral spinal fluid to constitute reliable empiric therapy for bacterial meningitis, and as the recommended drug of choice for gonococcal disease. Ceftazidime has increased activity against *P. aeruginosa*, but its current use is significantly limited due to the rapidly evolving group of extended-spectrum β-lactamases (ESBLs). ESBLs will hydrolyze third-generation cephalosporins and aztreonam, and are inhibited by clavulanic acid and increasing in frequency among *Enterobacteriaceae* (Paterson and Bonomo 2005).

The *fourth-generation cephalosporins* are extended-spectrum agents that have activity against most staphylococci (except MRSA), streptococci, and many Gram-negative organisms including isolates of *Serratia, Pseudomonas,* and *Enterobacter* spp. They also have a greater resistance to β-lactamases than third-generation cephalosporins. They do not have anaerobic activity, but can be used in the treatment of pneumonia and other Gram-negative infections. *Cefipime*, a broad-spectrum, anti-pseudomonal, fourth-generation, oxyimino-cephalosporin, has recently undergone significant scrutiny since meta-analyses identified that cefipime had a statistically significant (risk ratio 1.26, 95% CI 1.08–1.49) increase in mortality rates when compared with other antibiotics in randomized controlled clinical trials (Paul et al. 2006, Yahav et al. 2007). However, a review by the Food and Drug Administration (FDA) of 88 clinical trials concluded that: "data do not indicate a higher rate of death in cefepime-treated patients" (Leibovici et al. 2010). However, a Bayesian reappraisal of the FDA and Yahav meta-analysis data indicates that there is a 90.9% (by FDA trial meta-analysis), 80.8% (by FDA patient-level meta-analysis), and 99.2% (by Yahav meta-analysis) probability that cefepime raises mortality in neutropenic febrile patients. A similar harmful probability was observed with SSIs, but not with pneumonia, intra-abdominal infection, and urinary tract infections (Kalil 2011). Some have concluded that cefepime should be avoided in patients with neutropenic fever or SSIs. The FDA concludes that cefepime is an appropriate treatment option for patients with approved indications (Food and Drug Administration 2012a).

The *fifth-generation cephalosporins* include *ceftaroline* and *ceftobiprole*. Ceftaroline is the newest addition to the cephalosporin class of antibiotics (Steed and Rybak 2010, Poon et al. 2012). It is unique with activity against multidrug-resistant (MDR) *Staphylococcus aureus* which includes MRSA, vancomycin-intermediate *S. aureus* (VISA), heteroresistant VISA, and vancomycin-resistant *S. aureus, Streptococcus pneumoniae* (including drug-resistant strains), and respiratory Gram-negative pathogens. Ceftaroline exhibited a favorable safety and tolerability profile, consistent with other cephalosporins.

Two phase 3, multinational, randomized, double-blind, active-controlled clinical trials of identical design (CANVAS 1 and CANVAS 2) compared the effectiveness of ceftaroline with the combination of vancomycin and aztreonam in patients with complicated skin and skin structure infections (cSSSIs) (Corey et al. 2010a, Wilcox et al. 2010). The investigators concluded that the efficacy of ceftaroline (cure rate 85.9%) was noninferior to that of vancomycin and aztreonam (cure rate 85.5%) in the treatment of patients with cSSSIs (Corey et al. 2010b).

Two phase 3, multinational, randomized, double-blind, active-controlled clinical trials (FOCUS 1 and FOCUS 2) of similar noninferiority design compared the efficacy and tolerability of ceftaroline and ceftriaxone in the treatment of community-acquired pneumonia (CAP) (File et al. 2011, Low et al. 2011). The efficacy of ceftaroline was comparable to ceftriaxone in the treatment of CAP with equivalent cure rates in the clinically evaluable cohort (84.3% ceftaroline versus 77.7% ceftriaxone) in the combined analysis (File et al. 2010). Ceftaroline is an expanded-spectrum cephalosporin that is clinically effective for cSSSIs and community-acquired bacterial pneumonia, and it has distinctive activity against many MDR Gram-positive organisms.

The cephalosporin ceftobiprole was the first β-lactam antibiotic to have bactericidal activity against MRSA, as well as penicillin-resistant streptococci and a wide array of Gram-negative pathogens. It is highly active against both community-acquired and hospital-acquired forms of MRSA. In time-to-kill analysis, ceftobiprole was bactericidal at all concentrations tested (Leonard et al. 2008).

In a randomized, multicenter, global, double-blind trial comparing ceftobiprole with vancomycin plus ceftazidime in 729 clinically evaluable patients with cSSSIs (including diabetic foot infections), the clinical cure rate was 90.5% for ceftobiprole-treated and 90.2% for comparator-treated patients (95% CI –4.2, 4.9) (Noel et al. 2008a). In patients with MRSA infection, the clinical cure rate was 89.7% for ceftobiprole-treated and 86.1% for comparator-treated patients (95% CI –8.0, 19.7). Ceftobiprole was well tolerated, and the incidence of serious adverse events was similar in the two treatment groups.

A second global, randomized, double-blind trial compared the efficacy of ceftobiprole (500 mg every 12 h) against vancomycin (1 g every 12 h) in patients with cSSTIs caused by Gram-positive bacteria (Noel et al. 2008b). Of 559 clinically evaluable cases, 93.3% treated with ceftobiprole and 93.5% treated with vancomycin were cured (95% CI −4.4, 3.9). The cure rates for patients with MRSA infections were 91.8% (56/61) with ceftobiprole and 90.0% (54/60) with vancomycin (95% CI −8.4, 12.1). At least one adverse event was reported in 52% of the ceftobiprole-treated patients and 51% of the vancomycin-treated patients. The most common adverse events in ceftobiprole-treated patients were nausea (14%) and taste disturbance (8%). Discontinuation of the study drug because of adverse events occurred in 4% ($n = 17$) of the ceftobiprole-treated patients and 6% ($n = 22$) of the vancomycin-treated patients. Irregularities in the FDA review of clinical trial sites resulted in no approval of this drug for clinical use at present. The European Committee for Medicinal Products for Human Use (CHMP) has similarly concluded that ceftobiprole should not be authorized for use. Both Canada and Switzerland have discontinued the sale and use of ceftobiprole. Its clinical future is uncertain at this point.

Monobactams

Monobactams are monocyclic β-lactam compounds with a spectrum of antimicrobial activity against Gram-negative bacteria. Its mechanism of action is suppression of bacterial cell wall formation. It has no activity against Gram-positive or anaerobic bacteria. The only commercially available monobactam antibiotic is aztreonam. Aztreonam has no cross-hypersensitivity reactions with penicillin, and therefore it is commonly used for the treatment of infections in penicillin-allergic patients. Aztreonam is indicated for the treatment of intra-abdominal infections, lower respiratory tract infections, pelvic organ, and urogenital infections, and skin and soft-tissue infections. An additional antibiotic is required with aztreonam to cover Gram positives and anaerobes.

Carbapenems

Carbapenems are very broad-spectrum antibiotics that are structurally related to β-lactam antibiotics (Zhanel et al. 2007). The carbapenem class of antibiotics includes imipenem, meropenem, ertapenem, and doripenem. Carbapenems are used for serious Gram-negative infection (complicated abdominal infection, pneumonia) treatment because they provide enhanced Gram-negative and anaerobic coverage compared with other β-lactam antibiotics. The carbapenems are classified based on bacterial spectrum of activity:

1. Group 1 includes broad-spectrum carbapenems, with limited activity against non-fermentative Gram-negative bacilli, which are particularly suitable for community-acquired infections (e.g., ertapenem)

2. Group 2 includes broad-spectrum carbapenems, with activity against non-fermentative Gram-negative bacilli, which are particularly suitable for the treatment of nosocomial infections (e.g., imipenem, meropenem, doripenem).

A recent longitudinal study documented that the use of the group 2 carbapenems (imipenem and meropenem) was associated with significantly increased emergence of *P. aeruginosa* resistance, which was not identified with group 1 (ertapenem) carbapenem use. This study supports the preferential prescription of ertapenem when clinically appropriate (Carmeli et al. 2011). Similarly, results from 10 clinical trials evaluating the effect of ertapenem use on the susceptibility of *Pseudomonas* spp. to carbapenems confirmed that ertapenem use does not result in increased pseudomonas resistance (Nicolau et al. 2012).

Doripenem is the newest carbapenem to be FDA approved in 2007 for complicated intra-abdominal infections (doripenem vs imipenem) and complicated urinary tract infections (doripenem vs levofloxacin) and commercially released (Paterson and Depestel 2009). In addition, recent studies evaluated doripenem for the treatment of hospital-acquired pneumonia (HAP). The first randomized, open-labeled, phase 3 trial compared doripenem (500 mg i.v. every 6 h) with piperacillin/tazobactam (4.5 g i.v. every 6 h) for nosocomial or early onset (<5 days) ventilator-associated pneumonia (VAP) (Réa-Neto et al. 2008). Step-down therapy to oral levofloxacin was allowed after ≥72 h of study drug, for a complete treatment course of 7–14 days. The clinical cure rates in the clinically evaluable (CE) population were 81.3% (109/134) and 79.8% (95/119), and in the clinical modified intention-to-treat (cMITT) population were 69.5% (148/213) and 64.1% (134/209) in the doripenem and piperacillin/tazobactam arm, respectively (*p* is not significant). Overall microbiological cure rates were 84.5% for doripenem and 80.7% for piperacillin/tazobactam.

A second, randomized, open-label, phase 3 trial in patients solely with VAP compared doripenem (500 mg i.v. every 8 h) with imipenem (500 mg every 6 h or 1000 mg every 8 h) (Chastre et al. 2008). The clinical cure rates were 68.3% for doripenem versus 64.2% for imipenem and 59.0% for doripenem versus 57.8% for imipenem in the CE and cMITT populations, respectively. Doripenem met noninferiority criteria to imipenem for the treatment of VAP. In a subgroup analysis of patients with *P. aeruginosa*, there was a nonstatistically significant trend toward higher clinical cure rates with doripenem 80.0% versus imipenem 42.9%.

The US FDA (2012b) issued a statement regarding the early cessation of the clinical trial of doripenem in the treatment of VAP due to significant safety concerns. The study demonstrated excess mortality and a numerically poorer clinical cure rate among participants treated with doripenem compared with those treated with imipenem–cilastatin (**Table 2.5**). The FDA is reviewing the trial results. Of note, doripenem is not approved in the USA for the treatment of any type of pneumonia; it is, however, licensed for this indication in the European Union.

Table 2.5 Summary of clinical cure rates and all-cause 28-day mortality rate in doripenem clinical trial for ventilator-associated pneumonia.

Analysis population	Doripenem group (%)	Imipenem group (%)	Difference (%)	Two-sided 95% CI (%)
Clinical cure rates				
MITT	45.6	56.8	-11.2	-26.3 to 3.8
ME	49.1	66.1	-17	-34.7 to 0.8
All-cause 28-day mortality rate (MITT)	21.5	14.8	6.7	-5.0 to 18.5

From: www.fda.gov/Drugs/DrugSafety/ucm285883.htm
CI, confidence interval; ME, microbiologically evaluable; MITT, modified intent to treat.

A significant advantage of the carbapenems in the treatment of infections due to MDR Gram-negative bacteria is their stability to hydrolysis by many ESBLs. Carbapenems are therefore the antibiotic of choice for the treatment of ESBL-producing bacteria. But other mechanisms of resistance have been reported for carbapenems, and in vitro susceptibility testing must be performed on clinical isolates to determine whether these agents are appropriate in the clinical management of severe infections.

The recent report of a new type of carbapenem resistance gene (New Delhi metallo-β-lactamase 1 – *NDM-1*) poses a worldwide public health problem, and coordinated international surveillance is required (Yong et al. 2009). *NDM-1* was initially discovered in a strain of *Klebsiella pneumoniae* from a Swedish patient of Indian origin who traveled to New Delhi and acquired a urinary tract infection there. The original organism was found to be resistant to all antimicrobial agents tested except colistin (Kumarasamy et al. 2010). Molecular examination of the isolate revealed that it contained a novel metallo-β-lactamase that readily hydrolyzed penicillins, cephalosporins, and carbapenems (with the exception of aztreonam). The gene encoding this novel β-lactamase (which had not been known previously) was found on a large 180-kb resistance-conferring genetic element that was easily transferred to other *Enterobacteriaceae* and that contained a variety of other resistance determinants, including a gene encoding another broad-spectrum β-lactamase (*CMY-4*) and genes inactivating erythromycin, ciprofloxacin, rifampicin, and chloramphenicol. In addition, the genetic element encoded an efflux pump capable of causing additional antimicrobial resistance and growth promoters that insured the transcription of the genes contained in the genetic element (Moellering 2010).

The Clinical and Laboratory Standards Institute (2011) recently established revised criteria for the interpretation of sensitivity breakpoints for carbapenems (**Table 2.6**). This is an important change, because a number of clinical laboratories were having difficulties correctly identifying *Klebsiella pneumoniae* carbapenemase (KPC)-producing *Enterobacteriaceae*. Furthermore, utilizing the pre-2010 breakpoints, a significant percentage of KPC-producing organisms were identified as being susceptible to the carbapenem being tested, especially imipenem and meropenem. Based on MIC distributions presented to the committee, it became apparent that, by decreasing the carbapenem breakpoints to levels consistent with pharmacokinetic/

pharmacodynamic analyses, the vast majority of KPC-producing *Enterobacteriaceae* (>99%) would be reported as resistant to imipenem, meropenem, and ertapenem, and would diminish the need for clinical laboratories to perform the modified Hodge test to guide therapy.

◼ Colistin

The emergence of nosocomial infections due to MDR Gram-negative bacteria have led to the revival of forgotten antibiotics, such as the polymyxins. Colistin, mainly colistimethate sodium (polymyxin E), has been predominantly used as monotherapy or combination therapy in these MDR infections (Michalopoulos and Karatza 2010). Recent retrospective cohort studies document that the use of combination therapy (colistin–polymyxin B or tigecycline–carbapenem) for definitive therapy of KPC-producing *K. pneumoniae* bacteremia was associated with significantly improved survival (odds ratio 0.07, 95% CI 0.009–0.71, $p = 0.02$). The 28-day mortality was 13.3% in the combination therapy group compared with 57.8% in the monotherapy group (Hirsch and Tam 2010, Qureshi et al. 2012).

MDR Gram-negative bacteria (*Pseudomonas, Enterobacter, Acinetobacter* spp.) are increasingly common causes of VAP with limited antibiotic options for treatment. A systematic review and meta-regression documented that colistin may be as safe and efficacious as standard antibiotics for the treatment of VAP (Florescu et al. 2012). Aerosolized colistin is sometimes used as an adjunctive treatment of VAP due to MDR Gram-negative bacteria and is safe, although its efficacy (particularly its incremental benefit to systemic colistin treatment) is unclear (Michalopoulos et al. 2008). In patients with HAP or VAP, inhaled colistin should be used in a combined regimen with systemic antibiotics (Antoniu and Cojocarii 2012).

◼ Aminoglycosides

Aminoglycosides are experiencing resurgence in use because of the spread of MDR Gram-negative pathogens. Aminoglycosides are now commonly used in empiric antimicrobial regimens in critically ill patients and in life-threatening infections, as part of combination antimicrobial therapy to cover all possible Gram-negative causative pathogens. Aminoglycosides (gentamicin, tobramycin, amikacin, streptomycin) are bactericidal drugs that inhibit bacterial protein

Table 2.6 New carbapenem breakpoints for Enterobacteriaceae.

Drug	Minimum inhibitory concentration (µg/ml)			Standard dose used for breakpoint determination (mg)
	Susceptible	Intermediate	Resistant	
New carbapenem breakpoints				
Doripenem	≤1	2	≥4	500 every 8 h
Ertapenem	≤0.25	0.5	≥1	1 g every 24 h
Imipenem	≤1	2	≥4	500 every 6 h or 1 g every 8 h
Meropenem	≤1	2	≥4	500 every 6 h or 1 g every 8 h
Old carbapenem breakpoints				
Ertapenem	≤2	4	≥8	
Imipenem	≤4	8	≥16	
Meropenem	≤4	8	≥16	

Data from: Clinical and Laboratory Standards Institute. *Performance Standards for Antimicrobial Susceptibility Testing*. Twentieth Informational Supplement (June 2010 Update) M100-S20-U. CLSI, Wayne, PA, USA (2010).

synthesis by inhibiting the function of the 30-S subunit of the bacterial ribosome. Nephrotoxicity and ototoxicity are of significant concern with the use of aminoglycosides, but an additional risk is also under-dosing of aminoglycosides, which will impair efficacy. Optimization of aminoglycoside therapy therefore requires pharmacokinetic and pharmacodynamic dosing to minimize risk and maximize microbial killing and optimal patient outcomes (Drusano et al. 2007, Drusano and Louie 2011). Although once-daily aminoglycoside regimens may be appropriate for some patients, this strategy may not be adequate in critically ill patients and careful drug monitoring is required to both manage efficacy and limit toxicity (Conil et al. 2011).

Quinolones

The quinolones are synthetic analogs of nalidixic acid with a broad spectrum of activity. The action of all quinolones involves inhibition of bacterial DNA synthesis by blocking the enzyme DNA gyrase. The earlier quinolones (nalidixic acid, oxolinic acid, cinoxacin) did not achieve systemic antibacterial levels after oral intake and thus were useful only as urinary antiseptics. The fluoroquinolone derivatives (ciprofloxacin, levofloxacin, gemifloxacin, and moxifloxacin) have more potent antibacterial activity, achieve clinically useful levels in blood and tissues, and have low toxicity.

The spectrum of activity for quinolones is similar among the available agents. In general, these drugs have moderate-to-excellent activity against *Enterobacteriaceae* but are also active against other Gram-negative bacteria such as *Hemophilus, Neisseria, Moraxella, Brucella, Legionella, Salmonella, Shigella, Campylobacter, Yersinia, Vibrio,* and *Aeromonas* spp. Resistance to *E. coli* has significantly increased over the past decade, with some centers reporting up to 20–40% resistance. Ciprofloxacin and levofloxacin are the only quinolones with activity against *P. aeruginosa*, but the increasing resistance of *P. aeruginosa* to fluoroquinolones has limited their utility.

In general, the fluoroquinolones are less potent against Gram-positive than against Gram-negative organisms. Levofloxacin, gemifloxacin, and moxifloxacin have the best Gram-positive activity, including against pneumococci and strains of *S. aureus* and *S. epidermidis*, including some cases of MRSA. However, the emergence of resistant strains of staphylococci has limited the use of these drugs in infections caused by these organisms. Moxifloxacin demonstrates modest activity against many of the significant anaerobic pathogens, including *B. fragilis* and mouth anaerobes, and is approved for the treatment of intra-abdominal infection. However, increased rates of anaerobic resistance over time have been reported.

Quinolones may be used in the treatment of complicated intra-abdominal infections in combination with metronidazole for anaerobic coverage; however, the recent SIS/IDSA guidelines state: "because of increasing resistance of *Escherichia coli* to fluoroquinolones, local population susceptibility profiles and, if available, isolate susceptibility should be reviewed" (Solomkin et al. 2010a). Quinolones are also used in the treatment of complicated urinary tract infections and pyelonephritis, bacterial prostatitis, in combination with β-lactam antibiotics for febrile neutropenia and in some lower respiratory tract infections (although increasing rates of Gram-negative bacterial resistance have significantly limited their use).

Vancomycin and newer agents for MRSA infection

There are currently six antibiotics approved by the US FDA for the treatment of MRSA complicated skin and soft-tissue infections (cSSTIs): Vancomycin, linezolid, daptomycin, tigecycline, telavancin, and most recently ceftaroline. The two investigational glycopeptides, dalbavancin and oritavancin, are under investigation for treatment of cSSSIs, as is iclaprim, a diaminopyrimidine.

Vancomycin

Vancomycin, a bactericidal glycopeptide, emerged as an important antibiotic in the 1980s and 1990s with the rise of MRSA infections. Vancomycin has been the reference standard for treating MRSA infections because of its relatively safety, its durability against the development of resistance (fewer than 20 cases of *S. aureus* with overt vancomycin resistance worldwide), and – until recently – the lack of other approved alternatives for the treatment of MRSA (Liu et al. 2011).

However, vancomycin is being linked increasingly to clinical failures, possibly caused by underdosing, poor tissue penetration, loss of accessory gene-regulator function in the organism, slower bactericidal effect, escalation of vancomycin MICs, and reduced vancomycin susceptibility related to heteroresistant isolates (Haque et al. 2010, Howden et al. 2010, van Hal and Paterson 2011). In a single-center review of 288 patients who required surgical intervention for cSSTIs from 2000 to 2006, 100% of the MRSA isolates from SSTIs in 2003 had vancomycin MICs ≤0.5 μg/ml, whereas in 2006, 62% had vancomycin MICs ≤0.5 μg/ml, with 7% having an MIC of 1 μg/ml and 31% of 2 μg/ml (Awad et al. 2007).

Vancomycin has a relatively low rate of tissue penetration, typically between 10% and 20%, sometimes resulting in drug concentrations too low to be therapeutic (Daschner et al. 1987, Graziani et al. 1988, Cruciani et al. 1996). It also has delayed penetration into skin and soft tissues. Vancomycin concentrations in breast tissues were evaluated in 24 women undergoing reconstructive surgery after mastectomy for breast cancer. Patients were given a single prophylactic dose of vancomycin (1 g i.v.) 1–8 h before surgery, and tissue concentrations were measured by high-performance liquid chromatography. Vancomycin was not detectable in most patients at 1–3 h postdose (Luzzati et al. 2000). Vancomycin concentrations in serum, tissue, and sternal bone in patients receiving antimicrobial prophylaxis for coronary artery bypass surgery were also examined. The lowest drug concentrations (4.0–4.8 mg/g) were found in fat when the mean serum concentration was 55.1 ± 22.8 mg/ml. At 210 min after vancomycin dosing, the serum concentration decreased to 16.2 ± 4.6 mg/ml, with fat concentrations in the range 5.4–7.7 mg/g and skin concentrations 15.8–23.5 mg/g, thus documenting delayed tissue penetration (Kitzes-Cohen et al. 2000).

To overcome poor tissue penetration, a vancomycin loading dose of 25–30 mg/kg (actual body weight) is recommended in seriously ill patients. Continued dosing at 15–20 mg/kg per dose every 8–12 h, not to exceed 2 g per dose, in patients with normal renal function is recommended, or targeted vancomycin dosing aimed at pharmacodynamic targets with area under the curve (AUC)/MIC ratio >400. Vancomycin can trigger synergistic nephrotoxicity when administered in high doses or together with other nephrotoxic agents (Wong-Beringer et al. 2011), and can cause ototoxicity. In addition, it must be administered parenterally (except in colitis caused by *Clostridium difficile*), which requires skilled nursing time for intravenous catheter care, monitoring, and dosage adjustments.

Linezolid

After vancomycin, linezolid is the most studied treatment of MRSA infections. Linezolid, first in the class of oxazolidinones, offers broad-spectrum Gram-positive activity with 100% oral bioavailability. Linezolid is approved for the treatment of vancomycin-resistant *Enterococcus faecium* infections, cSSSIs, and nosocomial pneumonia caused by MSSA and MRSA, and uncomplicated SSSIs and CAPs caused by MSSA.

The 2008 LEADER surveillance program (initiated in 2004 to monitor emerging linezolid resistance in US medical centers) assessed more than 6113 clinical isolates from 57 medical centers throughout the USA, and reported that 99.64% of *S. aureus* isolates remain susceptible to linezolid (Farrell et al. 2009). Only 0.36% of sampled strains were nonsusceptible to linezolid, a slight decrease from 0.45% and 0.44% in 2006 and 2007, respectively. The nonsusceptible strains (n = 22) were *S. aureus* (n = 33), coagulase-negative staphylococci (n = 14), and *Enterococcus faecium* (n = 5), each with defined target mutations. These data document that linezolid activity sampled by the fifth year of the LEADER program showed sustained potency and spectrum (99.64% susceptibility levels). The nonsusceptible strain isolation rates remained stable and the plasmid-mediated ribosomal-based resistance mechanism that emerged in *S. aureus* and *S. epidermidis* strains in 2007 showed no evidence of dissemination or increased prevalence.

In an outbreak in the USA, 12 cases of linezolid-resistant *S. aureus* (LRSA, MIC >4 mg/l) were detected (Sanchez Garcia et al. 2010). All patients had been in an intensive care unit (ICU) for a prolonged period with prior broad-spectrum antibiotic use. The duration of linezolid before detection of LRSA was short (7.5 days). The overall mortality rate was 50%. Restriction of linezolid was required, as one of the measures, to effectively eradicate the outbreak.

The European linezolid surveillance network (ZAAPS program) reported its 8-year (2002–2009) linezolid susceptibility rates as >99.9, 99.7, and 99.6% for *S. aureus*, coagulase-negative staphylococci, and enterococci, respectively, and all streptococcal strains were susceptible. The ZAAPS program surveillance confirmed high, sustained levels of linezolid activity from 2002 to 2009, without evidence of MIC creep or escalating resistance in Gram-positive pathogens across monitored European nations (Ross et al. 2011).

Prior post-hoc analyses of clinical trials of nosocomial pneumonia and VAP have suggested that linezolid may yield significantly better clinical outcomes than vancomycin in patients with serious infections resulting from MRSA, but controversy still remains (Wunderink et al. 2003, Kollef et al. 2004). Two separate meta-analyses, one with eight trials (1641 patients) (Walkey et al. 2011) and one with nine trials (2329 patients) (Kalil et al. 2010) confirmed no evidence of superiority of linezolid over glycopeptide antibiotics for the treatment of nosocomial pneumonia.

A recent, prospective, double-blind multicenter trial compared linezolid (600 mg every 12 h) with vancomycin (15 mg/kg every 12 h) in hospitalized adult patients with MRSA pneumonia (n = 1184). Clinical success was higher in the linezolid cohort (57.6% vs 46.6%, 95% CI 0.5–21.6, p = 0.042). All-cause 60-day mortality rate was similar (linezolid 15.7%, vancomycin 17.0%). Nephrotoxicity was more frequent with vancomycin (18.2% vs 8.4% linezolid) (Wunderink et al. 2012). Limitations of this study include no serum vancomycin levels for 21% of patients, and day 3 trough levels <12.3 µg/ml for 52% of the remaining patients (Wolff and Mourvillier 2012). Additional limitations included unequal distribution of medical comorbidities between participants, more vancomycin-treated than linezolid-treated patients received mechanical ventilation at baseline (73.9% vs 66.9%) and had MRSA bacteremia (10.8% vs 5.2%) (Lahey 2012). The current pneumonia guidelines by the IDSA and American Thoracic Society (ATS) recommend either vancomycin or linezolid, with linezolid preferred in case of baseline renal failure or in non-responding patients and in patients with higher vancomycin MIC ≥2 mg/l (33 of 174 cases in this current study) (American Thoracic Society 2005, Torres 2012).

In the largest cSSSI trial to date, 1200 adult patients with suspected or proved MRSA were randomized to treatment with linezolid (intravenous or oral) or vancomycin (1 g every 12 h i.v.). Results showed significantly better clinical cure rates in patients treated with linezolid (94.4%) than in those treated with vancomycin (90.4%; p = 0.023) (Weigelt et al. 2005). For those with MRSA isolated at baseline in the modified intent-to-treat (mITT) and microbiologically evaluable (ME) populations, the clinical success (cure) rate was better for linezolid-treated patients than for the vancomycin-treated ones (MITT 92.0% vs 81.8%, p = 0.0114; ME 94.0% vs 83.6%, p = 0.0108) (Weigelt et al. 2006). The number of participants with MRSA at baseline was similar in the treatment groups. In this study, microbiologic eradication rates were better for linezolid (88.6%) versus vancomycin (66.9%, p <0.0001) in patients with confirmed MRSA. An earlier study in patients with MRSA-complicated surgical site infections also found that significantly more patients treated with linezolid experienced microbiologic success (87%) than did patients treated with vancomycin (48%; p = 0.0022) (Weigelt et al. 2004).

Most recently, a phase 4 clinical trial was designed to specifically examine the efficacy of linezolid versus appropriately weight-based dosing of vancomycin in the treatment of cSSSIs caused by culture-proven MRSA (Itani et al. 2010). MRSA was confirmed in 322 patients randomized to linezolid and 318 patients randomized to vancomycin. The rate of clinical success was similar in linezolid- and vancomycin-treated patients (p = 0.249). The rate of success was significantly higher in linezolid-treated patients in the mITT population (p = 0.048). The microbiologic success rate was higher for linezolid at the end of treatment (p = 0.001) and was similar at the end of the study (p = 0.127). Patients receiving linezolid had a significantly shorter length of stay and duration of intravenous therapy than patients receiving vancomycin. Both agents were well tolerated. Linezolid has a 100% bioavailable oral formulation, which shortens the length of hospital stay and duration of intravenous treatment compared with vancomycin.

A systematic review and meta-analysis of linezolid versus vancomycin for MRSA SSTIs included four trials and concluded that no difference was detected between the two treatments, but a trend toward higher effectiveness of linezolid was observed (Dodds and Hawke 2009). An additional meta-analysis included 5 trials with a total of 2652 patients and concluded that linezolid was more likely to consistently achieve microbiologic eradication in MRSA ME patients. But study limitations included an inability to assess for the effects of heteroresistance and appropriate vancomycin dosing on outcomes (Bounthavong and Hsu 2010). A third meta-analysis compared linezolid with vancomycin for the treatment of Gram-positive bacterial infections and concluded that linezolid was more effective than vancomycin in patients with cSSSIs (odds ratio 1.40, 95% CI 1.01–1.95); however, there was no difference in treatment success for patients with bacteremia or pneumonia (Beibei et al. 2010).

Thrombocytopenia is a potential complication of linezolid, and monitoring of complete blood counts is recommended, particularly in those requiring longer courses of therapy.

Daptomycin

Daptomycin, a cyclic lipopeptide available in intravenous form only, is a potent bactericidal agent (Owens et al. 2007). Daptomycin is FDA approved for the treatment of cSSSIs caused by Gram-positive pathogens and for bacteremia, but not for treatment of pneumonia. Daptomycin is also often used off-label to treat patients infected with vancomycin-resistant enterococci (VREs). Recently, however, the emergence of resistance to daptomycin during therapy threatens its usefulness. Whole genome sequencing and characterization of the cell envelope of a clinical pair of vancomycin-resistant *Enterococcus faecalis* isolates from the blood of a patient with fatal bacteremia documented that mutations in genes were responsible for the development of resistance to daptomycin during the treatment of VREs (Arias et al. 2011).

An analysis of 902 evaluable patients from two randomized, multinational trials demonstrated clinical equivalency between daptomycin and conventional antibiotics (vancomycin- or penicillinase-resistant penicillins) in the treatment of cSSSIs (Arbeit et al. 2004). Success rates in the clinically evaluable population were 83.4% for daptomycin-treated patients and 84.2% for comparator-treated patients (95% CI −4.0, 5.6). Only 64 patients with MRSA were evaluated microbiologically in the study cohort. Among the 64 patients with MRSA, the clinical success rates were 75.0% for daptomycin and 69.4% for the comparator drug (95% CI −28.5, 17.4). The frequency, distribution, and severity of adverse events were similar in the two treatment groups.

The efficacy of daptomycin in cSSTIs also has been examined in the Cubicin Outcomes Registry and Experience 2004 (CORE) Registry, a multicenter observational registry involving 45 institutions. A total of 165 patients were identified, including 145 with MRSA and 20 with MSSA cSSTIs, but without bacteremia, endocarditis, osteomyelitis, or other major infectious processes. Clinical success was achieved with daptomycin in 89.1% of patients overall, including 89.7% in patients with MRSA. Prior antibiotic therapy had been administered to 74.2% of patients and concomitant antibiotic therapy to 39.4% (Martone and Lamp 2006).

Another study examined daptomycin efficacy in 53 adult patients with cSSTIs at risk for MRSA infection compared with a matched retrospective cohort of 212 patients treated with vancomycin. The proportions of patients with clinical improvement or resolution of their infections on days 3 and 4 were 90% versus 70% and 98% versus 81% in the daptomycin and vancomycin groups, respectively (Davis et al. 2007).

The serum creatine phosphokinase (CPK) concentration should be monitored weekly during use of daptomycin, especially if high doses are given. Caution is necessary in patients previously treated with vancomycin, which may influence daptomycin susceptibility (Sakoulas et al. 2006). Clinical data from the retrospective daptomycin CORE registry confirmed that patients failing vancomycin were more likely to fail daptomycin salvage therapy compared with patients switched for other reasons ($p = 0.0009$). In an attempt to prevent resistance selection, higher doses of daptomycin (8 mg/kg) were associated with better therapeutic outcomes compared with lower doses (4–6 mg/kg) (Bassetti et al. 2010).

The FDA released a Drug and Safety Communication about daptomycin-induced acute eosinophilic pneumonia (AEP), characterized by new lung infiltrates and hypoxemia (FDA 2010c, Lal and Assimacopoulos 2010). Peripheral eosinophilia and rash may not be present, although eosinophilia was invariably detected in bronchoalveolar samples (Miller et al. 2010). The role of steroids is unclear but daptomycin should be withheld pending appropriate investigations in patients developing new infiltrates. Daptomycin rechallenge is not recommended. The incidence of daptomycin-induced AEP is small (determined from the FDA's Adverse Event Reporting System database) at approximately 0.43 per 10 000 patients treated.

Tigecycline

Tigecycline is the first agent of the glycylcycline class. Chemically similar to minocycline, tigecycline is better tolerated and more active against tetracycline-resistant strains (Boucher et al. 2000). Tigecycline is effective over a broader spectrum than many other agents, but does not cover *P. aeruginosa* or *Proteus* spp. In a study of more than 500 Gram-positive isolates, tigecycline inhibited all strains, including those resistant to other tetracyclines. Its coverage includes VREs, penicillin-resistant *S. pneumoniae*, and MRSA.

Tigecycline was first approved by the FDA in 2005 for use in cSSSIs and complicated intra-abdominal infections. Currently it is also approved for use in community-acquired bacterial pneumonia (CABP). Treatment begins with an initial dose of 100 mg i.v. followed by 50 mg i.v. every 12 h.

In two phase 3, double-blind studies of hospitalized patients with cSSSIs, tigecycline demonstrated clinical cure rates equivalent to those of vancomycin plus aztreonam among the 833 clinically evaluable patients (86.5% vs 88.6%, respectively; 95% CI −6.8, 2.7) (Ellis-Grosse et al. 2005). Among the 65 ME patients with MRSA infection, the eradication rates were 78.1% for tigecycline-treated patients and 75.8% for vancomycin-treated patients. More adverse events (AEs) related to the digestive tract were reported in the tigecycline group, and more rash, cardiovascular events, and liver enzyme increases were reported in the vancomycin/aztreonam group. In clinical trials, the most frequent side effects associated with tigecycline were nausea and vomiting.

A recent meta-analysis of eight randomized controlled trials ($n = 4651$) provides evidence that tigecycline monotherapy may be used as effectively as the comparison therapy for cSSSIs, complicated intra-abdominal infections, CAPs, and infections caused by MRSA and VRE. However, because of the high risk of mortality, AEs, and emergence of resistant isolates, prudence with the clinical use of tigecycline monotherapy in infections is required (Cai et al. 2011). The FDA Drug Safety Communication (FDA 2010d) reported an increased adjusted overall mortality rate of 0.6%, predominantly as a result of tigecycline use in the treatment of VAP and HAP, suggesting that alternative antibiotics should be considered in these serious infections.

Telavancin

Telavancin is a semisynthetic lipoglycopeptide with a dual mechanism of action: Inhibition of cell wall synthesis and disruption of membrane barrier function. It has a 7- to 9-h half-life, which allows once-daily dosing. Telavancin is approved for the treatment of cSSSIs caused by susceptible Gram-positive bacteria, including MRSA and MSSA. In two phase 2 trials for treatment of cSSTIs, similar clinical success rates were achieved in patients receiving telavancin or standard therapy for infections caused by *S. aureus* and MRSA (Stryjewski et al. 2005, 2006).

Two parallel, randomized, double-blind, active-control, phase 3 studies were conducted in patients aged ≥18 years who had cSSSIs caused by suspected or confirmed Gram-positive organisms (Stryjewski et al. 2008). Patients ($n = 1867$) were randomized to receive either telavancin (10 mg/kg i.v. every 24 h) or vancomycin (1 g i.v. every 12 h). In the clinically evaluable population; at 7–14 days after receipt of the last antibiotic dose, success was achieved in 88% and 87% of patients who received telavancin and vancomycin, respectively (95% CI −2.1, 4.6). MRSA was isolated at baseline in 579 clinically evaluable patients – the largest series to date. Among these patients, the cure rate was 91% among patients who received telavancin and 86% among patients who received vancomycin (95% CI −1.1, 9.3). Microbiologic eradication of MRSA was achieved in 90% of the telavancin group and 85% of the vancomycin group (95% CI −0.9, 9.8). This study confirmed that telavancin given once daily was at least as effective as vancomycin for the treatment of patients with cSSSIs, including those infected with MRSA.

A recent post-hoc analysis of the two phase 3 trials examined efficacy in different types of skin infections, and concluded that cure rates were similar for telavancin and vancomcyin including infections caused by MRSA and Panton–Valentine leukocidin (PVL)-positive strains of MRSA (Stryjewski et al. 2012).

Telavancin is also undergoing investigation for treatment of pneumonia. The global results of two phase 3 randomized, double-blind, clinical trials in patients ($n = 1503$) with nosocomial pneumonia (AT-TAIN-1 and ATTAIN-2) have recently been published (Rubinstein et al. 2011). The clinical evaluation of 654 patients (312 telavancin 10 mg/kg i.v. once daily, 342 vancomycin 1 g i.v. every 12 h, both groups treated with aztreonam) showed no outcome differences between groups. The subgroup analysis of patients with MRSA pneumonia with a vancomycin MIC of at least 1 µg/ml showed better results for telavancin (clinical response 87.1% vs 74.3%; $p = 0.03$). In a subgroup analysis of patients with VAP, there was a trend toward higher clinical cure rates with telavancin (80.3% vs 67.8%). However, treatment with telavancin was accompanied by a non-significant higher rate of renal dysfunction compared with vancomycin (16% vs 10%). The telavancin-associated renal dysfunction was restricted to patients with abnormal baseline renal function.

The European Commission approved telavancin for the treatment of adults with HAP, including VAP, known, or suspected, to be caused by MRSA. The FDA has not approved telavancin for pneumonia use in the USA.

Investigational semisynthetic glycopeptides

Two additional anti-MRSA intravenous glycopeptides are being evaluated: Dalbavancin and oritavancin.

Dalbavancin

The unique feature of dalbavancin is its extraordinarily long half-life (6–10 days), which allows once-weekly dosing. In a phase 3 trial, intravenous dalbavancin, administered on days 1 and 8, was compared with intravenous/oral linezolid, given twice daily for 14 days, in 660 clinically evaluable patients with cSSSIs; 88.9% of the dalbavancin-treated patients and 91.2% of the linezolid-treated patients had clinical success. The rates of MRSA eradication in 278 patients with confirmed MRSA cSSTIs were 91% in the dalbavancin group and 89% in the linezolid group. The safety profiles for the two agents were similar (Jauregui et al. 2005). Dalbavancin was similar to vancomycin in a phase 2 trial of the treatment of catheter-related bloodstream infection (Raad et al. 2005). Two new phase 3 studies are underway (Discover 1 and 2) for the treatment of acute bacterial skin and skin structure infections. It currently remains unapproved for use in the USA.

Oritavancin

Oritavancin is another broad-spectrum semisynthetic glycopeptide under development for the treatment of cSSTIs, catheter-related bloodstream infections, and nosocomial pneumonia. It has demonstrated activity against vancomycin-resistant strains of staphylococci and enterococci, and has a long half-life (100 h), which is expected to allow once-daily or every-other-day dosing. Two phase 3 trials for treatment of cSSSIs have been completed, with the primary endpoints reportedly being met in each. The drug has not been approved for use because of a lack of MRSA-specific data. Subsequently, two studies (SOLO I and SOLO II) are being conducted with completion expected in January 2013.

Iclaprim

Iclaprim is a synthetic diaminopyrimidine. It is a selective inhibitor of the enzyme dihydrofolate reductase (similar to trimethoprim), with bactericidal activity against MRSA and clinically important Gram-positive pathogens (Peppard and Schuenke 2008). Two phase 3 trials for the treatment of cSSSIs, comparing iclaprim with the comparator, linezolid, were conducted in 2007.

The multicenter, double-blind, randomized, active-control, parallel-assignment, phase 3 trial (ASSIST-1), compared IV iclaprim (0.8 mg/kg, $n = 250$) with IV linezolid (600 mg, $n = 247$), both administered for 10–14 days, in patients with cSSSI who had extensive cellulitis, abscesses, ulcers, burns, or wounds (Arpida 2012a). The primary objective was clinical cure rates of iclaprim versus linezolid. Secondary outcomes included clinical efficacy at the end of the trial and clinical outcomes of the ME and ITT populations. Approximately 70% of the pathogens isolated were *S. aureus*, 25% of which were MRSA. For the ME patients, the cure rates were 94.7% and 98.8% for iclaprim and linezolid, respectively. The overall clinical cure rate for the ITT population was 85.5% and 91.9% for iclaprim and linezolid, respectively. The clinically evaluable patients had cure rates of 93.8% and 99.1%, respectively.

A subsequent multicenter, double-blind, randomized, active-control, parallel-assignment, phase 3 clinical trial (ASSIST-2), was initiated in cSSSI patients with extensive cellulitis, abscesses, ulcers, burns, or wounds to compare intravenous iclaprim ($n = 251$) with intravenous linezolid ($n = 243$) (Arpida 2012b). The primary and secondary endpoints were the same as those in the ASSIST-1 trial. Preliminary analysis indicated overall clinical cure rates for the ITT population of 84.9% and 87.2% for iclaprim and linezolid, respectively. The most common baseline pathogen was *S. aureus* (approximately 60%), 50% of which were MRSA. The microbiological eradication rates for MSSA were 83.5% and 84.7% for iclaprim and linezolid, respectively, and 77.0% and 80.0% for MRSA, respectively. For patients with Gram-positive pathogen infections at baseline, the clinical cure rates were 83.3% and 85.9% for iclaprim and linezolid, respectively. In a preliminary analysis of the clinically evaluable population, the cure rates were 89.6% and 96.4% for iclaprim and linezolid, respectively. It has not been approved for use and clinical evaluation of this antibiotic continues.

Tedizolid (TR-701)

Tedizolid is the active moiety of the prodrug torezolid phosphate, a second-generation oxazolidinone with 4- to 16-fold greater potency than linezolid against Gram-positive species including MRSA. A double-blind phase 2 study evaluated three doses (200, 300, or 400 mg) of oral once-daily torezolid over 5–7 days for cSSSIs (Prokocimer et al. 2011). Cure rates in clinically evaluable patients were 98.2% at 200 mg, 94.4% at 300 mg, and 94.4% at 400 mg. Results of this study show a high degree of efficacy at all three dose levels with no safety issues. The phase 3 clinical trials in acute bacterial skin and skin structure infections confirmed non-inferiority comparing Tedizolid 200 mg daily for 6 days to Linezolid 600 mg twice daily for 10 days (http://www.triusrx.com/trius-therapeutics-tedizolid-results.php)

CONCLUSION

Inadequate treatment of severe infections in surgical patients contributes to in-hospital death and prolonged duration of hospitalization. Prompt, appropriate antimicrobial treatment of infections in surgical patients increases the chances of a successful outcome. The choice of antimicrobial agent for empiric treatment of surgical infections should be guided by a number of considerations, including the site and type of infection, presence of immunocompromised state or neutropenia, adequacy of source control, and risk factors for MDR bacteria. Patients with severe infection or comorbidities should be treated aggressively with empiric broad-spectrum antimicrobial therapy in appropriate dosing strategies, and then de-escalated to narrower-spectrum agents depending on the culture findings and clinical response. It is of paramount importance to obtain specimens for culture and antimicrobial susceptibilities given the high prevalence of MDR bacteria as causative pathogens in surgical infections. Surgeons must have a working knowledge of appropriate antimicrobial agents for surgical infections, particularly for use in acute bacterial skin infections and SSIs, complicated intra-abdominal infections, pneumonia, bacteremia, and urinary tract infections. There has been a significant increase in the number of antimicrobials that are FDA approved for the treatment of Gram-positive infections, but very few new Gram-negative antimicrobials are currently undergoing clinical trials. Antimicrobial stewardship is therefore necessary to retain the activity of our current antimicrobials for use in Gram-negative infections.

REFERENCES

American Thoracic Society. Guidelines for the management of adults with hospital-acquired, ventilator-associated, and healthcare-associated pneumonia. *Am J Respir Crit Care Med* 2005;**171**:388–416.

Antoniu SA, Cojocaru I. Inhaled colistin for lower respiratory tract infections. *Expert Opin Drug Deliv* 2012;**9**:333–42.

Arbeit RD, Maki D, Tally FP, et al. Daptomycin 98-01 and 99-01 Investigators. The safety and efficacy of daptomycin for the treatment of complicated skin and skin-structure infections. *Clin Infect Dis* 2004;**38**:1673–81.

Arias CA, Panesso D, McGrath DM, et al. Genetic basis for in vivo daptomycin resistance in enterococci. *N Engl J Med* 2011;**365**:892–900.

Arpida AG Arpida's Skin and Skin Structure Infection Study 1 (ASSIST-1). Phase 3 safety and efficacy study of IV iclaprim vs linezolid in cSSSI (ASSIST-1), 2012a. Available at: http://clinicaltrials.gov/ct2/show/NCT00299520?term=iclaprim+AND+skin&rank=1 (accessed March 1, 2012).

Arpida AG. Arpida's Skin and Skin Structure Infection Study 2 (ASSIST-2). Study of intravenous (IV) iclaprim versus linezolid in complicated skin and skin structure infections [cSSSI] (ASSIST-2), 2012b. Available at: http://clinicaltrials.gov/ct2/show/NCT00303550 (accessed March 1, 2012).

Awad SS, Elhabash SI, Lee L, et al. Increasing incidence of methicillin-resistant *Staphylococcus aureus* skin and soft-tissue infections: Reconsideration of empiric antimicrobial therapy. *Am J Surg* 2007;**194**:606–10.

Bassetti M, Nicco E, Ginocchio F, et al. High-dose daptomycin in documented *Staphylococcus aureus* infections. *Int J Antimicrob Agents* 2010;**36**:459–61.

Beibei L, Yun C, Mengli C, Nan B, Xuhong Y, Rui W. Linezolid versus vancomycin for the treatment of gram-positive bacterial infections: meta-analysis of randomised controlled trials. *Int J Antimicrob Agents* 2010;**35**:3–12.

Boucher HW, Wennersten CB, Eliopoulos GM. In vitro activities of the glycylcycline GAR-936 against Gram-positive bacteria. *Antimicrob Agents Chemother* 2000;**44**:2225–9.

Bounthavong M, Hsu DI. Efficacy and safety of linezolid in methicillin-resistant *Staphylococcus aureus* (MRSA) complicated skin and soft tissue infection (cSSTI): a meta-analysis. *Curr Med Res Opin* 2010;**26**:407–21.

Cai Y, Wang R, Liang B, Bai N, Liu Y. Systematic review and meta-analysis of the effectiveness and safety of tigecycline for treatment of infectious disease. *Antimicrob Agents Chemother* 2011;**55**:1162–72.

Carmeli Y, Lidji SK, Shabtai E, Navon-Venezia S, Schwaber MJ. The effects of group 1 versus group 2 carbapenems on imipenem-resistant *Pseudomonas aeruginosa*: an ecological study. *Diagn Microbiol Infect Dis* 2011;**70**:367–72.

Chastre J, Wunderink R, Prokocimer P, Lee M, Kaniga K, Friedland I. Efficacy and safety of intravenous infusion of doripenem versus imipenem in ventilator-associated pneumonia: A multicenter, randomized study. *Crit Care Med* 2008;**36**:1089–96.

Clinical and Laboratory Standards Institute. Rationale Document – Carbapenem Breakpoints for *Enterobacteriaceae*, 2011. Available at: www.clsi.org/Content/NavigationMenu/Committees/Microbiology/AST/RationaleDocuments/MicroAST_RationaleDocCarbapenemBreakpointsEnterobacteriaceae_2011.pdf (accessed April 1, 2012).

Conil JM, Georges B, Ruiz S, et al. Tobramycin disposition in ICU patients receiving a once daily regimen: population approach and dosage simulations. *Br J Clin Pharmacol* 2011;**71**:61–71.

Corey GR, Wilcox MH, Talbot GH, et al. CANVAS 1: the first Phase III, randomized, double-blind study evaluating ceftaroline fosamil for the treatment of patients with complicated skin and skin structure infections. *J Antimicrob Chemother* 2010a;**65**:iv41–51.

Corey GR, Wilcox M, Talbot GH, et al. Integrated analysis of CANVAS 1 and 2: phase 3, multicenter, randomized, double-blind studies to evaluate the safety and efficacy of ceftaroline versus vancomycin plus aztreonam in complicated skin and skin-structure infection. *Clin Infect Dis* 2010b;**51**:641–50.

Cruciani M, Gatti G, Lazzarini L, et al. Penetration of vancomycin into human lung tissue. *J Antimicrob Chemother* 1996;**38**:865–9.

Daschner FD, Frank U, Kümmel A, et al. Pharmacokinetcs of vancomycin in serum and tissue of patients undergoing open-heart surgery. *J Antimicrob Chemother* 1987;**19**:359–62.

Davis SL, McKinnon PS, Hall LM, et al. Daptomycin versus vancomycin for complicated skin and skin structure infections: Clinical and economic outcomes. *Pharmacotherapy* 2007;**27**:1611–18.

Dodds TJ, Hawke CI. Linezolid versus vancomycin for MRSA skin and soft tissue infections (systematic review and meta-analysis). *Aust N Z J Surg* 2009;**79**:629–35.

Drusano GL, Louie A. Optimization of aminoglycoside therapy. *Antimicrob Agents Chemother* 2011;**55**:2528–31.

Drusano GL, Ambrose PG, Bhavnani SM, Bertino JS, Nafziger AN, Louie A. Back to the future: using aminoglycosides again and how to dose them optimally. *Clin Infect Dis* 2007;**45**:753–60.

Ellis-Grosse EJ, Babinchak T, Dartois N, et al. Tigecycline 300 and 305 cSSSI Study Groups. The efficacy and safety of tigecycline in the treatment of skin and skin-structure infections: Results of 2 double-blind phase 3 comparison studies with vancomycin-aztreonam. *Clin Infect Dis* 2005;**41**(suppl 5):S341–53.

Farrell DJ, Mendes RE, Ross JE, Jones RN. Linezolid surveillance program results for 2008 (LEADER Program for 2008). *Diagn Microbiol Infect Dis* 2009;**65**:392–403.

File TM Jr, Low DE, Eckburg PB, et al. Integrated analysis of FOCUS 1 and FOCUS 2: randomized, double-blinded, multicenter phase 3 trials of the efficacy and safety of ceftaroline fosamil versus ceftriaxone in patients withcommunityacquired pneumonia. *Clin Infect Dis* 2010;**51**:1395–405.

File TM Jr, Low DE, Eckburg PB, et al. FOCUS 1: a randomized, doubleblinded, multicentre, Phase III trial of the efficacy and safety of ceftaroline fosamil versus ceftriaxone in community-acquired pneumonia. *J Antimicrob Chemother* 2011;**66**:iii19–32.

Florescu DF, Qiu F, McCartan MA, Mindru C, Fey PD, Kalil AC. What is the efficacy and safety of colistin for the treatment of ventilator-associated pneumonia? A systematic review and meta-regression. *Clin Infect Dis* 2012;**54**:670–80.

Food and Drug Administration. Information for Healthcare Professionals: Cefepime, 2012a. Available at: www.fda.gov/Drugs/DrugSafety/PostmarketDrugSafetyInformationforPatientsandProviders/DrugSafetyInformationforHeathcareProfessionals/ucm167254.htm (accessed March 1, 2012).

Food and Drug Administration. Statement on recently terminated clinical trial with doripenem, 2012b. www.fda.gov/Drugs/DrugSafety/ucm285883.htm (accessed March 1, 2012).

Food and Drug Administration. Drug Safety Communication. Eosinophilic pneumonia associated with the use of Cubicin (daptomycin), 2010c. Available at: www.fda.gov/Drugs/DrugSafety/PostmarketDrugSafetyInformationforPatientsandProviders/ucm220273 (accessed March 1, 2012)

Food and Drug Administration. Drug Safety Communication. Increased risk of death with Tygacil (tigecycline) compared to other antibiotics used to treat similar infections, 2010d. Available at: www.fda.gov/Drugs/DrugSafety/ucm224370.htm (accessed March 1, 2012).

Graziani AL, Lawson LA, Gibson GA, et al. Vancomycin concentrations in infected and noninfected human bone. *Antimicrob Agents Chemother* 1988;**32**:1320–2.

Haque NZ, Zuniga LC, Peyrani P, et al. Relationship of vancomycin minimum inhibitory concentration to mortality in patients with methicillin-resistant *Staphylococcus aureus* hospital-acquired, ventilator-associated, or health-care-associated pneumonia. *Chest* 2010;**138**:1356–62.

Hirsch EB, Tam VH. Detection and treatment options for *Klebsiella pneumoniae* carbapenemases (KPCs): an emerging cause of multidrug-resistant infection. *J Antimicrob Chemother* 2010;**65**:1119–25.

Howden BP, Davies JK, Johnson PD, et al. Reduced vancomycin susceptibility in *Staphylococcus aureus*, including vancomycin-intermediate and heterogeneous vancomycin-intermediate strains: resistance mechanisms, laboratory detection, and clinical implications. *Clin Microbiol Rev* 2010;**23**:99–139.

Huttner B, Jones M, Rubin MA, et al. Double trouble: how big a problem is redundant anaerobic antibiotic coverage in Veterans Affairs medical centres? *J Antimicrob Chemother* 2012; 67:1537–9.

Itani KM, Wilson SE, Awad SS, Jensen EH, Finn TS, Abramson MA. Ertapenem versus cefotetan prophylaxis in elective colorectal surgery. *N Engl J Med* 2006;**355**:2640–51.

Itani KM, Dryden MS, Bhattacharyya H, Kunkel MJ, Baruch AM, Weigelt JA. Efficacy and safety of linezolid versus vancomycin for the treatment of complicated skin and soft-tissue infections proven to be caused by methicillin-resistant *Staphylococcus aureus*. *Am J Surg* 2010;**199**:804–16.

Jauregui LE, Babazadeh S, Seltzer E, et al. Randomized, double-blind comparison of once-weekly dalbavancin versus twice-daily linezolid therapy for the treatment of complicated skin and skin structure infections. *Clin Infect Dis* 2005;**41**:1407–15.

Kitzes-Cohen R, Farin D, Piva G, et al. Pharmacokinetics of vancomycin administered as prophylaxis before cardiac surgery. *Therapeutic Drug Monit* 2000;**22**:661–7.

Kalil AC. Is cefepime safe for clinical use? A Bayesian viewpoint. *J Antimicrob Chemother* 2011;**66**:1207–9.

Kalil AC, Murthy MH, Hermsen ED, Neto FK, Sun J, Rupp ME. Linezolid versus vancomycin or teicoplanin for nosocomial pneumonia: a systematic review and meta-analysis. *Care Med* 2010;**38**:1802–8.

Kollef MH, Sherman G, Ward S, et al. Inadequate antimicrobial treatment of infections: a risk factor for hospital mortality among critically ill patients. *Chest* 1999;**115**:462–74.

Kollef MH, Rello J, Cammarata SK, et al. Clinical cure and survival in Gram-positive ventilator-associated pneumonia: Retrospective analysis of two double-blind studies comparing linezolid with vancomycin. *Intensive Care Med* 2004;**30**:388–94.

Kumar A, Roberts D, Wood KE, et al. Duration of hypotension before initiation of effective antimicrobial therapy is the critical determinant of survival in human septic shock. *Crit Care Med* 2006;**34**:1589–96.

Kumarasamy KK, Toleman MA, Walsh TR, et al. Emergence of a new antibiotic resistance mechanism in India, Pakistan, and the UK: a molecular, biological, and epidemiological study. *Lancet Infect Dis* 2010;**10**:597–602.

Lagacé-Wiens P, Rubinstein E. Adverse reactions to β-lactam antimicrobials. *Expert Opin Drug Saf* 2012; 11:381–99.

Lahey T. Questionable superiority of linezolid for MRSA nosocomial pneumonia: Watch where you step. *Clin Infect Dis* 2012; 55:159–60.

Lal Y, Assimacopoulos AP. Two cases of daptomycin-induced eosinophilic pneumonia and chronic pneumonitis. *Clin Infect Dis* 2010;**50**:737–40.

Leibovici L, Yahav D, Paul M. Excess mortality related to cefepime. *Lancet Infect Dis* 2010;**10**:293–4.

Leonard SN, Cheung CM, Rybak MJ. Evaluation of the activity of ceftobiprole, linezolid, vancomycin, and daptomycin against community-associated (CA-MRSA) and hospital-associated (HA-MRSA) methicillin-resistant Staphylococcus aureus. *Antimicrob Agents Chemother* 2008;**52**:2974–6.

Liu C, Bayer A, Cosgrove SE, et al. Clinical practice guidelines by the Infectious Diseases Society of America for the treatment of methicillin-resistant *Staphylococcus aureus* infections in adults and children. *Clin Infect Dis* 2011;**52**:e18–55.

Low DE, File TM Jr, Eckburg PB, et al. FOCUS 2: a randomized, double blinded, multicentre, Phase III trial of the efficacy and safety of ceftaroline fosamil versus ceftriaxone in community-acquired pneumonia. *J Antimicrob Chemother* 2011;**66**:iii33–44.

Luzzati R, Sanna A, Allegranzi B, et al. Pharmacokinetics and tissue penetration of vancomycin in patients undergoing prosthetic mammary surgery. *J Antimicrob Chemother* 2000;**45**:243–5.

Martone WJ, Lamp KC. Efficacy of daptomycin in skin and skin-structure infections due to methicillin-sensitive and -resistant *Staphylococcus aureus*: Results from the CORE Registry. *Curr Med Res Opin* 2006;**22**:2337–43.

The Medicines Company. Oritavancin versus IV vancomycin for the treatment of patients with acute bacterial skin and skin structure infection (SOLO I), 2012a. Available at: http://clinicaltrials.gov/ct2/show/NCT01252719 (accessed April 1, 2012).

The Medicines Company. Oritavancin versus IV vancomycin for the treatment of patients with acute bacterial skin and skin structure infection (SOLO II), 2012b. Available at: http://clinicaltrials.gov/ct2/show/NCT01252732?term=o ritavancin&rank=2 (accessed April 1, 2012).

Michalopoulos AS, Karatza DC. Multidrug-resistant Gram-negative infections: the use of colistin. *Expert Rev Anti Infect Ther* 2010;**8**:1009–17.

Michalopoulos A, Fotakis D, Virtzili S, et al. Aerosolized colistin as adjunctive treatment of ventilator-associated pneumonia due to multidrug-resistant Gram-negative bacteria: a prospective study. *Respir Med* 2008;**102**:407–12.

Miller BA, Gray A, Leblanc TW, et al. Acute eosinophilic pneumonia secondary to daptomycin: a report of three cases. *Clin Infect Dis* 2010;**50**:e63–8.

Moellering RC. NDM-1 – A cause for worldwide concern. *N Engl J Med* 2010;**363**:2377–9.

Napolitano LM. Perspectives in surgical infections: what does the future hold? *Surg Infect (Larchmt)* 2010;**11**:111–23.

Nicolau DP, Carmeli Y, Crank CW, et al. Carbapenem stewardship: does ertapenem affect Pseudomonas susceptibility to other carbapenems? A review of the evidence. *Int J Antimicrob Agents* 2012;**39**:11–15.

Noel GJ, Bush K, Bagchi P, et al. A randomized, double-blind trial comparing ceftobiprole medocaril with vancomycin plus ceftazidime for the treatment of patients with complicated skin and skin-structure infections. *Clin Infect Dis* 2008a;**46**:647–55.

Noel GJ, Strauss RS, Amsler K, et al. Results of a double-blind, randomized trial of ceftobiprole treatment of complicated skin and skin structure infections caused by Gram-positive bacteria. *Antimicrob Agents Chemother* 2008b;**52**:37–44.

Owens RC Jr, Lamp KC, Friedrich LV, Russo R. Postmarketing clinical experience in patients with skin and skin-structure infections treated with daptomycin. *Am J Med* 2007;**120**(10 suppl 1):S6–12.

Paterson DL, Bonomo RA. Extended-spectrum beta-lactamases: a clinical update. *Clin Microbiol Rev* 2005;**18**:657–86.

Paterson DL, Depestel DD. Doripenem. *Clin Infect Dis* 2009;**49**:291–8.

Paul M, Yahav D, Fraser A, Leibovici L. Empirical antibiotic monotherapy for febrile neutropenia: systematic review and meta-analysis of randomized controlled trials. *J Antimicrob Chemother* 2006;**57**:176–89.

Peppard WJ, Schuenke CD. Iclaprim, a diaminopyrimidine dihydrofolate reductase inhibitor for the potential treatment of antibiotic-resistant staphylococcal infections. *Curr Opin Invest Drugs* 2008;**9**:210–25.

Poon H, Chang MH, Fung HB. Ceftaroline fosamil: A cephalosporin with activity against Methicillin-resistant *Staphylococcus aureus*. *Clin Ther* 2012; 34:743–65..

Prokocimer P, Bien P, Surber J, et al. Phase 2, randomized, double-blind, dose-ranging study evaluating the safety, tolerability, population pharmacokinetics, and efficacy of oral torezolid phosphate in patients with complicated skin and skin structure infections. *Antimicrob Agents Chemother* 2011;**55**:583–92.

Qureshi ZA, Paterson DL, Potoski BA, et al. Treatment outcome of bacteremia due to KPC-producing *Klebsiella pneumoniae*: Superiority of combination antimicrobial regimens. *Antimicrob Agents Chemother* 2012;**56**:2108–13.

Raad I, Darouiche R, Vazquez J, et al. Efficacy and safety of weekly dalbavancin therapy for catheter-related bloodstream infection caused by Gram-positive pathogens. *Clin Infect Dis* 2005;**40**:374–80.

Réa-Neto A, Niederman M, Lobo SM, et al. Efficacy and safety of doripenem versus piperacillin/tazobactam in nosocomial pneumonia: a randomized, open-label, multicenter study. *Curr Med Res Opin* 2008;**24**:2113–26.

Ross JE, Farrell DJ, Mendes RE, Sader HS, Jones RN. Eight-year (2002–2009) summary of the linezolid (Zyvox® Annual Appraisal of Potency and Spectrum; ZAAPS) program in European countries. *J Chemother* 2011;**23**:71–6.

Rubinstein E, Lalani T, Corey GR, et al. Telavancin versus vancomycin for hospital-acquired pneumonia due to Gram-positive pathogens. *Clin Infect Dis* 2011;**52**:31–40.

Sakoulas G, Alder J, Thauvin-Eliopoulos C, et al. Induction of daptomycin heterogeneous susceptibility in *Staphylococcus aureus* by exposure to vancomycin. *Antimicrob Agents Chemother* 2006;**50**:1581–5.

Sanchez Garcia M, De la Torre MA, Morales G, et al. Clinical outbreak of linezolid-resistant *Staphylococcus aureus* in an intensive care unit. *JAMA* 2010;**303**:2260–4.

Solomkin JS, Mazuski JE, Bradley JS, et al. Diagnosis and management of complicated intra-abdominal infection in adults and children: guidelines by the Surgical Infection Society and the Infectious Diseases Society of America. *Surg Infect (Larchmt)* 2010a;**11**:79–109.

Solomkin JS, Mazuski JE, Bradley JS, et al. Diagnosis and management of complicated intra-abdominal infection in adults and children: guidelines by the Surgical Infection Society and the Infectious Diseases Society of America. *Clin Infect Dis* 2010b;**50**:133–64. Erratum in: *Clin Infect Dis* 2010;**50**:1695. Dosage error in article text.

Steed ME, Rybak MJ. Ceftaroline: a new cephalosporin with activity against resistant Gram-positive pathogens. *Pharmacotherapy* 2010;**30**:375–89.

Stryjewski ME, O'Riordan WD, Lau WK, et al., FAST Investigator Group. Telavancin versus standard therapy for treatment of complicated skin and soft-tissue infections due to Gram-positive bacteria. *Clin Infect Dis* 2005;**40**:1601–7.

Stryjewski ME, Chu VH, O'Riordan WD, et al., FAST 2 Investigator Group. Telavancin versus standard therapy for treatment of complicated skin and skin structure infections caused by Gram-positive bacteria: FAST 2 study. *Antimicrob Agents Chemother* 2006;**50**:862–7.

Stryjewski ME, Graham DR, Wilson SE, et al. on behalf of the Assessment of Telavancin in Complicated Skin and Skin-Structure Infections Study. Telavancin versus vancomycin for the treatment of complicated skin and skin-structure infections caused by Gram-positive organisms. *Clin Infect Dis* 2008;**46**:1683–93.

Stryjewski ME, Barriere SL, O'Riordan W, et al. Efficacy of telavancin in patients with specific types of complicated skin and skin structure infections. *J Antimicrob Chemother* 2012; 67:1496–502.

Torres A. Antibiotic treatment against methicillin-resistant *Staphylococcus aureus* hospital- and ventilator-acquired pneumonia: a step forward but the battle continues. [Editorial]. *Clin Infect Dis* 2012;**54**:630–2.

van Hal SJ, Paterson DL. Systematic review and meta-analysis of the significance of heterogeneous vancomycin-intermediate *Staphylococcus aureus* isolates. *Antimicrob Agents Chemother* 2011;**55**:405–10.

Walkey AJ, O'Donnell MR, Wiener RS. Linezolid vs glycopeptide antibiotics for the treatment of suspected methicillin-resistant *Staphylococcus aureus* nosocomial pneumonia: a meta-analysis of randomized controlled trials. *Chest* 2011;**139**:1148–55.

Weigelt J, Kaafarani HM, Itani KM, Swanson RN. Linezolid eradicates MRSA better than vancomycin from surgical-site infections. *Am J Surg* 2004;**188**:760–6.

Weigelt J, Itani K, Stevens D, et al., Linezolid CSSTI Study Group. Linezolid versus vancomycin in treatment of complicated skin and soft tissue infections. *Antimicrob Agents Chemother* 2005;**49**:2260–6.

Weigelt J, Itani K, Stevens D, Knirsch C. Is linezolid superior to vancomycin for complicated skin and soft tissue infections due to methicillin-resistant *Staphylococcus aureus*? *Antimicrob Agents Chemother* 2006;**50**:1910–11.

Wilcox MH, Corey GR, Talbot GH, et al. CANVAS 2: the second Phase III, randomized, double-blind study evaluating ceftaroline fosamil for the treatment of patients with complicated skin and skin structure infections. *J Antimicrob Chemother* 2010;**65**:iv53–65.

Wolff M, Mourvillier B. Linezolid for the treatment of nosocomial pneumonia due to methicillin-resistant *Staphylococcus aureus* (MRSA). *Clin Infect Dis* 2012; 55:160–1.

Wong-Beringer A, Joo J, Tse E, Beringer P. Vancomycin-associated nephrotoxicity: a critical appraisal of risk with high-dose therapy. *Int J Antimicrob Agents* 2011;**37**:95–101.

Wunderink RG, Rello J, Cammarata SK, et al. Linezolid vs vancomycin: Analysis of two double-blind studies of patients with methicillin-resistant *Staphylococcus aureus* nosocomial pneumonia. *Chest* 2003;**124**:1789–97.

Wunderink RG, Niederman MS, Kollef MH, et al. Linezolid in methicillin-resistant *Staphylococcus aureus* nosocomial pneumonia: a randomized, controlled study. *Clin Infect Dis* 2012;**54**:621–9.

Yahav D, Paul M, Fraser A, Sarid N, Leibovici L. Efficacy and safety of cefepime: a systematic review and meta-analysis. *Lancet Infect Dis* 2007;**7**:338–48.

Yong D, Toleman MA, Giske CG, et al. Characterization of a new metallo-β-lactamase gene, blaNDM-1, and a novel erythromycin esterase gene carried on a unique genetic structure in Klebsiella pneumoniae sequence type 14 from India. Antimicrob *Agents Chemother* 2009;**53**:5046–54.

Zaffiri L, Gardner J, Toledo-Pereyra LH. History of antibiotics. From salvarsan to cephalosporins. *J Invest Surg* 2012;**25**:67–77.

Zhanel GG, Wiebe R, Dilay L, et al. Comparative review of the carbapenems. *Drugs* 2007;**67**:1027–52.

Chapter 3 — Surgical immunology

William G. Cheadle, Ziad Kanaan, Adrian T. Billeter, Rebecca E. Barnett

■ INTRODUCTION

The human immune system consists of a highly complex and redundant arrangement of immune cells and secreted proteins that have evolved extensively over time. These cells and proteins are located throughout the body and include the bone marrow, thymus, liver, spleen, intestine, lymphatics, and various mucous membranes. Its role in defense of the host has been summarized as encounter, recognition, activation, deployment, discrimination, and regulation (**Table 3.1**). Intuitively, this system developed to recognize pathogens and defend the host against microbial invasion; however, products of tissue injury are now known to stimulate the immune system as well (Lotze et al. 2007). There are numerous pattern recognition receptors, both cell associated and secreted, that allow host recognition of various microbial pathogens and products of host tissue injury (Netea et al. 2004). Thus, pathogen- and danger-associated molecular patterns (PAMPs and DAMPs), which are products of pathogens and damaged host cells, respectively, can both stimulate an immune response that is mediated via these specific receptors. An excessive or unabated immune response may be associated with inappropriately vigorous systemic inflammation, which can lead to organ failure without infection. Discrimination of foreign pathogens from self-tissues is critical to avoid the immune system turning on the host and the potential 'horror autotoxicus' described by Paul Ehrlich over a century ago.

It has been known since antiquity that survival from an infectious disease often conferred lifetime immunity to it; however, Jenner was first to systematically vaccinate against microbes (smallpox virus) in the eighteenth century, which eventually led to eradication of this disease. Immunization against a variety of viral and bacterial diseases, and the development of antimicrobial therapy, have both reduced mortality from many common infectious diseases during the twentieth century. An increasingly immune-suppressed population has led to emergence of multi-resistant pathogens. A persistent inflammatory response in the setting of sepsis has also been associated with development of organ failure and mortality.

The immune system classification is now generally divided into innate and adaptive immunity. Components of the innate system include mechanical barriers such as the skin, and respiratory, genitourinary, and gastrointestinal tracts, as well as complement proteins, certain cytokines and inflammatory mediators, and the phagocytic process itself. These are activated with tissue injury or local infection, and can be directed against most foreign microbes regardless of whether the host has previously encountered such organisms. Mediators of such inflammation include histamine, kinins, and arachidonic acid metabolites. Tissue injury results in the release of histamine from mast cells, as well as bradykinin and kallikrein production, which act directly on vascular endothelium to transport cellular and protein elements of the immune system to the site of injury (Ley et al. 2007). Arachidonic acid is produced by breakdown of cellular membranes and the action of phospholipase A (Funk 2001). It is then degraded by either lipooxygenase to form leukotrienes or cyclooxygenase to form prostaglandins and thromboxanes. Most of these inflammatory mediators are formed quickly and locally, where their effect is maximal and short-lived. These mediators act in a paracrine fashion, and therefore serum measurements may not reflect local activity.

Phagocytosis is essential to eradication of most live invading microbial organisms and is carried out primarily by polymorphonuclear leukocytes (neutrophils) and cells of the mononuclear phagocyte system, which include tissue macrophages. This multistep process includes immune cellular adherence to the capillary endothelium, diapedesis to the site of inflammation via chemotaxis, possible prior opsonization of foreign antigens (mostly by complement or immunoglobulins), engulfment of the microbes into the cell, and finally microbial killing and degradation (**Figure 3.1**). The process is dependent on intrinsic cellular function for bacterial killing, but highly dependent on the surrounding milieu for most of the process. Immune cell necrosis amplifies the local immune response, whereas apoptosis, or programmed cell death, actually helps to resolve the inflammatory response (Wesche et al. 2005).

Cytokines are proteins by which cells communicate between themselves, usually in a paracrine fashion (**Table 3.2**). These proteins are involved in immune cell development and also help to regulate the overall immune and inflammatory response by activating other immune cells (Medzhitov 2007). Chemokines and growth factors are also cytokines with specific functions such as chemotaxis and augmentation of immune cell differentiation. Almost all cytokines interact with immune cells via specific receptors, although they shed receptors and may also bind cytokines in the intravascular space. There are 17 interleukins (IL-1 to IL-23) that have been well studied and regulate the immune response. Cytokines can also be produced by mononuclear cells in response to specific antigenic stimulation, e.g., tumor necrosis factor-α (TNFα) is produced by macrophages in response to antigenic stimuli, most notably endotoxin. Its production occurs rapidly and binding to soluble receptors has probably accounted for the inconsistency in its detection from the blood of patients in Gram-negative septic shock (Rittirsch et al. 2008). The interferons are a family of proteins that were initially described in the supernatant of virally infected cell cultures, which "interfered" with such viral superinfection. Interferon-γ is produced primarily by mononuclear cells and has been shown to increase class II histocompatibility antigens (HLA-DR, Ia) on the surface of monocyte/macrophages, which may amplify antigen recognition (Polk et al. 1992). T-helper cells have been divided into Th-1 and Th-2 subpopulations, both of which have distinct patterns of cytokine secretion that augment or inhibit various components of the

Table 3.1 Immune system classification.

Innate	Adaptive
Mechanical barriers	Macrophage/dendritic cell antigen presentation
Complement and coagulation cascades	T lymphocyte
Mediators, cytokines, chemokines	B lymphocyte and plasma cell (antibody production)
Inflammation	
Phagocytosis	

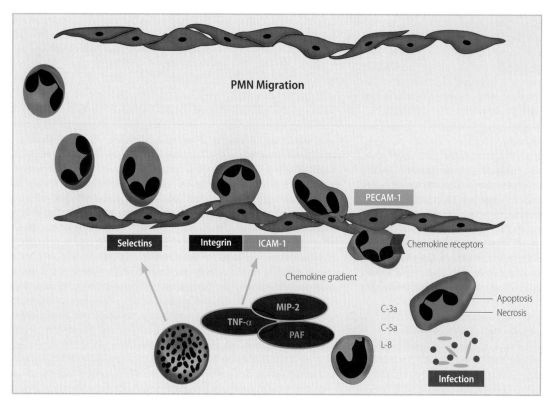

Figure 3.1 Neutrophil migration from the intravascular space into the interstitium at the site of infection. This migration is regulated by adhesion molecule expression and a chemokine gradient. The ultimate fate is either necrosis or apoptosis.

immune system. Th-1 cells secrete IL-2, IFN-γ, and TNFα which augment cell-mediated immunity by activating monocyte/macrophages, T cells, and natural killer (NK) cells. Th-2 cell secrete IL-4, -10, and -13 which activate B cells and aid in their maturation to plasma cells and antibody production. These cytokines are also anti-inflammatory and inhibit the actions of the Th-1 cytokines.

The complement cascade is a series of enzymatic cleavage reactions (**Figure 3.2**) that are triggered by either antigen–antibody complexes (classic pathway) or bacterial cell wall components (alternate pathway) (Ricklin et al. 2010). The complement system is highly conserved, indicating its early evolutionary development as a means of host defense. The latter pathway does not require prior exposure to a particular microbe, and represents a mechanism for immediate defense against microbial invasion. The membrane attack complex of complement is capable of direct bacterial lysis. Complement components recruit neutrophils to the site of infection by acting as chemoatttractants (C3a, C5a), and facilitate both phagocytosis and bacterial killing by opsonization of bacteria (C3b) and stimulation of neutrophil degranulation.

The specific immune system includes B (bursa-equivalent derived) and T (thymus derived) lymphocytes, and antigen-presenting cells such as macrophages and dendritic cells. Lymphocytes are formed from stem cells in the bone marrow, yolk sac, and liver, and then undergo differentiation into T cells by exposure to the thymus or continue to mature into B cells in the bone marrow. Foreign antigen recognition, uptake, degradation, and expression on the cell surface of macrophages or dendritic cells are the initial steps in the adaptive immune response. IL-1α is produced, and T-helper cells bind to the processed foreign antigen in contiguity with the class II histocompatibility antigen HLA-DR on the macrophage cell surface (Murphy 2011). The activated T-helper cell (CD4) then produces IL-2 which stimulates cytotoxic T-cell clonal expansion. Th-2 cells also bind to specific B cells that have been exposed to the same antigen.

This results in B-cell expansion by specific Th-2 cytokine production and maturation into plasma cells with subsequent antibody production. Antibodies produced are specific to the original foreign antigen, and memory B cells are then capable of an intense secondary response to a previously recognized antigen. The innate response may be augmented by antibody production, because phagocytosis proceeds more rapidly when microbes are opsonized and the process is receptor mediated.

BASIC CELLULAR IMMUNOLOGY

There is an overview in **Table 3.3**.

Monocyte, macrophages, and dendritic cells

Monocytes, macrophages, and dendritic cells are mononuclear granulocytic myeloid cells, which play a crucial role in the immune response. All three cell types can recognize PAMPs with their innate immune receptors, the so-called pathogen recognition receptors (PRRs), and an overview of the different classes of PRRs is provided in **Table 3.4**. Besides PAMPs, they can also recognize endogenous proteins such as heat shock proteins or high-mobility group protein B1 (HMGB1), which is released from host cells after tissue damage. These proteins are called alarmins and both PAMPs and alarmins are summarized as Danger Associated Molecular Patterns (DAMPs). Monocytes, macrophages, and dendritic cells have a high density of PRRs, and thus play a major role in the activation of the immune system after infection or tissue damage. These cells are considered the first line of defense and attract other cells of the innate immune systems such as granulocytes and new monocytes, and importantly dendritic cells, which are responsible for the activation and initiation of the adaptive immune system (Medzhitov 2007). Dysfunction of these cells occurs during

Table 3.2 Cytokines.

	Name	Function/Actions	Source
CSF	G-CSF	Stimulates neutrophil development and differentiation	Fibroblasts Monocytes
	GM-CSF	Stimulates myelomonocytic cell growth and differentiation, especially dendritic cells	Macrophages T cells
Interferons	IFN-α	Antiviral Increased MHC class I expression	Leukocytes Dendritic cells
	IFN-β	Antiviral Increased MHC class I expression	Fibroblasts
	IFN-γ	Monocyte/Macrophage activation Increased MHC II expression Promotes Ig class switch	T cells NK cells
Interleukins	IL-1β	Fever Monocyte/Macrophage activation T-cell activation	Monocytes/Macrophages Epithelial cells
	IL-2	T-cell proliferation	T cells
	IL-4	B-cell activation Induces IgE switch Induces Th2 differentiation	T cells Mast cells
	IL-5	Eosinophil growth and differentiation	T cells Mast cells
	IL-6	Fever Acute phase response T-cell growth and differentiation B-cell growth and differentiation	T cells Monocytes/Macrophages Endothelial cells
	IL-10	Suppresses monocyte, macrophage and dendritic cell functions	Monocytes
	IL-12	Activates NK cells Induces differentiation of CD4 T cells into Th1	Macrophages Dendritic cells
	IL-13	B cells growth and differentiation Inhibits monocyte/macrophage inflammatory cytokine production Inhibits Th1 cells Induces allergy/asthma	T cells
	IL-17	Induces strongly production of proinflammatory cytokines	Th17 T cells
Others	TNF-α	Promotes inflammation Endothelial cell activation	Monocytes/Macrophages NK cells T cells
	TGFβ1	Inhibits cells growth Anti-inflammatory properties Induces switch to IgA	Chondrocytes Monocytes/Macrophages T cells

G-CSF, Granulocyte colony-stimulating factor; GM-CSF, Granulocyte-macrophage colony-stimulating factor; IFN, Interferons; Ig, Immunoglobulin; IL, Interleukin; Nk, Natural killer; TGF, Transforming growth factor; Th, T-helper cell; TNF, Tumor necrosis factor.

sepsis and after trauma (Polk et al. 1986, Docke et al. 1997). Monocytes, macrophages, and dendritic cells have an array of common features: All of them express receptors of the innate immune systems such as toll-like receptors (TLRs), and they produce multiple cytokines and chemokines. All are capable of phagocytosis, antigen presentation in the development of the adaptive response, and secretion of various proteins. The types of cytokines and chemokines may vary among different subsets, and they are capable of presenting antigens to cells of the adaptive immune system such as B and T cells via the major histocompatibility complex II (MHC-II) (Gordon and Taylor 2005, Shi and Pamer 2011). The expression level of MHC II on the surface, such as HLA-DR, is widely accepted as a reliable marker for the functional state of the immune system, and several clinical trials aiming to restore HLA-DR expression in critically ill patients have been performed (Polk et al. 1992, Docke et al. 1997, Meisel et al. 2009).

All three of these cell types are derived from the multipotential hemopoietic stem cells, which differentiate into the common myeloid progenitor cell. This cell then develops into a myeloblast, which is the progenitor of the granulocyte and monocyte cell lines. There is not such a high plasticity, as previously believed, and all three cell types, despite having a related function, originate from different precursors, and cannot completely differentiate into each other. Monocytes, however, are capable of replenishing macrophages in tissues and can differentiate into some types of dendritic cells (Geissmann et al. 2010, Shi and Pamer 2011). It seems that the local environment influences the further development of monocytes, macrophages, and dendritic cells strongly (Murray et al. 2011). This differentiation depends on the expression of certain growth factor receptors and transcription factors such as PU.1 and MafB, which then activate the transcription of the cell-specific genes (Bakri et al. 2005).

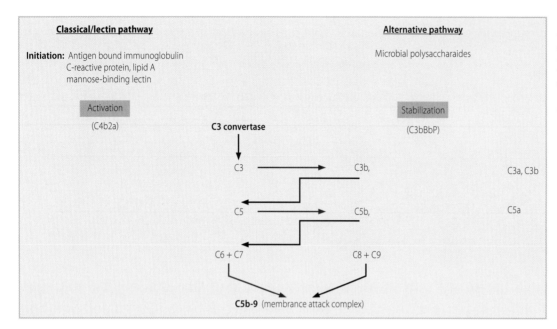

Figure 3.2 The complement cascade is activated by either antigen–antibody complexes or microbial products. C3b functions as an opsonin and C3a and C5a as chemokines. The membrane attack complex is directly lytic to microbes.

Monocytes

After production in the bone marrow, monocytes circulate in the blood, spleen, and bone marrow for several days. The spleen stores a considerable number of these cells (Shi and Pamer 2011). Under normal conditions they cannot proliferate outside the bone marrow. During infection, monocytes are released from both the bone marrow and the spleen, and become effector cells which produce cytokines as well as phagocytosing cell debris and toxic molecules (Gordon and Taylor 2005). The chemokine receptor CCR2 plays an important role in the release of monocytes from the bone marrow (Shi and Pamer 2011). These cells leave the bloodstream at the site of infection, during which time the endothelium expresses adhesion molecules; these allow the attachment of monocytes as well as their transmigration. Monocytes can then develop into inflammatory dendritic cells and tissue macrophages, depending on exposure to the local cytokine and growth factor milieu (Ziegler-Heitbrock 2007, Shi and Pamer 2011). Monocytes constitute 3–8% of the leukocytes in the blood, and about half are stored in the spleen to replenish monocytes that have left the bloodstream for sites of inflammation.

Monocytes are divided into three subgroups. The criteria are the expression of the surface markers CD14, CD16, HLA-DR, and CCR2 (a chemokine receptor), as well as the production of the cytokines TNFα and IL-10 (Ziegler-Heitbrock 2007, 2010, Shi and Pamer 2011).

- Classic monocyte: The hallmark is high expression of CD14, medium expression of HLA-DR and no expression of CD16 and CCR2. These monocytes produce both TNFα and IL-10, and seem to be the main cells that enter infectious sites and replenish tissue macrophages. These monocytes cannot re-enter the bloodstream once they are in the tissue (Belge et al. 2002).
- Non-classic monocyte (inflammatory monocyte, Tip-DC): The hallmark is high expression of CD16, HLA-DR, and CCR2, but low expression of CD14. It secretes more TNFα than the classic monocyte, but no IL-10. This monocyte subtype is believed to be the precursor of the inflammatory dendritic cell. These monocytes are capable of transmigrating through the endothelium in both directions, from blood to tissue and back into blood and lymph vessels. CD16+ cells expand during inflammatory states such as

sepsis, but also other systemic inflammatory disease. In addition, they have been associated with formation of thrombotic plaques (Fingerle et al. 1993, Mizuno et al. 2005, Kim et al. 2010).
- Intermediate monocyte: This has a high expression of CD14, but also expresses CD16 at a lower level. The cytokine production is not defined.

The current concept of monocyte development is that the classic monocyte differentiates first into the intermediate and then into the inflammatory monocyte (Ziegler-Heitbrock 2007, Shi and Pamer 2011). Furthermore, inflammatory monocytes are believed to be the precursor of inflammatory dendritic cells (Geissmann et al. 2010, Shi and Pamer 2011). Circulating monocytes have two main roles. Under normal conditions they replenish macrophages and dendritic cells in various different tissues. Under inflammatory conditions, blood monocytes are attracted to the site of inflammation and differentiate into macrophages. The main functions of monocytes are the production of cytokines, antigen presentation and phagocytosis.

Macrophages

Macrophages are found in almost all tissues and have different names depending on the tissue, i.e., Kupffer cells in the liver, histiocytes in the skin, alveolar macrophages in the lung and osteoclasts in the bone (Gordon and Taylor 2005). Macrophages develop from monocytes, which differentiate further after leaving the bloodstream, depending on the tissue that they enter. The role of tissue macrophages is twofold: Activation of the early, initial immune response in the case of infection or tissue damage, and phagocytosis of pathogens and cell debris. They actively patrol in healthy tissue with amoeboid movements as part of the immune surveillance and phagocytose debris of cells and potential pathogens (Medzhitov 2007). When macrophages recognize PAMPs, they produce proinflammatory cytokines such as TNFα, IL-1β, and IL-6, which serve as messengers between the immune cells and other tissues. The development and origin of certain macrophages such as microglia, dermal macrophages, and marginal zone macrophages in the spleen remain unclear (Geissmann et al. 2010). Current data suggest that these cells enter these tissues very early during embryogenesis, are able to replicate themselves, and are thus not dependent on monocytes from the blood.

Table 3.3 Cells of the immune system.

Name	Function	Contents/Secreted Cytokines	Surface Markers
Classic monocyte	Response to tissue injury Phagocytosis of pathogens Antigen presentation Induction of Th1 response Replacement of tissue macrophages	Proinflammatory cytokines: 　TNF-α, IL-1β, IL-6 T-cell stimulation: 　IL-12 Anti-inflammatory cytokines: 　IL-10, TGFβ	CD14 (high) HLA-DR CD33
Inflammatory monocyte (Tip-DC)	Response to tissue injury Antigen presentation Production of proinflammatory cytokines	Proinflammatory cytokines: 　TNF-α, IL-1β, IL-6 No production of IL-10	CD14 (low) CD16 HLA-DR (high) CCR2 CD33
Macrophage	Surveillance of tissues Phagocytosis of pathogens Induction of innate immune response Antigen presentation	Proinflammatory cytokines: 　TNF-α, IL-1, β IL-6 T-cell stimulation: 　IL-12 Anti-inflammatory cytokines: 　IL-10, TGFβ	CD14 CD16 HLA-DR CD11b
Dendritic cell – Myeloid dendritic cell (mDC) – Plasmacytoid dendritic cell (pDC)	Surveillance of tissues Antigen presentation in lymph node Induction of Th1 response Induction of adaptive immunity Antiviral response (pDC)	Proinflammatory cytokines: 　TNF-α, IL-1β IL-6 T-cell stimulation: 　IL-12 Anti-inflammatory cytokines: 　IL-10, TGFβ Antiviral response (pDC) 　IFN-α/β	HLA-DR CD85
Neutrophil	Response to tissue injury Phagocytosis of pathogens Antimicrobial Killing via release of granules and NETs Induction of adaptive immunity	Granule contents: 　Toxic oxygen derived products 　O_2^-, H_2O_2 O, OH, OCl⁻ 　Toxic nitrogen oxides NO 　Defensins cationic proteins 　Lysozyme acid hydrolases 　Lactoferrin and vitamin B_{12} binding protein Cytokines: 　Il-1, IL-6, IL-8 (CXCL-8), TNF-α GM-CSF	CD11 CD15 CD16 CD17 CD33
Mast cell	Response to tissue injury: 　IgE-dependent degranulation 　Complement-triggered release Production of: 　Lipid mediators (eicosanoids)	Granule contents: 　Serine-proteases 　Histamine 　Heparin 　Serotonin Lipid mediators: 　Thromboxane, prostaglandins, leukotriene Cytokines; 　TNF-α	CD117 CD23 (high)
B lymphocyte – Plasma cells – Memory cells	Humoral immune response: – Secretion of antibodies Development into memory B cells for fast response in second infection	Secreted by regulatory B cells: 　IL-10 or TGFβ-1 Secreted by effector B-cells: 　IL-2, IL-4, TNF-α, IL-6 (Be-2 cells) or IFN-γ, IL-12 and TNF-α (Be-1 cells)	CD45 CD19 CD45 CD20
T lymphocyte Helper T cells: Cytotoxic T cells:	Cytokines and growth factor production Lysis of virally infected cells, tumor cells and allografts	IL-4 IL-5 IL-10 IL-12	T cells: CD3 (T-cell receptor) Helper T cells: CD4 CD45 Cytotoxic T cells: CD8
Natural killer (NK) cells	Cytotoxic lymphocyte and part of the innate immune response: – Killing to tumor cells, non-self cells, and virus-infected cells – Secretion of perforin and granzyme to destroy target cells by apoptosis – Cytokine production	IL-3 IL-13 IL-21	CD8 – 80% of human NK cells CD16 (Fcγ RIII) CD56

GM-CSF, Granulocyte – macrophage colony-stimulating factor; IFN,.Interferons; Ig, Immunoglobulin; IL, Interleukin; NET, Neutrophil extracellular traps; NO, Nitric oxide; TGF, Transforming growth factor; TNF, Tumor necrosis factors.

Table 3.4 Pathogen recognition receptors.

Location	Receptor		Ligand	Source of ligand	Adaptor protein	Cell type
Cell Surface Receptors	Toll-like Receptors (TLR)	TLR 1	Triacyl lipopeptides	Bacteria	MyD88 MAL	Monocytes/Macrophages Dendritic cells B-cells
		TLR 2	Glyco- and lipopeptides Lipoteichoic acid Zymosan Heat Shock Protein 70	Bacteria Gram-positive bacteria Fungi Host cells	MyD88 MAL	Monocytes/Macrophages Dendritic cells Mast cells
		TLR 4	Lipopolysaccharide Heat shock proteins Fibrinogen Heparan sulfate HMGB1 Morphine and its derivates	Gram-negative bacteria Host cells Host cells Host cells Host cells	MyD88 MAL TRIF TRAM	Monocytes/Macrophages Dendritic cells Mast cells B lymphocytes
		TLR 5	Flagellin	Bacteria	MyD88	Monocytes/Macrophages Dendritic Cells
		TLR 6	Diacyl lipopeptides	Mycoplasma	MyD88	Monocytes/Macrophages Dendritic Cells
		TLR 10	Pili	Bacteria	MyD88	Monocytes/Macrophages B lymphocytes
	Receptor for Advanced Glycation Endproducts (RAGE)		Glycolysated protein HMGB1 S100	Host cells Host cells Host cells	?	Endothelial cells Pneumocytes Immune cells
	Scavenger Receptor		Lipopolysaccharide Lipoteichoic acid Oxidized lipoproteins	Bacteria		Monocytes/Macrophages
Cytosolic Receptors	Toll-like Receptors	TLR 3	Double-stranded RNA Poly I:C	Viruses Immunostimulants	TRIF	Dendritic cells B lymphocytes
		TLR 7	Single-stranded RNA	Viruses	MyD88	Monocytes/Macrophages Dendritic cells B lymphocytes
		TLR 8	Single-stranded RNA	Viruses	MyD88	Monocytes/Macrophages Dendritic cells Mast cells
		TLR 9	Unmethylated CpG DNA	Bacteria	MyD88	Monocytes/Macrophages Dendritic cells B lymphocytes
		TLR 11	Profilin	Toxoplasma gondii	MyD88	Monocytes/Macrophages
	NOD-like Receptors	NLRC 1 (NOD 1)	Peptido-glycan	Gram-negative bacteria	RIPK2	Mammalian cells
		NLRC 2 (NOD 2)	Muramyl dipeptide	Bacteria	RIPK2	Mammalian cells
		NLRP 3	Muramyl dipeptide Unmethylated CpG Double-stranded RNA Adenosine triphosphate Uric acid	Bacteria Bacteria Viruses Host cells Host cells	?	Mammalian cells
Secreted Receptors	Mannose-Binding Lectin		Certain sugar residues (Mannose, Glucose)	Gram-negative bacteria Fungi Viruses		Secreted by liver cells
	Complement Proteins	C3b	Mannose	Bacteria		Secreted by Liver cells Monoctyes/Macrophages Epithelial cells
	Pentraxin Proteins	Serum Amyloid A	Bacterial cell wall	Bacteria		Secreted by liver cells

Dendritic cells

In the current concept of the immune response, dendritic cells are considered the main antigen-presenting cells to B-and T cells (Geissman et al. 2010). Dendritic cells are also highly phagocytic cells and patrol tissues. On recognition of DAMPs, they leave the tissue, enter the lymphoid system, and present phagocytosed and processed antigens to B and T cells in the lymph nodes. The ability to enter and leave tissues, as well as the homing to lymphoid tissues, is one the key features of dendritic cells (Auffray et al. 2009). To activate B and T cells, dendritic cells express coactivating molecules, which are necessary for successful initiation of the adaptive immune response. Dendritic cells originate from the common dendritic cell precursor (CDP) and differentiate into two main types of dendritic cells: Classic and plasmacytoid dendritic cells. Classic dendritic cells patrol as immature cells through tissues and blood with a high phagocytic activity (Geissmann et al. 2010). After uptake of antigens, they develop into mature dendritic cells with high cytokine production and the ability to stimulate T cells. In addition, they are highly migratory and move into lymphoid organs to stimulate T and B cells. These cells are usually short-lived. Plasmacytoid dendritic cells are long-lived and mainly involved in the antiviral response by the production of large amounts of Interferon-α and -β (type I interferons, IFNs). However, they can also stimulate T cells and present antigens.

■ Function and regulation of monocytes, macrophages, and dendritic cells

The main function of all these three cells, monocytes, macrophages, and dendritic cells, is recognition of invading pathogens and tissue injury, and to respond to this danger by initiation of the immune response to clear the pathogens and restore homeostasis (Janeway and Medzhitov 2002). The key elements for this response are cytokine and chemokine production, antigen presentation, and phagocytosis. Monocytes, macrophages, and dendritic cells interact with other cells of the innate as well as the adaptive immune system.

Regulation of the function of monocytes, macrophages, and dendritic cells has been a focus of research in recent years. The first step of an immune response is the recognition of pathogens or tissue damage. For that purpose, monocytes are equipped with an array of several so-called PRRs (**Table 3.3**) (Medzhitov 2007). These receptors can be further divided into signaling molecules and phagocytosis receptors. Importantly, these receptors are constant and encoded in the genome, and are not rearranged as the receptors of the adaptive system (Janeway and Medzhitov 2002). For the early initiation of an innate immune response, the signaling PRRs are the most important. The best studied PPRs are the TLRs, which are extracellular receptors and able to recognize a wide variety of pathogen-associated molecules but also endogenous host proteins, which are typically released during tissue injury (Netea et al. 2004). Thirteen TLRs have been described, and the most studied is TLR-4. Other receptors include the receptor for advanced glycation endproducts (RAGE), which mainly recognizes endogenous proteins such as HMGB1, advanced glycation endproducts (AGE) or S-100, and the large group of NOD-like (nucleotide oligomerization domain) receptors. These are intracellular receptors and can recognize products of Gram-positive and Gram-negative bacterial cell walls, double-stranded RNA, or adenosine triphosphate (ATP). Importantly, the same molecule, e.g., glycopeptides or double-stranded RNA, can be recognized by several, different receptors and this overlap shows the tremendous redundancy of the immune system.

TLR-4 recognizes a broad range of pathogens and host-associated molecules such as lipopolysaccharide (LPS) or heat shock proteins. For the recognition of LPS additional proteins are required: LPS-binding protein (LBP), CD14, and lymphocyte antigen 96 (MD-2) (Guha and Mackman 2001). LBP is bound by CD14, which is a surface molecule with high density of monocytes. CD14 is anchored to the cell membrane by a glycosylphosphatidylinositol (GIP) anchor, has no intracellular domain, and is unable to signal directly. CD14 can be shed from the cell membrane or directly secreted by both monocytes and hepatocytes, and as such is a soluble receptor (Levine 2008). MD-2 is another surface molecule that seems necessary for recognition and response to LPS. The interplay of all these molecules, LBP, CD14, and MD-2, allows TLR-4 to recognize LPS and initiate the signaling cascade (Netea et al. 2004). TLR-4 is a transmembrane molecule but without a signaling domain. The main signaling molecule of TLR-4, and all other TLRs except TLR-3, is *MyD88* (myeloid differentiation primary response gene 88). In addition, TLR-4 can interact with three other signaling proteins (MAL, TRIF, TRAM). *MyD88* starts a cascade of signaling events (Li and Jiang 2010b, O'Neill et al. 2011). It interacts with *IRAK-1/2*, which in turn activates TRAF6. TRAF6 activates two different signaling pathways, the mitogen-activated protein kinases (MAPKs) and the nuclear factor-κB (NF-κB) pathway. Both are major signaling pathways and involved in response to stress such as radiation, ultraviolet light, temperature, or infection (Guha and Mackman 2001, Zhang and Dong 2005). The organization of these pathways is outlined in **Figure 3.3**.

Activation of both pathways results in production of cytokines as signaling molecules to coordinate the response of the whole organism, and also the production of defensive molecules such as complement; however, they also lead to expression of intracellular proteins, which may reduce intracellular damage (e.g., heat shock proteins) (Bianchi 2007). Interestingly, both pathways are not independent of each other. There is a broad cross-activation of both pathways, which is completed within minutes. This is possible because the molecules are preformed in the cytoplasm and are consecutively phosphorylated, which results in activation. The organization of both pathways is comparable in that they are both arrayed in several levels that lead to amplification, integration, and modulation of the incoming signal from several upstream receptors. It is important to consider that the response produced by cytokines results in feedforward and feedback mechanisms, which modulate the immune response. The receptors for TNFα and IL-1β, for example, signal through the same pathways as the TLRs (Hu et al. 2008). Other cytokines such as IL-6 and IL-10 use the JAK-STAT signaling system (Murray 2007). These signaling systems have a high level of interaction leading to either suppression or priming of one of the receptor systems. Interferon-γ, for example, can suppress IL-10 signaling. The exact mechanisms by which these signaling cascades lead to their response and how these responses are regulated remain largely unknown (Murray 2007, Murray and Wynn 2011).

Once activated, the different arms of the MAPK pathway are deactivated by dephosphorylation by specific phosphates, the group of dual specificity phosphatases (DUSPs) also known as MAPK-phosphatases (MKPs). (Patterson et al. 2009). These proteins have been recently discovered and so far 30 proteins containing the phosphatase domain have been described in whole genome studies. However, only 11 of those contain a MAPK-binding domain. These phosphatases are upregulated upon activation of the MAPK pathway within 30 min to 1 h by the same stimulus, which activates the MAPK pathway. A certain DUSP is specific for the molecule, which it can inactivate. DUSP 1, for example, inactivates p38 and JNK, but can inactivate Erk only marginally. Of note, the specificity of inactivation investigated

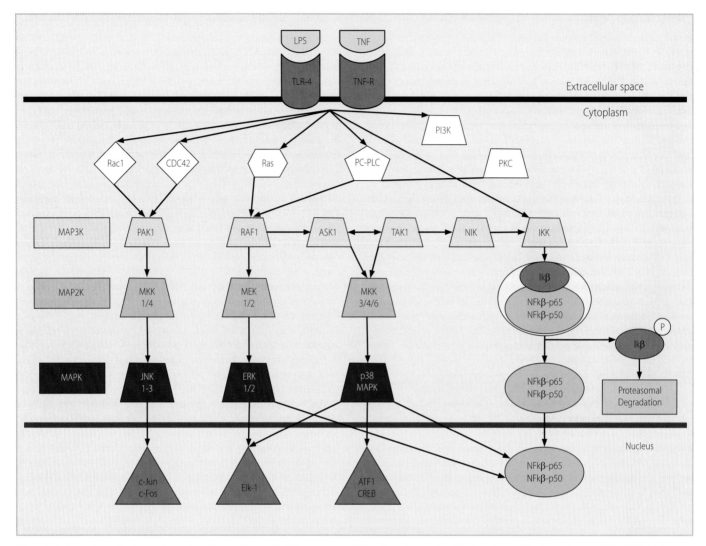

Figure 3.3 Overview of inflammatory signaling pathways. Toll-like receptor 4 (TLR-4) activates the NF-kB pathway. The key activator of NF-kB is inhibitory k kinase (IKK), which phosphorylates the Inhibitory k protein β, leading to its degradation. The NF-kB complex (p50 and p65 subunits) can then translocate into the nucleus and start transcription of inflammatory genes. TLR-4 can also activate the mitogen-activated protein kinase (MAPK) pathway, which consists of the JNK, Erk, and p38 arms. The MPAK pathway activates several different transcription factors such as c-Jun/c-Fos or Elk-1. MAPK leads to the transcription of proinflammatory cytokine and IL-10 mRNA.

in in vitro models differs remarkably from the specificity observed in animal models.

Inactivation of NF-κB is slightly different. After degradation of the inhibitory kappa protein (Ikα) or Ikβ and subsequent migration of the p50/p65complex into the nucleus, where it acts as transcription factor, Ikα/Ikβ are constitutively re-expressed and inactivate the p50/p65 complex (Karin and Ben-Neriah 2000). As a result of the activation of the MAPK pathway, common transcription factors such as PU1, CREB (cAMP response element-binding protein), and c-Myc are activated. The p65 and p50 subunits of NF-κB are transcription factors themselves. These factors then initiate transcription of mRNA for various cytokines, chemokines, and other proteins and enzymes involved in the immune response. However, as an immediate response, preformed proteins are activated such as heat shock proteins, or preformed cytokines are secreted without the delay of transcription and translation. The secretion of preformed cytokines followed by the secretion of newly produced cytokines allows a very fast response to any kind of infection or tissue damage.

The activation of these pathways by alarmins leads to production of proinflammatory cytokines such as TNFα, IL-1β, and IL-6. In addition, chemokines such as macrophage migration inhibitory factor (MIF) and IL-8 are produced and secreted. Of note, surface receptors such as HLA-DR and proteolytic enzymes are also upregulated. Following this early proinflammatory response is a delayed, counter-regulatory response, which aims to inhibit the production of proinflammatory products. One of the key cytokines in this anti-inflammatory response is IL-10. The same pathways (NF-κB and MAPK) that are responsible for the production of pro-inflammatory cytokines are responsible for the induction of IL-10 (Saraiva and O'Garra 2010). In the MAPK pathway, it seems that the Erk arm is crucial for the induction of IL-10.

It is important to note that this response pattern of sequential phases is highly reproducible and uniform in the innate immune response. In addition, cytokines in the circulation or local tissue modulate these response patterns. Some cytokine receptors signal through NF-κB and MAPK, and this leads to a highly complex intracellular response with synergistic, but also sometimes contrary, signals. The phosphorylation or dephosphorylation of these pathways is the principal means by which the immediate response functions; however, different amounts of these signaling proteins can alter the overall response profoundly. The organization of these pathways at several levels and the diverse nature of these interactions allow fine-tuning and adaptation in response to changes in the environment. The discovery of the role of micro-RNAs in the immune response can explain the mechanisms of this fine-tuning.

◼ Role of micro-RNAs in regulation of monocyte function

Monocytes/macrophages serve here as an example of cells in which the role of micro-RNAs has been described most extensively thus far. Mature micro-RNAs are short, single-stranded, 20- to 22-nucleotide-long RNA molecules, folded in a characteristic hairpin structure, which protects the mRNA from cleavage and degradation. Therefore, micro-RNAs are very stable molecules and can be found even in stored, paraffin-fixed tissue samples. Micro-RNAs are part of the non-coding RNA family, to which ribosomal RNA (rRNA), translational RNA (tRNA), and silencing RNA also belong. Micro-RNAs can inhibit protein translation in three different ways by binding to the 3'-untranslated region (UTR) of the mRNA: First, they suppress protein translation via the RISC or, rarely, the RNA-induced silencing complex (RISC) can activate other proteins, which splice the mRNA directly. The third way was discovered recently and is called the mRNA decay. Here, the poly(A) tail is degraded (dead-enylation) and the 'cap' of mRNA is subsequently removed, resulting in rapid mRNA degradation. All three mechanisms result in decreased protein production. Of note, the mRNA level is not necessarily reduced despite reduced protein expression.

Several micro-RNAs have been reported to modulate the TLR signaling pathway. The best-described are miRNA-155 and -146a. As outlined in **Figures 3.4** and **3.5**, virtually every level of the signaling pathways, but also the production of cytokines, is believed to be modulated by micro-RNAs. MiRNA-155 is easily upregulated in endotoxin shock after TLR-4 activation, and seems essential for an adequate immune response. Once upregulated, miR-155 targets negative regulators of the inflammatory response such as SOCS1 (suppressor of cytokine signaling 1) and SH2 domain-containing inositol 5'-phosphatase 1 (SHIP), which act on the signaling transducers of the TLR family and inhibit proinflammatory signals. Interestingly, miR-155 acts also as a negative regulator by reducing *MyD88* or *TAB2*, an activator of the MAPK-pathway. in a later phase of the response.

The anti-inflammatory cytokine IL-10 downregulates miR-155, supporting its primary proinflammatory role. Both miR-146a and miR-125b have been shown to inhibit TNFα and production of other proinflammatory cytokines (Tili et al. 2007, Bhaumik et al. 2009); miR-125b directly binds TNFα and suppresses TNFα protein production. Other cytokines are also subject to profound regulation by micro-RNAs such as IL-6 (Sun et al. 2011). Murphy et al. (2010) recently demonstrated that miR-125b is involved in the regulation of NF-κB activity by decreasing NF-κB activation. MiR-146a is upregulated on exposure of cells to LPS but also to IL-10 and seems to act as a major anti-inflammatory micro-RNA; it also targets upstream signaling molecules of the TLRs such as IRAK1/2 and TRAF6, and inhibits proinflammatory signals from the TLRs (Hou et al. 2009). Due to its anti-inflammatory features, miR-146a plays a crucial role in endotoxin tolerance, whereas miR-146a is upregulated after the first LPS exposure and consecutively protects the host from the second LPS hit and reduces the TNFα levels (Nahid et al. 2009, 2010). In addition, miR-146a is predicted to bind proteins of the MAPK-signaling cascade.

Micro-RNAs are also involved in regulation of the inflammatory signaling cascades, e.g., miR-15a and -16, which are expressed as

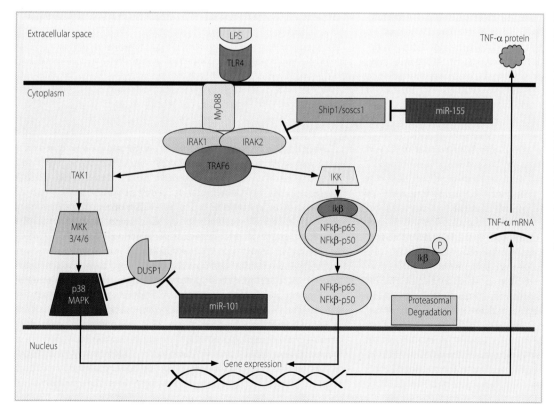

Figure 3.4 In the proinflammatory phase, two micro-RNAs (miRNA-155 and -101) play an important role by inhibiting the production of negative regulators of the toll-like receptor-signaling pathway such as SHIP1/SOCS1 and DUSP1 (aka MKP1). In this situation, the effect of the micro-RNAs is immediate, because these proteins SHIP1/SOCS1 and DUSP1 are newly produced after monocyte activation. This inhibition of negative regulators leads to an enhanced inflammatory response. Only the p38-arm of the MAPK pathway is shown here.

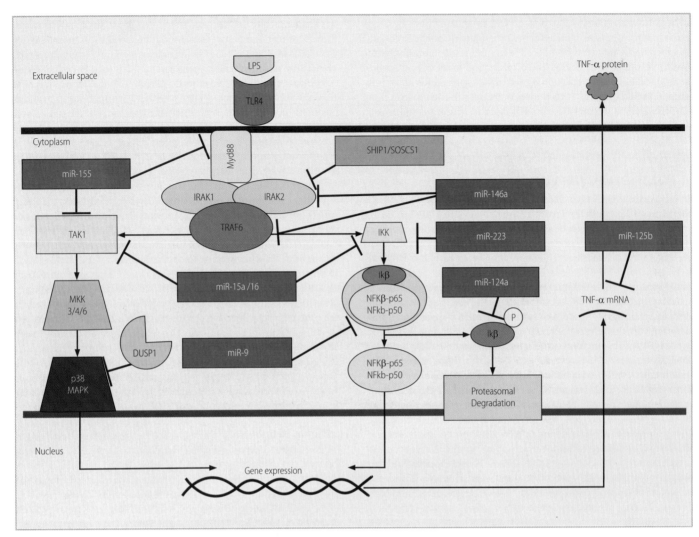

Figure 3.5 In the counterinflammatory phase of the monocyte/macrophage response, several micro-RNAs act on virtually every level of the signaling pathways and inhibit the production of signaling proteins. As these signaling proteins exist at the time of activation of the cells, the effect of micro-RNAs is delayed because they can inhibit only the new production of these signaling proteins. MiRNA-146a plays an important role because it inhibits the central activating complex for the NF-kB and MAPK pathway consisting of IRAK-1 and -2 and TRAF6. MiRNA-155 plays a dual role in the inflammatory response: It first has a proinflammatory effect by inhibiting the production of SHIP1/SOCS1, but has in the secondary phase an inhibiting effect by downregulation of the central signaling pathway of almost all toll-like receptors, MyD88.

a cluster, are critical regulators of both the NF-κB and the MAPK pathways, and Li et al. showed that they target IKKα, one of the activators of NF-κB (Li et al. 2010a). Another study revealed that both micro-RNAs (15a and 16) act on the MAPK pathway, especially on the MAP3 kinases, which are responsible for the cross-activation of the NF-κB pathway, such as TAK1 (Roccaro et al. 2009). MiR-124a and -223 also influence IKKβ, exemplifying the redundant role of several micro-RNAs in regulating the same gene (Lindenblatt et al. 2009). It has also been shown that miR-9 regulates NF-κB activation, but not by inhibiting the inhibitory protein. It directly acts on the p50 subunit of NF-κB (Bazzoni et al. 2009). In addition to the direct regulation of the signaling proteins, the negative regulator of the MAPK signaling, the DUSPs, are also regulated by micro-RNAs. MiR-101 has been shown to control DUSP-1 directly (Zhu et al. 2010). MiR-101 is upregulated early upon activation of the TLRs, but it is downregulated by the PI3K-Akt pathway, an important anti-inflammatory signaling pathway.

Besides the regulation of the signaling cascade, micro-RNAs have also been shown to directly downregulate specific protein receptors, which recognize the DAMPs. Let-7i, for example, directly downregulates TLR-4 (Chen et al. 2007). Furthermore, miRNA-21 has been shown to induce IL-10 expression by a complex feedback mechanism, which is already induced on LPS stimulation of TLR-4 (Sheedy et al. 2010). These data draw an intensively regulated network of proteins and their activation but also gene expressions with post-transcriptional modification (mRNAs and micro-RNAs), which affect each other, resulting in the final response to inflammation – measured as systemic cytokines. It seems that micro-RNAs are especially important for the switch from pro- to the counter-regulatory phase of the immune response. Based on their profound impact on cell function, micro-RNAs offer opportunities as diagnostic and probably therapeutic targets. Some micro-RNAs have been described as marker for sepsis, potentially with prognostic capabilities in humans (Vasilescu et al. 2009, Wang et al. 2010).

Polymorphonuclear leukocytes (neutrophils)

Neutrophils, similar to all other cellular components of the blood, are derived from pluripotent hemopoietic stem cells in the bone marrow, which then give rise to myeloid and subsequent granulocyte progenitors. These granulocytes or polymorphonuclear leukocytes (PMNs) include neutrophils, basophils, and eosinophils. Neutrophils, similar to other granulocytes, are distinctive for their multilobed nucleus and granules; they are the most abundant granulocyte and are found mostly dormant in the blood, although they are not present in normal healthy living tissue. They have a key role in the innate immune response due to their ability to recognize, ingest (phagocytose), and destroy pathogens without the aid of the adaptive immune response. Congenital or acquired deficiencies of neutrophil function lead to life-threatening infections.

Neutrophils are short lived (8–20 h), although their lifespan can be extended by cytokines (IL-6, IFN-β, and granulocyte–macrophage colony-stimulating factor [GM-CSF]), hypoxia and microbial products to enhance function at sites of infection (El Kebir and Filep 2010).

Neutrophils contain three different subsets of granules, or stores of proteins that kill microbes and digest tissues, based on the characteristic granule proteins (Borregaard 2010). Primary or azurophil granules contain myeloperoxidase (MPO), secondary or specific granules contain lactoferrin, and tertiary ones contain gelatinase. Azurophilic granules are considered the most potent, containing many antimicrobial peptides including lytic enzymes and defensins, presumed to work by making pores in bacterial membranes. Specific or secretory granules are important early in inflammation, easily mobilized, and contain multiple membrane-associated receptors, including those mediating endothelial attachment and complement receptors involved in host–pathogen interactions (Nordenfelt and Tapper 2011). Gelatinase granules contain enzymes to degrade the extracellular matrix and receptors for direct migration when the neutrophil has migrated into the tissues.

Neutrophil migration

Neutrophils are the first blood cell attracted to the site of infection in large numbers as the early part of the innate immune response, beginning in minutes. They are attracted by chemoattractants, including complement fragments C3a and C5a, and CXCL8 (previously known as IL-8). CXCL8 is produced by macrophages and dendritic cells in response to infection, and binds to CXCR receptors 1 and 2, causing mobilization, activation, and degranulation of neutrophils.

Bacterial formylated peptides (fMLP) also act as chemoattractants for neutrophils. PMNs possess the fMLP receptor, which is a G-protein-coupled receptor similar to complement and chemokine receptors.

Leukocytes usually flow in the center of small vessels where flow is fastest (see Figure 3.1). However, vessel dilation in areas of inflammation, with resulting decreased flow rates, allow the leukocytes to interact with the endothelium. A change in the adhesion molecules on both neutrophils and endothelial cells, in response to infection, leads to the recruitment of large numbers of circulating neutrophils. Neutrophil movement across the endothelial wall of blood vessels (extravasation) occurs mostly in postcapillary venules, where there is a sufficiently thin wall and flow can continue around the adherent neutrophils (Silva 2011). The first stage of neutrophil extravasation is the expression of P-selectin on endothelial cells in response to leukotriene B$_4$ (LTB$_4$), TNFα, IL-1β, IL-17, C5a, or histamine, which also leads to the later expression of E-selectin (after exposure to TNFα or LPS) (Ley et al. 2007). Selectins recognize sulfated sialyl Lewis that

is exposed on the tips of leukocyte microvilli, and reversibly bind, leading to rolling along the vessel wall. Integrins LFA-1 and CRB bind the intercellular adhesion molecules ICAM-1 (induced by TNFα) and ICAM-2. This usually results in a weak binding, but a conformational change induced by CXCL8 increases adhesion, and the firmly attached neutrophil stops rolling along the endothelial wall.

There are two routes for transendothelial migration: Transcellular (20%) whereby neutrophils penetrate the individual endothelial cell, or paracellular (80%), whereby the neutrophils diapedese between endothelial cells (Borregaard 2010).

Further interactions between integrins and Ig-related molecules PECAM or CD31, which is expressed on neutrophils and the intracellular junction of endothelial cells, allow the neutrophil to squeeze between endothelial cells, and then penetrate the basement membrane with the help of matrix metalloproteinases that break down the extracellular matrix of the basement membrane. Tissue migration then occurs under the influence of chemokine concentration gradients produced at the site of infection and bound to proteoglycans in the extracellular matrix. Neutrophils that have migrated into tissues are more active than the dormant blood-circulating population, and are able to recruit additional inflammatory cells via necrosis and CXCL8 production (Borregaard 2010).

Pathogen recognition

PMNs recognize pathogens via cell-surface receptors, and can also discriminate the host from pathogens. PRRs recognize PAMPs present on extra- and intracellular microbes and include TLRs, NOD-like receptors, and Dectin-1. Neutrophils are activated by the detection of pathogen and tissue damage via PRRs. Some pathogens, notably *Staphylococcus epidermidis*, are able to shield themselves from the phagocyte receptor by coating themselves with a thick polysaccharide capsule (biofilm). Activated neutrophils release soluble pattern recognition molecules that enhance phagocytosis, activate complement, and regulate inflammation. Complement facilitates the uptake and destruction of pathogens by phagocytic cells, because specific complement receptors (CRs) recognize bound complement components and complement-coated particles are more efficiently taken up by phagocytes. CR3 receptor engagement on neutrophils induces phagocytosis. C5a acts directly on neutrophils and macrophages to increase vessel wall adherence, migration toward sites of antigen deposition, increasing the ability to ingest pathogens and upregulating the expression of CR1 and -3 on the cell surface.

Phagocytosis and microbial killing

Neutrophils eliminate many pathogens by phagocytosis, where the cell wall is extended around the target to internalize it in a membrane-bound vacuole or phagosome. Phagocytosis is initiated by a phagocytic receptor which interacts with IgG, among other proteins to initiate particle uptake (Nordenfelt and Tapper 2011). Neutrophils exhibit more rapid rates of phagocytosis and higher intensity of oxidative respiratory response than macrophages. This is likely due to the secretion of preformed granules, enhancing the speed of efficient pathogen killing. One of the key features of neutrophils is the generation of reactive oxygen species (ROS) by activation of the NADPH oxidase complex within the phagosome. This occurs after the fusion of granule contents with phagosomes and/or the plasma membrane, and to a greater extent in neutrophils than in macrophages. NADPH oxidase activation induces molecular oxygen reduction to the superoxide anion, which is transformed into ROS, including hydrogen peroxide, hydroxyl radicals, and hypochlorous acid (see Table 3.2) by myeloperoxidase. The generation of ROS also affects the local pH, as does bicarbonate, ion transport, and exchange systems. Phagosomal pH is often determined by vacuolar-type ATPase (V-ATPase) activity, with increasing acidification with recruitment of increasing number of V-ATPases, although this is more important in macrophages, because neutrophils tend to have a more neutral pH, which does not seem to impair antimicrobial activity and changes in pH are more likely to come from the oxidative burst. Necrotic neutrophils contribute a major component of pus (especially in extracellular pyogenic bacteria) and amplify local inflammation as opposed to apoptotic neutrophils, which do not incite an inflammatory response.

Other cell signaling

Neutrophils in tissues produce agents that attract additional neutrophils and macrophages, and regulate their activity. Macrophages and neutrophils cooperate to potentiate antimicrobial effector functions and accelerate the resolution of infection-associated inflammation via apoptosis (Silva 2011). Neutrophils also produce cytokines involved in the survival, maturation, and differentiation of both B and T cells, and can increase the cytokine production of NK cells via ROS generation and granule content release (Mantovani et al. 2011). Through contact dependent interactions, neutrophils may also induce the maturation of monocyte-derived dendritic cells in vitro, via CD18. These dendritic cells acquire the ability to induce T-cell proliferation, with a Th-1 propensity. Activated neutrophils are also able to migrate to lymph nodes after antigen capture, to influence the available lymphocyte population and the adaptive immune response.

Neutrophil extracellular traps

The short lifespan of resting neutrophils can be prolonged when recruited to sites of infection, but apoptosis spontaneously occurs after 24–28 hours and may be accelerated by pathogens (Silva 2011). Macrophage and neutrophil cooperation continues in the resolution phase when apoptotic and non-apoptotic neutrophils are removed by macrophages. Neutrophils may express 'eat-me' signals as a pro-clearance mechanism before they release cytotoxic and immunogenic components through "open autolysis." Macrophages may even induce apoptosis of neutrophils through secreted molecules or direct cell interactions. The apoptosis of neutrophils and ingestion by macrophages are important to the resolution of the local inflammatory response (Serhan et al. 2008). Neutrophils are very cytotoxic, especially when they lyse, hence the need for regulation due to the risk of collateral tissue damage. Macrophage phagocytosis not only protects host tissues, but also allows the granules of the neutrophil to be added to its arsenal of antimicrobial activity, enhancing its own effector function. In addition this reduces neutrophil necrosis and downregulates the production of G-CSF to limit local neutrophil activation and bone marrow release. Neutrophils are also able to phagocytose apoptotic neutrophils, usually after exposure to activating substances such as LPS or IFN-γ (Nordenfelt and Tapper 2011). This enhances the resolution of inflammation, because the neutrophils are present in greater numbers than macrophages. Neutrophils contribute to the synthesis of resolvins, lipid mediators of the resolution phase of inflammation, which are able to inhibit neutrophil activation. In the resolution stage of inflammation, neutrophils also aid by blocking and scavenging cytokines and chemokines (Mantovani et al. 2011).

Formation of neutrophil extracellular traps (NETs) is an alternative to death by necrosis or apoptosis. During necrosis, the nuclei swell and the chromatin is dissolved, and large strands of decondensed DNA are extruded from the cell, carrying with them proteins from the cytosol, granules, and chromatin (histones) (Borregaard 2010). NET proteins are primarily the cationic bactericidal proteins: Histones, defensins, elastase, proteinase 3, lactoferrin, and MPO. The mechanism of formation is not yet completely known but depends on hydrogen peroxide generated by NADPH oxidase and further metabolized by MPO. NETs also contain some neutrophil-derived pattern recognition molecules (PRMs) with antibody-like properties. NETs act to trap microorganisms such as *Eschericha coli* and *Staphylococcus aureus*, and allow interactions with their associated granular proteins to facilitate elimination. NETs are cleared by DNA-ases, a strategy of some bacteria such as *Streptococcus pyogenes* and *Streptococcus pneumoniae* which are known to cause necrotizing fasciitis, but these DNAases can damage the surrounding tissues, likely having a proinflammatory role.

Clinical implications from PMN-mediated lung injury

The balance of neutrophil recruitment and activation during inflammation is important because the mechanisms by which these cells can destroy pathogens via ROS and proteases can also inflict damage on the host tissues. Acute respiratory distress syndrome (ARDS) can occur as a complication of pneumonia or as a consequence of trauma or sepsis, where there is failure of oxygen transfer between the alveolar sac and the pulmonary circulation. Neutrophil activation and sequestration in the alveolar capillaries, correlate with the severity of gas exchange and protein leak (Segel et al. 2011). The release of neutrophil elastase, defensins, and ROS causes local damage to the epithelium increasing paracellular permeability and fluid leakage, which occurs in the acute lung injury associated with ARDS. Neutrophil-derived proteinases also inhibit surfactant activity, worsening the decreased gas exchange. There is also a decrease in neutrophil apoptosis proportional to the severity of the sepsis.

Mast cells, basophils, and eosinophils

These granulocytes all have a multitude of granules which contain compounds that amplify the local innate immune response, including histamine, chemokines, leukotrienes, prostaglandins, and interleukins. These cells have Fc receptors for IgE, and mediate inflammation by causing intense vasodilation, capillary leak, and neutrophil accumulation after degranulation and mediator release (Kawakami and Galli 2002). Mast cells also metabolize arachidonic acid to produce additional prostaglandins and leukotrienes, in addition to those existing in preformed granules. Eosinophils also have compounds (oxides) that are directly lytic to extracellular pathogens, notably parasites. Mast cells are mostly located in tissues underlying skin and mucous membranes, whereas basophils circulate in the vascular compartments. Complement components C3a and C5a also trigger mast cell degranulation.

LYMPHOCYTES
T cells

When hemopoietic progenitor cells migrate to the fetal thymus, they acquire the phenotypic characteristics of T cells under the influence of thymic hormones. CD2 and CD3 (TCR) are the major markers retained on all peripheral T cells, which consist of α and β chains ($\alpha\beta$ T cells). Other T lymphocytes include natural killer T cells, which express the NK1.1 molecule, similar to NK cells and $\gamma\delta$ T cells, the TCR of which is composed of these different chains. These two subpopulations can bind antigens directly or via other MHC molecules, and are often located in submucosal tissues. Two major types of T cells exist and they are classified based on the expression of the cell surface proteins CD4 or CD8. CD4 defines a T-helper (Th) subset, which differentiates in the molecules they secrete (cytokines). CD8 defines a cytotoxic-suppressor cell (Tc or Ts) subset. Th-17 cells produce IL-17 which augments inflammation via PMN recruitment and stimulation of pro-inflammatory cytokine production.

Th cells (CD4+ T lymphocytes)

These cells enhance both humoral and cell-mediated immunity, and consist of two distinct subtypes of Th cells with different functions (Th-1 and Th-2), which are mutually inhibitory through their patterns of cytokine secretion:

- **Th-1 lymphocytes**: These are primarily made in response to microbes that infect or activate macrophages and NK cells, and in response to viruses. The Th-1 cell's function is to promote cytotoxic T-cell (CD8+ cell) responses and the delayed-type hypersensitivity response. Th-1 lymphocytes produce cytokines such as IFN-γ, lymphotoxin, and tumor necrosis factor-β (TNFβ). Cytokines produced by Th-1 lymphocytes activate macrophages, enabling them to kill microbes in phagolysosomes, release inflammatory cytokines to promote inflammation, recruit phagocytes, and increase expression of MHC molecules and cofactors for T-lymphocyte activation. In addition, these Th-1-produced cytokines stimulate B lymphocytes to produce complement-binding and -opsonizing antibody molecules for enhanced attachment of microbes to phagocytes during phagocytosis.
- **Th-2 lymphocytes**: These lymphocytes are primarily made in response to helminths, allergens, and extracellular microbes and toxins. Th-2 lymphocytes produce cytokines such as IL-4, IL-5, and IL-13. The cytokines produced by Th-2 lymphocytes stimulate:
    - B lymphocytes to produce immunoglobulin E (IgE). IgE serves as an opsonizing antibody to bind eosinophils to helminths and triggers mast cells to release mediators of inflammation.
    - B lymphocytes to produce a subclass of the antibody IgG that is able to neutralize microbes and toxins.

Cytokines produced by Th-2 cells mainly include IL-4, IL-5, IL-6, IL-10, and IL-13. Th-2 cells stimulate B lymphocytes to proliferate and differentiate into antibody-producing cells. In general, the activation and proliferation of Th cells depends on the co-recognition of specific antigenic peptides and MHC class II molecules on antigen-presenting cells (APCs) such as macrophages, dendritic cells, or B cells. In turn, the activated Th cells produce cytokines, differentiation factors, and inflammatory cytokines.

■ Regulatory T cells (T$_{reg}$)

This subpopulation actually inhibits many immune functions and includes cells within $\alpha\beta$, NK, and $\gamma\delta$ T-cell populations. These have a particularly important function in the developing thymus to suppress cells that recognize self, thus preventing the development of autoimmunity and allergy. These cells also produce several cytokines including IL-4, -10, -21, and -22, and transforming growth factor (TGF) β. Collectively T$_{reg}$ cells stimulate T and NK cells, promote mast cell growth, but inhibit Th-1 cells and macrophages. TGFβ actually inhibits

T cells as well, so T$_{reg}$ function is determined primarily by their cytokine secretion profile.

■ Killer cells

Cytotoxic T cells are mostly CD8+ cells and are part of the cell-mediated immune response directed primarily against virus-infected cells or tumor cells by apoptosis. Cytotoxic T cells act by recognizing foreign antigen peptide in contiguity with MHC class I molecules and specific surface TCRs. Activation of the cells can also occur through CD40–CD ligand interactions and IL-2 is necessary for T-cell function. Target cell destruction occurs by initial adhesion of the cytotoxic T cell, subsequent release of toxic cytoplasmic granules, and finally target cell apoptosis. A portion of cytotoxic T cells becomes a memory population capable of rapid recognition and deployment.

NK cells represent around 10–15% of lymphocytes in the peripheral circulation. They kill certain tumor cells (without damaging normal tissues) and defend the host against viral infection (Sun and Lanier 2011). Unlike T cells, NK cells recognize foreign antigen that does not have to be presented on MHC molecules. NK cells also mediate ADCC toxicity and secrete several proinflammatory cytokines. This allows NK cells to kill antibody-coated target cells. NK cells are usually activated by IFN-y and IL-2 and also induce target cell apoptosis.

■ B lymphocytes
Differentiation and types of B cells

B lymphocytes terminally differentiate into plasma B cells. These cells secrete large amounts of immunoglobulin (antibodies) in response to antigenic stimulation. There are two major subtypes of B lymphocytes: CD5+ cells which produce IgM antibody to soluble polysaccharides and self-antigens. They are stimulated by non-specific cytokines from Th cells, and CD5– cells, which produce IgG, IgA, or IgE antibody specific to individual protein antigens, and bacterial LPSs. These cells require direct physical interaction with specific Th cells. Memory B cells are produced after primary exposure to an antigen. They produce antibody with increased affinity for its antigen because of somatic mutation of Ig genes. Mature B cells have both surface IgM and IgD which serve as the B-cell receptor and bind antigen. B cells can also present antigen to Th cells via class II MHC. Generally, B cells respond to two types of antigens: (1) T-cell-independent antigens activate B cells in the absence of CD4+ Th cells. These antigens are usually composed of polysaccharides or carbohydrates with repeating structures. (2) T-cell-dependent antigens (almost all protein antigens) that require B- and T-cell interaction. The T cell then drives B cells to switch antibody classes (class switching) via direct contact and cytokine secretion.

B cells play an important role in immune responses through antibody production, APC function, and cytokine secretion (Johnson 1999). Immunoglobulins are secreted by B cells and these are Y-shaped proteins consisting of two identical light (L) and two identical heavy (H) chains, which are held together by disulfide bridges. Both the low-molecular-weight L and the high-molecular-weight H chains have constant and variable regions. These regions are subdivided into segments called domains. The L chain has one variable and one constant domain whereas H chains have one variable and three or four constant domains. The variable domains are responsible for antigen binding and the constant chains are responsible for other functions. Differences in the amino acids in the constant region divide the L chain into a κ or λ type. Two important peptides of the immunoglobulins are the Fab fragment containing the antigen-binding sites, and the Fc fragment, which is involved in specifically assigned functions such as complement fixation, attachment to cells, and placental transfer.

Development and function of B cells

B-cell development is a highly regulated process whereby functional peripheral subsets are produced from hemopoietic stem cells, in the fetal liver before birth and in the bone marrow afterward. If stem cells remain in the bone marrow, they acquire the phenotypic CD markers characteristic of the stages of B-cell differentiation (Johnson 1999). A membrane-bound, epitope-specific, antigenic receptor that is a monomeric immunoglobulin M (IgM) antibody distinguishes the B-cell antigenic receptor from that of the T cell. There are specific B-cell homing areas that primarily exist in the splenic follicles and red pulp, the lymph nodes, and mucosal-associated tissues. Partial maturation in the thymus and bone marrow *in utero* is followed by migration to and seeding of the peripheral lymphoid tissues. After birth, the T and B cells differentiate further and gain immune competency under antigenic stimuli.

Naïve B cells in the bone marrow are generally divided into three subsets, B-1 B cells, follicular B cells, and marginal zone (MZ) B cells (Allman and Pillai 2008). Cells of the follicular and MZ subsets vary in terms of their location, ability to migrate, and the likelihood that they will be activated in a T-dependent or a T-independent fashion. In addition to the well-recognized role of peripheral B cells in mediating humoral immune responses, B cells can also secrete cytokines and have the potential to present antigen to naïve T cells. Some of the functions of B cells that are less well understood include the potential role of some B-cell populations as regulatory cells inhibiting tissue-specific inflammation, the potential role of activated cytokine-producing B cells in the activation of T cells that drive inflammation, and the possible role of B cells in the induction of tertiary lymphoid organs at sites of disease-related inflammation.

Naïve, mature, follicular B cells occupy two niches during their re-circulatory paths. Once they mature and are able to re-circulate in the spleen or bone marrow, they migrate repeatedly through the blood and the lymph to B-cell homing areas of lymph nodes, Peyer patches, and the spleen. Naïve follicular B cells residing in the "follicular niche" may thus present T-dependent antigens to activated T cells. The "follicular niche" therefore represents the major site at which re-circulating B cells mediate T-dependent immune responses to protein antigens. Apart from homing in on their "follicular niche," follicular B cells also migrate to the bone marrow where they form discrete collections around vascular sinusoids (Cariappa et al. 2005, 2007). This "perisinusoidal niche" is made up of the same re-circulating B cells that reside in follicles. Perisinusoidal B cells can be activated by blood-borne microbes in a T-cell-independent manner, and differentiate into IgM-secreting, antibody-forming cells (AFCs), but they are unable to induce antibody immunodeficiency, possibly because they are not architecturally configured to readily interact with helper T cells which are relatively scarce in this compartment.

MZ B cells are considered to be innate-like cells that can be induced to differentiate into short-lived plasma cells (Allman and Pillai 2008). MZ B cells can also mediate the transport of antigen in immune complexes into splenic follicles, may be involved in T-dependent B-cell responses, and may participate in immune responses to lipid antigens. MZ B cells can also transport antigen in immune complexes from the vicinity of the marginal sinus to follicular B cells in the splenic follicle (Ferguson et al. 2004, Cinamon et al. 2008). In human lymph nodes, B cells located in the outer extrafollicular rim have also long been called MZ B cells. These human cells with an IgM+ memory B-cell phenotype could potentially also play a role in antigen capture and transport into

lymph node B-cell follicles, in a manner analogous to that postulated for mouse splenic MZ B cells. In addition to their important role in T-independent responses, MZ B cells may also participate in T-cell-dependent immune responses to protein and lipid antigens.

▊ IMMUNOGLOBULINS

There are mainly five classes of immunoglobulins: IgG, IgM, IgA, IgE, and IgD. These are identified by differences in the heavy chains and the γ H chain is expressed on IgG, the α on IgA, the μ on IgM, the ε on IgE, and the δ on IgD.

- **IgG** is composed of two L chains and two H chains. IgG has the highest serum levels of all the other four classes of immunoglobulins and a half-life of 18–25 days. IgG is the only maternal immunoglobulin that crosses the placental barrier and confers immunity. It is specifically produced during the secondary immune response. IgG adheres to cells that possess a receptor for the Fc fragment from IgG (Fcγ), is bound by staphylococcal protein A, fixes and activates complement (resulting an enzymatic reaction that leads to cell lysis), and mediates placental passage of maternal antibody to the fetus. There are four subtypes with varying capabilities to activate complement or affinity to the Fc receptor on phagocytic cells.

- **IgM** mainly exists in two structural forms: A monomer (one four-chain Y structure) synthesized by and retained on the membrane of B cells as an antigen receptor and a pentamer secreted after antigen and cytokine activation of plasma cells. The pentameric IgM molecule has five Y-shaped molecules joined by a J chain and is the major immunoglobulin produced by the primary antibody response. IgM has ten binding sites, giving it the highest avidity for antigen, and its five chains with Fc complement-binding sites also make it the most efficient complement-binding activating immunoglobulin. IgM is the first to be produced in infancy and possibly in the fetus *in utero* as a defense against infection.

- **IgA** exists in three main forms: A monomer, a dimer, and a dimer plus secretory piece. IgA is the main immunoglobulin used in secretions such as milk colostrum, saliva, tears, and respiratory and intestinal mucus. IgA prevents the attachment of microorganisms to mucous membranes. It is secreted as a dimer with the monomeric forms joined by a J chain and a secretory piece called sIgA, which is added during the passage through the mucosa. This secretory piece protects IgA from proteolysis.

- **IgE** is present in very low concentrations in serum because its Fc region can bind avidly to mast cells and basophils and trigger the release of their granules. The binding of antigen to these IgE-sensitized cells triggers the release of vasoactive amines (mainly histamine). This can result in a local (hives) or systemic reaction (anaphylaxis). IgE provides protection against parasites but is also response for immune hypersensitive (allergic) reactions in some individuals.

- **IgD** is found on the membranes of 15% of newborns and 5% of adult peripheral blood lymphocytes together with IgM. IgD is very low in serum and is known to function in antigen recognition because it is primarily found bound to the membrane of mature B cells.

▊ THE INNATE IMMUNE RESPONSE

An innate immune system can be found in all animal and plants. It responds in a uniform, reproducible way to the same stimulus and is not capable of building a memory like the adaptive system. The key factor in the innate immune system is the recognition of certain, common molecular patterns, the DAMPs, which derive directly from pathogens (PAMPs), or are released from host cells upon tissue injury (alarmins) as an indirect sign of danger. These DAMPs are recognized by PRRs (see Table 3.4). The response of the cells of the innate system lead to a whole cascade of events, which aim to clear the infection and repair damaged tissue. The importance of the innate immune system is underlined by the fact that there are very few survivable gene defects in this system. The barrier function of skin or mucosa and other passive defense mechanisms such as tears or cilia movements are an important first line of defense and help prevent the invasion of pathogens into tissues. Besides the cellular part of the innate immune response, the complement system also contributes to clearance of pathogens by directly killing bacteria, increasing phagocytosis, or attracting additional leukocytes to the site of infection. Of note, there are several intersections between the innate and adaptive system, which lead to enhancement of the response of both systems.

Sequence of events

The response of the innate immune system has two aspects. The first focuses on containment and clearance of the local infection; the second aspect is to focus the body's metabolism on supporting the clearance of infection. The local control of the infection is discussed first. An overview of the different steps and processes in the local innate immune response at the site of infection is given in **Figure 3.6**. The first step is recognition of DAMPs by PRRs, which are mainly found on macrophages, monocytes, and dendritic cells. The activation of these cells leads to the secretion of cytokines and chemokines. At the site of infection, cytokines activate the endothelium, which is the principal signal for leukocytes in the blood to exit the bloodstream. The influx of cells at the infectious site follows a typical and reproducible pattern. The first cells are the PMNs such as granulocytes, which are followed

by monocytes and lymphocytes. In addition, the activation of the complement and coagulation system supports the inflammation process. The complement system can be activated in two ways, the classic and alternative pathways. The activated complement can opsonize bacteria for more efficient phagocytosis, act as chemoattractants for leukocytes, or destroy bacteria directly by formation of the membrane attack complex (MAC). The injury of blood vessels leads to the initiation of the coagulation cascade, which results in clotting arteries and capillaries. Both systems support the overall goal of bacterial clearance synergistically. The coagulation system contains the infection and prevents the spreading of bacteria by occluding the blood flow from the tissue; the complement system kills bacteria and attracts immune cells (de Jong et al. 2010). It is now known that there is a considerable cross-reactivity between the complement and coagulation system, but also PRRs and cells of the innate and adaptive immune system, meaning that activated proteinases of the complement system can activate the coagulation cascade and vice versa (Amara et al. 2010, Ricklin et al. 2010). This allows the activation of both systems at the same time by one stimulus and therefore a faster coordinated response.

All these different events are together responsible for the clinical picture of inflammation of swelling, redness, heat, and pain. Derivates of arachidonic acid such as prostaglandins and leukotrienes are produced during inflammation and lead to vasodilation and platelet activation at the site of infection (Basu 2010). The increased blood flow is responsible for the heat and redness, which is seen clinically, but it also brings a higher number of leukocytes to the tissue. Increased permeability of the endothelium leads to exudation of plasma proteins and facilitates the transmigration of leukocytes trough the endothelium. This increased permeability is visible as swelling of the infected site. Pain results from the activation of nerve endings by several of the secreted substances such as leukotrienes and others.

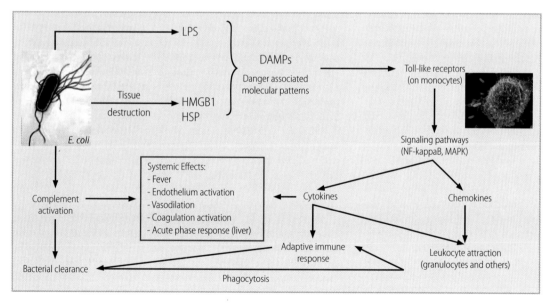

Figure 3.6 The innate immune system can be activated by either pathogen-associated molecular patterns (PAMPs) such as lipopolysaccharide (LPS) or by endogenous proteins (alarmins) such as HMGB1 or heat shock proteins. These danger-associated molecular patterns (DAMPs) are recognized by innate immune receptors (pattern recognition receptors [PRRs]), which are found in high density on monocytes, macrophages, and dendritic cells. Activation of these cells leads to the production of cytokines (TNF-α, IL-1α, IL-6) and chemokines (CCL2, MIP), leading to attraction of other immune cells such as granulocytes and lymphocytes via endothelium activation. The interplay of these cells, supported by the complement system and coagulation system, leads to the clearance of the pathogen. Cytokines are also responsible for the systemic response of the body such as fever and the induction of the acute phase response by the liver.

Role of endothelium

The trigger signals for leukocytes to enter a site of infection are the expression of adhesion molecules on activated endothelial cells, as previously described. The endothelium is activated by cytokines leading to the expression of several different adhesion molecules such as selectins and integrins, allowing migration to occur along a chemokine gradient. There are several subgroups of these adhesion molecules described and it seems that they are specialized for a certain step in leukocyte transmigration (see Figure 3.1). However, there is a certain degree of redundancy among these molecules and blocking of one subgroup alone is usually not sufficient to prevent extravasation of leukocytes. Selectins and other adhesion molecules such as ICAM-1 and -2 or VCAM-1 are mainly expressed on the endothelium, whereas integrins such as LFA-1 or CD11a/b are expressed on leukocytes. Chemokines are a large group of proteins, which serve as attractants for immune cells. They are divided into two groups of CC and CXC chemokines, based on their amino acid sequence at the N-terminus (Laing et al. 2004). Examples of chemokines are MIF and monocyte chemoattractant protein 1 (MCP-1), also known as CCL2. The nomenclature for chemokines and their receptor is standardized. CC or CXC stands for the type of chemokine, R stands for receptor, and L for ligand. Therefore, CCR2 is the receptor for CCL2.

Role of granulocytes and macrophages

Granulocytes are the first cells entering an infected site and their main role is phagocytosis and microbial killing. The fluid consisting of bacteria and dead neutrophils is clinically described as pus. Tissue macrophages and mainly monocytes from the bloodstream, which differentiate into macrophages, are responsible for the phagocytosis of neutrophil debris and remaining bacteria. Macrophages and monocytes form a wall of mononuclear cells around the pus and an abscess is generated, which has a collagen wall and its own blood supply via angiogenesis. Resolution of this structure is often via extrusion in animals, but requires drainage in humans. The initial goal of the inflammatory process is to contain the infection that occurs by clotting of outflowing vessels, as well as abscess formation. There is a continual replacement of PMNs via neovascularization of the abscess.

Other cell types

In addition to phagocytes such as granulocytes and monocytes/macrophages, which are mainly responsible for the defense of bacteria, certain lymphocyte subsets are also considered to be part of the innate immune system. NK cells play an important role in first-line antiviral and anti-tumor response. NK cells are an exception among immune cells because they do not need to be activated by DAMPs or cytokines. NK cells check the expression of inhibitory receptors on host T cells, such as MHC-I. If the appropriate amounts of inhibitory receptors are expressed, NK cells do not lyse the host T cell or induce apoptosis. Virally infected cells and tumor cells fail to express MHC-I and are therefore lysed by patrolling NK cells. Besides the first-line defense against virally infected cells and tumor cells, NK cells produce also large amounts of cytokines when stimulated by cytokines. A rare subtype of T cells, γδ T cells, is also believed to have surveillance and early response capabilities. The TCR of these cells consists of a γδ chain instead of αβ chains with a limited capacity to recognize antigens. These cells are believed to recognize alarmins such as heat shock protein and other uncommon antigens such as lipids. In addition,

they seem to be capable of phagocytosis, which was believed to be an exclusive feature of cells of the myeloid lineage such as granulocytes and monocytes (Wu et al. 2009).

Resolution of inflammation

The resolution of the inflammatory process is now known to be an active process. In this concept, granulocytes and especially macrophages produce lipid mediators, which inhibit the influx of granulocytes but attract monocytes, which are non-phlogistic (non-inflammatory) (Serhan et al. 2008). These monocytes differentiate into macrophages with a high phagocytic capacity, but they do not produce proinflammatory cytokines or chemokines. Instead they secrete high amounts of IL-10 and TGFβ. In addition, the efflux of immune cells through the lymphatic systems in increased. The lipid mediators involved in this process are mainly derived from essential omega-3 fatty acids. Only one of the described lipid mediators, lipoxin, is derived from a non-essential fatty acid (arachidonic acid). Intravenous administration of these lipid mediators has been shown to increase survival in a sepsis model and might offer an avenue for future therapeutic interventions (Spite et al. 2009).

Regulation of innate response

All these above-mentioned processes are tightly regulated with a wide variety of cytokines and other mechanisms such as the autonomous nervous system. The initiation of the immune response is based on proinflammatory cytokines such as TNFα, IL-1β, and IL-6. These cytokines are initially secreted primarily by monocytes, macrophages, and dendritic cells, but later reinforced by Th cells. The differentiation of naïve T cells to Th cells relies on IL-12, which is produced by monocytes, macrophages, and dendritic cells. HMGB1 is a recently described protein that has cytokine-like properties (de Jong et al. 2010). It was first discovered as a DNA-binding protein but is now considered to be a crucial signaling molecule. It is released from necrotic cells, but, more importantly, actively secreted and then recognized by several receptors (TLR-2, -4, and RAGE). It seems that the release of HMGB1 is the key activator of the systemic response to tissue injury after trauma (Levy et al. 2007), but it is also increased during sepsis, probably due to phagocytosis of increased apoptosis of lymphocytes in the spleen by macrophages, which then release HMGB1 (Huston et al. 2008). Of note, HMGB1 alone without co-stimulatory factors such as cytokines or PAMPs seems to be incapable of inducing a cytokine response, but it strongly amplifies the production of proinflammatory cytokines (Hreggvidsdottir et al. 2009).

Besides proinflammatory cytokines, there are also anti-inflammatory cytokines such as IL-10 and TGFβ, which have an inhibiting effect on immune cells. Production of these cytokines are delayed, and produced after stimulation of the cells within a few hours. The main purpose of this counterinflammatory response is to avoid damage to the host by an exaggerated proinflammatory immune response. Despite being important to the counter-regulatory response, the mechanisms that lead to the production of IL-10 are not very well understood.

Autonomic nervous system and sex hormones

The autonomic nerves system clearly influences the immune response and the overall effect is similar to other effects of the sympathetic and parasympathetic system: The sympathetic system has proinflammatory properties whereas the parasympathetic system has anti-inflammatory actions. Immune cells are equipped with adrenergic and acetylcholine receptors. Catecholamines from the adrenal medulla are also produced from macrophages, and enhance the production of proinflammatory cytokines via NF-κB-dependent mechanisms (Flierl et al. 2007). Exhaustion of the adrenal glands during sepsis may also, therefore, affect the immune response. In contrast, the vagal system has anti-inflammatory properties via acetylcholine receptors (Tracey 2009). Stimulation of the vagus nerve has been shown to reduce the production of proinflammatory cytokines and HMGB1, but also increases survival. The main effector organ of this neuroinflammatory reflex in animal models seems to be the spleen; however, vagal stimulation of the gut abrogates burn induced (sterile) lung injury, which is mediated by TLR-4 (Krzyzaniak et al. 2011a, 2011b). In addition, sex hormones, mainly estrogen, also modulate the response to infection and tissue injury. It is a well-described phenomenon that women of reproductive age have a better survival and fewer complications after trauma and sepsis (Wichmann et al. 1996, Zellweger et al. 1997, Angele 2000). In humans, the data are controversial. It seems that premenopausal women have fewer infectious complications than men, but the mortality in women is higher once the complication has occurred (May et al. 2008). Of note, estradiol levels in both genders are associated with mortality in critically ill and trauma patients.

Apoptosis of immune cells

A very effective way to regulate the immune response is the induction of apoptosis of effector cells. The deletion of self-recognizing T cells in the thymus is the principal way by which the immune system selects non-self-attacking T cells. However, uncontrolled apoptosis or even necrosis of immune cells gained interest in recent years and seems to contribute to immune-dysfunction in sepsis. The increased apoptosis of lymphocytes subsets and monocytes is believed to contribute to the unresponsiveness of the immune system in late sepsis (Hotchkiss et al. 2005, Pelekanou et al. 2009). The reason for the increased apoptosis is not clear. Several cytokines such as TNFα and other cytokines, Fas ligand, and intracellular events can induce the activation of the caspase system, leading to apoptosis. Recently, an unknown, early, circulating factor, which has higher levels in non-survivors of sepsis, has been shown to induce apoptosis in monocytes and lymphocytes. As apoptosis is believed to contribute heavily to the immune dysfunction in sepsis, the reduction of apoptosis in immune cells offers interesting therapeutic possibilities (Ayala et al. 2008).

Systemic effects of inflammatory mediators

All these different processes such as vasodilation, increased permeability, adhesion, and transmigration of leukocytes, activation of the complement and coagulation cascade, as well as production of ROS together are essential for local control of an infection. However, if these processes do not remain locally and spread through the whole organism, they are detrimental and can kill it. The clinical picture associated with uncontrolled systemic inflammation is described as the systemic inflammatory response syndrome (SIRS) and all the symptoms can be attributed to the same mechanisms, which are locally very helpful to control infections but systemically cause problems. Systemic vasodilation leads to hypotension, increased endothelial permeability leads to interstitial fluid, ROS formation leads to tissue damage, and activation of the coagulation systems leads to microthrombi, which ultimately lead to hypoxia of the tissue followed by necrosis. Two organ

systems, in which these processes have been clinically well described and remain major challenges, are ARDS and liver injury. Several cytokines such as TNFα mimic the clinical picture of sepsis when given systemically and the blockade of TNFα was shown to improve survival in experimental sepsis (Tracey et al. 1987). However, blockade of several cytokines or their receptors in septic patients did not lower 30-day mortality (Abraham et al. 1995). Therefore, new approaches were investigated. The close and largely not understood interactions of the immune cells, complement, and coagulation system make the discovery for new drugs very challenging.

Acute phase response

Local infections also have systemic effects, which are induced mainly by cytokines. The whole body response to infection is called the acute phase response. The function of this acute phase response is to support the clearance of infection. Acute phase proteins are secreted by the liver and opsonize bacteria such as C-reactive protein (CRP) and serum amyloid A (SAA); others, such as coagulation factors, aim to contain the infection localized and should prevent the spread of the infection. CRP and SAA can also be considered PRRs because they recognize phosphorylcholine, a very common part of bacterial cell walls. Other proteins such as albumin or transferrin have decreased production. In addition, the metabolism shifts to a catabolic state, which supplies the immune cells with necessary substrates such as glucose and amino acids. This catabolic state typically manifests as weight loss in patients with chronic infections.

THE ADAPTIVE IMMUNE RESPONSE

Adaptive immunity consists of all responses that lead to the development of specific antibodies and antigen-specific lymphocytes. To fulfill this, many cells work together to produce this complex immune response (**Figure 3.7**). This includes antigen-presenting cells (APCs), T cells, and B cells that interact together in the central lymphoid (thymus and bone marrow) and the peripheral lymphoid (e.g., spleen, lymph nodes, tonsils) organs to produce the two main types of adaptive immunity, humoral and cell-mediated immunity. Humoral immunity is primarily mediated by antibodies, which neutralize microorganisms and toxins and remove antigens in the body fluids through phagocytosis or lysis. Cell-mediated immunity (CMI) is mediated by cytotoxic T cells, NK cells, and macrophages, and is responsible for killing microorganisms inside body cells as well as eradicating abnormal host T cells (e.g., cancer cells). Cells of the adaptive immunity (both humoral and cell mediated) include the B and T lymphocytes, which represent 30% of the circulating leukocytes. Adaptive (acquired) immunity takes several days to become protective, is designed to remove a specific antigen, and is the specific immunity that one develops throughout life.

Humoral immunity

This response to specific pathogens involves the production of antibody molecules in response to an antigen and is mediated by B lymphocytes, which circulate throughout the host including body fluids. The production of these antibodies takes place in several stages. If antigen entry is intravenous, the antigen is phagocytosed or pinocytosed in the spleen. However, if antigen entry is other than intravenous, the antigen moves to the lymph node draining the site

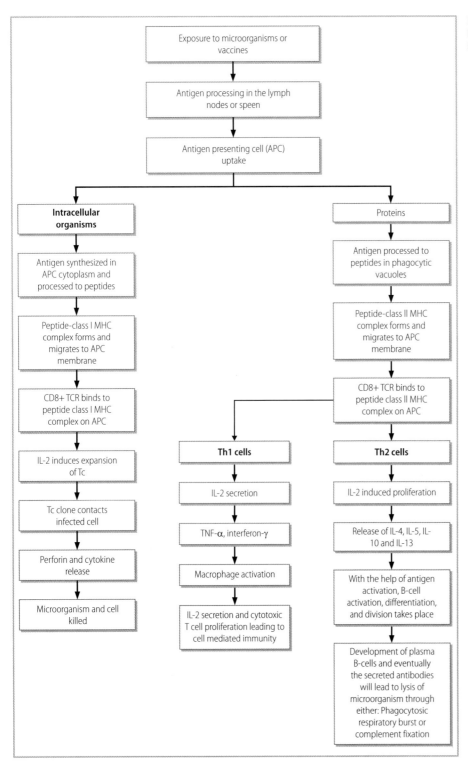

Figure 3.7 Schematic summary outlining the humoral and cell-mediated arms of the adaptive immune response.

of entry. In the lymph nodes or spleen, the antigen encounters the T cell, B cell, APC triad, and is initially processed by the APC. As a result, antigen processing brings about the activation of T cells. For viruses and intracellular parasite antigens, these antigens are synthesized endogenously within the APC cytoplasm and endocytoplasmic reticulum, and then processed to peptides by proteasomes. The resulting peptides bind to the heavy chains of MHC-I molecules and migrate to the APC membrane, where they are presented to CD8+ cells. For exogenous protein antigens, these antigens are phagocytosed by the APCs from the extracellular environment by pinocytosis and are processed in acidic endosomal vacuoles. The processed peptides will eventually bind to the cleft in MHC-II molecules and are transported into the cell membrane, where they are presented to CD4+ T cells.

■ Activation of T and B cells
Exogenous protein antigens

After being transported to the APC cell membrane, the antigenic peptide–MHC-II complex is presented to CD4+ Th cells. The Th-1 cell response then develops as the specific CD4+ Th-1 cell clone differentiates, divides logarithmically, and secretes IL-2, IFN-γ, and TNFα. IL-2 is necessary for T- and B-cell transformation, whereas IFN-γ is a potent macrophage and NK-cell activator and also enhances cell-mediated immunity. IFN-γ also triggers HLA antigen presentation by endothelial cells and downregulates IL-4 synthesis by Th-2 cells; thus, it can also suppress antibody formation. TNFα activates macrophages, stimulates the acute phase response, and synergizes with IL-1 in inducing this response. The Th-2 cell response develops after antigen activation and stimulation by IL-2, and the CD4+ Th-2 cell responds by transforming, differentiating, and dividing logarithmically, while secreting IL-4, IL-5, IL-10, and IL-13. IL-4 promotes the development of antibody synthesis by stimulating B-cell differentiation and downregulates IFN-γ by Th-1 cells, thus suppressing cell-mediated immunity. In addition, IL-4 is significant in the switch to IgE production. IL-5 functions in synergy with IL-4 and IL-2 to help B-cell differentiation, facilitate IgA synthesis, and stimulate the growth and differentiation of eosinophils. IL-10, similar to IL-4, inhibits Th-1 cell release of IFN-γ and IL-2, thereby negating macrophage activation by IFN-γ. IL-13 mimics IL-4 actions and inhibits Th-1 cytokine release.

B-cell response

Antigens are recognized by B cells with the appropriate membrane-bound IgM that is specific for that antigen. The binding of antigen along with stimuli from the T-cell cytokines IL-2 and IL-4 triggers differentiation of that specific B-cell clone into large blast cells, and logarithmic division follows. IL-5 continues the process, during which the B cell acquires the cytoplasmic machinery necessary for antibody synthesis. The heavy and light chains are then synthesized, assembled, and promoted by IL-6, and will undergo terminal differentiation into a plasma cell and secrete IgM. Subsequent gene rearrangements result in a switch to IgG, IgA, and IgE synthesis and secretion. IL-4 and IFN-γ influence the switch to IgG, TGFβ influences the switch to IgA, and IL-4 influences the switch to IgE. The binding of CD40 on the B cell to its ligand on the Th cell (CD40L) is necessary for switching to occur. Memory B cells of all classes are generated independently of the plasma cell lineage and migrate to various lymphoid tissues, where they have an extended survival. A secondary response occurs when further exposure to the same antigen results in a shorter induction period to antibody synthesis, more rapid class switching from IgM to IgG, increased IgG with antibodies of higher affinity, and a predominant IgA synthesis in mucosal tissues.

■ Cell-mediated immunity

This type of response involves the production of cytotoxic T lymphocytes, activated macrophages, activated NK cells, and cytokines in response to an antigen and is mediated by T lymphocytes. CMI is directed against intracellular microorganisms and aberrant, endogenous cells (tumor cells). Immune reactivity is affected by cytotoxic T cells, macrophages, and NK cells on direct contact with the target T cell. This reactivity is transferable to normal, non-sensitized hosts with sensitized effector cells. No antibodies are involved except in ADCC reactions. The effector cells, in these cases, are linked to the target T cells by an antibody bridge, with the Fab protein binding to the specific membrane antigen on the target T cell, and the Fc portion binding to the Fc receptor on an activated effector cell. There are multiple types of CMI and these include reaction to infectious agents (tuberculin test), granulomatous reactions, and contact dermatitis. Although CMI is basically a defense mechanism against foreign substances, cells in the vicinity of antigen deposition, as well as those harboring microorganisms, are damaged if the inflammatory response induced is excessive. This is caused by the magnified inflammatory response induced by activated macrophages, cytotoxic T (Tc) lymphocytes, and NK cells.

■ CONCLUSION

The immune system is a complex and highly redundant system of cells and proteins working together to defend the body from invading pathogens. It is made up of two distinct parts, the innate and adaptive systems, which overlap considerably to protect the body from infections. For surgical infections, the innate system seems to be of more importance because of the fast and immediate response to a very broad variety of pathogens. The adaptive system needs several days to be engaged. However, it provides a very good protection against re-infection with the same pathogen because of its memory cells.

Major trauma and surgical stress can compromise the immune system, with patients becoming anergic and unable to respond to immunological insults post-surgery (immune paralysis) due to cellular dysfunction. The mechanisms of this unresponsiveness (anergy) are unclear, but involve defects in cell-mediated adaptive immunity. Modulation of signaling pathways by micro-RNAs in cells of the innate system such as monocytes, macrophages, and dendritic cells or counterinflammatory cells of the adaptive system such as Treg cells might play a role.

Influencing the immune response by a variety of strategies including anti-TNFα antibodies and stimulation by IFN-γ has not lead to improvement of clinical outcomes thus far. This finding reinforces the complex nature of the immune system and our lack of understanding of the principal mechanisms. There are several new avenues of research, which might improve the care of surgical patients with infections such as the modulation of lymphocyte apoptosis, micro-RNA expression, and strategies to promote resolution of inflammation.

■ REFERENCES

Abraham E, Wunderink R, Silverman H, et al. Efficacy and safety of monoclonal antibody to human tumor necrosis factor alpha in patients with sepsis syndrome. A randomized, controlled, double-blind, multicenter clinical trial. TNF-alpha MAb Sepsis Study Group. *JAMA* 1995;**273**:934–41.

Allman D, Pillai S. Peripheral B cell subsets. *Curr Opin Immunol* 2008;**20**:149–57.

Amara U, Flierl MA, Rittirsch D, et al. Molecular intercommunication between the complement and coagulation systems. *Journal of immunology* 2010;**185**:5628–36.

Angele MK, Schwacha MG, Ayala A, Chaudry IH. Effect of gender and sex hormones on immune responses following shock. *Shock* 2000;**14**:81–90.

Auffray C, Sieweke MH, Geissmann F. Blood monocytes: development, heterogeneity, and relationship with dendritic cells. *Annu Rev Immunol* 2009;**27**:669–92.

Ayala A, Perl M, Venet F, Lomas-Neira J, Swan R, Chung CS. Apoptosis in sepsis: mechanisms, clinical impact and potential therapeutic targets. *Curr Pharmaceutical Design* 2008;**14**:1853–9.

Bakri Y, Sarrazin S, Mayer UP, et al. Balance of MafB and PU.1 specifies alternative macrophage or dendritic cell fate. *Blood* 2005;**105**:2707–16.

Basu S. Bioactive eicosanoids: role of prostaglandin F(2alpha) and F-isoprostanes in inflammation and oxidative stress related pathology. *Mol Cells* 2010;**30**:383–91.

Bazzoni F, Rossato M, Fabbri M, et al. Induction and regulatory function of miR-9 in human monocytes and neutrophils exposed to proinflammatory signals. *Proc Natl Acad Sci U S A* 2009;**106**:5282–7.

Belge KU, Dayyani F, Horelt A, et al. The proinflammatory CD14+CD16+DR++ monocytes are a major source of TNF. *J Immunol* 2002;**168**:3536–42.

Bhaumik D, Scott GK, Schokrpur S, et al. MicroRNAs miR-146a/b negatively modulate the senescence-associated inflammatory mediators IL-6 and IL-8. *Aging (Albany NY)* 2009;**1**:402–11.

Bianchi ME. DAMPs, PAMPs and alarmins: all we need to know about danger. *J Leukoc Biol* 2007;**81**:1–5.

Borregaard N. Neutrophils, from marrow to microbes. *Immunity* 2010;**33**:657–70.

Cariappa A, Mazo IB, Chase C, et al. Perisinusoidal B cells in the bone marrow participate in T-independent responses to blood-borne microbes. *Immunity* 2005;**23**:397–407.

Cariappa A, Chase C, Liu H, Russell P, Pillai S. Naive recirculating B cells mature simultaneously in the spleen and bone marrow. *Blood* 2007;**109**:2339–45.

Chen XM, Splinter PL, O'Hara SP, LaRusso NF. A cellular micro-RNA, let-7i, regulates Toll-like receptor 4 expression and contributes to cholangiocyte immune responses against Cryptosporidium parvum infection. *J Biol Chem* 2007;**282**:28929–38.

Cinamon G, Zachariah MA, Lam OM, Foss FW Jr, Cyster JG. Follicular shuttling of marginal zone B cells facilitates antigen transport. *Nat Immunol* 2008;**9**:54–62.

de Jong HK, van der Poll T, Wiersinga WJ. The systemic pro-inflammatory response in sepsis. *J Innate Immun* 2010;**2**:422–30.

Docke WD, Randow F, Syrbe U, et al. Monocyte deactivation in septic patients: restoration by IFN-gamma treatment. *Nat Med* 1997;**3**:678–81.

El Kebir D, Filep JG. Role of neutrophil apoptosis in the resolution of inflammation. *Scientific World J* 2010;**10**:1731–48.

Ferguson AR, Youd ME, Corley RB. Marginal zone B cells transport and deposit IgM-containing immune complexes onto follicular dendritic cells. *Int Immunol* 2004;**16**:1411–22.

Fingerle G, Pforte A, Passlick B, Blumenstein M, Strobel M, Ziegler-Heitbrock HW. The novel subset of CD14+/CD16+ blood monocytes is expanded in sepsis patients. *Blood* 1993;**82**:3170–6.

Flierl MA, Rittirsch D, Nadeau BA, et al. Phagocyte-derived catecholamines enhance acute inflammatory injury. *Nature* 2007;**449**:721–5.

Funk CD. Prostaglandins and leukotrienes: advances in eicosanoid biology. *Science* 2001;**294**:1871–5.

Geissmann F, Manz MG, Jung S, Sieweke MH, Merad M, Ley K. Development of monocytes, macrophages, and dendritic cells. *Science* 2010;**327**:656–61.

Gordon S, Taylor PR. Monocyte and macrophage heterogeneity. *Nat Rev Immunol* 2005;**5**:953–64.

Guha M, Mackman N. LPS induction of gene expression in human monocytes. *Cell Signal* 2001;**13**:85–94.

Hotchkiss RS, Osmon SB, Chang KC, Wagner TH, Coopersmith CM, Karl IE. Accelerated lymphocyte death in sepsis occurs by both the death receptor and mitochondrial pathways. *J Immunol* 2005;**174**:5110–8.

Hou J, Wang P, Lin L, et al. MicroRNA-146a feedback inhibits RIG-I-dependent Type I IFN production in macrophages by targeting TRAF6, IRAK1, and IRAK2. *J Immunol* 2009;**183**:2150–8.

Hreggvidsdottir HS, Ostberg T, Wahamaa H, et al. The alarmin HMGB1 acts in synergy with endogenous and exogenous danger signals to promote inflammation. *J Leukoc Biol* 2009;**86**:655–62.

Hu X, Chakravarty SD, Ivashkiv LB. Regulation of interferon and Toll-like receptor signaling during macrophage activation by opposing feedforward and feedback inhibition mechanisms. *Immunol Rev* 2008;**226**:41–56.

Huston JM, Wang H, Ochani M, et al. Splenectomy protects against sepsis lethality and reduces serum HMGB1 levels. *J Immunol* 2008;**181**:3535–9.

Janeway CA Jr, Medzhitov R. Innate immune recognition. *Annu Rev Immunol* 2002;**20**:197–216.

Johnson AG. *High Yield Immunology*. Philadelphia, PA: Lippincott, Williams & Wilkins, 1999.

Karin M, Ben-Neriah Y. Phosphorylation meets ubiquitination: the control of NF-kB activity. *Annu Rev Immunol* 2000;**18**:621–63.

Kawakami T, Galli SJ. Regulation of mast-cell and basophil function and survival by IgE. *Nat Rev Immunol* 2002;**2**:773–86.

Kim OY, Monsel A, Bertrand M, Coriat P, Cavaillon JM, Adib-Conquy M. Differential down-regulation of HLA-DR on monocyte subpopulations during systemic inflammation. *Crit Care* 2010;**14**:R61.

Krzyzaniak M, Cheadle G, Peterson C, et al. Burn-induced acute lung injury requires a functional Toll-like receptor 4. *Shock* 2011a;**36**:24–9.

Krzyzaniak MJ, Peterson CY, Cheadle G, et al. Efferent vagal nerve stimulation attenuates acute lung injury following burn: The importance of the gut-lung axis. *Surgery* 2011b;**150**:379–89.

Laing KJ, Secombes CJ. Chemokines. *Developmental and comparative immunology* 2004;**28**:443–60.

Levine SJ. Molecular mechanisms of soluble cytokine receptor generation. *J Biol Chem* 2008;**283**:14177–81.

Levy RM, Mollen KP, Prince JM, et al. Systemic inflammation and remote organ injury following trauma require HMGB1. *Am J Physiol Regul integr Comp physiol* 2007;**293**:R1538–44.

Ley K, Laudanna C, Cybulsky MI, Nourshargh S. Getting to the site of inflammation: the leukocyte adhesion cascade updated. *Nat Rev Immunol* 2007;**7**:678–89.

Li T, Morgan MJ, Choksi S, Zhang Y, Kim YS, Liu ZG. MicroRNAs modulate the noncanonical transcription factor NF-kappaB pathway by regulating expression of the kinase IKKalpha during macrophage differentiation. *Nat Immunol* 2010a;**11**:799–805.

Li X, Jiang S, Tapping RI. Toll-like receptor signaling in cell proliferation and survival. *Cytokine* 2010b;**49**:1–9.

Lindenblatt C, Schulze-Osthoff K, Totzke G. IkappaBzeta expression is regulated by miR-124a. *Cell Cycle* 2009;**8**:2019–23.

Lotze MT, Zeh HJ, Rubartelli A, Sparvero LJ, et al. The grateful dead: damage-associated molecular pattern molecules and reduction/oxidation regulate immunity. *Immunol Rev* 2007;**220**:60–81.

Mantovani A, Cassatella MA, Costantini C, Jaillon S. Neutrophils in the activation and regulation of innate and adaptive immunity. *Nat Rev Immunol* 2011;**11**:519–31.

May AK, Dossett LA, Norris PR, et al. Estradiol is associated with mortality in critically ill trauma and surgical patients. *Crit Care Med* 2008;**36**:62–8.

Medzhitov R. Recognition of microorganisms and activation of the immune response. *Nature* 2007;**449**:819–26.

Meisel C, Schefold JC, Pschowski R, et al. Granulocyte-macrophage colony-stimulating factor to reverse sepsis-associated immunosuppression: a double-blind, randomized, placebo-controlled multicenter trial. *Am J Respir Crit Care Med* 2009;**180**:640–8.

Mizuno K, Toma T, Tsukiji H, et al. Selective expansion of CD16highCCR2- subpopulation of circulating monocytes with preferential production of haem oxygenase (HO)-1 in response to acute inflammation. *Clin Exp Immunol* 2005;**142**:461–70.

Murphy AJ, Guyre PM, Pioli PA. Estradiol suppresses NF-kappaB activation through coordinated regulation of let-7a and miR-125b in primary human macrophages. *J Immunol* 2010;**184**:5029–37.

Murphy K. *Janeway's Immunobiology*, 8th edn. New York: Garland Science, 2011.

Murray BW, Cipher DJ, Pham T, Anthony T. The impact of surgical site infection on the development of incisional hernia and small bowel obstruction in colorectal surgery. *Am J Surg* 2011;**202**:558–60.

Murray PJ. The JAK-STAT signaling pathway: input and output integration. *J Immunol* 2007;**178**:2623–9.

Murray PJ, Wynn TA. Protective and pathogenic functions of macrophage subsets. *Nat Rev Immunol* 2011;**11**:723–37.

Nahid MA, Pauley KM, Satoh M, Chan EK. miR-146a is critical for endotoxin-induced tolerance: Implication in innate immunity. *J Biol Chem* 2009;**284**:34590–9.

Nahid MA, Satoh M, Chan EK. Mechanistic role of microRNA-146a in endotoxin-Induced differential cross-regulation of TLR signaling. *J Immunol* 2010;**186**:1723–34.

Netea MG, van der Graaf C, Van der Meer JW, Kullberg BJ. Toll-like receptors and the host defense against microbial pathogens: bringing specificity to the innate-immune system. *J Leukoc Biol* 2004;**75**:749–55.

Nordenfelt P, Tapper H. Phagosome dynamics during phagocytosis by neutrophils. *J Leukoc Biol* 2011;**90**:271–84.

O'Neill LA, Sheedy FJ, McCoy CE. MicroRNAs: the fine-tuners of Toll-like receptor signalling. *Nat Rev Immunol* 2011;**11**:163–75.

Patterson KI, Brummer T, O'Brien PM, Daly RJ. Dual-specificity phosphatases: critical regulators with diverse cellular targets. *Biochem J* 2009;**418**:475–89.

Pelekanou A, Tsangaris I, Kotsaki A, et al. Decrease of CD4-lymphocytes and apoptosis of CD14-monocytes are characteristic alterations in sepsis caused by ventilator-associated pneumonia: results from an observational study. *Crit Care* 2009;**13**:R172.

Polk HC Jr, George CD, Wellhausen SR, et al. A systematic study of host defense processes in badly injured patients. *Ann Surg* 1986;**204**:282–99.

Polk HC Jr, Cheadle WG, Livingston DH, et al. A randomized prospective clinical trial to determine the efficacy of interferon-gamma in severely injured patients. *Am J Surg* 1992;**163**:191–6.

Ricklin D, Hajishengallis G, Yang K, Lambris JD. Complement: a key system for immune surveillance and homeostasis. *Nat Immunol* 2010;**11**:785–97.

Rittirsch D, Flierl MA, Ward PA. Harmful molecular mechanisms in sepsis. *Nat Rev Immunol* 2008;**8**:776–87.

Roccaro AM, Sacco A, Thompson B, et al. MicroRNAs 15a and 16 regulate tumor proliferation in multiple myeloma. *Blood* 2009;**113**:6669–80.

Saraiva M, O'Garra A. The regulation of IL-10 production by immune cells. *Nat Rev Immunol* 2010;**10**:170–81.

Segel GB, Halterman MW, Lichtman MA. The paradox of the neutrophil's role in tissue injury. *J Leukoc Biol* 2011;**89**:359–72.

Serhan CN, Chiang N, Van Dyke TE. Resolving inflammation: dual anti-inflammatory and pro-resolution lipid mediators. *Nat Rev Immunol* 2008;**8**:349–61.

Sheedy FJ, Palsson-McDermott E, Hennessy EJ, et al. Negative regulation of TLR4 via targeting of the proinflammatory tumor suppressor PDCD4 by the microRNA miR-21. *Nat Rev Immunol* 2010;**11**:141–7.

Shi C, Pamer EG. Monocyte recruitment during infection and inflammation. *Nat Rev Immunol* 2011;**11**:762–74.

Silva MT. Macrophage phagocytosis of neutrophils at inflammatory/infectious foci: a cooperative mechanism in the control of infection and infectious inflammation. *J Leukoc Biol* 2011;**89**:675–83.

Spite M, Norling LV, Summers L, et al. Resolvin D2 is a potent regulator of leukocytes and controls microbial sepsis. *Nature* 2009;**461**:1287–91.

Sun JC, Lanier LL. NK cell development, homeostasis and function: parallels with CD8 T cells. *Nat Rev Immunol* 2011;**11**:645–57.

Sun Y, Varambally S, Maher CA, et al. Targeting of microRNA-142–3p in dendritic cells regulates endotoxin-induced mortality. *Blood* 2011;**117**:6172–83.

Tili E, Michaille JJ, Cimino A, et al. Modulation of miR-155 and miR-125b levels following lipopolysaccharide/TNF-alpha stimulation and their possible roles in regulating the response to endotoxin shock. *J Immunol* 2007;**179**:5082–9.

Tracey KJ. Reflex control of immunity. *Nat Rev Immunol* 2009;**9**:418–28.

Tracey KJ, Fong Y, Hesse DG, et al. Anti-cachectin/TNF monoclonal antibodies prevent septic shock during lethal bacteraemia. *Nature* 1987;**330**:662–4.

Vasilescu C, Rossi S, Shimizu M, et al. MicroRNA fingerprints identify miR-150 as a plasma prognostic marker in patients with sepsis. *PLoS One* 2009;**4**:e7405.

Wang JF, Yu ML, Yu G, et al. Serum miR-146a and miR-223 as potential new biomarkers for sepsis. *Biochem Biophys Res Commun* 2010;**394**:184–8.

Wesche DE, Lomas-Neira JL, Perl M, Chung CS, Ayala A. Leukocyte apoptosis and its significance in sepsis and shock. *J Leukoc Biol* 2005;**78**:325–37.

Wichmann MW, Zellweger R, DeMaso CM, Ayala A, Chaudry IH. Enhanced immune responses in females, as opposed to decreased responses in males following haemorrhagic shock and resuscitation. *Cytokine* 1996;**8**:853–63.

Wu Y, Wu W, Wong WM, et al. Human gamma delta T cells: a lymphoid lineage cell capable of professional phagocytosis. *J Immunol* 2009;**183**:5622–9.

Zellweger R, Wichmann MW, Ayala A, Stein S, DeMaso CM, Chaudry IH. Females in proestrus state maintain splenic immune functions and tolerate sepsis better than males. *Crit Care Med* 1997;**25**:106–10.

Zhang YL, Dong C. MAP kinases in immune responses. *Cell Mol Immunol* 2005;**2**:20–7.

Zhu QY, Liu Q, Chen JX, Lan K, Ge BX. MicroRNA-101 targets MAPK phosphatase-1 to regulate the activation of MAPKs in macrophages. *J Immunol* 2010;**185**:7435–42.

Ziegler-Heitbrock L. The CD14+ CD16+ blood monocytes: their role in infection and inflammation. *J Leukoc Biol* 2007;**81**:584–92.

Ziegler-Heitbrock L, Ancuta P, Crowe S, et al. Nomenclature of monocytes and dendritic cells in blood. *Blood* 2010;**116**:e74–80.

Chapter 4 Surgical site infections

Donald E. Fry

Infection at the surgical site (SSI) continues to be a major problem. With the introduction of the germ theory of disease, Joseph Lister, in the 1860s, introduced antiseptics into surgical practice in the hopes of killing bacteria that might contact the open wound. As the twentieth century emerged, surgeons developed dedicated operating rooms within hospitals and adopted a code of infection control behaviors to reduce the likelihood of SSI. Surgical gowns and drapes, facemasks, hand scrubbing, and surgical gloves were all introduced in the hopes of minimizing infection. Sterilization of surgical instruments and sophisticated air-handling systems were similarly introduced to avoid environmental introduction of potential pathogens. Although the infection control practices of the operating room have favorably impacted rates for most operations, the complexity of surgical interventions and the vulnerability of patients due to an expanded array of comorbidities make the frequency and severity of SSIs a continued complication of care. In addition to patient morbidity, preventable SSIs are a recognized major economic cost of surgical care (Fry 2002).

Bacteria are ubiquitously distributed in our environment. They colonize the skin of patients and healthcare providers alike. The human aerodigestive tract is a rich source of bacteria. The air and floor in the operating room are a source of bacteria. It is likely that bacteria can be cultured from every open surgical wound at the completion of the procedure. Yet every wound does not get infected.

SSI is the result of a complex interaction of the microbes that contaminate the wound, the local environment of the wound, and the multifaceted components of the human host defense. In most circumstances the effectiveness of host defense and the preventive measures that are employed result in the absence of infection. In a minority of cases infection occurs for reasons that are suspected by the clinician. In an occasional case SSI occurs without any plausible clinical explanation. This chapter explores the multiple interactions of the pathogen and the host to provide a context for understanding and preventing SSI.

PATHOPHYSIOLOGY OF SSI

An SSI is the sustained local activation of the human inflammatory response due to the proliferation of microorganisms at the site of a surgical procedure. The determinants that are responsible for SSI are illustrated in **Figure 4.1**. The clinical variables that favor the emergence of an SSI are the inoculum of bacteria in the surgical site, the virulence characteristics of the bacterial contaminant, and the local tissue and

environment conditions that are present within the contaminated wound tissues. The innate and adaptive immune responses of the host (see Chapter 3) are designed to eradicate the bacterial contaminants of the wound, and prevent SSI as an outcome. Each of the determinants in **Figure 4.1** is individually discussed. It must be understood that there are additive and synergistic relationships among these major determinants.

Inoculum of contamination

Among all of the clinical variables associated with SSI, the inoculum of bacteria in the incision and soft tissues of the operation is the best recognized. Most of the preventive strategies that are subsequently discussed are designed to reduce the quantity of bacteria that access the surgical site. The clinical variables that govern the inoculum of bacteria at the surgical site are the intrinsic colonization of the anatomic structure that is being entered at the time of surgery, and the presence of contamination or infection that may already exist within the patient at the time of the procedure. The microbial burden that can be anticipated with a given operation is the basis for the American College of Surgeons' wound classification system (Culver et al. 1991).

Clean operations

A clean operation does not enter a normally colonized anatomic structure, nor is there any pre-existent infection. Although the skin is penetrated by the surgical incision, under elective circumstances the number of cutaneous bacteria to enter the wound from this source is manageable. This presumes that cutaneous colonization can be reduced by antibacterial skin preparation before the start of surgery and that appropriate infection control practices are employed. Clean operations include elective breast surgery, cutaneous level operations, and even inguinal hernias. Inguinal hernias are in close proximity to the groin and perineum with heavier cutaneous colonization, but elective surgery with adequate local skin preparation should have observed infection rates that are commonly reported as less than 2%. Craniotomies, total joint replacements, and vascular procedures are more complex examples of clean operations. As coronary artery bypass procedures may have additional groin incisions with increased local colonization, infection rates may be higher than in other clean procedures.

Clean-contaminated operations

Clean-contaminated operations are elective operations that enter into normally colonized anatomic areas. Elective resections of the colon, hysterectomy, and oropharyngeal resections are prototypical

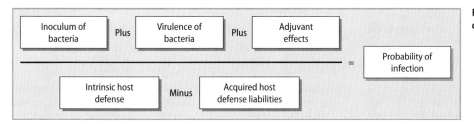

Figure 4.1 A simple equation of the determinants of infection of a surgical site.

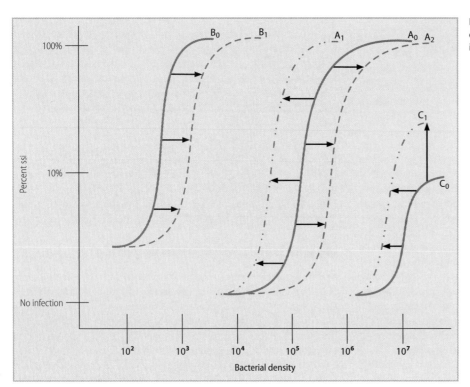

Figure 4.2 The relationship between the inocula of bacteria in the wound and the probability of infection.

clean-contaminated operations. The human colon has about 10^6–10^7 bacteria per gram of content at the cecum, and this increases to nearly 10^{12} organisms per gram in the rectum (Ahmed et al. 2007). Vaginal colonization may be 10^8 bacteria/ml during hysterectomy (Redondo-Lopez et al. 1990). Although the density of microbial colonization is less in the upper gastrointestinal and biliary tract, oropharynx, and lung, these are all considered clean-contaminated procedures. SSIs have been correlated with the microbial density in the anatomic area entered by the procedure. Reported infection rates vary from 3% in open biliary procedures to 20% in open colon resections (Itani et al. 2006).

Contaminated operations

Contaminated operations have overt contamination during the conduct of an elective procedure, or are emergency procedures where the conventional control of the elective surgical setting is lost. Spillage of intestinal contents during an elective colon operation is an example. A trauma laparotomy, any abdominal reoperation, emergency cesarean sections, and emergency open heart procedures constitute circumstances where the urgency of surgical intervention results in higher SSI rates. SSI rates commonly exceed 20% in contaminated procedures. Infections are often polymicrobial and include cutaneous and enteric pathogens.

Dirty operations

Massive contamination may be present to give the presumption that infection is eminent, or infection may already be present. A perforated viscus, a penetrating injury of the colon with fecal contamination, or repair of a perforated esophagus are all dirty procedures. The density and diversity of microbes at the surgical site are great. The surgical sites are likely to have an SSI at the completion of the procedure without specific and dramatic preventive measures (e.g., delayed primary closure).

The traditional threshold for the microbial inoculum to result in infection has been defined as 10^5 bacteria/g tissue. This has been derived from laboratory experiments where variable inocula of bacteria have been introduced into the soft tissues of healthy animals (Robson et al. 1973). In **Figure 4.2**, the experimental curve in a normal host for a hypothetical bacterial pathogen (e.g., *Staphylococcus aureus*) is illustrated by the line labeled A_0. When the inoculum of bacteria is <10^4, no infection occurs. When the bacterial density approaches 10^6, infection is almost uniformly present. Thus, the wound classification adopted by the American College of Surgeons is a descriptive effort to estimate the wound inoculum by identification of the primary source of contamination. Clean wounds have a low inoculum and a low infection rate. Operations with gross spillage or active infection have high concentrations of bacteria and higher infection rate.

■ Virulence of contamination

As discussed in Chapter 1, there are many secreted and structural elements that account for the virulence of bacteria. Different strains within a species can have vastly different virulence profiles. These different virulence characteristics modify the number of microbial contaminants in a surgical incision that result in infection. In **Figure 4.2**, line B_0 illustrates an organism with unusual bacterial virulence (e.g., *Streptococcus pyogenes*). Clinical infection rates are observed with an inoculum less than a conventional pathogen, illustrated in A_0. Conversely, line C_0 in **Figure 4.2** illustrates the infection-to-inoculum relationship of a very low virulence bacterial organism, such as *Enterococcus faecalis*. Very high inocula are usually necessary for infections with low virulence pathogens.

■ Environment of the surgical site

At the time of his death, Louis Pasteur is alleged to have said: "the microbe is nothing, the terrain is everything." So it is with the surgical site. Every incision has bacteria that can be cultured, but the conditions of the surgical site dramatically affect whether infection occurs.

The surgeon and the techniques employed in handling the tissue of the incision dictate whether wound contaminants result in SSI.

Hematoma and free hemoglobin enhance the virulence of bacteria. Hemoglobin is a substrate to support the proliferation of microbes. The ferric iron is a key element for supporting bacterial growth (Polk and Miles 1971), and the metabolism of selected organisms in a hemoglobin environment may actually create a degradation product that retards specific leukocyte function (Pruett et al. 1984).

Other adjuvant effects are numerous. Tissue trauma, dead tissue, and foreign bodies within the surgical site promote infection. Crushed tissue from over-exuberant retraction or indiscrete use of tissue clamps leaves dead tissue where bacterial contaminants may reside and proliferate. Inappropriate use of electrocautery similarly leaves islands of dead tissue. Foreign bodies such as suture (especially non-absorbable braided materials), meshes, and other prostheses serve an important purpose in the operation, but represent surfaces for microbial attachment that are poorly handled by host defense mechanisms. Obesity and incisional dead space yield poorly perfused adipose tissue and reservoirs of serum, blood, and bacteria in the dependent portion of the incision that foster infection.

The net effect of adjuvant variables is illustrated in Figure 4.2. Line A_1 represents a complete shift to the left of the relationship between the required inoculum of bacteria and the probability of infection due to an adverse local environment from adjuvant factors for a given level of bacterial contamination. Line C_1 illustrates the shift to the left in the infection:inoculum relationship and its impact upon low virulence organisms. It is obvious that the primary responsibility of the surgeon in the prevention of SSI is effective intraoperative management of local environmental variables.

Innate and acquired host defense

Effective or suboptimal host responses are poorly defined but real determinants of SSI. There is genetic variability in the efficiency of the host response among patients. Chronic granulomatous disease of childhood illustrates the genetic absence of intracellular killing capacity of the neutrophil. Although this example is an extreme one, it is more likely that pathogen recognition, leukocyte responsiveness, cytokine responses, and other innate elements follow a pattern of normal variation that result in selected individuals being more vulnerable to infection when compared with the population mean. Although the pursuit of methods to enhance the responsiveness of the host to resist postoperative infection continues, the reality is that we cannot efficiently measure the genetic predisposition of the patient to develop an infection. It is likely that the hypothetical relationship of the infection:inoculum ratio (see line A_0, Figure 4.2) should actually have a 95% confidence interval for each point to illustrate the variability of the population under this theoretical ideal circumstance.

However, acquired conditions can be measured and monitored, and evidence demonstrates that the host is more vulnerable to postoperative infections when specific conditions exist (Anderson 2011). Shock, hypoxemia, anemia, and multisystem trauma have an acute suppressive effect upon the innate host response, with increased rates of SSI and other infections. Hypoalbuminemia, chronic renal failure, acute and chronic alcoholism, chronic lung disease, chronic tobacco use, and chronic liver disease each increase the risk for infection. Diabetes increases infection risk probably due to the systemic immunosuppression of hyperglycemia. Steroid treatment and transfusion are clearly associated with increased SSI rates. Advancing age is an independent factor in a suboptimal host response. With reference to Figure 4.2, the shift to the left seen with line A_1 and

C_1 could be ascribed to increased susceptibility of the host to SSI from acquired immunosuppression as a result of the aforementioned conditions and diseases.

DIAGNOSIS AND SURVEILLANCE OF SSI

Diagnosis of SSI

SSI occurs when the microbes at the surgical site are proliferating and invading the adjacent normal host tissues. The host inflammatory responses to invading microbes are the classic signs and symptoms of redness, warmth, swelling, and pain at the surgical site. For most surgeons, the defining moment of an SSI is the discharge of pus at the incision.

However, many issues surrounding the diagnosis and interpretation of an SSI remain poorly defined and controversial. An infection can be declared from the above criteria, but be of trivial clinical consequence with no increase in the duration of hospitalization or costs of care (Fry et al. 2012). A single stitch sinus may innocently drain a small amount (<1–2 ml) of turbid fluid, the suture is spontaneously expelled, and the small site of disruption heals spontaneously without additional sequelae or clinical intervention. In another setting, a wound seroma is spontaneously discharged from the wound, only to have it cultured and a small number of *Staphylococcus epidermidis* are recovered. This wound proceeds to uneventful healing, but such events are labeled an SSI. A third setting may be the marked erythema about the incision with some palpable induration in the subcutaneous tissue. The erythema may relate to foreign body reaction due to staples in the skin and not bacterial infection. No wound discharge is identified. The patient is started on oral antibiotics and sent home. Are these described conditions an SSI?

To provide some direction, the Centers for Disease Control (CDC) of Atlanta have provided detailed definitions for SSI (**Box 4.1**). An important consideration in the CDC definitions is that SSIs are categorized into three types: Superficial, deep, and organ/space (Mangram et al. 1999). In general, little controversy exists about the occurrence or clinical significance of a deep or organ/space infection. Most of the debate surrounds the occurrence and the relevance of the superficial SSIs. The CDC definitions allow the frequency of SSIs to be standardized for evaluation by surgeons and hospital surveillance personnel.

Surveillance

Effective surveillance is a critical component of any quality improvement program in surgical care. Only with effective surveillance can rates of SSI be known, and progress in prevention occur or outbreaks be identified. Surveillance methods are controversial because the more intense the effort, the more expensive the process and the higher the rates of SSI. As an increasing number of SSIs are not identified until after discharge, the post-discharge surveillance program is costly and logistically difficult. As a result of the expense and logistical issues, many hospitals use surveillance nurses or wound managers for inpatient evaluation, and then depend on self-reporting either by patients or physicians for post-discharge events.

An important part of any surveillance program is risk assessment, and the SSI rates need to be correlated with the patient risk profile. Overall SSI rates without classification of patient risk become an incomplete assessment. Hospital-wide infection rates without

Box 4.1 Details the recommended definitions of surgical site infection by the Centers for Disease Control (Horan et al. 1992).

Superficial incisional surgical site infection (SSI): Infection occurs within 30 days of the operation and infection involves only skin or subcutaneous tissue of the incision and at least one of the following:

1. Purulent drainage, with or without laboratory confirmation, from the superficial incision
2. Organisms isolated from an aseptically obtained culture of fluid or tissue from the superficial incision
3. At least one of the following signs or symptoms of infection: pain or tenderness, localized swelling, redness, or heat, and superficial incision is deliberately opened by surgeon, unless incision is culture negative
4. Diagnosis of superficial incisional SSI by the surgeon or attending physician

Do not report the following conditions as SSI:

1. Stitch abscess (minimal inflammation and discharge confined to the points of suture penetration)
2. Infection of an episiotomy or newborn circumcision site
3. Infected burn wound
4. Incisional SSI that extends into the fascial and muscle layers (see deep incisional SSI)

Deep incisional SSI: Infection occurs within 30 days of the operation if no implant[a] is left in place or within 1 year if implant is in place and the infection appears to be related to the operation and infection involves deep soft tissues (e.g., fascial and muscle layers) of the incision and at least one of the following:

1. Purulent drainage from the deep incision but not from the organ/space component of the surgical site
2. A deep incision spontaneously dehisces or is deliberately opened by a surgeon when the patient has at least one of the following signs or symptoms: Fever (>38°C), localized pain, or tenderness, unless site is culture negative
3. An abscess or other evidence of infection involving the deep incision is found on direct examination, during reoperation, or by histopathological or radiological examination
4. Diagnosis of a deep incisional SSI by a surgeon or attending physician

Notes:

1. Report infection that involves both superficial and deep incision sites as deep incisional SSI
2. Report an organ/space SSI that drains through the incision as a deep incisional SSI

Organ/space SSI: Infection occurs within 30 days of the operation if no implant[a] is left in place or within 1 year if implant is in place, and the infection appears to be related to the operation and infection involves any part of the anatomy (e.g., organs or spaces), other than the incision, which was opened or manipulated during an operation and at least one of the following:

1. Purulent drainage from a drain that is placed through a stab wound[b] into the organ/space
2. Organisms isolated from an aseptically obtained culture of fluid or tissue in the organ/space
3. An abscess or other evidence of infection involving the organ/space that is found on direct examination, during reoperation, or by histopathological or radiological examination
4. Diagnosis of an organ/space SSI by a surgeon or attending physician

[a]National Nosocomial Infection Surveillance definition: A non-human-derived implantable foreign body (e.g., prosthetic heart valve, non-human vascular graft, mechanical heart, or hip prosthesis) that is permanently placed in a patient during surgery.
[b]If the area around a stab wound becomes infected, it is not an SSI. It is considered a skin or soft tissue infection, depending on its depth.

stratification are not of value because gross rates are dictated by the risk profile of the patients.

Several different classification systems have been used to stratify risk. The American College of Surgeons' (ACS's) classification system identified previously uses only the likely quantity of bacterial contamination and does not employ any patient risk assessment.

In 1985, the Study of the Efficacy of Nosocomial Infection Control (SENIC) project was undertaken to bring more variables into the prediction model (Haley et al. 1985). Four variables were found to be of significance for SSI prediction:

1. Abdominal operations
2. Operations lasting >2 h
3. Surgical sites that were the ACS classification of contaminated or dirty
4. More than two discharge diagnoses at the conclusion of hospitalization.

A further modification of the SENIC model was undertaken by the CDC in the early 1990s as part of the National Nosocomial Infection Surveillance (NNIS) system (Culver et al. 1991). The NNIS system used only three clinical variables and developed a point system of 0–3 for classification of infection risk. A point is assigned for each of the three variables. Those patients with none of the three risk factors are assigned a score of zero. The three variables are (1) ACS contaminated or dirty classification, (2) the American Society of Anesthesiology (ASA 2012) score ≥3, and (3) patients where the operation lasted longer than the 75th percentile for operations of that type. The ASA score is a subjective scale from 1 to 6 by anesthesiologists for overall assessment of the patient risk. An ASA score of 1 is a patient with no comorbidities and ASA 2 is a patient with mild systemic disease. ASA 3 and above all have major systemic disease or diseases that pose a major threat for complications or death. Operations exceeding the 75th percentile in duration are illustrated in **Table 4.1** (Edwards et al. 2008). NNIS has been renamed the National Healthcare Safety Network (NHSN) but the scoring system for risk of SSI remains much the same (Centers for Disease Control 2012).

Despite all of the discussion about risk stratification and surveillance, there remain problems with the interpretation of SSI surveillance data. First, NNIS (now NHSN) risk categories are lacking in detail. There are many details of the patient (e.g., age, selected chronic diseases, selected laboratory studies) that could enhance the accuracy of the prediction model. The variables of NNIS risk assignment were derived by incomplete modeling. Second, the transformation of all disciplines in surgery to minimally invasive strategies has reduced SSI rates. This means that any decline in SSIs may not reflect improvements of infection control, but are rather the consequences of changes in surgical strategy. NHSN now recommends that 1 point be removed from the risk score if the procedure is done by a minimally invasive technique. Third, post-discharge rates of infection escape surveillance and are commonly not accurate.

A better system is needed that reports SSI as a function of *patient risk* and the *severity* of the SSI. We cannot interpret the results of

Table 4.1 Identifying the cut point in minutes of the 75th percentile and the respective surgical site infection (SSI) rates for operations in National Healthcare Safety Network categories 0 and 1, and the infection rates in categories 2 and 3.

Procedure	Cut point (min)	SSI infection rate (0 or 1) (%)	SSI infection rate (2 or 3) (%)
Abdominal aortic aneurysm repair	217	2.1	6.5
Appendix surgery	81	1.2	3.5
Bile duct, liver, or pancreatic surgery	321	8.1	13.7
Cardiac surgery	306	1.1	1.8
Colon surgery	187	5.0	7.3
Craniotomy	225	2.2	4.7
Cesarean section	56	1.8	3.8
Kidney transplantation	237	3.7	6.6
Ovarian surgery	183	0.4	1.4
Thoracic surgery	188	0.8	2.0

cancer care without knowing the stage of the patient at the time of treatment! Why should we not apply the same criteria to SSI? If the NNIS classification of risk were paired with the CDC definitions of infection severity in Box 4.1, then a 3 × 4 matrix of SSIs with true clinical meaning could be generated (**Table 4.2**). Reporting of SSIs at present by simply counting all events the same without regard for risk or severity cannot be interpreted and provides little foundation for improvement strategies.

PREVENTION OF SSI

SSIs are always viewed as preventable infections in patient care. Preventive methods are employed before, during, and after the surgical event.

Preoperative methods
Prehospitalization cleansing

Reduction of the cutaneous colonization at the surgical incision site is commonly initiated before the patient enters the hospital or ambulatory surgical center. A common practice has been to have the patient scrub the surgical site with antiseptic soap on one or multiple

Table 4.2 The types of clinical scenarios that would be identified by combining the National Healthcare Safety Network (NHSN) classification of patient risk with the Centers for Disease Control (CDC) measure of severity of surgical site infection (SSI).

NHSN risk index	CDC defined severity of infection		
	Superficial (S_1)	Deep (S_2)	Organ/Space (S_3)
0 (N_0)	N_0S_1 A 35-year-old patient (ASA 1) has transient serous discharge that is culture positive from an inguinal hernia procedure that lasted 60 min. Local drainage is all that is required	N_0S_2 A 55-year-old man (ASA 2) has a wound abscess of hernia incision requiring complete opening of the wound 3 days after 78 min elective repair of inguinal hernia	N_0S_3 64-year-old (ASA 2) patient has an infected hip replacement prosthesis 4 days after a 2.5-h total hip arthroplasty. The prosthesis has to be removed
1 (N_1)	N_1S_1 A 60-year-old (ASA 2) patient has a superficial surgical wound infection 4 days after a 6-h laparotomy for small bowel obstruction. The wound is spontaneously closed 72 h after local drainage	N_1S_2 A 57-year-old man (ASA 2) has an emergency sigmoid colectomy for fecal peritonitis secondary to perforative diverticulitis. The incision is opened for a wound abscess to the fascia on postoperative day 7	N_1S_3 A 63-year-old patient (ASA 4) with severe chronic lung disease has a large pelvic abscess requiring drainage and prolonged antibiotics on postoperative day 5 after a 2-h total abdominal hysterectomy
2 (N_2)	N_2S_1 A 63 year old (ASA 3) has a superficial SSI 10 days after a multilevel laminectomy which requires drainage only and no antibiotics	N_2S_2 A 64-year-old patient (ASA 4) has the whole incision opened to the mesh after a 5-h ventral hernia repair. The cultures grow MRSA. An additional 12 days of hospitalization and antibiotics are required	N_2S_3 A 48-year-old (ASA 3) morbidly obese (480 lb, 216 kg) patient has a wound evisceration from a subfascial abscess after an elective 4.5-h roux-en-Y gastric bypass
3 (N_3)	N_3S_1 A 37 year old (ASA 5) has an exploratory laparotomy for a gunshot wound to the colon, pancreas, and left renal vein/artery; profound shock. He has a 5-cm area of locally drained, superficial wound infection on day 5	N_3S_2 An 83 year old (ASA 4) undergoes subtotal gastrectomy for perforated gastric carcinoma that has a deep SSI requiring opening of the entire wound on day 6 after a 5.5-h subtotal gastrectomy	N_3S_3 A 68 year old (ASA 4) with severe congestive heart failure, aortic insufficiency, and staphylococcal endocarditis has a postoperative sternal infection with mediastinitis 5 days after a 7-h aortic valve replacement

ASA, American Society of Anesthesiologists.

occasions preoperatively. Chlorhexidine, povidone–iodine, or isopropyl alcohol applications to the site are also used. None has been clearly documented to reduce the frequency of SSIs. Whole body baths and showers with conventional soaps or any of the aforementioned antiseptics have also been advocated, but the most recent analysis has not shown a reduction in SSIs, even though cultures before the operation have demonstrated a reduction in bacterial counts (Webster and Osborne 2007). Chlorhexidine has been demonstrated to bind to skin proteins and to have a sustained antibacterial action. This observation has raised the issue that repeated localized scrubs or whole body bathing over several days before surgery may be preferable to a single scrub on the day before the procedure (Edmiston et al. 2008).

Surveillance cultures

A very recently popularized technique in the preoperative period is *screening cultures of the nasopharynx* of the patient. This method has been shown to identify patients with colonization by specific pathogens, particularly meticillin-resistant *Staphylococcus aureus* (MRSA). MRSA colonization has been associated with increased rates of infection. Screening with preoperative cultures has been used for decontamination (e.g., mupiricin) of positive patients, changing the systemic antibiotics used for prevention, or deferring the actual timing of the surgical procedure. Some studies have demonstrated reduced infection rates with preoperative decontamination, and others have not. Consistent effectiveness has not been demonstrated (Simor 2011).

An interesting feature of surveillance cultures is that hospital workers have similar rates of MRSA colonization as the population in general, even when working in environments (e.g., intensive care units) with frequent exposure to the pathogen (Ibarra et al. 2008). Thus, an interpretation of those patients with positive MRSA colonization may be that it is the phenotype of a host that carries pathogenic bacteria, and not necessarily an environmentally acquired risk factor. MRSA decontamination may reduce MRSA SSIs, but not change rates from all pathogens in a vulnerable population. With the increased prevalence of community-associated MRSA, which is approaching 20% of elective patients, the effectiveness of this surveillance methodology deserves continued evaluation.

Preoperative hospitalization

The duration of preoperative hospitalization is associated with increased rates of SSIs. Cruse and Foord (1980) identified a twofold increase in SSIs with 4 days of preoperative hospitalization and a fourfold increase with 7 preoperative days. More recently, Vogel et al. (2010) have similarly noted increases in SSIs with the duration of preoperative hospitalization in cardiac, colon, and lung operations.

Several hypotheses explain these observations. Hospitalization is associated with colonization of the patient with hospital-associated microflora, and these organisms are more resistant to conventional preventive antibiotics. Days of preoperative hospitalization are probably a surrogate marker for the severity of the patient's medical and surgical condition, because routine surgical cases are usually on the same or first day of admission to the hospital. Extended preoperative inpatient assessment is a risk factor for increased surgical morbidity. Similarly, the patient who has been hospitalized, discharged, and then re-hospitalized has both exposure to hospital microflora and likely complications of prior care that will increase SSI rates for subsequent surgery.

Preoperative nursing home patients

Nursing homes are a concentrated collection of chronically ill patients who have high rates of clinical infections and antibiotic utilization.

Hence, nursing home patients harbor resistant profiles of bacterial colonization. Elective or emergency operations for these patients require consideration for preventive antibiotic choices (discussed subsequently) that are different from those conventionally employed.

Prior antibiotics

Antibiotic administration results in changes in the patient's microbial colonization. Oral antibiotics for streptococcal pharyngitis or for a community-acquired urinary tract infection result in changes in the patient's cutaneous and gastrointestinal colonization. Similar to prior inpatient care, ambulatory antibiotics will likely impact the probability of SSIs. Deferral of elective procedures, if practical, because of recent antibiotic use is appropriate.

■ Intraoperative methods
Hair removal

Removal of hair at the surgical site has been part of surgical lore as a technique that reduces SSIs. Many patients have limited hair at the surgical site and the majority opinion would be that no hair removal is necessary for prevention of SSIs. For cranial, inguinal, and operations on hirsute males, hair removal may be desirable because of logistical issues at the surgical site.

Although hair removal has not been shown to reduce SSIs, the methods employed in removal have been documented to increase them. Removal the night before surgery with either a razor or elective clippers has been associated with increased SSIs (Cruse and Foord 1980). Cutaneous abrasions from early hair removal are colonized with bacteria and increased wound contamination. Even straight razors used at the time of surgery have been implicated with increased infections (Alexander et al. 1983). Electric clippers are the preferred method but only in the operating room immediately before preparation of the surgical site. Loose clipped-hair pieces are potential foreign bodies in the surgical wound and should be mechanically removed. Depilatory creams have been used for hair removal but little evidence supports this practice. Hypersensitivity reactions to depilatory creams may be a legitimate reason to not use them.

Skin antiseptics

The mechanical cleansing of the skin at the surgical site is performed with a number of antiseptic soaps. No evidence favors one over another, nor is there a scientific basis for defining the duration of the scrub. The traditional mechanical scrub is initiated at the central area of the proposed incision and the scrubbing action continues in a concentric fashion. The scrub is repeated with the circular action always moving from the cleanest area toward the more contaminated perimeter.

A topical antiseptic solution is then applied over the mechanically scrubbed area. Isopropyl alcohol, chlorhexidine gluconate, and povidone–iodine solutions all have antibacterial action and have been used. Isopropyl alcohol is a potent antiseptic but presents a risk of flammability. Povidone–iodine must be permitted to dry to have optimal antibacterial action. Chlorhexidine has been a preferred topical antiseptic in other skin preparation studies.

A recent clinical trial compared a hybrid antiseptic solution of chlorhexidine and isopropyl alcohol together with povidone–iodine alone. A statistically significant reduction ($p = 0.004$) in SSIs was seen with the hybrid solution (9.5%) when compared with povidone–iodine (16.1%) (Darouiche et al. 2010). It is unclear whether the addition of isopropyl alcohol to the chlorhexidine solution is better than either chlorhexidine or isopropyl alcohol alone. The addition of isopropyl alcohol may have similar effects to povidone–iodine. Future studies to examine the choice of topical antiseptics will be required to answer these questions. As skin colonization is only one variable to account for SSIs, such studies will likely require rigorous control, standardization of case selection (e.g., only clean operations), and large numbers of cases.

Air-handling systems

Air-borne bacteria exist in the operating room. Although air-borne bacteria have been a concern for causing SSIs, there are no solid scientific data to demonstrate whether significant contamination of the surgical site occurs from this source. Air-handling systems are used in all hospitals and guidelines require that the operating room air must be exchanged and filtered at specified intervals of time.

The ultraviolet (UV) light clinical trial of the 1960s provided insight into the role of air-borne contaminants and SSIs (Ad Hoc Committee of the Committee on Trauma 1964). UV light was demonstrated to reduce bacterial fall out in the operating room but did not impact on SSI rates except for refined-clean surgical procedures. This study concluded that conventional air-handling systems were sufficient to control air-borne bacteria.

Nevertheless, concern remains in those clean operations where infection is infrequent but the consequences are especially catastrophic (e.g., total joint replacement). Charnley (1972) popularized laminar-flow air management for the operating room and provided personal experience of its efficacy. However, clinical trials have not demonstrated benefit. Although some continue to advocate and use laminar flow, the expense and lack of documented efficacy have limited general use.

Operating room traffic

Personnel movements in and out of the operating room are an expected event during procedures. Circulating nurses, technicians, anesthesiology personnel, and surgical spectators are anticipated in most cases. Bacterial "fall out" can be documented by placing culture plates about the operating room, and seeing the increased number of bacteria that are recovered as a function of people entering and leaving the operating theater (Adams and Fry 1984). Contaminants may be on the footwear and clothing of those entering, and air currents are created which render floor contaminants "air borne." Restricting operating room traffic has not been scientifically proven to reduce SSIs, and selected movements into and about the operating room environment are necessary. In clean operations, a low-cost method of reducing air-borne contamination is to restrict unnecessary operating room traffic.

Adhesive drapes/wound sealants

Even with vigorous scrubbing of the surgical site and use of topical antiseptics, residual bacteria remain within the hair follicles and pores of the skin. Furthermore, the number of bacteria on the skin surface will increase as lengthy procedures unfold. As it is impractical to re-scrub and re-apply antiseptics at intervals during lengthy procedures, alternative methods have been explored to partition the residual colonization of the skin from accessing the open wound.

Adhesive drapes placed over the surgical site have been used for >40 years. More recent modifications of the adhesive drape have antiseptics (e.g., povidone–iodine) on the cutaneous surface. Two studies have demonstrated that the traditional adhesive drape actually increases SSIs (Paskin and Lerner 1969, Cruse and Foord 1980). Increased SSIs are likely due to increased microbial proliferation from perspiration and a "green house" effect beneath the synthetic drape. The antiseptic-coated drapes need objective study.

An alternative to the adhesive drape is the wound sealant (Towfigh et al. 2008). This cyanoacrylate preparation is applied over the proposed surgical site after scrubbing and antiseptic application. The sealant is permitted to dry and then the operation commences. This process seals residual bacteria in the skin. Unlike the adhesive drapes discussed above, the sealant does not have microbial proliferation under the cyanoacrylate. Actual microbial counts within the wound have been reduced with use of the sealant, but actual reductions in SSIs remains to be documented. Importantly, adhesive drapes and sealants have value only for those procedures where the skin is the major source of surgical site contamination.

Technical considerations

As identified above, adjuvant factors at the surgical site increase SSIs. Control of many of these adjuvant factors is by the surgeon. Effective hemostasis, parsimony in the use of suture materials in the wound, and the avoidance of excessive use of the electrocautery are all important considerations. Avoidance of excessive local tissue trauma to the wound edges can also be of value. Adherence to accepted principles of technique in the operating room can be easily forgotten, with dire consequences for the patient.

Topical antibiotics at the surgical site have been an attractive method to potentially reduce SSIs (Lord et al. 1983). Experimental methods in the laboratory have demonstrated benefits of topical antibiotics, but clinical trials demonstrating superiority to the use of systemic antibiotics have not been identified. Recently Alexander et al. (2009) have reported effectiveness of a topical application of antibiotic solution into the surgical wound of patients undergoing bariatric surgery. The antibiotic solution is introduced via a closed suction catheter system at the completion of the procedures, retained within the surgical wound for 2 h, and then completely evacuated. Compared with historical controls, the improvement in SSI rates has been dramatic. This or similar methods deserve additional clinical evaluation.

Drains

No one area of surgical practice defies any meaningful analytical evaluation such as the use of drains in the surgical incision at the end of the procedure. There are passive drains, sump drains, and closed suction drains. The patient populations who have received drains have been heterogeneous and are usually selected based on the biases of the operating surgeon. Drains that exit the wound through the incision itself are likely to increase SSI rates (Cruse and Foord 1980). Closed suction drains exiting via a separate stab wound have the intellectual appeal of removing the residual bloody drainage that collects in the dependent portion of the wound, especially in obese patients. The use of drainage systems at the surgical site requires more scientific rigor before recommendations in practice can be made.

Delayed primary closure

In selected operations, the surgeon is confronted with severe contamination or pyogenic infection during the procedure. These circumstances have the clinical appearance of virtual certainty that infection will occur at the surgical site because of the magnitude of the contamination. Delayed primary closure is a potentially useful method to avoid invasive infection of the surgical site (Bernard and Cole 1963).

Preventive antibiotics

The introduction of antibiotics into the clinical practice of medicine and surgery brought the expectation that antibiotics for prevention would reduce SSIs. Expectations lapsed into disillusionment as early clinical trials of preventive antibiotics failed for several reasons. First, surgical cases were poorly stratified. Clean and clean-contaminated cases were indiscriminately mixed and no limits were placed on the risk profile of patients entered into the clinical trials, e.g., inguinal hernia repairs were randomized with colon resections. Second, the timing of antibiotic administration was not standardized. The drugs were generally given after the operation and for a sustained period of time into the postoperative period. By the end of the 1950s, preventive antibiotics were viewed as not having any clinical value for surgical patients.

The reason for the failure of preventive antibiotics in these early trials was elucidated by experimental studies of cutaneous infection. Miles et al. (1957) demonstrated that the antibiotic needed to be in the tissue at the time of microbial contamination if effectiveness was to be seen. Burke (1961) similarly demonstrated the importance of pre-incisional administration of the antibiotic in a surgically relevant animal model to achieve drug presence at the time of the surgical incision. From these experimental models it was demonstrated that the antibiotic had to be in the incised tissue before contamination, it needed to have activity against the likely pathogens to be encountered, and systemic antibiotics given after contamination had little or no impact on the natural history of infection.

Clinical trials then followed that documented the principles that were defined in the experimental studies. Bernard and Cole (1964) used benzylpenicillin, meticillin, and chloramphenicol in three intravenous doses, given preoperatively, intraoperatively, and postoperatively in abdominal surgery patients. Two-thirds of the patients were gastric and pancreaticobiliary operations and a third were intestinal operations. Patients receiving the antibiotics had an 8% infection rate at the surgical site whereas placebo managed controls had a 27% SSI rate. Polk and Lopez-Mayor (1969) used cephaloridine (intramuscularly) preoperatively with two postoperative doses compared with placebos in only gastrointestinal resection, of which 50% were colon operations. Placebo patients had a 29% SSI rate, whereas patients receiving antibiotics had only 6% SSIs.

The principles proposed in the early studies were further validated by Stone et al. (1976) in two separate studies. In a four-arm clinical trial, multiple preoperative doses of the preventive antibiotic (cefazolin) yielded the same result as a single preoperative dose in patients undergoing gastric, biliary and colon surgery. Antibiotics not started until after the operation had the same infection rate as those receiving only the placebo. Furthermore, in a subsequent study with a different antibiotic (cefamandole), the same types of surgical patients as in the previous study received only the perioperative three doses, but were compared with patients who received an additional 5 postoperative days of the antibiotic (Stone et al. 1979). No improvement in SSI rates was seen by extending the preventive antibiotic duration into the postoperative period.

Gastrointestinal, biliary, and colonic procedures were the focus of the above-cited early studies because SSI rates were highest in these cases. Subsequent studies followed in hysterectomy, trauma, peripheral vascular surgery, orthopedic surgery, and even hernia and breast surgery. Some procedures such as coronary artery bypass grafting have limited placebo-controlled evidence to validate the use of preventive antibiotics, but the principles appear to apply across all patients and all surgical procedures. The general philosophy has been that preventive antibiotics should be used in surgical procedures where infections are frequent (e.g., colon surgery) or when the consequences of infection are particularly severe such as total joint replacement, heart valve replacement, and peripheral vascular procedures. In terms of the inoculum and the probability of infection, preventive antibiotics shift the relationship to the right in Figure 4.2 from A_0 to A_1 for conventional pathogens, and B_0 to B_1 for pathogens of increased virulence.

Principle 1: The antibiotic must be in the tissues of the surgical site at the time of contamination

This is a foundation principle that has been repeatedly confirmed. The antibiotic needs to be at appropriate concentrations throughout the duration of the whole procedure. If the antibiotic has a short half-life ($t_{\frac{1}{2}}$) and is administered too early before the incision is made, the patient may have insufficient antibiotic through the entire procedure. Short $t_{\frac{1}{2}}$ antibiotics, such as cephalothin ($t_{\frac{1}{2}}$ = 30 min), are rapidly eliminated and have been shown not to prevent SSIs in longer procedures such as colon resection (Burdon et al. 1977). Early administration before the incision may result in a reduced period of antibacterial coverage for the surgical site (Shapiro et al. 1982). Hence, it has been recommended that the preventive antibiotic be administered within 60 min of the surgical incision (Bratzler et al. 2005). Of course, if a long $t_{\frac{1}{2}}$ antibiotic is used then administration 2 h preoperatively will be less of a liability than a short $t_{\frac{1}{2}}$ drug would be. The appropriate preventive antibiotic choices based on the recommendations of Bratzler et al. (2005) are identified in **Table 4.3**.

The duration of the operation is also a variable in maintaining adequate antibiotic in the tissues of the surgical site. Antibiotic is being eliminated during the course of the operation and procedures longer than 4 h will exceed 1–2 h $t_{\frac{1}{2}}$ antibiotic concentrations at the surgical wound. Although not well studied, it is advisable to redose the preventive antibiotic at an interval of about 2 $t_{\frac{1}{2}}$ (Fry and Pitcher 1990). Thus, cefazolin with a $t_{\frac{1}{2}}$ of 1.8 h should be re-dosed at about 3.5 h after the time of the initial dose. Better studies are needed for the issue of re-dosing preventive antibiotics during the procedure.

The body mass of the patient is another important consideration in maintaining adequate antibiotic concentration at the surgical site. Almost all studies have used a single dose for all adult patients with little or no consideration for the patient's size. Patients with a body mass index (BMI) ≥ 30 kg/m^2 will have larger volumes of distribution than smaller patients, and this will likely influence the concentration of drug at the surgical site (Pevzner et al. 2011). Large BMI patients should receive larger preoperative antibiotic doses.

Multiple trauma patients requiring emergency surgical intervention with blood loss and an expanded volume of distribution will likely have increased requirements for antibiotic dosing to maintain appropriate tissue concentrations during operations (Reed et al. 1992).

Principle 2: The antibiotic must have antimicrobial activity against the pathogens likely to be encountered

Different operations are at risk for infections from different bacteria encountered at surgery. Skin incisions by definition mean that the skin microflora of *Staphylococcus aureus* and *Staphylococcus epidermidis* are likely pathogens. For clean operations, the skin colonists are the major bacterial risk; nafcillin or cefazolin is the logical choice for preventive antibiotics. Biliary tract operations will most likely encounter *Escherichia coli* or *Klebsiella pneumoniae*, and these pathogens make cefazolin or a synthetic penicillin/β-lactamase inhibitor combination a good choice. Female genital tract operations require coverage for enteric Gram-negative bacteria and obligate anaerobes. The human colon harbors *E. coli* and *Bacteroides fragilis* as target organisms for coverage. The microbiology of SSIs reflects the colonization of the transgressed anatomic structures and the selected antibiotic must target those potential pathogens.

Patients exposed to the healthcare environment before elective operations can be expected to have colonization with resistant microbes not ordinarily seen. Prior antibiotics will increase the presence of *S. epidermidis* on the skin and will replace ordinary species with resistant Gram-negative rods on mucous membrane surfaces. The selection of a preventive antibiotic regimen must be expanded into the Gram-negative range for patients from nursing homes or those with prolonged preoperative hospitalization. Without surveillance cultures of the patient from the nursing home environment, the selection of an antibiotic(s) can be very difficult to predict.

The emergence of the community-associated MRSA (CA-MRSA) has also changed the selection of suitable antibiotics for prevention, especially in clean operations. MRSA has traditionally been of concern in SSIs only when patients have recently or currently been hospitalized. However, the CA-MRSA is currently responsible for most *S. aureus* infections that occur in the community, and the frequency of colonization with this organism creates concern about whether conventional preventive antibiotics (e.g., cefazolin, nafcillin) are adequate.

Finkelstein et al. (2002) examined vancomycin versus cefazolin for the prevention of SSIs in cardiac surgical patients in an institution that was deemed to have high rates of MRSA infections (3% of cardiac admissions). In a randomized trial of 885 patients, 9.2% of all patients had SSI. Patients that received vancomycin had higher rates of meticillin-sensitive *S. aureus* (MSSA), whereas patients receiving cefazolin had higher rates of MRSA infection. Comparison of the overall SSI rate was no different between the two study groups. The results indicate that patients in high MRSA infection environments are colonized with both sensitive and resistant strains of *S. aureus*, and that infection in the vulnerable host occurred with the pathogen not covered by the preventive antibiotic used. It also appears that vancomycin is less effective against MSSA than cefazolin, which poses a real problem in the use of vancomycin for the prevention of clean wound infections. Unfortunately, vancomycin is currently the only drug with evidence for prevention of MRSA infections after clean operations.

Thus, coverage of MRSA in major elective clean operations appears to be warranted when (1) the hospital has a high prevalence of MRSA infections, (2) the patient has documented colonization with MRSA, (3) the patient has had treatment with a β-lactam antibiotic in the period of timing leading up to the procedure and colonization with MRSA is presumed, or (4) the patient has had a significant exposure to the healthcare environment before the procedure (hospitalization or nursing home). This potentially leaves the patient vulnerable to infection from MSSA. Some are recommending that additional antibiotics (e.g., cefazolin) for coverage of MSSA be used with vancomycin in the clinical settings identified above. There are no clinical trials to validate the addition of MSSA coverage to vancomycin.

Principle 3: Continued antibiotic administration after wound closure has no impact on the frequency of SSIs

It has been counterintuitive for surgeons to accept that antibiotics given after wound closure do not reduce infection rates. Yet all the clinical studies have failed to demonstrate any benefit from extending the duration of drug administration. In general surgery, McDonald et al. (1998) have demonstrated no reduction in SSI rates by extending postoperative antibiotics beyond the time of surgery in an extensive meta-analysis of 25 clinical trials. Song and Glenny (1998) have confirmed the same observation in an extensive review of elective colon surgery. Similar studies have been done in total joint replacement, cardiac surgery, hysterectomy, trauma laparotomy, and open fractures with no benefit demonstrated from extension of the postoperative antibiotics.

The lack of benefit of postoperative preventive antibiotics is illustrated in **Figure 4.3**. First, during the operation the human inflammatory cascade is activated within the surgical site, which includes the coagulation cascade and the formation of tissue edema. The acute endproduct of the inflammatory response is the formation of fibrin over the wound surface. Fibrin deposition begins at the start of the operation and continues throughout. As bacteria contaminate the surgical site from all potential sources, these microbes are encased within the dynamically forming fibrin matrix. A critical consideration in antibiotic effectiveness is that the antibiotic be present and is entrapped within the matrix as the fibrin is formed. The density of the mature fibrin matrix is poorly penetrated if at all by antibiotics given after it has formed. Subsequently administered drugs will not access the bacterial contaminants within. Then as the wound surfaces are closed, the potential interface between the apposed wound surfaces is promptly filled with fibrin. This fibrin serves as the scaffolding for the subsequent deposition of collagen as part of wound healing.

Table 4.3 The recommended prophylactic antibiotic regimens by the Surgical Care Improvement Project.

Procedure	Approved antibiotics	Approved for β-lactam allergic patients
Coronary artery bypass graft, other cardiac surgery, or peripheral vascular surgery	Cefazolin, cefuroxime, or vancomycin	Vancomycin or clindamycin
Hysterectomy	Cefotetan, or cefazolin, or cefoxitin, or cefuroxime, or ampicillin/sulbactam	Clindamycin or metronidazole
Hip or knee arthroplasty	Cefazolin, or Cefuroxime, or Vancomycin	Vancomycin, or Clindamycin
Colon resection	Cefotetan, cefoxitin, ampicillin/sulbactam, or ertapenem **Drug Combinations** Cefazolin or cefuroxime with metronidazole Clindamycin with aminoglycoside Clindamycin with quinolone Clindamycin with aztreonam Aminoglycoside with metronidazole Quinolone with metronidazole	Clindamycin with aminoglycoside Clindamycin with quinolone Aminoglycoside with metronidazole Quinolone with metronidazole

Unfortunately, microbes wedged into this wound matrix will not make contact with systemic antibiotics given after closure, and systemic antibiotics administered after wound closure do not make contact with the potential microbial pathogens within the surgical site.

A second consideration in the failure of postoperatively administered antibiotics is that edema continues in the tissues after wound closure. Edema can be viewed as an obligatory response of the host to provide aqueous conduits for leukocytes to navigate through the dense extracellular tissues and access would-be pathogens. Millions of years of evolution did not anticipate that surgeons would be closing wounds, and accordingly the continued formation of edema after wound closure creates increased hydrostatic pressure about the wound. Thus, not only is the fibrin matrix of the wound interface poorly penetrated by antibiotics, but also the wound itself is functionally ischemic from increased hydrostatic pressure about its perimeter. Simply stated, postoperatively administered antibiotics do not access the microbial contaminants of the surgical site!

A common justification for the continuation of postoperative antibiotics is coverage of various tubes and interventions that are used in patient care. Wound drains, chest tubes, mediastinal tubes, intravenous catheters, Foley catheters, endotracheal tubes, and others are recognized as potential avenues for microbial entrance into the host. Some surgeons insist on the continuation of systemic antibiotics to "cover" these alternative routes for microbial contamination despite no evidence to support this use.

Continuing antibiotics to cover drains and tubes ignores the concept of the "decisive period" as proposed by Miles et al. (1957). Antibiotics can provide prevention only if the period of bacterial contamination at a site is temporally limited, e.g., the duration of a surgical procedures. During this decisive period, the colonization of the host is stable and the pathogens have a stable and predictable sensitivity to the antibiotics that are employed. However, if systemic antibiotics are administered across multiple generation times of the bacteria, then the character of the colonization of the patient changes. Sensitive bacteria are eliminated and the proliferation of resistant species remaining, from either the original colonization of the patient or species acquired from the hospital environment, results in resistant bacteria. The charade of using prolonged preventive antibiotics is not only ineffectiveness in the prevention of infection, but also the substitution of resistant colonization for subsequent pathogens.

The negative consequences for the patient of extending preventive antibiotics into the postoperative period are real. Needless antibiotics are expensive to purchase and expensive to deliver. As noted above, multiple days of postoperative systemic antibiotics change the patient's colonization to resistant forms and also create epidemiological resistance in the hospital environment. Finally, excess preventive antibiotics result in increased drug complications, especially with the epidemic increase in *Clostridium difficile* infections (see Chapter 11). Prolongation of systemic antibiotics after wound closure cannot be justified.

■ Preoperative colon preparation

The colon is the largest repository of bacteria in the human body. Elective colon surgery is associated with higher infection rates than elective procedures at any other anatomic site. In a review, Poth (1982) identified that before the use of contemporary preventive measures, an SSI rate of >80% and a perioperative mortality rate >10% were seen in elective colon surgery in the 1930s.

Early surgical efforts to reduce SSIs in colon surgery included the use of the mechanical bowel preparation (MBP). Although the full magnitude of the microbial density has not been fully appreciated

since the 1930s, there has always been the intuitive idea that purging the colon of stool should prevent infection after colon resection. Studies from the 1930s demonstrated no reduction in SSIs with mechanical preparation alone.

When antibiotics emerged as potential therapy for patients in the late 1930s, there was considerable interest in using oral antibiotics to reduce infection after colon surgery. This concept was to give poorly absorbed oral antibiotics after a complete MBP of the colon in the preoperative period to reduce the microbial contamination of the surgical site. The major impetus for adding oral antibiotics to the MBP was because mechanical preparation alone has been recognized since the 1930s not to reduce SSI rates after colon surgery.

The early efforts to use oral antibiotics failed to demonstrate efficacy of this method. Numerous sulfanilamide derivatives and oral aminoglycosides were initially used, but none demonstrated in prospective trials a reduction in SSIs through three decades of clinical research. During this entire period of time, improved MBP was explored because complete colonic evacuation was considered essential for the reduction of stool bulk, but also to facilitate antibiotic delivery to the mucosal surface of the colon.

Finally, in 1974 a randomized clinical trial demonstrated significance in the use of the oral antibiotic bowel preparation (Washington et al. 1974). Patients were randomized to three groups after complete MBP. One group received oral neomycin alone, a second group received oral neomycin plus tetracycline, and a third group received only oral placebo. No patients received systemic antibiotics. The combination of oral neomycin and tetracycline reduced SSI rates by nearly 90%. Neomycin alone resulted in no reduction in SSI rates. The rationale of the antibiotic combination was that the neomycin covered the aerobic gut bacteria, whereas tetracycline covered the anaerobic species.

A subsequent study evaluated the use of neomycin and erythromycin versus a placebo in elective colon surgery within Veterans Administration hospitals (Clarke et al. 1977). Erythromycin was chosen because of superior anaerobic coverage compared with tetracycline which was used previously. All patients received a complete 3-day MBP before the oral antibiotics were started. SSI rates were 35% in placebo patients but only 9% in those patients receiving the oral antibiotics.

Thus, during the 1970s the concept of preventive systemic antibiotics and the oral antibiotic bowel preparation evolved independently as strategies to reduce SSI rates after elective colon surgery. Conceptually, systemic preventive antibiotics provided a "safety net" to control bacterial contaminants within the surgical wound, whereas the oral antibiotic bowel preparation reduced the number of contaminants that escaped from the colon and into the surgical site.

As the two preventive strategies had different mechanisms of prevention, several studies examined the utility of both methods together. In 2002 (Lewis 2002), a definitive study had patients who were randomized to receive the oral antibiotic bowel preparation of oral neomycin and metronidazole versus MBP alone, with the patients in both arms of the clinical trial receiving the systemic antibiotics amikacin and metronidazole preoperatively. The results demonstrated that patients receiving only the systemic antibiotics (and MBP) had an SSI rate of 16%, whereas patients receiving both systemic antibiotics and the oral antibiotic bowel preparation had an SSI rate of 7%. Furthermore, a meta-analysis of 13 individual studies demonstrated a significant reduction of SSI rates ($p < 0.0001$) in favor of oral antibiotics and systemic antibiotics together versus systemic antibiotics alone. Similarly, separate studies have demonstrated that the combination of oral and systemic antibiotics is superior to just oral antibiotics (Englesby et al. 2010).

The evidence indicates that the oral antibiotic bowel preparation with MBP is a significant method to reduce SSIs, in addition to the use of systemic preventive antibiotics. However, this method continues to have many unanswered questions that need to be addressed.

What is the optimal MBP?

Very different mechanical preparations have been used individually and in concert to clear the colon of all fecal content. Clear liquid diets (commonly for many days preoperatively), castor oil, magnesium salts, sodium phosphate, and other oral cathartics or purgatives have been used. Sequential enemas with multiple agents have also been used usually together with various oral cathartics. The ongoing issues have been the duration necessary to cleanse the colon preoperatively, the thoroughness of the result, and the necessity for significant patient discomfort to achieve effective MBP.

In recent years the use of polyethylene glycol solutions has been popular for MBP. The polyethylene glycol solution can give a rapid and complete cleansing of the colon, but requires patient compliance and perseverance in the ingestion of 4 l of solution over a 4- to 6-h period of time. Poor compliance and suboptimal colon preparation are issues, especially among elderly patients undergoing preparation as an outpatient. Thus, dissatisfaction with available MBP regimens means that improved alternatives need to be developed.

Although MBP itself has not been shown to reduce SSIs, a further consideration is whether the composition of the MBP may actually have an influence. Itani et al. (2007) have shown an apparent reduction of SSIs when sodium phosphate MBP was compared with polyethylene glycol. Experimental research studies by Long et al. (2008) have demonstrated that maintenance of normal phosphate concentrations modulate the virulence of Gram-negative bacteria. Hypophosphatemia enhances Gram-negative bacterial virulence. Mobilization of phosphate from the mucosal surface of the colon to the extracellular reservoir may be an important consequence of the physiological stress response. Although not conclusively proven, phosphate-containing MBP may be an important addition to the oral antibiotic preparation and needs further clinical evaluation. The concept that electrolyte and macromolecules that are not antibiotics could have attenuation effects on microbial virulence opens an entirely new direction in MBP.

What is the best oral antibiotic choice?

The basic premise of the oral antibiotic bowel preparation is that the drug(s) have activity against the target pathogens of the colon, and that they be poorly absorbed or not at all to achieve intraluminal effects. Neomycin has been commonly used but is suspect as to the extent of its antimicrobial activity because of the anaerobic intraluminal environment of the colon, and the requirement for aminoglycoside antibiotics to have oxygen availability for biological activity. Erythromycin does have very good anaerobic activity and significant aerobic Gram-negative activity as well. It does have some systemic absorption, and is also associated with gastrointestinal motility disorders. Tetracycline has less anaerobic activity than erythromycin and is also absorbed to a greater degree. Metronidazole has superb anaerobic activity but is also absorbed. As vast numbers of antibiotics have been evaluated for parenteral use, it is likely that minimally absorbed oral alternatives can be identified.

What is the best timing for oral antibiotic administration?

Current evidence indicates that the oral antibiotics should be administered in three divided doses over the 10- to 20-h time span before the operation. Oral antibiotics must not be given until the MBP is complete or undissolved drug will pass through the colon with no antimicrobial effect. Oral antibiotics given too close to the time of the operation (e.g., <8 h before the incision) will not have had ample time to reach the entire length of the colon and not had sufficient time to reduce microbial concentrations on the mucosal surface. In the original study by Washington et al. (1974), the antibiotics were given >48 h before the incision and it should be noted that the SSI rates in the antibiotic arm of the trial were quite low (5%). Studies in the early years of investigating oral antibiotics started the drugs for 2 days before the operation, based on experimental observations of the duration necessary to achieve optimum antimicrobial effect. Thus, additional investigation is necessary to define the timing and duration of oral antibiotic administration. The timing and duration will also need to be determined by the specific antibiotic strategy that is employed because the total administration may need to be adjusted for the specific drug that is used.

Is C. difficile infection increased with the oral antibiotic bowel preparation?

The emergence of *C. difficile* infection (CDI) as a complication of inpatient care is associated with the administration of systemic antibiotics. This is thought to be in large part the disruption of the normal microflora of the colon (see Chapter 11). One retrospective study has demonstrated an increased rate of CDI with the oral antibiotic bowel preparation (Wren et al. 2005), whereas another did not (Krapohl et al. 2011). Additional studies need to examine the frequency of CDI after the oral antibiotic bowel preparation, and particularly focus on its association with the specific antibiotics used. Prolongation of systemic preventive antibiotics into the postoperative period becomes especially problematic when the oral antibiotic bowel preparation has been used because this will impact the recolonization process postoperatively. The use of postoperative probiotics or prebiotics needs to be evaluated in the postoperative colon resection patient who has received both the oral antibiotic bowel preparation and systemic antibiotics for prevention.

■ Physiologic/Metabolic methods
Supplemental oxygen

A substantial volume of experimental studies has demonstrated the benefits of increased oxygen availability in the prevention of infection after soft-tissue contamination with bacteria. Molecular oxygen availability is a critical variable in the intracellular killing function of phagocytic cells and enhanced synthesis of reactive oxygen intermediates, and may be beneficial for other cellular pathways (e.g., chemotaxis efficiency).

Greif et al. (2000) demonstrated a 50% reduction in SSI rates when supplemental oxygen was administered during and immediately after elective colon surgery. The supplemented patients received 80% inhaled oxygen and had documented partial O_2 pressure (PO_2) of 40 kPa (>300 mmHg) during and after the operation. Control patients had 30% inhaled oxygen and normal intraoperative PO_2 values. Importantly, supplemented patients received a vastly larger amount of crystalloid solution (7 l versus 2 l) to expand the extracellular water volume to facilitate oxygen delivery.

Pryor et al. (2004) reported a randomized clinical trial with supplemental oxygen in general surgery laparotomy patients, which had exactly the opposite effect. Supplemented patients had a statistically significant increase in SSIs. Supplemented patients received 80% inhaled oxygen during the procedure whereas control participants received 35%. No supplemental perioperative crystalloid solutions were used. A third trial by Belda et al. (2005), with many of the same investigators from the Greif study and using the same protocol, again demonstrated a 40% reduction in SSIs in general surgery patients.

Thus, there are conflicting clinical data about supplemental oxygen and many questions remain. How could increased oxygen be deleterious in the short term? What is the percentage of inhaled oxygen necessary to achieve a beneficial effect? What should be the time span for oxygen delivery. Should it be only during the procedure, or should it be extended after the operation? Oxygen supplementation remains of uncertain value until additional clinical trials have been completed.

Normothermia

Maintenance of core body temperature has been a desired goal in surgical patients. Intraoperative hypothermia is a commonly recognized event from conduction heat loss during open thoracotomy and laparotomy procedures. The major concern has traditionally focused on the association of coagulopathy with the decline in core body temperature. The threshold for intraoperative hypothermia has been poorly defined, but it has generally not been a source of concern in elective operations until the core temperature declines <35°C.

Kurz et al. (1996) reported on the effects of a reduced core body temperature in patients undergoing elective colon surgery. The intervention group of patients had core temperatures ≥36.5°C whereas control patients had no body temperature intervention until the temperature reached ≤34.5°C. The final difference between groups was 1.8°C. Maintenance of core body temperature ≥36.5°C resulted in a 70% reduction in SSIs. Of interest, patients with the higher core temperature nearly had a lower probability of receiving a transfusion ($p = 0.054$).

It is likely that maintenance of physiological core body temperature is of value to the patient undergoing surgical intervention, although this solitary study has not confirmed this conclusion. Experimental evidence would identify global effects of hypothermia on leukocyte migration and other biochemical processes of the innate host response. Additional studies in other surgical procedures are necessary.

Glycemic control

Decades of diabetes research have led to the conclusion that hyperglycemia is associated with increased infections. Hyperglycemia appears to have a host of different effects on the innate host defense mechanisms and correcting the hyperglycemic state restores the normal host response. This negative effect on leukocytes and potentially other components does not appear to be specific to the patient with diabetes but applies to hyperglycemia secondary to any clinical cause in patient care.

The benefits of glycemic control in the prevention of infection in surgical patients have been demonstrated in open-heart cardiac surgical patients (Furnary et al. 1999). These authors demonstrated that maintenance of blood sugar during and after operation <200 mg% resulted in a statistically lower rate of sternal infections. This benefit was true for patients who were either diabetic or non-diabetic. Latham et al. (2001) confirmed an increasing odds ratio of SSIs in cardiac surgical patients because the blood sugar increased above the 200 mg% threshold.

Multiple issues now confront the desirability and benefit of glucose control for the prevention of SSIs and other surgical infections. The Furnary study has demonstrated benefits by keeping the blood glucose below the 200 mg% threshold. Whether additional improvements in SSI rates can be achieved with lower thresholds of blood glucose

remain to be defined. Can other types of operations benefit from glycemic control? Finally, an important feature of glycemic control is having real-time methods to measure blood glucose rather than the episodic measurement and insulin response method that currently characterizes management. Safe blood glucose management <200 mg% is problematic at present, and future applications of lower thresholds will require better quantitative methods for glucose monitoring.

Postoperative prevention

Prevention, before and during the surgical procedure, has been documented as of value in the prevention of SSIs. However, there is little that can be identified to change the outcome of the surgical site after the operation. Once closure of the surgical site has been completed, a fibrin matrix seals the wound space very promptly (**Figure 4.3**). Wound dressings offer limited if any protection. Topical salves and antibiotic creams influence colonization only around the skin of wound closure, not where infection will occur. Continuation of postoperative systemic antibiotics is certainly not of any value!

Optimization of the physiology of the patient may offer an opportunity for postoperative prevention. Oxygen supplementation, core body temperature control, and glycemic control extended into the postoperative period may offer benefit. There is a lack of current evidence. Restoration of homeostasis in the surgical patient is likely to have some benefit and not have downside risks. Future investigations need to explore the postoperative benefits of physiological control and SSI rates.

MANAGEMENT OF SSIs

Despite application of preventive measures, SSIs still occur. Each infection will have unique characteristics with respect to the patient and the bacteriology of the infection. Therapy of an SSI must be individualized to the specifics of each event. The foundation principles for management of these infections include drainage and debridement of the focus of infection, removal of foreign bodies, antibiotic management if needed, and local wound care.

Drain and debride the Infection

The staples or sutures of the infected area of the wound are removed. Visible pus is evacuated. Pus that extends the length of the incision, or the presence of erythema and induration across most of the wound length, requires complete opening. If sinus tracts are present, additional opening of the tissues will be required. Initial assessment dictates

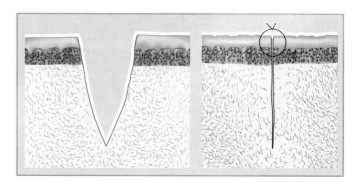

Figure 4.3 The fibrin layer on the wound interface and the presence of the fibrin matrix in the closed wound. Note the "halo" of edema about the closed wound and the potential consequences of increased tissue hydrostatic pressure and ischemia of the interface.

the need for local or even general anesthesia to achieve complete drainage. All necrotic tissue and fibrinous debris should be removed, often by sharp dissection. Dark eschar and cutaneous necrosis must be removed. The wound will require careful daily inspection after the initial drainage because specific pathogens and specific patient comorbidities may make additional drainage necessary.

Cultures of pus and infected tissue are necessary. Although drainage without cultures was reasonable for those localized staphylococcal infections in the past, the era of CA-MRSA makes cultures a requirement to guide antibiotic therapy.

Removal of foreign bodies

Suture materials in the wound are generally removed, except for those at the fascial level. If necrotic fascia is present, then the associated sutures will need removal. Infected mesh is debrided and removed with only that mesh that is firmly incorporated into adjacent tissues preserved. The removal of orthopedic hardware or vascular grafts is usually required in most of these infections, and efforts to salvage these prostheses require clinical judgment by the treating surgeon.

Antimicrobial management

Antimicrobial treatment of the open, infected wound may be required. It must be emphasized that drainage and debridement of most SSIs will be sufficient. Topical agents are commonly employed but have not been well studied for efficacy (Drosou et al. 2003). Topical povidone–iodine, Dakin solution, and others have been employed. Topical antiseptics in open wounds may be toxic to the host tissues and to phagocytic cells (Lineweaver et al. 1985). Use of topical agents commonly employed in burn wound management, such as silver sulfadiazine and mafenide, may be useful in the opened wound where evidence of invasive infection exists about the perimeter tissues.

Evidence of severe inflammation, tissue necrosis, presence of prosthetic materials, and immunosuppression of the host justifies systemic antibiotics. Empirical choices of antibiotics are based on suspected pathogens, and therapy is de-escalated as culture results are available or clinical resolution of the infection is observed. MSSA infections are best covered with nafcillin or a first-generation cephalosporin (e.g., cefazolin). CA-MRSA may be treated with trimethoprim–sulfamethoxazole in most cases, and hospital-acquired MRSA will require vancomycin, linezolid, or daptomycin. Polymicrobial infections will require Gram-negative coverage and suspected infections after colonic contamination may benefit from metronidazole for anaerobic coverage. In general, the effectively drained and debrided wound may require only a short course (e.g., 48 h) of antibiotic coverage, although MRSA infections in particular may require longer duration.

Wound management

The infected wound that has been opened requires daily, bedside debridement. Loosely packed, coarse gauze that is moist with saline is preferred, with the frequency of dressing changes as necessary (at least daily). Dressings should not be permitted to completely dry because this creates neoeschar in desiccated tissues and fosters the continuation of local infection. Wounds should not be packed tightly, lest this functionally converts an open wound to a closed one.

Negative pressure-assisted closure devices are often deployed in the large open wound. These have generally been useful for secondary closure and preparing large surfaces for skin grafting. A secondary benefit has been to protect the open wound from secondary contamination in circumstances such as abdominal wall stomas. It can be said that support for negative pressure devices is largely anecdotal and little has been determined by clinical trials.

■ REFERENCES

Adams R, Fry DE. Surgical suite reconstruction: infection control. *Assoc Oper Room Nurses J* 1984;39:868–76.

Ad Hoc Committee of the Committee on Trauma, Division Medical Sciences, NAS-NRC. Postoperative wound infections: The influence of ultraviolet irradiation of the operating room and of various other factors. *Ann Surg* 1964;**160**(suppl):1–192.

Ahmed S, Macfarlane GT, Fite A, et al. Mucosa-associated bacterial density in relation to human terminal ileum and colonic biopsy samples. *Appl Environ Microbiol* 2007;**73**:7435–42.

Alexander JW, Fischer JE, Boyajian M, et al. The influence of hair-removal methods on wound infection. *Arch Surg* 1983;**118**:347–52.

Alexander JW, Rahn R, Goodman HR: Prevention of surgical site infections by an infusion of topical antibiotics in morbidly obese patients. *Surg Infect* 2009;**10**:53–7.

American Society of Anesthesiologists. ASA physical status classification system, 2012. Available at: www.asahq.org/Home/For-Members/Clinical-Information/ASA-Physical-Status-Classification-System (accessed May 16, 2012).

Anderson DJ. Surgical site infections. *Infect Dis Clin North Am* 2011;**25**:135–53.

Belda FJ, Aguilera L, Garcia de la Asuncion J, et al. Supplemental perioperative oxygen and the risk of surgical wound infection: a randomized controlled trial. *JAMA* 2005;**294**:2035–2042.

Bernard HR, Cole WR. Wound infections following potentially contaminated operations. Effect of delayed primary closure of the skin and subcutaneous tissue. *JAMA* 1963;**184**:290–2.

Bernard HR, Cole WR. The prophylaxis of surgical infection: the effect of prophylactic antimicrobial drugs on the incidence of infection following potentially contaminated operations. *Surgery* 1964;**56**:151–7.

Bratzler DW, Houck PM, Richards C, et al. Use of antimicrobial prophylaxis for major surgery: baseline results from the National Surgical Infection Prevention Project. *Arch Surg* 2005;**140**:174–82.

Burdon JGW, Morris PJ, Hunt P, Watts JM. A trial of cephalothin sodium in colon surgery to prevent wound infection. *Arch Surg* 1977;**112**:1169–73.

Burke JF. The effective period of preventive antibiotic action in experimental incisions and dermal lesions. *Surgery* 1961;**50**:161–8.

Centers of Disease Control and Prevention. National Healthcare Safety Network, 2012. Available at: www.cdc.gov/nhsn (accessed May 16, 2012).

Charnley J. Postoperative infection after total hip replacement with special reference to air contamination in the operating room. *Clin Orthop Relat Res* 1972;**87**:167–87.

Clarke JS, Condon RE, Bartlett JG, et al. Preoperative oral antibiotics reduce septic complications of colon operations: results of prospective, randomized, double-blind clinical study. *Ann Surg* 1977;**186**:251–9.

Cruse PJ, Foord R. The epidemiology of wound infection: a 10-year prospective study of 62,939 wounds, *Surg Clin North Am* 1980;**60**:27–40.

Culver DH, Horan TC, Gaynes RP, et al. Surgical wound infection rates by wound class, operative procedure, and patient risk index, *Am J Med* 1991;**91**(suppl 3B):152S–7S.

Darouiche RO, Wall MJ Jr, Itani KMF, et al. Chlorhexidine–alcohol versus povidone–iodine for surgical-site antisepsis. *N Engl J Med* 2010;**362**:18–26.

Drosou A, Falabella A, Kirsner RS. Antiseptics on wounds: an area of controversy. *Wounds* 2003;**15**:149–66.

Edmiston CE Jr, Krepel CJ, Seabrook GR, et al. Preoperative shower revisited: can high topical antiseptic levels be achieved on the skin surface before surgical admission? *J Am Coll Surg* 2008;**207**:233–9.

Edwards JR, Peterson KD, Andrus ML, et al. National Healthcare Safety Network (NHSN) report, data summary for 2006 through 2007. *Am J Infect Control* 2008;**36**:609–26.

Englesby MJ, Luchtefeld MA, Kubus J, et al. A statewide assessment of surgical site infection (SSI) following colectomy: The role of oral antibiotics. *Ann Surg* 2010;**252**:514–19.

Finkelstein R, Rabino G, Mashiah T, et al. Vancomycin versus cefazolin prophylaxis for cardiac surgery in the setting of a high prevalence of methicillin-resistant staphylococcal infections. *J Thorac Cardiovasc Surg* 2002;**123**:326–32.

Fry DE. The economic costs of surgical site infection. *Surg Infect* 2002;**3**(suppl 1): S37–43.

Fry DE, Pine M, Jones BL, Meimban RJ. Control charts to identify adverse outcomes in elective colon resection. *Am J Surg* 2012;**203**:392–6.

Fry DE, Pitcher DE. Antibiotic pharmacokinetics in surgery. *Arch Surg* 1990;**125**:1490–92

Furnary AP, Zerr KJ, Grunkemeier GL, Starr A. Continuous intravenous insulin infusion reduces the incidence of deep sternal wound infection in diabetic patients after cardiac surgical procedures, *Ann Thorac Surg* 1999;**67**:352–360.

Greif R, Akca O, Horn EP, et al. Supplemental perioperative oxygen to reduce the incidence of surgical wound infection. *N Engl J Med* 2000;**342**:161–7.

Haley RW, Culver DH, Morgan WM, et al. Identifying patients at high risk of surgical wound infection: A simple multivariate index of patient susceptibility and wound contamination, *Am J Epidemiol* 1985;**121**:206–15.

Horan TC, Gaynes RP, Martone WJ, et al. CDC definitions of nosocomial surgical site infections, 1992: a modification of CDC definitions of surgical wound infections. *Infect Control Hosp Epidemiol* 1992;**13**:606–8.

Ibarra M, Flatt T, Van Maele D, et al. Prevalence of methicillin-resistant Staphylococcus aureus nasal carriage in healthcare workers. *Pediatr Infect Dis J* 2008;**27**:1109–11.

Itani KMF, Wilson SE, Awad SS, et al. Ertapenem versus cefotetan prophylaxis in elective colorectal surgery. *N Engl J Med* 2006;**355**:2640–51.

Itani KMF, Wilson SE, Awad SS, et al. Polyethylene glycol versus sodium phosphate mechanical bowel preparation in elective colorectal surgery. *Am J Surg* 2007;**193**:190–94.

Krapohl GL, Phillips LR, Campbell DA Jr, et al. Bowel preparation for colectomy and risk of Clostridium difficile infection. *Dis Colon Rectum* 2011;**54**:810–17.

Kurz A, Sessler DI, Lenhardt R. Perioperative normothermia to reduce the incidence of surgical wound infection and shorten hospitalization, *N Engl J Med* 1996;**334**:1209–15.

Latham R, Lancaster AD, Covington JF, et al. The association of diabetes and glucose control with surgical-site infections among cardiothoracic surgery patients. *Infect Control Hosp Epidemiol* 2001;**22**:607–12.

Lewis RT. Oral versus systemic antibiotic prophylaxis in elective colon surgery: a randomized study and meta-analysis send a message from the 1990s. *Can J Surg* 2002;**45**:173–80.

Lineweaver W, Howard R, Soucy D, et al. Topical antimicrobial toxicity. *Arch Surg* 1985;**120**:267–70.

Long J, Zaborina O, Holbrook C, et al. Depletion of intestinal phosphate after operative injury activates the virulence of *P. aeruginosa* causing lethal gut-derived sepsis. *Surgery* 2008;**144**:189–97.

Lord JW Jr, LaRaja RD, Daliana M, Gordon MT. Prophylactic antibiotic wound irrigation in gastric, biliary, and colonic surgery. *Am J Surg* 1983;**145**:209–12.

McDonald M, Grabsch E, Marshall C, Forbes A. Single- versus multiple-dose antimicrobial prophylaxis for major surgery: a systematic review. *Aust N Z J Surg* 1998;**68**:388–96.

Mangram AJ, Horan TC, Pearson ML, et al. Guideline for prevention of surgical site infection, 1999. *Infect Control Hosp Epidemiol* 1999;**20**:247–78.

Miles AA, Miles EM, Burke J. The value and duration of defence reactions of the skin to primary lodgement of bacteria. *Br J Exp Pathol* 1957;**38**:79–96.

Paskin DL, Lerner HJ. A prospective study of wound infections. *Am Surg* 1969;**35**:627–9.

Pevzner L, Swank M, Krepel C, et al. Effects of maternal obesity on tissue concentrations of prophylactic cefazolin during cesarean delivery. *Obstet Gynecol* 2011;**117**:877–82.

Polk HC Jr, Lopez-Mayor JF. Postoperative wound infection: a prospective study of determinant factors and prevention. *Surgery* 1969;**66**:97–103.

Polk HC Jr, Miles AA. Enhancement of bacterial infection by ferric iron: kinetics, mechanisms, and surgical significance. *Surgery* 1971;**70**:71–7.

Poth EJ. Historical development of intestinal antisepsis. *World J Surg* 1982;**6**:153–9.

Pruett TL, Rotstein OD, Fiegel VD, Sorenson JJ, Nelson RD, Simmons RL. Mechanism of the adjuvant effect of hemoglobin in experimental peritonitis: VIII. A leukotoxin is produced by Escherichia coli metabolism in hemoglobin. *Surgery* 1984;**96**:375–83.

Pryor KO, Fahey TJ, 3rd, Lien CA, Goldstein PA. Surgical site infection and the routine use of perioperative hyperoxia in a general surgical population: a randomized controlled trial. *JAMA.* 2004;**291**:79–87.

Robson MC, Krizek TJ, Heggers JP. Biology of surgical infection. *Curr Probl Surg* 1973;1–62.

Redondo-Lopez V, Cook RL, Sobel JD. Emerging role of lactobacilli in the control and maintenance of the vaginal bacterial microflora. *Rev Infect Dis* 1990;**12**:856–72.

Reed RL 2nd, Ericsson CD, Wu A, et al. The pharmacokinetics of prophylactic antibiotics in trauma. *J Trauma* 1992;**32**:21–7.

Shapiro M, Muñoz A, Tager IB, et al. Risk factors for infection at the operative site after abdominal or vaginal hysterectomy. *N Engl J Med* 1982;**307**:1661–6.

Simor AE. Staphylococcal decolonization: an effective strategy for prevention of infection? *Lancet Infect Dis* 2011;**11**:952–62.

Song R, Glenny AM. Antimicrobial prophylaxis in colorectal surgery: a systematic review of randomized controlled trials. *Br J Surg* 1998;**85**:1232–44.

Stone HH, Hooper CA, Kolb LD, et al. Antibiotic prophylaxis in gastric, biliary and colonic surgery. *Ann Surg* 1976;**184**:443–52.

Stone HH, Haney BB, Kolb LD, et al. Prophylactic and preventive antibiotic therapy: timing, duration and economics. *Ann Surg* 1979;**189**:691–9.

Towfigh S, Cheadle WG, Lowry SF, et al. Significant reduction in incidence of wound contamination by skin flora through use of microbial sealant. *Arch Surg* 2008;**143**:885–91.

Vogel TR, Dombrovskiy VY, Lowry SF. In-hospital delay of elective surgery for high volume procedures: the impact on infectious complications. *J Am Coll Surg* 2010;**211**:784–90.

Washington JA II, Dearing WH, Judd ES, Elveback LR. Effect of preoperative antibiotic regimen on development of infection after intestinal surgery: prospective, randomized, double-blind study. *Ann Surg* 1974;**180**:567–71.

Webster J, Osborne S. Preoperative bathing or showering with skin antiseptics to prevent surgical site infection. *Cochrane Database Syst Rev* 2007;(2):CD004985.

Wren SM, Ahmed N, Jamal A, Safadi BY. Preoperative oral antibiotics in colorectal surgery increase the rate of Clostridium difficile colitis. *Arch Surg* 2005;**140**:752–6.

Chapter 5

Skin, skin structure, and soft-tissue infections

Donald E. Fry

Skin, skin structure, and related soft-tissue infections (SSSTIs) are common clinical problems. SSSTIs are the most common cause for emergency department visits by patients, and these infections are one of the most common causes for outpatient and inpatient antibiotic administration. They are secondary to bacteria that normally colonize the skin or bacteria that are carried into the underlying tissues by penetrating injury. The spectrum of infections may vary from limited areas of spontaneous cellulitis to widely invasive and life-threatening necrotizing soft-tissue infection. Understanding the full scope of these infections is very important for correct diagnosis and treatment of SSSTIs.

ANATOMY OF THE SKIN

Human skin is a water-impervious envelope that constitutes the primary barrier between the host and noxious challenges from the environment. It consists of the epidermis, dermis, and subcutaneous layers (**Figure 5.1**). The basal cells of the skin rest on the basement

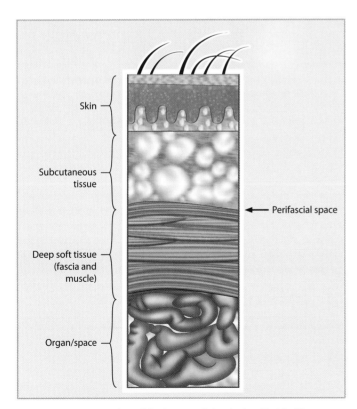

Figure 5.1 A cross-section of the human abdominal wall with skin, subcutaneous tissue, muscle, and abdominal contents. The perifascial space is that potential space on the surface of the investing muscle that anteriorly contacts the subcutaneous fat, and posteriorly contacts the underlying muscle.

membrane of the epidermis, and are the cell population that undergoes active mitosis to replace losses from skin injury and sloughed superficial layers of the epidermis. Mature daughter cells are progressively displaced toward the surface and undergo progressive desiccation until they become the stratum corneum layer of the superficial epidermis. Effete cells are then sloughed as part of the dynamic replacement of skin. Beneath the basement membrane of the epidermis is the dermal layer of the skin, which contains the hair follicle, cutaneous vasculature, and sensory nerves, all of which are in a dense collagen matrix that gives the overall skin its tensile strength. Beneath the dermis is the subcutaneous tissue, which exists between the inferior surface of the dermis and extends for a variable depth to the anterior surface of the investing muscle fascia.

Skin has structures and functions other than being a barrier that serve the host. Hair follicles arise from the dermis via specialized pores, and are abundant on the head or absent on volar surfaces. Small muscle fibers are attached at the base of the follicle for piloerection. Sebaceous glands communicate into the pores of the hair follicle, and provide lubrication for the hair follicle and epidermal surface. Apocrine sweat glands share the pore of the hair follicle. A separate pore structure exists for the eccrine sweat glands which originate in the dermis and communicate to the surface of the epidermis for purposes of sweat production and thermoregulatory control for the host. The dermis also contains the sensory nerves that recognize pain and other noxious stimuli. The rich arteriolar, venular, and lymphatic channels in the dermis deliver nutrients and provide exit channels for the perfusion of the total skin structures. Beneath the dermis is the subcutaneous layer which is primarily made of adipocytes and a loose collagen structure. The subcutaneous tissue is largely a warehouse for fat stores, but may also have a secondary role in providing thermal insulation. A larger physiological and metabolic role of the subcutaneous adipocytes is being identified (Frayn et al. 2003). The subcutaneous fat tissues rest on the surface of the dense collagen layer of investing fascia. Although the fascia is not part of the skin, the blood and lymphatic channels that serve the skin penetrate through and course over the surface of this investing fascia.

An important cell population that should be considered as part of the "anatomy" of the skin is the microbial colonization (**Table 5.1**). The skin has up to 10^6 bacteria per gram of tissue (Greene 1996), although specific environmental conditions may increase or decrease microbial colonization (**Table 5.2**). These microbial colonists are present on the surface of the stratum corneum, and within the various pores and crevices of the skin. Anaerobic colonists are present which reflects the low oxidation–reduction potential in selected areas of the cutaneous histology. Indigenous bacteria are present in all humans, but the microflora in any host will reflect those transient microbes acquired from environmental exposure. The composition and concentration of the colonization of the skin at the time of an injury of the epidermis are clinical variables that assume major importance in whether infection or uneventful healing will be a consequence.

A symbiotic relationship ordinarily exists between skin colonization and host cells. Bacteria provide a "housekeeping" function by digesting

Table 5.1 Normal skin microflora.

Normal skin microflora	Commentary
Staphylococcus aureus	Have demonstrated an increased tendency to be community-associated meticillin-resistant organisms. Cutaneous colonization has been correlated with nasopharyngeal carriage
Staphylococcus epidermidis	*S. epidermidis* is one of many coagulase-negative staphylococcal colonists of the skin, but of these it is most commonly associated with clinical infection but also as a contaminant of blood cultures
Peptococci	Includes *Peptococcus anaerobius*, *P. saccharolyticus*, *P. constellatus*, *P. magnus*. Also a colon and genitourinary colonist. Periodically appears in polymicrobial soft tissue infections
Corynebacterium spp.	*C. lipohilicus* and *C. minutissimum* are species among many of the skin. These are anaerobic Gram-positive rods. They are common colonists of sebaceous glands and are collectively referred to as diphtheroids on cultures
Micrococci	A common Gram-positive coccus of the skin that is rarely seen in clinical infection. It has the unique quality of an extraordinarily thick cell wall that may represent half of the mass of the cell
Brevibacterium spp.	Numerous species that colonize the skin and are associated with foot odor
Gram-negative rods	*E. coli*, and *Klebsiella*, *Enterobacter*, *Proteus*, and even *Acinetobacter* spp. are colonists of the perineum and intertriginous areas
Transient colonization	Streptococci and all flora of the mouth and gastrointestinal tract can be transient colonists of the skin. Hospital environments promote the acquisition of highly resistant hospital-based microflora on the skin of patients

Table 5.2 The numerous environmental factors that influence the qualitative and quantitative character of human skin colonization.

Environmental factor	Commentary
Climate	Higher environmental temperature and increased humidity of the environment together increases bacterial density. Different geographic areas will have different qualitative and quantitative cutaneous colonization
Occlusive dressings	The "green house" effect may increase bacteria counts by 10^4 organisms/g (Aly 1982)
Body location	Intertriginous areas have higher counts. Head and neck with oral colonists; perineum with colonic colonization. Hands and feet with transient flora. Upper arms with lowest colonization
Hospitalization	Transient colonization with healthcare-associated pathogens, commonly resistant gram positive and gram negative species.
Antimicrobial	Systemic antibiotics quickly eliminate colonization by sensitive species that are replaced by other resistant or transient colonization
Medications	Estrogens, corticosteroids and others affect the composition and quantity of microbial colonization
Age	Infants and children carry more potentially pathogenic bacteria; adults higher *Propionibacterium* spp. reflecting higher skin lipid content (Somerville 1969)
Gender	Males have higher skin counts and larger numbers of species likely due to greater sweat production
Occupation	Sun exposure, hospital workers, and other occupations with unique environments will influence colonization
Soap and detergent exposure	Medicated soaps will reduce microbial counts as does the mechanical process of cleansing
Ultraviolet light	Reduces surface colonization
Bacterial adherence	Unique adherence properties of randomly encounter bacteria will affect the transient skin colonization (Nobbs et al. 2009)

unwanted surface debris and eliminating dead cells. The density of microbial colonization is regulated by the sloughing of the cornified layer of skin, but also by the dynamic movement of sweat and sebaceous products that prevents excessive colonization of the pore structures of the skin. The sequestration of bacteria within the pore structure of the skin, due to excessive sebaceum, external contaminants, clusters of exfoliated cells that have not been expelled, and epidermal/dermal edema that narrows pore diameter, creates a situation for microbial accumulation, proliferation, and invasive infection.

Other anatomic peculiarities of the skin are important in understanding the genesis of specific infectious events. Disruption of the dermal vascular structures from penetrating or crush injury will create ischemic islands of skin tissue. Remote radiation treatment impairs the efficiency of lymphatic function and will be associated with increased spontaneous infections due to cutaneous edema. Penetrating injury into the subcutaneous fat tissues will introduce bacteria into an environment of poor vascularity where inflammatory responses are slow to respond. Another vulnerability is the potential space that exists between the subcutaneous fat and the surface of the muscle fascia. This potential "perifascial" space permits the rapid dissemination of bacterial infection but also exposes vascular inflow to the overlying tissues to the potential of thrombosis and necrosis of tissues dependent on these nutrient routes (see Figure 5.1).

COMMON SKIN AND SKIN STRUCTURE INFECTIONS

Cellulitis

Cellulitis is the most common SSSTI. Cellulitis may occur following superficial cuts, abrasions, and small burns. It may occur in areas of lymphedema and of prior radiation therapy. Cellulitis may occur as a spontaneous event without any local injury or provocation. This infection is known to affect the skin at any anatomic site on the body.

Cellulitis affects the full thickness of the skin and extends into the subcutaneous tissues

The diagnosis of cellulitis is a clinical one and thus appreciation of its clinical appearance is vitally important. Cellulitis is a superficial spreading infection that is characterized by advancing erythema from an epicenter of origin. The epicenter is commonly the injury site that has disrupted the integrity of the epidermis, or the epicenter may be an infection originating from one of the anatomic pores of the skin. The infection involves both the epidermis and the dermis, with the attendant inflammatory response of the host causing vasodilation of the microcirculation, and the resultant characteristic blanching erythema. The infection has palpable tenderness over the clearly defined areas of erythema, but palpable induration is usually identified only around the epicenter of the infection. The central site of injury or puncture may appear clinically innocent, may have a serous-to-purulent drainage, and local skin necrosis or sloughing may be seen. Bullae indicate an especially severe cellulitis infection or may indicate that a deeper necrotizing infection is actually present.

Gram-positive organisms predominate as the pathogens of cellulitis. Most are secondary to *Streptococcus pyogenes*, and a smaller number to *Staphylococcus aureus* (Gunderson and Martinello 2012). Only a very small percentage is due to other bacteria when the infection originates from a community source. Wounds from rural or farm environments will demonstrate Gram-negative or polymicrobial pathogens. When infections are due to staphylococci or Gram-negative organisms, the central infection about the injury site is usually pyogenic with only a limited perimeter of cellulitis identified. In general, streptococci are the pathogens of the typical spreading erythematous infection of cellulitis.

The merits of cultures remain a problematic issue in the management of these infections. Blanching erythema with minimal drainage at the injury site is most always *Streptococcus pyogenes* and most clinicians will provide treatment in the absence of culturing the injury site. However, genuinely purulent drainage or evidence of necrosis/eschar at the injury site raises the issue of community-associated meticillin-resistant *Staphylococcus aureus* (CA-MRSA) as the pathogen. Cultures are important in this setting and tissue biopsy for culture may be required to obtain accurate identification of the pathogen. SSSTIs receiving antibiotic therapy that do not promptly respond should also have cultures of available drainage.

The treatment of cellulitic infections is oral antibiotics. Penicillin has maintained activity against *Strep. pyogenes* and is the appropriate choice for non-allergic patients. Clindamycin is an appropriate choice for the penicillin-allergic patient. The broad sensitivity of streptococci allows any number of antibiotics as choices for a successful outcome in treatment. Occasionally, a limited area of infection may be drained or debrided with superficial cellulitic streptococcal infections. Antibiotic choices for staphylococcal infections are dictated by the sensitivity of the pathogen. Meticillin-sensitive *Staph. aureus* (MSSA) is treated with an oral penicillin (dicloxacillin) or cephalosporin (cephalexin). CA-MRSA is commonly treated with trimethoprim–sulfamethoxazole or clindamycin. Patients with severe CA-MRSA infections may be hospitalized and require parenteral vancomycin therapy.

Erysipelas

A unique variant of a superficial spreading infection of the skin is erysipelas. As opposed to those infections defined as cellulitis, erysipelas is confined to the epidermis and dermis of the skin. This infection typically occurs in those aged >60 or in very young children. It follows a cutaneous injury that may be very minor in nature and is sometimes difficult to discern. The extremities and the head/neck are the most common anatomic sites of erysipelas. Predisposing factors include diabetes, alcoholism, and lymphedema secondary to venous insufficiency or prior surgical interventions (e.g., mastectomy). This infection is most often due to *Strep. pyogenes* but may be caused by other streptococci.

The diagnosis is made by the identification of the typical advancing red rash with a clear line of demarcation about the perimeter. It has the typical signs of inflammation and is quite painful. A peau d'orange appearance can be seen from the skin edema. Lymphadenitis and lymphangitis may be observed. The patients will usually demonstrate a systemic toxemia from the infection, although blood cultures are not dependably positive for diagnosis. In advanced cases, blistering and bullae will be observed in the central areas of the infection.

Antibiotic therapy alone is the treatment for erysipelas. Penicillin, clindamycin, or even quinolones have been used for treatment. Severe infections or those occurring with compromised hosts may require hospitalization and parenteral therapy.

Pyogenic SSSTIs

Pyogenic infections of the skin and skin structures cover a broad collection of different infections. Impetigo, furuncles, and carbuncles are the various terms employed to cover the array of differently presenting infections that have the common feature of being abscesses involving the skin structures. They have the common denominator of having *Staph. aureus* as the most frequent pathogen.

Impetigo is the skin infection of children that arises from non-follicular, small abscess collections of the skin. The disease begins as cutaneous blisters which suppurate, drain, and form cutaneous crusts. The infections are commonly cause by staphylococci, but may be secondary to *Strep. pyogenes*. Effective treatment for many cases is to cleanse the skin and remove crusts, and then use topical antibiotics (e.g., bacitracin). More extensive disease is treated with systemic antibiotics that cover staphylococci. CA-MRSA has been implicated and may need coverage based on clinical suspicion.

The more common pyogenic infection of the skin begins in the hair follicle due to stasis of sebum and microbial proliferation. This is usually *Staph. aureus*. These infections are commonly referred to as boils or furuncles. Local inflammation and edema may result in the occlusion of adjacent follicular units, and a carbuncle is the result of multiple confluent furuncles. Regardless of nomenclature, these cutaneous abscesses can reach several centimeters in diameter. The diagnosis is purely a clinical one with a fluctuant central area, apparent pus beneath the intact epidermis, and a perimeter of induration and erythema. Spontaneous drainage may have already begun at the time of presentation.

Drainage of the abscess is the treatment. In most cases, this will be sufficient (Rajendran et al. 2007). Anti-staphylococcal antibiotic therapy is reserved for only the most severe infections when the pathogen is MSSA. The prevalence of CA-MRSA now makes cultures necessary, and antibiotic therapy is unavoidable in this circumstance. The cutaneous lesions of CA-MRSA infection are commonly associated with a black eschar which may have limited or no suppuration, and is commonly reported by patients to be an insect bite. Treatment is with trimethoprim–sulfamethoxazole or clindamycin. Severe CA-MRSA cutaneous infections may require hospitalization and vancomycin treatment.

Other variations on this theme may be the inoculation of the skin and adjacent soft tissues from scrapes, puncture wounds, or even infected bites. Infections from wounds or self-administration of drugs are likewise seen. These pyogenic infections will have characteristics that are shared with furunculosis but may have an extensive associated degree of cellulitis, lymphadenitis, and lymphangitis. The treatment remains local drainage and antibiotic therapy for most cases. CA-MRSA infections are common in these infections and cultures are necessary. Unusual clinical circumstances such as farm-associated soft-tissue injuries will have Gram-negative and even anaerobic pathogens involved in the soft-tissue infection. Cultures are essential with unusual mechanisms of injury.

Human and animal bite infections

Animal bites are common events and are a potential source of infections of the extremity (Talan et al. 1999). Acute wounds are best handled by local cleansing and irrigation. Continued cleansing and occlusive dressings are employed to avoid secondary contamination, and perhaps topical antibiotic ointment may be of value. A single parenteral antibiotic dose at the time of presentation and injury management makes practical sense. However, sustained systemic antibiotics for post-injury prophylaxis have not worked in any other clinical setting of surgical or traumatic injury of the soft tissues and are not likely to be of any benefit in this circumstance (Medeiros and Saconato 2001).

When patients present with established infection after animal bites, the same principles of local debridement and drainage apply as would be uses for any other soft-tissue infection. Dog and cat bites are associated with *Pasteurella* spp. infection, but are identified with multiple other pathogens. *Staph. aureus*, and *Bacteroides*, *Fusobacterium*, *Capnocytophaga*, and *Porphyromonas* spp. are also recognized pathogens. Treatment for these infections should be with oral amoxicillin–clavulanate. Patients with β-lactam allergy may receive doxycycline, trimethoprim–sulfamethoxazole, or a combination of a fluoroquinolone and clindamycin. Severe infections requiring hospitalization may need intravenous cefoxitin, ampicillin–sulbactam, or even a carbapenem to effectively cover all pathogens.

A related infection from domestic animals is cat-scratch infection. The pathogen is a *Bartonella* spp., usually *B. henselae*. Infections are identified from 3 days to 4 weeks after injury. Culture documentation of the pathogen is difficult and frequently assumed to be present with a suggestive clinical history. Four weeks of oral therapy is recommended with azithromycin (Bass et al. 1999).

Human bites or hand lacerations from tooth injuries during fist-fights pose another unique microbial challenge (Talan et al. 2003). Streptococci, *Staph. aureus*, and *Eikenella corrodens* are the most common pathogens. *Fusobacterium*, *Peptostreptococcus*, *Provotella*, and *Porphyromonas* spp. are also seen. Oral antibiotic therapy for established infection is with amoxicillin–clavulanate. Inpatient treatment with cefoxitin or ampicillin–sulbactam is recommended.

Hydradenitis suppurativa

Hydradenitis suppurative (HS) is a chronic bacterial and inflammatory disease of the apocrine sweat glands (Jemec 2012). The apocrine sweat glands drain into the pilosebaceous unit, as opposed to the more common eccrine sweat glands which open independently on to the skin. The apocrine glands occur in selected areas, especially in the axilla, perineum, and pubic areas, and about the areola of the breast. The apocrine glands are in a deeper location within the skin structure than eccrine glands. Occlusion of the drainage system of the apocrine sweat gland leads to stasis, microbial proliferation within the gland–follicle complex, and a local inflammatory response. Local infection

and abscess are the result. The process can be viewed as similar to that of facial acne, except that the sebaceous glands of the face do not have the apocrine sweat gland apparatus. Acne also has a typical pathogen of *Propionibacterium acres* as an inciting pathogen, which is also different from HS. HS seldom occurs before adolescence and occurs most commonly over the ages 25–40. It is more common in women. It has been clinically associated with obesity, tobacco use, and tropical climates. It affects 1% of adults.

Pathogens associated with HS have been *Staph. aureus*, non-group A streptococci, and an array of Gram-negative rods. Pathogens are commonly Gram-positive skin colonists in the axilla and Gram negatives in the groin, perianal region, and perineum. Repeated courses of antibiotics may change the identified pathogen over time. Although infectious pathogens are associated with the disease, many feel that the disease represents a functional impairment of the epithelial cells of the pilosebaceous unit which leads to the abnormal sinus tracts of the illness (Kurokawa et al. 2002).

Tissue damage and local scarring result in fibrotic occlusion to apocrine and sebaceous glandular products, which in turn results in chronic recurrent infections and soft-tissue disfigurement. Sinus tracts develop as alternative drainage passages for glandular secretions that have normal egress routes obstructed. Sinus and fistula tracts develop between adjacent glands and lead to the large fibrous abscesses that are seen in advanced disease. The spectrum of HS can be mild and effectively managed medically whereas advanced diseased with matted clusters of interdigitated abscesses, sinus tracts, and chronic drainage require the surgical option.

The diagnosis of HS is made by recognition of the typical physical findings. Typically there is a delay in patient presentation so initial assessment may not reflect the duration of disease. Inflammatory intradermal lesions are palpable and occur in clusters. They have variable tenderness and may be only a few millimeters to several centimeters in diameter. The inflammatory lesions are cutaneous abscesses that are in variable states of evolution and eventually suppurate and drain. Fluctuance is not common because of the chronic fibrosis and loss of tissue elasticity that occur in the skin and adjacent subcutaneous fat. The lesions become chronic with periodic exacerbations from acute infection.

As the HS occurs across a continuum of mild to extremely severe disease, treatment needs to be individualized for each patient. Sitz baths, heating pads, maintenance of a dry local environment, avoidance of tight-fitting clothing, and antibiotic therapy are components of medical management. Antibiotic therapy commonly consists of tetracycline, clindamycin, or a combination of clindamycin with rifampin (Jemec 2012). Tobacco cessation and weight reduction are recommended. Local incision and drainage of individual abscesses are commonly employed, but recurrent local infection is then generally observed.

Other treatments have been employed. Intralesional injection of steroids, systemic isotretinoin, and anti-androgenic therapies has been used. Laser treatments and even external beam radiation have also been used. Recent trials have examined anti-tumor necrosis factor, monoclonal antibody treatments with mixed results.

Surgical management is the option for advanced disease and is usually chosen when disease is far advanced and patients are fatigued from sustained and poorly successful conservative measures. Adequate excision of all affected tissues is essential. Retained, diseased glands will result in recurrence. Wound management is problematic. Primary closure with split-thickness skin grafts is commonly used. Flap closures are used for large tissue defects. Staged procedures have been used when extensive excisions are required and chronic suppuration is present. The role of negative pressure dressings is not well defined for these cases, but may have a role in preparation of the excised wound for subsequent closure.

NECROTIZING SOFT-TISSUE INFECTION

SSSTIs infrequently evolve in rapid order into a life-threatening necrotizing soft-tissue infection (NSTI). NSTI occurs when either the infection in a conventional SSSTI progresses vertically toward the investing muscle fascia, or the injury itself penetrates to the level of fascia, or through the fascia, and carries contaminants into deep tissues. Areas of skin with shallow subcutaneous tissues (olecranon or patellar surfaces) can be especially vulnerable to vertical extension of infection to the fascial level. Established infection at the level of the perifascial space (see Figure 5.1) progresses laterally in a rapid fashion. The relative avascularity of the perifascial space and the minimal perfusion of the overlying fat tissue and underlying collagen of the fascia permit rapid progression of the infection. When injury violates the muscle fascia, infection within and over the surface of the muscle may similarly extend in a lateral direction. Usually either necrotic muscle from the initial injury, or hematoma, or introduced foreign bodies are present to allow the initiation of the infectious event. Toxin-producing pathogens such as *Clostridium perfringens* or *Strep. pyogenes* are cytotoxic and result in direct tissue necrosis or thromboses of the microcirculation. Dead muscle tissue becomes the nutrient resource for sustained microbial replication, additional toxin production, and extended necrosis. The extension of infection above the fascia results in thrombosis of the perforating nutrient blood vessels to the overlying skin and subcutaneous tissues. The progression of infection is far greater than the physical evidence indicates on observation. With deep myofasciitis, muscle necrosis may be extensive and the patient will manifest extreme toxemia from the systemic inflammatory response syndrome but not have dramatic external visual evidence of NSTI.

The characteristic finding of the NSTI patient is *pain and tenderness that is out of proportion to the inciting injury*. Minor cuts, punctures, abrasions, or burns that result in severe complaints of pain in a wider perimeter (5–10 cm) about the injury, and similarly have palpable tenderness within this described perimeter, must be considered as being NSTI. In patients with a relatively shallow depth of subcutaneous tissue and an infection superficial to the investing muscle fascia, there will be induration that is palpable, and the discriminating examiner may even be about to palpate the leading edge of the advancing induration. However, if the infection is beneath the fascia, then induration cannot be appreciated. Severe pain with passive movements will be evidence of muscle necrosis, which will evolve into signs of extremity compartment syndrome. Soft-tissue crepitus leads to the diagnosis of 'gas gangrene.' Soft-tissue crepitus is often associated with *C. perfringens*, but may exist with streptococcal NSTI and even with infections where aerobic Gram negatives or obligate anaerobes are present. Conventional radiographs of the soft tissue may demonstrate the presence of air, and computed tomography (CT) or magnetic resonance imaging (MRI) may identify evidence of severe edema within the muscle. The most critical issue in the diagnosis of NSTI is that the clinician has a high index of suspicion. Exaggerated clinical symptoms within 24–48 h of an apparently minor wound must stimulate thoughts of NSTI.

NSTIs are associated with common risk factors (**Box 5.1**). Any comorbid condition that is associated with reduced perfusion or

Box 5.1 Risk factors for necrotizing soft tissue

Infection
Diabetes
Age >65 years
Alcoholism/Cirrhosis
Cardiac disease
Chronic lung disease
Cancer diagnosis
Chronic renal failure
Intravenous drug abuse
Postoperative status
HIV disease
Chronic corticosteroid therapy
Clinical immunosuppression
APACHE score ≥15
Pre-existent shock or sepsis

reduced oxygen delivery to tissues will be associated with NSTIs after skin or soft-tissue injury (Mills et al. 2010, Huang et al. 2011, Tunovic et al. 2012). Congestive heart failure, chronic lung disease, and peripheral vascular disease are the most notable associations. Other chronic diseases of renal failure, liver failure, and HIV infections are associated conditions. Diabetes and obesity are identified as risks in virtually every published series of NSTI cases. Corticosteroid treatment is noted for both an association with NSTI, but also with delayed symptoms in the evaluation of the disease. Nevertheless, 30% or more of NSTIs appears in patients without apparent immunocompromise or predisposing risk factors, and likely reflect pathogens of unusual virulence characteristics.

The microbiology of NSTIs has high variability between reports. In a report consistent with this author's experience, polymicrobial infections were 2.5 times more common than monomicrobial infection (Bernal et al. 2012). However, another recent report from a geographically different area of the USA demonstrated a nearly equal frequency of polymicrobial to monomicrobial infection (Kao et al. 2011). As a general rule, monomicrobial infections seem to complicate lesser injuries to the skin and soft tissues, whereas polymicrobial infections are more commonly seen after major tissue injuries and at the surgical site of major operations. Mortality rates of monomicrobial infections appear to be higher with clostridial myonecrosis at >50%, streptococcal at 20–30%, and polymicrobial infections in the 10% range (Das et al. 2011, Tunovic et al. 2012). An effort to aggregate all reported series of necrotizing fasciitis over nearly 30 years has identified a 24% overall mortality rate (May et al. 2009). As discussed, mortality rates for general description of any one subgroup of NSTIs are very difficult because each case has a unique risk and microbiology that make generalizations very difficult (McHenry et al. 1995).

Regardless of risk factors, microbiology and other issues in care, it is essential that debridement must remove all necrotic tissues and those perimeter tissues that have striking evidence of invasive infection (Wong et al. 2008). The surgical field should have clearly viable and bleeding tissues at the time of completion. Efforts to save marginally viable tissue or those that may appear viable but have evidence of induration and erythema will result only in major necrotic tissues on subsequent debridements. Patients should be returned for daily debridements until a completely viable wound has been identified.

Clostridial NSTIs

Clostridial myonecrosis is the least common but most deadly of the NSTIs. It is commonly associated with *C. perfringens* as the responsible pathogen, although *C. septicum*, *C. sordellii*, and other clostridia have been identified with NSTIs (Stevens et al. 2012). The wounding process can lead to clostridial NSTIs when the wounding device is laden with clostridial spores. Clostridial spore colonization of human skin is a very unlikely source to lead to this clinical infection. Local tissue necrosis and/or hematoma provides the substrate and environment for the obligate anaerobe to transform into the vegetative state from the spores. Exotoxins result in necrosis of adjacent muscle tissue, microbial replication in invasion of the dead (and very anaerobic) muscle, and microbial replication produces additional toxin. Fatal infection can evolve within 24 h of injury because the toxic products of inflammatory cytokines, necrotic tissue, and the systemic distribution of clostridial toxins generate a profound clinical syndrome of systemic inflammatory response syndrome (SIRS) and septic shock.

Among clostridial SSSTIs, an occasional infection will be seen that is confined to the skin and subcutaneous fat and is superficial to the muscle fascia. These infections are far less virulent than those characterized by myonecrosis. These lesser infections result when spore contamination is confined to the subcutaneous fat, and associated hematoma/non-viable tissues are superficial to the muscle fascia. Subsequent toxin production does not have the same pathological consequences in adipose tissue as is seen in muscle. These superficial "clostridial cellulitis" infections will usually have more common clinical evidence of cutaneous erythema and induration than is seen with the true myonecrosis infection. Palpable crepitus is usually present and therapeutic intervention is far more easily achieved. The patients exhibit a far less severe picture of systemic inflammation. As infection within the subcutaneous tissue commonly accompanies the more severe myonecrosis, only exploration of the area will clearly define the limits of the infection.

When the clinical criteria of pain and tenderness are present about the injury site, timely clinical intervention is essential. Streptococcal myonecrosis has a clinical picture that is very similar to clostridial NSTIs and, in the immunosuppressed host, other pathogens can mimic the clostridial infection syndrome. When NSTI is present, preoperative definition of the specific organism is not as important as surgical debridement.

Typical findings of clostridial myonecrosis are important to recognize but all are seldom present. Palpable crepitus is commonly present. Drainage at the site of injury will often have the "dish water" appearance of an anaerobic infection. Leukocytosis or leukopenia may be present with white cell counts being very high or very low, leukopenia of <2000/mm³ being a poor prognostic finding. Laboratory evidence of an increased serum creatinine and elevated hepatic enzymes is a common finding. Respiratory failure and coagulopathy emerge rapidly. Cultures of the drainage, excised tissue, and blood will usually demonstrate clostridial bacteremia, but results will not be available until after the patient's fate has been dictated by therapeutic intervention. The identification of Gram-positive rods by the Gram stain of wound drainage provides ample evidence to identify this organism prospectively (**Figure 5.2**).

The treatment for clostridial NSTIs is prompt and aggressive debridement of necrotic tissues. Black muscle is completely excised as is the overlying dead fascia. Muscle that does not bleed or contract is presumed to be dead and debrided. Overlying skin and subcutaneous tissue may or may not be viable, and excision of these superficial tissues requires clinical judgment. In this author's judgment,

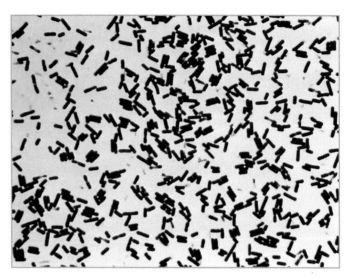

Figure 5.2   A photomicrograph of Clostridium perfringens, 1000 x magnification. (From the Public Health Image Library, Centers for Disease Control – courtesy of CDC/Don Stalons.)

successful initial intervention (defined as patient survival for 24 h) requires reoperation within 24 h for re-debridement and cleansing of fibrinous debris. Re-debridement in the operating room every 24 h is necessary until all tissue is identified as viable at reoperation.

Systemic antibiotics will not manage the infection that is established in dead tissue and has not been successfully debrided. However, aggressive systemic antibiotics may slow the advance of the pathogens into uninfected tissues and hopefully provides some benefit for the attendant clostridial bacteremia of these cases (**Table 5.3**). High-dose intravenous benzylpenicillin (24 MU/24 h) and clindamycin (1200–1500 mg/8 h) are the antibiotic combination of choice. *C. perfringens* and the other clostridia are sensitive to the cell wall activity of penicillin, and clindamycin as a protein synthesis inhibitor is considered effective in the inhibition of toxin production.

An important aspect of care for these patients is the use of aggressive support measures. The patients all have an expanded volume of distribution and sequestered extracellular water in systemic edema. Intravascular volume expansion with crystalloid solutions (e.g., lactated Ringer solution) is important, and the hemolytic and blood loss consequences of the disease and its management may require red blood cell replacement. Colloidal solutions are ordinarily withheld until there is evidence that "third spacing" of fluids has stopped. As coagulopathy is a usual accompaniment to clostridial NSTI, coagulation factors may be necessary even during the hyperacute phases of management. Supportive management of cardiac output (catecholamines), renal output (volume support), and systemic oxygenation (ventilator support) is essential for patient survival.

Hyperbaric oxygenation has been proposed and advocated for the treatment of clostridial NSTIs (Kaide and Khandelwal 2008). Thorough oxygenation of all tissues will presumably kill or retard the advance of this aggressive NSTI. Despite testimonial evidence, studies of hyperbaric oxygen have many shortcomings, not the least of which is that control patients have not received increased oxygen delivery under normobaric conditions (Fry 2005). Dead tissue remains dead tissue and it is unlikely that hyperbaric oxygen reaches or has therapeutic effect within dead necrotic muscle. Hyperbaric oxygen has severe vasoconstrictive effects, and will result in increased ventricular afterload for the patient with tenuous cardiac reserve. Finally, the

Table 5.3 The antibiotic choices, doses, and rationale for each of the pathogens of necrotizing soft tissue infection.

Target pathogen	Antibiotic choice	Rationale
Clostridium myonecrosis	Penicillin 2 MU every 2 h; clindamycin 1200–1500 mg every 6–8 h. If penicillin allergic, use vancomycin 30 mg/kg daily in two doses	Aggressive dosing necessary because of the expanded volume of distribution identified with the systemic inflammatory response of these patients. Clindamycin reduces toxin production
Streptococcus pyogenes	Penicillin 2 MU every 2 h; clindamycin 1200–1500 mg every 6–8 h. If penicillin allergic, use vancomycin 30 mg/kg daily in two doses	Aggressive dosing necessary because of the expanded volume of distribution identified with the systemic inflammatory response of these patients. Clindamycin reduces toxin production
Meticillin-sensitive *Staphylococcus aureus* (MSSA)	Nafcillin 1–2 g every 4 h or cefazolin 1–2 g every 6–8 h	Aggressive dosing is recommended because of the expanded volume of distribution seen in these patients. Dosing should be de-escalated once the systemic inflammatory response is improving
Meticillin-resistant *Staphylococcus aureus* (MRSA)	Vancomycin 30 mg/kg per day in two doses; or linezolid 600 mg every 12 h, or daptomycin 6 mg/kg daily	Presumptive coverage of MRSA is employed if sensitivities are not known and then de-escalated if MSSA.
Polymicrobial infection: Use all three if cultures are not available		
Gram-positive coverage	Vancomycin 30 mg/kg per day in two doses; or linezolid 600 mg every 12 h, or daptomycin 6 mg/kg daily	Presumptive coverage of MRSA is employed if sensitivities are not known and then de-escalated if MSSA
Gram-negative coverage	Piperacillin/Tazobactam 3.375–4.5 g every 6 h; or imipenem 1 g every 8 h; or meropenem 1 g every 8 h	Treatment will need modification after culture and sensitivity results are available
Anaerobic coverage	Clindamycin 1200–1500 mg every 6–8 h	This is the preferred choice because of anaerobic coverage, but because of toxic inhibition if Gram positives are present

hyperbaric chamber becomes logistically problematic for the patient on ventilator support. Hyperbaric oxygen remains of controversial value, and requires more evidence to support its routine use.

Other therapies have been proposed for *C. perfringens* infections. Some consideration has been given to a vaccine not unlike the one that has been successfully used for the prevention of tetanus infection (Titball 2009). Efforts at vaccine development have been unsuccessful. The scope of an immunization program cannot be justified when considering the infrequency of this infection. Immunoglobulin for neutralization of the cytotoxins of clostridia has been considered but has not been successfully employed in patient care.

Finally, some special consideration should be given to clinical circumstances that are unique to *C. septicum* and *C. sordellii* infections (Stevens et al. 2012). *C. septicum* bacteremia and NSTIs have been identified without any physical injury present at the site of the infection. These *C. septicum* metastatic infections are associated with colon cancers, diverticulitis, and other pathological circumstances in the gastrointestinal tract. Spontaneous myonecrosis should be a consideration in patients that develop acute and painful soft-tissue illnesses with systemic toxemia, but no injury at the location. Those patients fortunate enough to survive these *C. septicum* infections need to have a gastrointestinal evaluation to define the source of the bacteria. Similarly, one may see a metastatic myonecrosis infection in association with severe myometrial infection after medical or self-induced interruption of pregnancy with infections due to *C. sordellii*.

Streptococcal NSTIs

Strep. pyogenes is a common pathogen for soft-tissue infections after relatively minor skin injuries. Most pursue an indolent course and require minimal or no treatment. A very select minority of these infections result in streptococcal NSTIs, which may be the result of rapidly invasive infection within the perifascial space and cause necrosis of the skin and subcutaneous tissues, but leave the muscle fascia and underlying muscle viable. When the wounding process violates the fascia, a rapidly advancing myonecrosis can be seen that has visual features in common with the clostridial myonecrosis described earlier. Whether the infection is within the perifascial space or in the muscle itself, the progression of the infection is rapid and requires prompt recognition by the clinician if intervention is to be effective.

Any breech or injury to the epidermis has the potential to result in streptococcal NSTIs. "Paper cuts" of the finger and tangential abrasions of the skin at any site can yield streptococcal NSTIs. Scratching of pruritic chickenpox vesicles by children, with presumed streptococci from the mouth, have been associated with streptococcal NSTIs (Waldhausen et al. 1996). Inguinal hernia incisions (Sistla et al. 2011) and trochar sites from laparoscopic procedures have also been seen (Bharathan and Hanson 2010). Anatomically, streptococcal NSTIs occur most commonly on the extremities and the truck. Similar to all NSTIs, they occur least frequently in the head–neck areas, although these latter infections are often spectacular in severity and appearance, and are reported in the literature. Why most SSSTIs due to streptococci prove to be innocuous, and selected others become life-threatening NSTIs remains an unanswered question. The answer lies in either the impaired effective of the host, or the random encounter of an unusually virulent strain of *Strep. pyogenes*.

Streptococcal NSTIs can occur via metastatic seeding of an injury site from a remote source. Soft-tissue contusions, subcutaneous or muscle hematomas, and chronic joint effusions can all be receptive sites for blood-borne seeding and NSTIs without any disruption of the skin over the site of the acute or chronic injury. Remote sites of innocent cellulitis or even asymptomatic pharyngeal colonization is thought to result in hematogenous seeding of a distant location. This author has witnessed metastatic NSTIs when the patient has presented with infection at one site, only to develop metastatic streptococcal infection at a distant infiltrated intravenous catheter location.

Streptococcal NSTIs can be a difficult diagnosis to appreciate in the early phases, and are commonly not recognized by inexperienced clinicians. The characteristic rule of NSTIs is pain and tenderness out of proportion to the inciting injury, and never is that rule more valid than when *Strep. pyogenes* is the putative pathogen. When an NSTI is superficial to the muscle fascia, a rapidly developing cellulitis is seen in the skin. Commonly, bullae and sloughing of skin will be seen at the wound site, although not within the first few hours of the infection. Clinical evidence of lymphadenitis or lymphangitis may be present with extremity infections. The cellulitis changes can be observed to advance several centimeters within a 30- to 60-min period of time. Nevertheless, the extent of the advancing cellulitis underestimates the progression of the infection at the perifascial level. With streptococcal myonecrosis, the overt findings of cellulitis, bullae, and sloughing are absent until late in the progression of the infection. Only with the rapid advance of pain, tenderness, and SIRS will the diagnosis be made. Crepitus may be present in a minority of cases. Dramatic leukocytosis in the early phases of streptococcal NSTI evolves into leukopenia as the infection progresses. Pulmonary, renal, and hepatic failure evolves quickly. Coagulopathy is usually present and may lead to disseminated intravascular coagulation. Cultures of infected tissues and blood are almost always positive but results will not be available in a clinically relevant period of time. The Gram stain of the drainage at the injury site will often identify Gram-positive cocci in chains (**Figure 5.3**).

Similar to clostridial NSTIs, streptococcal NSTIs are a clinical diagnosis that requires prompt surgical intervention. Debridement of the infection must be liberal and aggressive. The subcutaneous fat will be necrotic and the perifascial space will weep with a tan-colored, thin-consistency, exudative fluid. The exudate lacks a purulent character except at the area adjacent to the site of injury. It has been this author's experience that the skin and subcutaneous tissue will need to be excised in all areas above the extent of the tan exudate and induration of the fascial layer. When myonecrosis is present then all obviously dead, non-contracting, and non-bleeding muscle is excised. Debridement must proceed with the full understanding that the

patient's life depends on the effectiveness of the surgical intervention. The effort to conserve tissue in the interest of future reconstruction is a risky proposition. The patient is returned to the operating room for additional wound inspection every 24 h until no necrotic tissue is identified. Clinical deterioration after debridement may necessitate an earlier return to the operating room for additional debridement.

Extremity streptococcal NSTIs are the site of infection in over 50% of these cases, and they invariably result in questions about the necessity of amputation. When infection involves only the skin and subcutaneous tissue of the extremity, then the extremity can be salvaged. When muscle groups of the leg or arm are necrotic, then amputation is necessary. In questionable cases, the issue of amputation may or may not be resolved until the second or third reoperation.

The combination of high-dose benzylpenicillin and clindamycin is the antibiotic of choice in doses similar to those used for clostridial NSTIs (see Table 5.3). Streptococci are very sensitive to benzylpenicillin, but rapidly multiplying streptococci will demonstrate the "Eagle effect" (Eagle 1949). High density of streptococci in tissue as are seen in NSTI will be less influenced by antibiotics and may have reduced expression of penicillin-binding proteins among rapidly dividing bacterial cells. The addition of clindamycin reduces the rapidity of replication and reduces toxin production (Bisno and Stevens 1996). With penicillin-allergic patients, clindamycin remains the choice and a second drug (e.g., vancomycin or quinolone) may be added. The systemic edema of the streptococcal NSTI patient is extensive and generalized and requires aggressive dosing to achieve therapeutic effect.

Supportive care of the streptococcal NSTI patient is vitally important. Many of these patients demonstrate a toxic shock-like syndrome, which is felt to be secondary to the production of superantigens by the pathogen (see Chapter 1; Stevens 1995). Volume support is essential during the acute phase of the infection, and catecholamine support for maintenance of the systemic circulation is commonly needed. Resolution of elevated creatinine levels and increased concentrations of liver enzymes reflect clinical resolution of the infection. Prolonged ventilatory support may be required for many days after clinical resolution of the infection and for many days after antibiotic therapy has been discontinued. Nosocomial pneumonia becomes a risk from hospital-acquired bacteria for the NSTI patient that requires prolonged ventilator support.

Similar to clostridial NSTI, the use of intravenous immunoglobulin and hyperbaric oxygen has been proposed for the treatment of streptococcal NSTIs. Some evidence supports the use of immunoglobulin for severe streptococcal infections (Darenberg et al. 2003), especially when administered early in the natural history of the infection. Additional studies are needed for the evaluation of intravenous immunoglobulin. Similar to clostridial NSTI, there is little objective evidence to support the use of hyperbaric oxygen with streptococcal infection.

The overall outcome for patients with streptococcal NSTIs remains, with an overall mortality rate in the range of 25% (Davies et al. 1996). No one institution has a large experience and this 25% figure is certainly an estimate. The morbidity of the disease involves reconstruction and rehabilitation for the major loss of tissue that is necessary to achieve survival for these patients. Improved public awareness and physician recognition of the disease are necessary for improvement in clinical outcomes.

■ Staphylococcal NSTIs

Traditionally, *Staph. aureus* has been a common pathogen of pyogenic bacterial infections of the skin and soft tissues but an

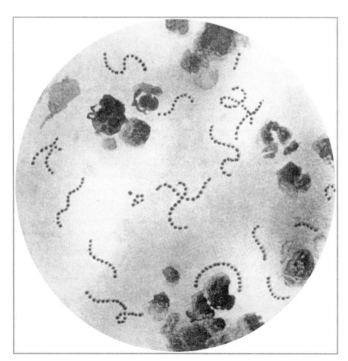

Figure 5.3 A photomicrograph of Streptococcus pyogenes, 900 x magnification. (From the Public Health Image Library, Centers for Disease Control – courtesy of CDC.)

infrequent pathogen of NSTIs. Even when infection occurs in the perifascial space or muscle, the coagulase-positive *Staph. aureus* infection has been largely of a pyogenic character and not the rapidly expanding infection of NSTIs. The presence of the Panton–Valentine leukocidin and other virulence characteristics of CA-MRSA have changed the behavior of staphylococci, and NSTIs have become a more frequent event (Miller et al. 2005). Since the major publication by Miller et al., the numbers of individual cases and small series that have identified staphylococcal NSTIs have escalated at a very rapid rate. Staphylococcal NSTIs are usually seen in patients with major medical comorbidities such as diabetes, hepatitis C, intravenous drug abuse, and HIV infection. Similar to streptococcal NSTIs, all anatomic areas appear to be vulnerable to this aggressive staphylococcal infection. Unlike streptococcal infection, the staphylococcal infection has a lower mortality rate but typically a very high morbidity rate.

Staphylococcal NSTIs usually evolve from conventional SSSTIs. The unattended pyogenic infection may become vertically invasive into the subcutaneous fat, where the perifascial plane is entered and lateral progression of the infection proceeds. The primary infection site will have a pyogenic character but may exhibit only the black eschar that is commonly associated with CA-MRSA. An advancing cellulitis is identified emanating from the epicenter of the infection, but it does not characteristically have the rapidly spreading cellulitis seen in streptococcal NSTIs. The cellulitis adjacent to the area of the wound and eschar may not blanch, reflecting thrombosis of the intradermal vasculature secondary to the effects of coagulase. The induration of the soft tissues to physical examination is more pronounced than streptococcal infection. The progression of staphylococcal NSTIs can still be clinically rapid, but not in the same order of magnitude seen with streptococcal or clostridial NSTIs. Similar to streptococcal NSTIs, staphylococci have been identified with metastatic seeding to injured soft-tissue sites without an open injury to the soft tissue (Kim et al. 2010).

An important NSTI with staphylococci is seen in the diabetic fetid foot infection. These infections begin with ulceration of toes and the plantar surface of the feet in patients with diabetes and advanced neuropathy and peripheral vascular disease. The chronic neuropathic and ischemic tissue, combined with the effects of hyperglycemia, results in repeated infections in these chronic ulcers. Infection in the diabetic foot ulcer has been demonstrated initially to be with *Staph. aureus* and the persistence of this infection, which burrows into the several soft-tissue planes of the foot, is an indolent variation of a necrotizing infection. These patients undergo repeated hospitalizations and multiple courses of antibiotics. Ultimately the infection becomes polymicrobial with Gram-negative and even anaerobic bacteria. MRSA is commonly a continued participant in this polymicrobial infection. Ascending infection in the lower extremity results in severe and aggressive local necrosis, cellulitis, lymphadenitis, and lymphangitis. Amputation is a common outcome when distal ulcers, infection, and the diabetes itself are neglected.

With staphylococcal NSTIs, establishing a bacterial diagnosis is important. The clinical presentation is highly variable and these NSTIs can mimic streptococcal infections at times and appear much like the polymicrobial NSTIs discussed below. The Gram stain of the exudates will commonly be of value in the identification of the grape-like clusters of Gram-positive cocci (**Figure 5.4**). Blood cultures are infrequently positive with staphylococcal NSTIs. Cultures of the wound purulence and tissue biopsies will identify the pathogen, but more

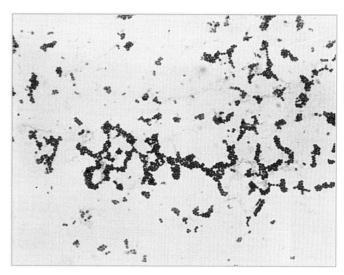

Figure 5.4 A photomicrograph of Staphylococcus aureus, 250 x magnification. (From the Public Health Image Library, Centers for Disease Control – courtesy of CDC/Richard Facklam, PhD; http://phil.cdc.gov/phil/details.asp.)

importantly give the sensitivity patterns of the specific staphylococcal pathogen. MSSA, CA-MRSA, and healthcare-associated MRSA each have unique sensitivities that are important in choosing antimicrobial therapy. In complex infections and in the fetid foot, deep tissue samples are best for yielding dependable culture results. Selected patients will have different levels of sensitivity to vancomycin, which is becoming an increasing problem in the selection of therapy for these patients.

The principles of treating the staphylococcal NSTI are the same as for all of these infections. Adequate local debridement, which results in only viable tissue remaining, is essential. Repeat debridements are often necessary depending on the severity of the infection. Bedside debridement on a daily basis is useful. Eradication of dead tissue is the objective, whether done by repeated debridements under general anesthesia or debridement performed at the bedside. Many topical antibacterial agents have been used to treat these infections at the completion of debridement. Mafenide acetate solution or silver sulfadiazine is preferred.

Systemic antibiotics are important components for the treatment of staphylococcal NSTIs (see Table 5.3). Although MSSA infection may principally respond to drainage and debridement alone, it needs appropriate antibiotic coverage (see Chapter 2). Staphylococcal NSTIs will require inpatient antibiotic therapy and vancomycin remains the drug of choice for most patients. Linezolid as an inhibitor of protein synthesis may offer the advantages of suppressing toxic production by these organisms. Oral agents may be used in selected patients and trimethoprim–sulfamethoxazole or clindamycin may be chosen for CA-MRSA infections that are sensitive. Antibiotics are continued until local evidence of inflammation has resolved and granulation tissue is identified in the wound. Because of risks from the complication of bacterial endocarditis, systemic drug therapy may be continued for up to 4 weeks in those patients with bacteremia during the infection.

As with other pathogens of NSTIs, interest in staphylococcal vaccines and antibody treatments focused on specific virulence factors (e.g., PVL) is under study. The constantly changing antigenic and virulence factors of *Staph. aureus* make successful immune-based therapies a worthy but difficult goal (Proctor 2012).

Polymicrobial NSTIs

Over 50% of NSTIs are polymicrobial infections, and may include any combination of Gram-positive, Gram-negative, or anaerobic pathogens. Polymicrobial NSTIs are most frequently seen in major soft-tissue traumatic injuries and at surgical sites where massive contamination or active infection has been encountered. The scenario with large traumatic wounds includes devitalized tissue, foreign bodies, soft-tissue hematoma, and varying degrees of microbial contamination from the injury. Invasive polymicrobial NSTIs commonly follow when the acute debridement of the injury site has been suboptimal, or the magnitude of the contamination makes infection a probable outcome. The celiotomy incision for trauma surgery or an acute perforated viscus results in the surgical site being subjected to a large inoculum of microbes, which reflect the character of the viscus that was disrupted. Colon disruptions are most notable in this regard because of the large inocula of colonic microflora that contaminate the surgical site.

The pathogens that have been identified in polymicrobial NSTIs are detailed in **Table 5.4**. This list is certainly incomplete because virtually every human pathogen has been reported as part of these infections. Meleney's gangrene was one of the originally reported polymicrobial NSTIs and consisted of staphylococci and anaerobic streptococci. NSTIs after colon disruption are commonly Gram-negative rods (e.g., *Escherichia coli*) and colonic anaerobes (e.g., *Bacteroides fragilis*). Four or more pathogens may be recovered from the infection before specific antibiotic therapy is begun (Elliott et al. 2000, Ustin and Malangoni 2011). It is likely that anaerobes are under-reported in several reported clinical series because of inefficiency in culturing these organisms. The synergistic relationship between aerobic and anaerobic bacteria likely contributes to the invasive perifascial infection seen in

polymicrobial NSTIs. Among patients with large, open traumatic, or surgical wounds, the duration of hospitalization and influence of systemic antibiotic therapy result in healthcare-associated pathogens such as *Pseudomonas aeruginosa, Staph. epidermidis*, MRSA, *Enterococcus* spp., and *Acinetobacter baumanii* as resultant pathogens in the sustained infection.

Appropriate attention to the acute injury wound and to the celiotomy wound with massive contamination can reduce the frequency and severity of polymicrobial NSTIs. Dead tissue must be debrided, foreign bodies are removed, and hematoma is evacuated. Broad-spectrum preoperative antibiotics are employed for prevention but are likely to be of only limited value in the massively contaminated wound. The traumatic wound requires daily vigilance because continued debridement is usually necessary. Traumatic wounds should not be closed primarily. Similarly, delayed primary closure or secondary closure is the choice for management of the contaminated celiotomy wound. Prevention of desiccation of the large open wound requires frequent dressing changes with saline-moist gauze. Evidence to support any one topical antimicrobial in these wounds is not available. Negative pressure dressings can be useful in preparing large tissue defects for subsequent reconstruction, and for secondary closure of celiotomy wounds.

The diagnosis of polymicrobial NSTI requires a high index of suspicion. Traumatic wounds can be quite complex and invasive infection along lateral fascial planes can escape immediate recognition. Furthermore, the trauma patient or patient with a perforated abdominal viscus has many reasons to have leukocytosis, fever, and evidence of systemic inflammation.

These infections are generally indolent compared with the monomicrobial NSTIs, although the rapidity of advancing infection is highly variable. Careful inspection of the wound, identification of evidence of new cellulitic changes, recognition of new exudates that are expressed from the fascial margins, and pain and tenderness beyond the perimeter of the open wound are all important findings. Crepitus can be seen in polymicrobial NSTIs but cannot be depended on as a reliable finding. Crepitus is often evidence of advanced infection which may have been overlooked earlier. Once the diagnosis of infection has been made, good cultures at the site are essential. The best cultures are actual biopsies of the infected tissues that are promptly submitted to the clinical laboratory.

The treatment of these polymicrobial NSTIs is similar to those infections from other pathogens. Debridement of non-viable tissue is essential and reoperation to re-debride the site of infection is essential. Antibiotic therapy is very broad spectrum because presumptive therapy will need to cover the Gram-positive, Gram-negative, and anaerobic possibilities (see Table 5.3). De-escalation of therapy is important to avoid sustained treatment that is in excess of the patient's needs.

OTHER PATHOGENS

This discussion has focused on the four major bacterial groups that are associated with NSTIs. It must be emphasized that, with a vulnerable host and microbial contamination that reaches the critical area of the perifascial area, literally any human pathogen can be the agent for NSTIs. *Vibrio* spp. after injuries in salt water (Hong et al. 2012), *Aeromonas hydrophila* (Park et al. 2011), *Bacillus cereus* as a seemingly random event (Hutchens et al. 2010), and even fungi (Harada and Lau 2007) have all been implicated in NSTIs. The clinical presentation and the anatomic distribution of these unusual pathogens appear to follow the same pattern as those microbes that are more commonly associated with these infections.

Table 5.4 Pathogens of polymicrobial NSTIs

Aerobic species	Anaerobic species
Gram-positive bacteria	
Staphylococcus aureus	*Bacteroides* spp.
Coagulase-negative staphylococci	*Clostridium* spp.
Enterococcus spp.	*Peptostreptococcus* spp.
Streptococcus pyogenes	*Peptococcus* spp.
Non-group A streptococci	*Corynebacterium* spp.
Gram-negative bacteria	Prevotella spp.
Escherichia coli	*Fusobacterium* spp.
Klebsiella spp.	*Veillonella* spp.
Enterobacter spp.	
Serratia spp.	
Pseudomonas spp.	
Proteus spp.	**Fungi**
Acinetobacter spp.	*Candida* spp.
Aeromonas spp.	*Aspergillus* spp.
Citrobacter spp.	*Mucor* spp.
Vibrio spp.	
Eikenella corrodens	

CONCLUSION

The complexity and the clinical variability of NSTIs appear to be increasing. The number of publications reporting individual or small series of cases is escalating at a rapid rate. Improvement in the overall results of care requires greater public awareness and increased physician sensitivity to the diagnosis of this overall constellation of pathogens and clinical presentations that represent NSTIs. A foundation has been established to help achieve the goals of more public attention to this problem and better care for these patients (National Necrotizing Fasciitis Foundation – www. nnff.org).

REFERENCES

Aly R. Effect of occlusion of microbial population and physical skin conditions. *Semin Dermatol* 1982;**1**:137–42.

Bharathan R, Hanson M. Diagnostic laparoscopy complicated by group A streptococcal necrotizing fasciitis. *J Minim Invasive Gynecol* 2010;**17**:121–3.

Bass JW, Freitas BC, Freitas AD, et al. Prospective randomized double blind placebo-controlled evaluation of azithromycin for treatment of cat-scratch disease. *Pediatr Infect Dis J* 1998;**17**:447–52.

Bisno AL, Stevens DL. Streptococcal infections of skin and soft tissues. *N Engl J Med* 1996;**334**:240–5.

Bernal NP, Latenser BA, Born JM, Liao J. Trends in 393 necrotizing acute soft tissue infection patients 2000–2008. *Burns* 2012;**38**:252–60.

Darenberg J, Ihendyane N, Sjölin J, et al., the Streptig Study Group. Intravenous Immunoglobulin G therapy in streptococcal toxic shock syndrome: a European randomized, double-blind, placebo-controlled trial. *Clin Infect Dis* 2003;**37**:333–40.

Das DK, Baker MG, Venugopal K. Increasing incidence of necrotizing fasciitis in New Zealand: a nationwide study over the period 1990 to 2006. *J Infect* 2011;**63**:429–33.

Davies HD, McGeer A, Schwartz B, et al. Invasive group A streptococcal infection in Ontario, Canada. Ontario Group A streptococcal study group. *New Engl J Med* 1996;**335**:547–54.

Eagle H. The effect of the size of the inoculum and the age of the infection on the curative dose of penicillin in experimental infections with streptococci, pneumococci, and *Treponema pallidum*. *J Exp Med* 1949;**90**:595–607.

Elliott D, Kufera JA, Myers RA:The microbiology of necrotizing soft tissue infections. *Am J Surg* 2000;**179**:361–6.

Frayn KN, Karpe F, Fielding BA, et al. Integrative physiology of human adipose tissue. *Int J Obes Relat Metab Disord* 2003;**27**:875–88.

Fry DE. The story of hyperbaric oxygen continues. *Am J Surg* 2005;**189**:467–8.

Greene JN. The microbiology of colonization, including techniques for assessing and measuring colonization. *Infect Control Hosp Epidemiol* 1996;**17**:114–18.

Gunderson CG, Martinello RA. A systematic review of bacteremias in cellulitis and erysipelas. *J Infect* 2012;**64**:148–55.

Harada AS, Lau W. Successful treatment and limb salvage of mucor necrotizing fasciitis after kidney transplantation with posaconazole. *Hawaii Med J* 2007;**66**:68–71.

Hong GL, Lu CJ, Lu ZQ, et al. Surgical treatment of 19 cases with vibrio necrotising fasciitis. *Burns* 2012;**38**:290–5.

Huang KF, Hung MH, Lin YS, et al. Independent predictors of mortality for necrotizing fasciitis: a retrospective analysis in a single institution. *J Trauma* 2011;**71**:467–73;

Hutchens A, Gupte A, McAuliffe PF, et al. *Bacillus cereus* necrotizing fasciitis in a patient with end-stage liver disease. *Surg Infect (Larchmt)* 2010;**11**:469–74.

Jemec GBE. Hidradenitis suppurativa. *N Engl J Med* 2012;**366**:158–64.

Kaide CG, Khandelwal S. Hyperbaric oxygen: applications in infectious disease. *Emerg Med Clin* North Am 2008;**26**:571–95.

Kao LS, Lew DF, Arab SN, et al. Local variations in the epidemiology, microbiology, and outcomes of necrotizing soft-tissue infections: a multicenter study. *Am J Surg* 2011;**202**:139–45.

Kim HJ, Kim DH, Ko DH. Coagulase-positive staphylococcal necrotizing fasciitis subsequent to shoulder sprain in a healthy woman. *Clin Orthop Surg* 2010;**2**:256–9.

Kurokawa I, Nishijima S, Kusumoto, et al. Immunohistochemical study of cytokeratins in hidradenitis suppurativa (acne inversa). *J Int Med Res* 2002;**30**:131–6.

May AK, Stafford RE, Bulger EM, et al. Treatment of complicated skin and soft tissue infections. *Surg Infect* 2009;**10**:467–99.

McHenry CR, Piotrowski JJ, Petrinic D, Malangoni MA. Determinants of mortality for necrotizing soft-tissue infections. *Ann Surg* 1995;**221**: 558–63.

Medeiros I, Saconato H. Antibiotic prophylaxis for mammalian bites. *Cochrane Database Syst Rev* 2001;CD001738.

Miller LG, Perdreau-Remington F, Rieg G, et al. Necrotizing fasciitis caused by community-associated methicillin-resistant Staphylococcus aureus in Los Angeles. *N Engl J Med* 2005;**352**:1445–53.

Mills MK, Faraklas I, Davis C, et al. Outcomes from treatment of necrotizing soft-tissue infections: results from the National Surgical Quality Improvement Program database. *Am J Surg* 2010;**200**:790–6.

Nobbs AH, Lamont RJ, Jenkinson HF. Streptococcus adherence and colonization. *Microb Mol Biol Rev* 2009;**73**:407–50.

Park SY, Nam HM, Park K, Park SD. *Aeromonas hydrophila* sepsis mimicking *Vibrio vulnificus* infection. *Ann Dermatol* 2011;**23**(suppl 1):S25–9.

Proctor RA. Challenges for a universal *Staphylococcus aureus* vaccine. *Clin Infect Dis* 2012;**54**:1179–86.

Rajendran PM, Young D, Maurer T, et al. Randomized, double-blind, placebo-controlled trial of cephalexin for treatment of uncomplicated skin abscesses in a population at risk for community-acquired methicillin-resistant *Staphylococcus aureus* infection. *Antimicrob Agents Chemther* 2007;**51**:4044–8.

Sistla SC, Sankar G, Sistla S. Fatal necrotizing fasciitis following elective inguinal hernia repair. *Hernia* 2011;**15**:75–7.

Somerville DA. The normal flora of the skin in different age groups. *Br J Dermatol* 1969;**81**:248–58.

Stevens DL. Streptococcal toxic-shock syndrome: spectrum of disease, pathogenesis, and new concepts in treatment. *Emerg Infect Dis* 1995;**1**:69–78.

Stevens DL, Aldape MJ, Bryant AE. Life-threatening clostridial infections. *Anaerobe* 2012;**18**:254–9.

Talan DA, Citron DM, Abrahamian FM, et al. Bacteriologic analysis of infected dog and cat bites. Emergency Medicine Animal Bite Infection Study Group. *N Engl J Med* 1999;**340**: 85–92.

Talan DA, Abrahamian FM, Moran GJ, et al. Clinical presentation and bacteriologic analysis of infected human bites in patients presenting to emergency departments. *Clin Infect Dis* 2003;**37**:1481–9.

Titball RW. Clostridium perfringens vaccines. *Vaccine* 2009;**27** (suppl 4):D44–7.

Tunovic E, Gawaziuk J, Bzura T, et al. Necrotizing fasciitis: a six-year experience. *J Burn Care Res* 2012;**33**:93–100.

Ustin JS, Malangoni MA. Necrotizing soft-tissue infections. *Crit Care Med* 2011;**39**:2156–62.

Waldhausen JH, Holterman MJ, Sawin RS. Surgical implications of necrotizing fasciitis in children with chickenpox. *J Pediatr Surg* 1996;**31**:1138–41.

Wong CH, Yam AK, Tan AB, Song C. Approach to debridement in necrotizing fasciitis. *Am J Surg* 2008;**196**:19–24.

Chapter 6 Intra-abdominal infections

John E. Mazuski

■ INTRODUCTION AND DEFINITIONS

Intra-abdominal infections (IAIs) are common. They arise from a number of different sources. Usually, they are caused by enteric bacteria and other microorganisms normally found within the lumen of a hollow viscus.

These infections can be classified as uncomplicated or complicated. Uncomplicated IAIs are those that do not extend beyond the wall of the hollow viscus, although they are at risk of doing so if left untreated. Acute appendicitis is an example of an uncomplicated IAI. In contrast, complicated IAIs are those in which the infection extends into the peritoneal cavity or another normally sterile area of the abdomen. Thus, perforated appendicitis is an example of a complicated IAI (Marshall 2004, Blot and De Waele 2005, Solomkin et al. 2010).

Management of most complicated IAIs requires an invasive procedure to control the source of the infection. This has sometimes been used as a surrogate definition of a complicated IAI (Solomkin et al. 1992). However, a source control procedure may not be utilized to treat certain localized complicated infections, such as complicated diverticulitis; thus, the definition of a complicated IAI should not be strictly based on this operational criterion.

Many complicated IAIs are characterized by inflammation of the peritoneal cavity, or peritonitis. Others are described as an intra-abdominal abscess, within either the peritoneal cavity or the retroperitoneal tissues, or occasionally as an intra-abdominal phlegmon. Peritonitis itself has been described as primary, secondary, or tertiary.

■ Primary and catheter-related peritonitis

Primary peritonitis is inflammation or infection of the peritoneal cavity that occurs in the absence of overt perforation or leakage from the gastrointestinal tract (Blot and De Waele 2005). In the past, primary peritonitis due to streptococci or pneumococci was relatively common. In the current era, the most common type of primary peritonitis is "spontaneous bacterial peritonitis," which typically occurs in patients with ascites due to hepatic cirrhosis. The microorganisms that most frequently cause this disorder are *Enterobacteriaceae* (Strauss and Caly 2006). It is likely that at least some of these infections occur as a result of translocation of these microorganisms through the wall of the gut into the peritoneal cavity.

Peritonitis associated with devices that access the peritoneal cavity, such as peritoneal dialysis catheters, has become an increasingly common problem. As with primary peritonitis, these infections occur in the absence of any violation of the gastrointestinal tract. Microorganisms colonizing the skin can produce these infections, with the catheter providing a portal of entry into the peritoneal cavity. Thus, staphylococci are frequent causes of this type of peritonitis, although infections due to *Enterobacteriaceae* are also common (Faber and Yee 2006).

Both primary and catheter-associated peritonitis are typically monomicrobial infections. They are treated medically with intravenous antibiotics or, in some cases of catheter-associated peritonitis, with topical antibiotics administered through the device itself. Unless catheter removal is needed, source control is not a major consideration in the treatment of these forms of peritonitis. These disorders are not considered further.

■ Secondary peritonitis

Secondary peritonitis is the IAI most frequently treated surgically. Most cases of secondary peritonitis are polymicrobial, involving a variety of microorganisms normally found within the gastrointestinal tract. Generally, secondary peritonitis is the result of an overt perforation somewhere in the gastrointestinal tract, which allows direct access of contaminants to the peritoneal cavity. However, secondary peritonitis may also occur with ischemia or necrosis of a portion of the intestine. In this case, microorganisms access the peritoneal cavity by invading through the wall of the intestine.

■ Tertiary peritonitis

As opposed to primary and secondary peritonitis, there is no generally accepted definition of tertiary peritonitis. It is often defined as any peritoneal infection observed after initial treatment of secondary peritonitis. However, tertiary peritonitis is described here as a late infection that occurs only after several serial attempts have been made to control an IAI. Typically, tertiary peritonitis is a diffuse, poorly localized process. The microbial agents associated with this disorder tend to be nosocomial organisms, which are more resistant to common antimicrobial agents than those producing secondary peritonitis (Nathens et al. 1998, Buijk and Bruining 2002). Most patients with tertiary peritonitis have significant impairment of host defenses, which allows microorganisms of relatively low pathogenic potential to proliferate and produce the disease process. Tertiary peritonitis is the most lethal type of IAI.

■ Intra-abdominal abscess

Intra-abdominal abscesses are localized collections of fluid containing inflammatory cells and microorganisms. They characteristically occur in dependent areas of the peritoneal cavity such as the pelvis, subphrenic spaces, subhepatic space, right and left paracolic gutters, and lesser sac. Intra-abdominal abscesses may also develop at other sites within the peritoneal cavity, such as between loops of bowel, as well as in the retroperitoneum (Altemeier et al. 1973).

As with secondary peritonitis, most intra-abdominal abscesses originate after perforation of a hollow viscus. An intra-abdominal abscess results from localization of the peritoneal infection by the host over a period of days. The microbiology of secondary peritonitis and intra-abdominal abscess is generally quite similar. Abscesses can also develop in solid organs, such as the liver and spleen, but resulting from hematogenous dissemination of bacteria rather than from intraperitoneal pathogens.

Intra-abdominal phlegmon

An intra-abdominal phlegmon is a frequently described type of IAI, but the entity has been very poorly characterized. In general, an intra-abdominal phlegmon is a solid inflammatory mass that infiltrates into adjacent tissues of the abdominal cavity. Intestinal loops and other structures may become incorporated into this inflammatory mass. Although small collections of fluid may be present within the mass, these do not constitute most of the volume of the mass. This provides some distinction between an intra-abdominal phlegmon and an abscess, but this distinction may be somewhat arbitrary. There are clearly examples in which an intra-abdominal phlegmon evolves into an intra-abdominal abscess over time, although the frequency with which this occurs is unknown.

Similar to an intra-abdominal abscess, an intra-abdominal phlegmon is generally the result of a hollow viscus perforation. However, the result of this is an intense inflammatory and fibrotic reaction, usually confined to a discrete area within the abdominal cavity or retroperitoneum. The reason why a phlegmon rather than an abscess develops in a given patient is unclear.

PATHOPHYSIOLOGY

The pathophysiology of IAIs has been studied using experimental models of peritonitis developing after hollow viscus injury. These experimental data relate to the pathophysiology of secondary peritonitis and intra-abdominal abscess development, and may not necessarily be relevant to the pathophysiology of other types of IAIs, such as postoperative infections.

There is a fairly stereotypical response that follows contamination of the peritoneal cavity with gastrointestinal content from a hollow viscus, which is a reaction to both the chemical irritants and microbiological agents released as a result of the perforation. The various host defense mechanisms invoked serve to limit the spread of these agents and reduce the likelihood of the development of an overt infection.

First, there is rapid mechanical clearance of contaminated fluid from the peritoneal cavity. Fluid within the peritoneal cavity is in constant circulation due to diaphragmatic contraction and relaxation. Contaminated fluid comes into contact with the undersurface of the diaphragm relatively quickly. There, specialized stomata take up that fluid into lymphatic vessels, where it is distributed to larger lymphatics and lymph nodes in the mediastinum. This mechanical clearance results in the rapid removal of a significant portion of extravasated fluid and its associated pathogenic microorganisms.

An inflammatory reaction also develops relatively rapidly in response to contamination of the peritoneal cavity. Chemical and biological irritants, particularly microbial molecules, are recognized by pattern recognition receptors of resident macrophages and other proinflammatory cells present within the peritoneal cavity. This results in release of signals that attract large numbers of inflammatory cells into the peritoneal cavity. Early on, these are primarily polymorphonuclear leukocytes, but after 1 or 2 days, mononuclear leukocytes come to predominate. These cells may directly phagocytose pathogenic microorganisms or other particulate matter. In addition, this early inflammatory reaction triggers the development of the specific immune response, as well as subsequent phases of wound healing.

Sequestration is another key component of the host response that serves to limit the extent of the infection. This process occurs at both the microscopic and the macroscopic level. Microscopic sequestration involves production of fibrin and other macromolecules that entrap microorganisms and facilitate their disposal. Fibrin production and deposition play a key role in the development of macroscopic sequestration. These adhesive molecules promote the binding of various surfaces covered by parietal or visceral peritoneum to each other. Thus, the omentum, mesentery, bowel loops, and abdominal wall all adhere together in the area of most intense inflammation. This restricts the access of pathogens or other irritants to other areas of the abdomen. This process also may result in the sealing of some perforations of the gastrointestinal tract (Cheadle and Spain 2003).

The end result of sequestration and the inflammatory reaction may be a contained intra-abdominal abscess, with a phlegmon as a potential intermediate stage in this evolution. The development of an intra-abdominal abscess may actually represent a successful host response, because the infection has been localized. When host defense mechanisms are ineffective, a much more virulent infection may ensue. An example of this is the highly lethal diffuse disease process characterized as tertiary peritonitis. Thus, standard host defense mechanisms play a key role in promoting survival and recovery after peritoneal contamination.

SOURCES OF IAIs

A variety of different types of infections are collectively grouped together as IAIs. As already indicated, these infections can be described as uncomplicated or complicated. However, some processes described as uncomplicated IAIs are not initially infections, e.g., acute cholecystitis is initially an inflammatory process induced by obstruction or ischemia, and not by microbial invasion.

Beyond this gross division of IAIs into uncomplicated and complicated varieties, the site from which an infection develops will have a significant impact on its clinical characteristics and management. The source of an IAI will influence its microbiology, because the site of perforation within the gastrointestinal tract will determine the quantity and type of microbial contamination that occurs. Similarly, the source of infection may also determine the degree to which a particular infection spreads, depending on whether the perforation is into the free peritoneal cavity, or the mesentery or retroperitoneum.

The types of IAIs and their associated sources vary with the age of the patient. In the neonatal period, necrotizing enterocolitis is the most common entity producing an IAI (Brook 2003, Blakely et al. 2008). During childhood, appendicitis is the predominate type encountered. Appendicitis persists as the major source of IAIs throughout early adulthood, although infections arising in the gallbladder become increasingly more frequent. However, development of a complicated IAI due to perforation of the gallbladder is relatively unusual. During the later decades of life, infections arising from the colon due to diverticular disease or malignancy increase progressively in numbers, and surpass the appendix as the most frequent cause of a complicated infection in those age groups (Podnos et al. 2002).

Appendicitis

Overall, appendicitis is the most frequently encountered IAI. In the developed world, the incidence had been reported to be 75–140 cases per 100 000 patients per year (Körner et al. 1997, Al-Omran et al. 2003). More recent data suggest that rates have been increasing over the past 10–15 years, possibly in association with increased use of imaging studies to make the diagnosis (Livingston et al. 2007). In the developing world, somewhat lower rates have been reported, but these also appear to be increasing (Oguntola et al. 2010). There is a male-to-female predominance of approximately 1.4–1.5:1. The peak incidence occurs in the second decade of life, but appendicitis occurs in all age groups. In association with changes in demographic trends, increased numbers of middle-aged and elderly patients are being treated for this disease (Harbrecht et al. 2011).

Acute appendicitis has long been assumed to be due to obstruction of the appendiceal lumen, subsequent distension of the appendix with inflammatory fluid and mucus, bacterial overgrowth within the lumen, and eventual gangrene and perforation as the end result. This concept has been challenged. Non-obstructive etiologies can clearly give rise to appendicitis, and actual obstruction of the appendiceal lumen as the initiating factor may be relatively uncommon. The supposition that acute appendicitis, once initiated, will inexorably progress to perforation has also been challenged. Spontaneous regression of appendiceal inflammation may be a much more common process than is generally appreciated, making many cases self-limited (Mason 2008).

Appendicitis can be considered either an uncomplicated or a complicated IAI, depending on its stage. Acute, non-perforated appendicitis is an uncomplicated IAI, whereas perforated appendicitis is a complicated infection. Gangrenous appendicitis is somewhat more difficult to classify; however, unless microorganisms are isolated from inflammatory fluid outside the appendix, it should be considered an uncomplicated infection. Perforated appendicitis rarely results in generalized peritonitis; if present, this is usually seen at the extremes of age. More often, perforated appendicitis presents with localized peritonitis in the right lower quadrant, with the inflammatory process being limited by the ileocecal mesentery, adjacent loops of bowel, and omentum. If the disease process progresses for several days, an appendiceal phlegmon or periappendiceal abscess may develop.

Large and small bowel perforation

Next to the appendix, the colon is the most common source of an IAI. In developed countries, diverticular disease causes most IAIs related to a colonic source. Other colonic processes leading to IAIs include perforated colonic malignancy, iatrogenic or traumatic injury, foreign body perforation, ischemic colitis, inflammatory bowel disease, and stercoral perforation. IAIs from a colonic source tend to occur in older patients. Not surprisingly, mortality from these infections tends to be higher than from other types of IAIs. This is particularly true for infections developing from a colonic process other than diverticular disease (Mosdell et al. 1991).

IAIs arising from a small bowel source are much less common than those arising from a colonic source. There is no predominant etiology of small bowel perforation. Crohn disease causes frequent perforations of the small bowel, but this process may be limited to localized abscess or fistula formation. Perforations of the small bowel due to abdominal trauma may result in an IAI if not treated expeditiously within 12 h. Necrosis of the small bowel leading to peritonitis with or without overt perforation may be due to vascular compromise or a low-flow state. Vasculitis may give rise to a discrete focus of necrosis and resultant perforation. Perforation may also be related to a Meckel diverticulum or a primary or metastatic small bowel tumor. Certain infectious diseases, such as tuberculosis or cytomegalovirus infection, lead to perforations of the distal small bowel. Finally, many IAIs arising from the small bowel are postoperative infections.

Gastroduodenal perforation

Gastroduodenal perforations are responsible for a minority of the complicated IAIs. In one population-based survey, 9% of cases of secondary bacterial peritonitis not associated with prior surgery were due to such perforations (Mosdell et al. 1991). Although peptic ulcer disease is the most common cause of an acute gastroduodenal perforation, the incidence of this is decreasing, possibly as a result of widespread use of proton pump inhibitors and other agents for reducing gastric acid production (Hermansson et al. 2009, Wang et al. 2010). The incidence of gastric perforation has not decreased as rapidly as has the rate of duodenal perforation (Wang et al. 2010). Gastroduodenal malignancies may present with an acute perforation, but benign diseases are responsible for a far higher proportion of these perforations. Iatrogenic perforations, due to endoscopic or surgical therapy, may also cause these infections. The amount of microbial contamination of the peritoneal cavity produced by a gastroduodenal perforation tends to be quite low in patients with normal acid production. Arbitrarily, such patients are considered to have peritoneal contamination, and not a complicated IAI, if they undergo a source control procedure within 24 h of the perforation.

Biliary disease

The gallbladder and the biliary tree are frequent sources of IAI. Infections arising in the gallbladder are much more common than those developing in the bile ducts. Acute cholecystitis leads to most of the intra-abdominal infections developing from the gallbladder. Acute cholecystitis is not synonymous with an infection of the gallbladder. Bacteria are isolated from the bile of only 40–50% of patients with acute calculous cholecystitis (Csendes et al. 1996, Yoshida et al. 2007). Acute cholecystitis may evolve into a complicated IAI. Perforation of the gallbladder occurs in a small percentage of patients who develop cholecystitis, and accounts for approximately 5% of all complicated IAIs (Mosdell et al. 1991).

Acute cholangitis may develop with obstruction of the major biliary ducts. Although biliary calculi are the most common cause of this obstruction, extrinsic compression due to neoplasms or inflammatory masses, biliary strictures, and occlusion of drains or stents placed into the biliary system may all lead to acute cholangitis. Perforation of the biliary tree is very uncommon in the absence of gallbladder disease, and is usually associated with leakage from a biliary–biliary or biliary–enteric anastomosis. Acute cholangitis is frequently associated with bacteremia or frank septicemia. The onset of disease is usually quite acute, and systemic symptoms and signs such as fever, chills, and hypotension predominate over abdominal symptoms and signs.

Pancreatic and peripancreatic infection

IAIs related to the pancreas generally develop in the setting of severe acute pancreatitis. There are several different types of pancreatic or peripancreatic infections that can be included in this category, including infected pancreatic pseudocysts, pancreatic abscesses, or infected pancreatic necrosis (Loveday et al. 2008). Infected pancreatic necrosis is among the most lethal. The reported mortality rate is approximately 30%, which is considerably higher than the mortality rate secondary to necrotizing pancreatitis alone (Banks and Freeman 2006). The high mortality may be due to the inherent difficulty in surgically managing these infections, but it has also been suggested that infection is a marker for the severity of pancreatitis, and not necessarily an independent risk factor for mortality (Büchler et al. 2000, Bourgaux et al. 2007).

Postoperative IAIs

The numbers of patients with postoperative IAI have increased in concert with the number and complexity of abdominal procedures. Approximately 15–20% of complicated IAIs occur postoperatively (Pacelli et al. 1996, Kologlu et al. 2001). Gastroduodenal and colon procedures are those most frequently associated with these infections. The mortality rate for postoperative IAIs is around 30% (Mulier et al. 2003). The microbial pathogens producing these nosocomial infections are somewhat different to those involved with most community-acquired infections.

MICROBIOLOGY

Most IAIs are caused by microorganisms normally present in the gastrointestinal tract, whereas blood-borne pathogens may produce some less common infections, such as splenic or hepatic abscesses. The types and numbers of microorganisms present within the lumen of the gastrointestinal tract vary greatly in different areas of the gut. As a general principle, the numbers of microorganisms and the prevalence of Gram-negative *Enterobacteriaceae* and anaerobic organisms increase in frequency from the stomach to the distal colon. In the normal individual, the stomach and proximal small intestine contain fewer than 10^3–10^4 organisms per gram of contents. These are primarily streptococci or lactobacilli (Savage 1977, Tappenden and Deutsch 2007). However, in critically ill and other hospitalized patients, the stomach and duodenum may become heavily colonized with *Enterobacteriaceae, Pseudomonas* spp., enterococci and other Gram-positive cocci, and yeasts (Marshall et al. 1993, Reddy et al. 2008). In the more distal small intestine, Gram-negative enteric aerobic/facultative anaerobic bacilli become increasingly prevalent, although Gram-positive cocci continue to be present. In the terminal ileum, bacterial counts may reach 10^7–10^8 organisms/g contents; significant numbers of anaerobic organisms are present in addition to the aerobic Gram-negative bacilli and Gram-positive cocci. In the colon, obligate anaerobic microorganisms come to predominate as much as 100- to 1000-fold over the aerobic microorganisms. Bacterial counts reach 10^{10}–10^{11} microorganisms/g contents (Savage 1977, Tappenden and Deutsch 2007). In the presence of intestinal obstruction or intestinal dysmotility, this pattern of colonic flora becomes prevalent in more proximal portions of the small intestine as well.

The actual pathogens responsible for an IAI reflect the gastrointestinal flora at the source of the infection. Thus, the most common pathogens are enteric Gram-negative bacilli, Gram-positive cocci, and anaerobic microorganisms. These infections are nearly always polymicrobial (**Box 6.1**). In fact, 5–10 isolates can be obtained from clinical samples analyzed in research laboratories; however, few of these microorganisms are actually identified by most clinical laboratories (Brook 2002, Roehrborn et al. 2003, Goldstein and Snydman 2004).

The most common microorganism isolated from IAI is *Escherichia coli*. This organism is identified in at least 50% of specimens obtained with these infections. (Brook 2002, Goldstein and Snydman 2004). *Klebsiella* spp. is probably the next most common Gram-negative aerobic organism found, although it is encountered much less frequently than *E. coli*. Other enteric Gram-negative bacilli, such as *Enterobacter* spp. may also be identified. *Pseudomonas aeruginosa* is associated with nosocomial infections, but can also be isolated occasionally from patients with community-acquired IAIs.

Along with Gram-negative bacilli, aerobic Gram-positive cocci are commonly isolated from IAIs. These are predominately *viridians*-type

---

Box 6.1 Common pathogens in intra-abdominal infection.

Community-acquired infection
Gram-negative bacilli:
  Escherichia coli, Klebsiella spp.
  Enterobacter spp., *Pseudomonas aeruginosa* – infrequently isolated
Gram-positive cocci:
  Streptococcus milleri group
  Enterococci – infrequently isolated
Anaerobic bacteria
  Bacteroides fragilis, other *B. fragilis* group, peptostreptococci, peptococci, eubacteria, *Fusobacterium* spp., *Clostridium* spp.

Postoperative infection (limited prior antimicrobial exposure)
Gram-negative bacilli:
  Escherichia coli, Klebsiella spp., *Enterobacter* spp., *Pseudomonas aeruginosa*
Gram-positive cocci:
  Enterococcus faecalis
Anaerobic bacteria
  Bacteroides fragilis, other *B. fragilis* group – less frequently isolated
Fungi:
  Candida albicans – infrequently isolated

Healthcare-associated infection (significant prior antimicrobial exposure)
Gram-negative bacilli:
  E. coli, Klebsiella spp., *Enterobacter* spp., *Pseudomonas aeruginosa, Acinetobacter* spp.
Gram-positive cocci
  Enterococcus faecium, including vancomycin-resistant *E. facecium*
  Staphylococcus aureus, including meticillin-resistant *S. aureus*
  Coagulase-negative staphylococci
Anaerobic bacteria
  Bacteroides fragilis, other *B. fragilis* group – infrequently isolated
Fungi:
  Candida albicans
  Non-*C. albicans* spp.

---

streptococci, described as the *Streptococcus milleri* group (Goldstein and Snydman 2004); species that are components of this group include *S. anginosus, S. constellatus*, and *S. intermedius* (Verrall 1986). Although much attention has been paid to the role of enterococcal organisms in IAIs, these are isolated much less frequently than the *S. milleri* group streptococci. Enterococci are encountered in only 10–20% of peritoneal cultures (Waites et al. 2006). When enterococci are isolated in patients with community-acquired IAIs, it is most commonly a penicillin-susceptible strain of *E. faecalis* (Teppler et al. 2002). *Enterococcus faecium*, which is generally resistant to penicillins and may become resistant to vancomycin, is increasingly encountered as a component of healthcare-associated IAIs. The pathogenic role of enterococci, particularly in the setting of community-acquired IAIs, remains controversial.

Obligate anaerobic organisms are important in the pathogenesis of most IAIs, particularly those arising from a lower gastrointestinal source. *Bacteroides fragilis* is isolated from a third to a half of cultures.

Other members of the *B. fragilis* group, including *B. thetaiotaomicron*, *B distasonis*, *B. vulgatus*, *B. ovatus*, and *B. uniformis*, are also encountered. Other anaerobic bacteria that contribute to these infections include peptostreptococci, peptococci, eubacteria, and *Fusobacterium* and *Clostridium* spp., among others (Goldstein 2002).

Fungal microorganisms are isolated from less than 10% of patient IAIs. Almost all are *Candida* spp., most frequently *C. albicans*, although non-*C. albicans* spp. are also encountered. These yeasts play relatively little role in the pathogenesis of community-acquired IAIs, but have a greater role in healthcare-associated infections.

Microbiology of healthcare-associated IAIs

The standard microbial flora of IAIs is altered in patients with prior exposure to the healthcare setting, with regard to both the microbial species and the susceptibility profiles (see Box 6.1). There is a shift in the relative frequency of various Gram-negative isolates. *E. coli* tends to be isolated less frequently, but *Enterobacter* and *Pseudomonas* spp. more frequently. A similar shift is seen in Gram-positive organisms. Streptococci are less likely, but enterococci are identified more frequently. Anaerobic bacteria are isolated less frequently in patients with healthcare-associated IAIs, and may play less of a role in these infections because of prior treatment. *C. albicans* and non-*C. albicans* spp. are identified more commonly in healthcare-associated IAIs. Patients who have recurrent gastrointestinal perforations, e.g., after surgical procedures or pancreatic infections, are at increased risk for candidal infections (Calandra et al. 1989). Colonization of the upper gastrointestinal tract with *Candida* spp. becomes more common in critically ill patients (Sandven et al. 2001).

Patients with tertiary peritonitis exhibit the most resistant types of IAI pathogens. The most common pathogens isolated in these patients include multiply resistant, Gram-negative pathogens, such as *Pseudomonas* and *Acinetobacter* spp., enterococci, including vancomycin-resistant *E. faecium*, coagulase-negative staphylococci, meticillin-resistant *Staphylococcus aureus* (MRSA), and fungal organisms (Trick et al. 2002, DeLisle and Perl 2003, Pfaller et al. 2005).

Susceptibilities of common pathogens

Antimicrobial resistance has become increasingly common among pathogens involved in community-acquired IAIs. For *E. coli*, in vitro resistance to ampicillin/sulbactam is commonplace, occurring in at least 45% of strains cultured from IAIs. These resistant strains are recovered at approximately the same frequency in all parts of the world (Chow et al. 2005). *E. coli* resistance to fluoroquinolones has also become common, particularly in Latin America and south Asia, and is increasing elsewhere (Hsuch and Hawley 2007, Coque et al. 2008, Ko and Hsueh 2009). Probably the most ominous change is the emergence in the community of strains of *Enterobacteriaceae*, including *E. coli*, *Klebsiella* spp., and *Enterobacter* spp. with resistance to several β-lactam antibiotics. These strains typically carry plasmids that encode for one of a variety of different extended-spectrum β-lactamases. Such strains have become widespread in Latin America and south Asia. Most of these strains remain susceptible to carbapenems; however, some strains of *Enterobacteriaceae*, particularly those carrying the New Delhi metallo-β-lactamase, are resistant to essentially all β-lactam antibiotics, including carbapenems (Dupont 2007, Coque et al. 2008, Gupta et al. 2011).

Increasing resistance to antibiotics such as clindamycin and cefotetan is frequently seen in strains of *B. fragilis* and other anaerobic species (Snydman et al. 1999, Aldridge et al. 2001, Mazuski et al. 2002b). However, it is uncertain if this increased resistance is of clinical importance except in the small subgroup of patients who have anaerobic bacteremia. MRSA is increasingly encountered throughout the world (Chua et al. 2011), but is infrequent in community-acquired infections.

DIAGNOSIS

An IAI is suspected in most patients on the basis of a constellation of abdominal symptoms and signs. The most frequent symptom is abdominal pain, which is present in most patients. Pain is typically of relatively recent onset, but of variable severity, quality, and radiation. Symptoms of gastrointestinal dysfunction, such as anorexia, nausea, vomiting, diarrhea, or constipation, are frequently observed, but are generally non-specific in character. Many patients present with systemic signs of inflammation, such as fever, tachycardia, and tachypnea, but these may be absent in severely ill patients.

The abdominal exam is generally abnormal. Most often, there is some degree of abdominal tenderness, which may range from mild and poorly localized to severe and localized to one part of the abdomen, or generalized to the entire abdomen. Rebound tenderness and voluntary or involuntary guarding is variably elicited.

Basic laboratory examinations, although non-specific, are frequently utilized in the diagnostic evaluation of patients with suspected IAIs. Leukocytosis with a neutrophilia is observed in many patients. Blood chemistry studies, such as serum bilirubin or other liver function tests for patients with suspected hepatobiliary disease, or amylase or lipase with suspected pancreatitis, can be valuable in selected patients.

It is not necessary to obtain blood cultures in suspected IAIs. Only 0–5% of patients will have positive blood (Solomkin et al. 2010). However, higher rates of bacteremia are observed in critically ill patients with IAIs. It is recommended that routine blood cultures be acquired in such patients when they present with severe sepsis or septic shock (Wagner et al. 1996).

For most patients, the history, physical exam, and basic laboratory studies will establish the presence of an IAI. Clinical diagnoses of appendicitis, cholecystitis, or diverticulitis can frequently be made on the basis of their characteristic symptoms and signs. For the diagnosis of appendicitis, scoring systems have been devised that integrate various symptoms, signs, and laboratory findings into a single score. Although these scoring systems appear to have good sensitivity and specificity, their utility for clinical practice has not been universally accepted (Alvarado 1986, Urban and Fishman 2000, Doria et al. 2006, Bundy et al. 2007).

Ultimately, however, clinical diagnoses will not always be accurate. More importantly, many patients will not present in a classic manner for IAIs. The diagnosis may be particularly obscure in certain patient groups, such as elderly people, those receiving corticosteroids or other immunosuppressive therapies, and those with an unreliable examination due to a neurological problem such as dementia or a prior spinal cord injury. Thus, further confirmatory testing is employed in many patients to establish the presence of an IAI.

A number of different imaging procedures are used. Standard radiographic views of the chest and abdomen may reveal free abdominal air or other findings of IAIs, but these are often inconclusive. Ultrasonography and computed tomography (CT) of the abdomen are the principal imaging modalities of diagnostic value. Ultrasonography is the technique of choice for suspected hepatobiliary disease. It is also of use in pelvic sources of gynecological infection in women.

If there is good technical expertise available, ultrasonography can also be used to establish the diagnosis of appendicitis.

However, for most suspected IAIs, CT of the abdomen has become the preferred imaging modality (Anaya and Nathens 2003). There is a large body of literature comparing ultrasonography and CT for the diagnosis of appendicitis. In a meta-analysis of this literature, it was found that the sensitivity and specificity of CT was superior to that of ultrasonography for diagnosing appendicitis in both children and adults (Wacha et al. 1999).

Other considerations play a role in the decision to use one or other of these techniques. Avoidance of ionizing radiation may be desirable in the diagnostic evaluation of children and pregnant women. Also, any decision on the imaging modality includes local availability of CT and ultrasonography, as well as access to technical expertise in their performance and interpretation.

MANAGEMENT OF IAIs

The three fundamental principles for managing patients with IAIs are:
1. Physiological resuscitation and support
2. Interventional procedures to control the source of the infection
3. Antimicrobial therapy to treat the residual infection remaining after a source control procedure.

Application of these principles will vary according to the patient's acuity and associated underlying medical comorbidities. Thus, an assessment of patient risk factors may be useful in selecting the specific therapeutic approach for a given patient.

Patient risk assessment

Risk factors for treatment failure and death in patients with IAIs have been evaluated in a number of multivariate analyses. Identified risk factors include those related to patient characteristics as well as those that are related more to the infection itself. Patient-related risk factors include a higher APACHE II (Acute Physiology and Chronic Health Evaluation II) score, advanced age, hypoalbuminemia, hypocholesterolemia, malnutrition, significant cardiovascular, hepatic, or renal disease, malignancy, and corticosteroid therapy (Mazuski et al. 2002b). Among these, the APACHE II score has been the most consistent predictor of treatment failure and death. The individual components of the APACHE II score include measures of the host response to the infection as well as underlying comorbidities. However, this score is somewhat problematic to calculate and subject to significant interobserver variation. It is also a general marker of illness, and its utility for tailoring specific therapeutic interventions in patients with IAIs seems limited.

Risk factors that pertain more directly to the characteristics of the IAI might be more useful for the selection of specific treatment modalities. Surprisingly, the source of infection has not proven to be a reliable predictor of outcome, although one relatively large study identified a non-appendiceal source of infection as an independent risk factor for severe sepsis (Anaya and Nathens 2003). The Mannheim peritonitis index, a measure of how widespread an IAI is within the peritoneal cavity, has been found to be an independent risk factor (Pacelli et al. 1996). However, most importantly, several studies have found that failure to achieve adequate source control at the time of the initial intervention is a very strong predictor of an adverse outcome (Wacha et al. 1999). Thus, it appears important that an optimal operative or other source control procedure be performed as part of the early therapy in IAIs.

Risk factors may also relate to the type of microbial pathogens involved in an IAIs. The presence of certain resistant microorganisms, such as enterococci, has been associated with an increased risk of treatment failure (Hopkins et al. 1993, Christou et al. 1996, Sitges-Serra et al. 2002). Furthermore, the use of an inadequate initial empirical antimicrobial regimen, defined as one that did not provide coverage of one or more of the microorganisms eventually isolated from the infected site, has also been found to be an independent predictor of treatment failure and death (Montravers et al. 1996, Krobot et al. 2004, Sturkenboom et al. 2005). Thus, the choice of the initial empirical antimicrobial therapy appears to play a role in determining clinical outcome. Stratification of patients based on the absence of presence of a healthcare-associated infection, and thereby the likelihood of encountering resistant organisms, has been recommended as a means of selecting specific antimicrobial therapy.

Physiological resuscitation and support

Correction of physiological abnormalities associated with IAIs is a fundamental principle in management. The goal is to improve tissue perfusion, such that delivery of endogenous mediators of host defense as well as exogenous antimicrobial agents to inflamed and infected tissues is optimized. Enhancement of systemic perfusion should also allow the patient to better withstand the physiological challenges inherent in source control procedures, thereby improving outcomes. None the less, physiological resuscitation and support are not an end in themselves, and attempts to correct these physiological abnormalities without also addressing source control and antimicrobial therapy will lead to treatment failure.

The degree to which a patient with an IAI demonstrates severe sepsis or septic shock can be used to assess that patient's need for aggressive physiological resuscitation and support. Criteria have been established to define patients with sepsis, severe sepsis, and septic shock (**Box 6.2**) (Bone et al. 1992). Although these criteria are not highly sensitive or specific, they provide a basis on which to stratify patients according to severity of illness. Another option is to use the serum lactic acid concentration as a marker of severity. This measurement is usually readily available, and can be used not only to stratify patients according to risk, but also to monitor their response to therapy (Bakker et al. 1991, Shapiro et al. 2005, Arnold et al. 2009, Jones et al. 2010).

Most patients with IAIs will have some depletion of intravascular volume and extracellular fluid due to poor oral intake, increased insensible water loss due to fever, extracellular fluid losses from vomiting or diarrhea, and sequestration of fluid within the bowel or in the peritoneal cavity. Thus, administration of isotonic intravenous fluids is generally indicated in these patients. For patients with severe sepsis or septic shock, more aggressive resuscitation is recommended. Early goal-directed therapy during the first 6 h of recognition of the infection is a reasonable approach for administration of intravenous fluids, as well as selective use of vasopressor agents and inotropic support in these patients (Rivers et al. 2001). Early goal-directed therapy is included in the Sepsis Resuscitation Bundle, a component of The Surviving Sepsis Campaign guidelines for managing septic shock (Dellinger et al. 2008).

Source control

Interventions to control the source of an IAI include drainage of infected fluid collections, debridement of infected tissue, and procedures to contain further microbial contamination. The eventual goal of source control is to re-establish normal anatomy and function. In patients with uncomplicated IAIs, the source control procedure

Box 6.2 Criteria for sepsis, severe sepsis, and septic shock (based on Bone et al. 1992).

Systemic inflammatory response syndrome (SIRS)
Two or more of the following:
Temperature >38°C or <36°C
Heart rate >90 beats/min
Respiratory rate >20 breaths/min or $PaCO_2$ <32 mmHg (4.26 kPa)
White blood cell count >12 000/mm^3, <4000/ mm^3, or with >10% immature forms

Sepsis
The presence of an infection with two of more SIRS criteria

Severe sepsis:
Sepsis associated with organ dysfunction, hypoperfusion, or hypotension
Hypoperfusion and perfusion abnormalities including, but not limited to:
　Lactic acidosis
　Oliguria
　Acute alteration in mental status

Septic shock
Sepsis-induced hypotension unresponsive despite adequate fluid resuscitation
Perfusion abnormalities including, but not limited to:
　Lactic acidosis
　Oliguria
　Acute alteration in mental status

should result in full control of the site of infection. In patients with complicated IAIs, this procedure does not entirely eliminate the infection, but should serve to sufficiently limit it such that subsequent antimicrobial therapy will lead to its complete resolution.

A number of treatment modalities are utilized for source control. Patients with circumscribed abscesses or other infected fluid collections can be treated with percutaneous drainage, provided that a safe route of access to the infection is available (Akinci et al. 2005, Theisen et al. 2005). Minimally invasive procedures are employed in many patients for the treatment of uncomplicated IAIs, such as acute appendicitis (Cueto et al. 2006, Sauerland et al. 2010). Minimally invasive procedures are also being increasingly used in patients with complicated IAIs, although this is less widespread. For many patients, open surgical procedures are still utilized, particularly when the infectious process is not well localized or there is necrotic tissue that needs to be debrided.

In patients with complicated IAIs, the source control procedure provides the opportunity for obtaining cultures of the infected peritoneal fluid. There is some disagreement as to the utility of such cultures. For individual patients with a community-acquired IAI, routine cultures appear to have relatively little value, particularly for those with perforated appendicitis (Dougherty 1997, Bilik et al. 1998, Kokoska et al. 1999). However, even though these cultures may be considered optional for the individual patient, their use is recommended as part of an overall surveillance program for resistant pathogens within a community. As a result of the greater potential for resistant organisms in patients with healthcare-associated IAIs, routine cultures are recommended.

The timing of source control interventions in patients with IAIs is also a matter of controversy. It had been customary for such procedures to be carried out promptly at the time of diagnosis. However, with the increasing use of less invasive but more technically complex procedures, a delay in performing source control to ensure availability of adequate technical expertise and resources has become more common. For patients with diffuse peritonitis or with ongoing hemodynamic instability, source control should be undertaken as soon as feasible, even if ongoing physiological resuscitation needs to be provided simultaneously. For hemodynamically stable patients with localized infections, a delay in performing source control can be considered if the availability of additional resources is likely to improve patient outcome. If such a delay is to be contemplated, adequate antimicrobial therapy must be provided and the patient needs to be carefully monitored for any evidence of deterioration.

Many of the details about source control procedures are determined by the specific organ that is involved in the infection. A full summary of all these operative procedures and options is beyond the scope of this chapter. Rather, some of the trends and controversies related to source control will be highlighted by considering the management of appendicitis, localized intra-abdominal fluid collections, and diffuse, generalized peritoneal infections.

Source control for appendicitis

The management of appendicitis has undergone significant changes over the past two decades. Appendectomy had been considered the treatment of choice for nearly all patients with suspected appendicitis for nearly a century. The primary exception to this was for children who presented with a periappendiceal abscess, in whom drainage followed by interval appendectomy was considered a reasonable approach (Mason 2008).

In the past, nonsurgical management of acute appendicitis was described as an option to be used only if surgical treatment was completely unavailable (Adams 1990). However, deliberate use of this approach in the treatment of patients with acute appendicitis has been investigated in several prospective randomized controlled trials. In these trials, nonsurgical management of appendicitis using antibiotics alone was compared with mandatory surgical treatment (Eriksson and Granström 1995, Styrud et al. 2006, Hansson et al. 2009, Malik and Bari 2009). Despite the availability of these data on over 700 randomized patients, various authors have come to different conclusions about nonsurgical management (Varadhan et al. 2010, Ansaloni et al. 2011, Liu and Fogg 2011). The combined data indicate that appendectomy was avoided in approximately 58% of the patients in these trials. Appendicitis subsequently recurred in around 14% of patients who were initially managed nonsurgically. There was no apparent increase in perforation as a result of a delay in surgical management in the patients who failed antibiotic treatment alone. Overall complication rates were significantly higher in patients randomized to initial surgical management (Ansaloni et al. 2011).

Although these data indicate that nonsurgical management of acute appendicitis using antibiotic therapy alone is a relatively safe option, there are also extensive data attesting to the general safety of appendectomy. The overall mortality rate in patients undergoing surgical management of non-perforated appendicitis was estimated to be 0.8/1000 in a Swedish database, although the rate increased to >10/1000 in patients aged ≥70 years (Blomqvist et al. 2001). Another long-term study of the Swedish population found that an operation for small bowel obstruction had been performed in only 0.75% of patients who had undergone appendectomy after 30 years, although this rate was approximately 3.6-fold higher than that observed in matched control patients who had not undergone appendectomy (Andersson 2001). Currently, it would appear that both a traditional surgical and nonsurgical approach using only antibiotics are viable options for treating patients with acute non-perforated appendicitis.

The approach to perforated appendicitis has also undergone significant evolution. Nonsurgical management of perforated appendicitis, particularly for those patients who present with a periappendiceal phlegmon, has become increasingly accepted. This has been estimated to occur in 3.8% of patients with appendicitis (Andersson and Petzold 2007). Primary surgical therapy of such patients may necessitate a larger procedure, such as a ileocecectomy or right hemicolectomy, rather than simple appendectomy. There are only very small prospective randomized controlled trials evaluating this approach; most of the data are retrospective and uncontrolled. In one meta-analysis comparing initial nonsurgical management of patients with a periappendiceal mass with an initial surgical approach, the failure rate with the nonsurgical approach was only 7.2%. Utilization of nonsurgical management was associated with a nearly threefold decrease in complication rates. Recurrent appendicitis was identified in only 7% of patients. As the risk of morbidity of routine interval appendectomy was greater than the risk of recurrent appendicitis, these authors recommended against routine interval appendectomy. The finding that patients with a periappendiceal mass or phlegmon had fewer complications with an initial nonsurgical approach was validated in a second meta-analysis as well (Simillis et al. 2010).

Laparoscopic appendectomy is now widely used for the treatment of appendicitis. The use of this technique has been supported by a large body of evidence. Compared with patients treated with open appendectomy, patients treated with laparoscopic appendectomy have a decreased rate of surgical site infection, decreased pain, a decreased length of hospitalization, and an earlier return to normal activities. The rate of postoperative intra-abdominal abscess is higher, however, in patients undergoing laparoscopic appendectomy. Young female patients, obese patients, and those needing to return to employment appear to be those who benefit most from use of the laparoscopic approach (Sauerland et al. 2010).

Overall, current management of patients with appendicitis exemplifies a trend toward using less invasive procedures for, and even complete deferral of source control interventions in, selected groups of patients. Utilization of these approaches appears to result in decreased patient morbidity. None the less, these approaches may not produce similar results if applied to other patients with IAIs. Overall morbidity and mortality related to appendicitis are low because the patients are generally young and previously healthy. In contrast, other types of intra-abdominal infections are more lethal and morbid than appendicitis, and the patients who sustain them typically have fewer physiological reserves than patients with appendicitis (Merlino et al. 2001).

Source control for infected intra-abdominal fluid collections

The use of percutaneous drainage techniques for treating patients with localized infected intra-abdominal abscesses and other fluid collections is another example where less invasive procedures have come to be the predominant approach to source control. The continued advancement of techniques has made it possible to approach many fluid collections that hitherto required a surgical procedure for treatment (Maher et al. 2004). Percutaneous drainage is routinely used for treating both the spontaneous abscess that develops

after an acute process such as appendicitis or diverticulitis, as well as the iatrogenic abscess that forms after an abdominal procedure. The presence of localized extraluminal air or fluid around the site of perforation or leak is not a contraindication to the placement of a percutaneous catheter. Overall success rates for percutaneous procedures range from 80% to 92%, and complication rates are low. Many failures of initial percutaneous drainage can be salvaged by subsequent catheter drainage procedures (Akinci et al. 2005, Theisen et al. 2005).

The success of percutaneous drainage is related to both the size of the abscess and its complexity. In one study, the best success occurred with a unilocular fluid collection containing no more than 200 ml fluid and with no fistulous connection to the bowel or other intra-abdominal organ. However, patient characteristics also influenced outcome after percutaneous drainage procedures; severity of illness, as assessed by APACHE-III scores, increased the risk of failure, regardless of the abscess characteristics (Betsch et al. 2002).

Source control for generalized peritonitis

It has generally been recommended that patients with generalized peritonitis undergo expeditious source control. However, many of these patients are at high risk for an adverse outcome due to significant physiological compromise. Thus, there is an interest in utilizing less invasive, less morbid procedures for source control in such patients as well, even if the intervention is just a temporizing measure (Fry 2003).

One example of a less invasive intervention for patients with generalized peritonitis is the use in laparoscopic lavage and drainage as treatment for patients with perforated diverticulitis. One review of such patients, most of whom had generalized purulent peritonitis, found a reoperation rate of only 2.4% during the initial treatment period, and a mortality rate of only 1.4% (Alamili et al. 2009). As this approach has not been evaluated in controlled trials, these results should be considered preliminary.

Damage control laparotomy is another potential approach that can be utilized to avoid an extensive procedure at the time of the initial intervention in severely ill patients with generalized peritonitis (Subramanian et al. 2010). The principles of this approach have been adapted from experience gained in patients with severe abdominal trauma (Waibel and Rotondo 2010). During the initial intervention, only the essential procedures necessary to control bleeding or ongoing peritoneal contamination are performed. Thus, a diseased portion of bowel may be resected, but an anastomosis or stoma is not placed. The fascia is left open to facilitate subsequent, definitive procedures, which are undertaken after the patient has reached physiological stability.

There are certain indications for which a planned, repeat laparotomy has gained acceptance. Planned re-laparotomy is utilized when the source of the infection cannot be controlled with a single procedure, when bowel or other hollow viscus continuity cannot be safely restored at the time of the initial procedure, there is a potential for ongoing intestinal ischemia such that re-laparotomy is needed to establish the viability of the remaining bowel, and there is significant visceral edema that could lead to an abdominal compartment syndrome if primary fascial closure were performed (Schein 2003).

For patients with generalized peritonitis who do not have one of these indications, however, there is no consensus as to the utility of planned re-laparotomy. A prospective randomized controlled trial compared patients with severe secondary peritonitis who were treated with planned re-laparotomy versus those who underwent repeat laparotomy only if there was a clinical indication ("on-demand laparotomy"). Only 42% of patients in the latter group actually underwent repeat laparotomy. Overall, there was no evidence of a clinical benefit for patients undergoing mandatory re-laparotomy, and this approach resulted in a longer hospital and intensive care lengths of stay as well as higher costs (Van Ruler et al. 2007).

Thus, use of less invasive procedures may be an option for the management of severely ill patients with IAIs, just as it is has become for the treatment of less severely ill patients. The use of temporizing measures may be of benefit in these patients with significant compromise of vital organs. However, these approaches need to undertaken with some caution because inadequate source control is associated with a substantially increased risk of an adverse clinical outcome. When managing any patient with limited or deferred source control, the patient should be carefully monitored. A potentially life-saving procedure is undertaken expeditiously if the patient's clinical trajectory declines. Carefully performed, adequately controlled research studies are needed to better understand which patients might best be treated with approaches featuring limited or deferred source control interventions.

■ Antimicrobial therapy

Antimicrobial therapy is part of the general therapeutic armamentarium for the treatment of patients with IAIs. The effectiveness of antimicrobial therapy is dependent on the presence of a functioning host defense system, which is ultimately responsible for the clearance of microbial pathogens and toxins.

Antimicrobial therapy is used for both prophylactic and thera-peutic purposes when managing an IAI, although it may be difficult to distinguish between these two purposes. Prophylactic use of antimicrobial agents is generally advocated for the prevention of surgical site infection in patients undergoing surgical procedures classified as clean contaminated, contaminated, or dirty infected. This applies to virtually every patient with an IAI. For patients with complicated IAI, the therapeutic aim of antimicrobial agents is to eradicate pathogenic microorganisms that remain after a source control procedure. For selected patients in whom a primary source control is not performed, the antimicrobial regimen is purely therapeutic, since it plays a definitive role along with the host response in controlling the infection.

The general principle underlying antimicrobial therapy for IAIs is to use agents effective against the aerobic/facultative anaerobic Gram-negative bacilli and aerobic Gram-positive cocci. For most IAIs, except for some that arise in the upper gastrointestinal tract or hepatobiliary tree, the antibiotic regimen should also cover obligate anaerobic organisms (Wong et al. 2005, Solomkin et al. 2010). Several studies have shown that failure rates increase if anaerobic coverage is not included (Edelsberg et al. 2008).

Selection of a specific antimicrobial regimen should be based on stratification of the patient according to risk of an adverse outcome. Different regimens have been recommended for patients with community-acquired and health care-associated IAIs. In addition, within the category of community-acquired infections, different agents are recommended according to the severity of the illness (Solomkin et al. 2010). Thus, no single antimicrobial regimen is preferred for all patients. Use of a regimen that inadequately covers the pathogens may result in treatment failure, but use of an excessively broad regimen may lead to collateral damage through selection of resistant bacteria and superinfecting pathogens.

Antimicrobial therapy for mild-to-moderate community-acquired IAIs

For less severely ill patients with community-acquired IAIs, antimicrobial therapy should be relatively narrow spectrum, directed against Gram-negative *Enterobacteriaceae*, particularly *E. coli*, streptococci, and usually obligate anaerobic microorganisms. In general, activity of the regimen against *Pseudomonas* spp., enterococci, and fungal organisms is not necessary. The safety of using narrower-spectrum as opposed to broader-spectrum agents in these patients is established. Recommended agents for the treatment of patients with community-acquired IAIs of mild-to-moderate severity are shown in **Table 6.1**.

Selection of the specific antimicrobial regimen for a given patient would ideally be based on considerations of efficacy and toxicity. However, there are very few data to indicate that one regimen is more effective than another (Mazuski et al. 2002a, Solomkin et al. 2003, Wong et al. 2005). The relative efficacy of aminoglycoside-based regimens, which at one time were considered the "gold standard" for IAIs, was challenged in one meta-analysis (Bailey et al. 2002). These regimens are no longer considered first-line agents for empirical treatment.

Changing microbial susceptibilities would be expected to have an impact on the efficacy of different antimicrobial regimens. This is reflected in newer recommendations about antimicrobial regimens for IAIs. The widespread resistance of *E. coli* to ampicillin/sulbactam throughout the world led to this antibiotic being removed from recommended agents. Resistance of *E. coli* to fluoroquinolones has led to caution in their use if the local prevalence of resistance is >10–20%. The emergence of *Enterobacteriaceae* in the community with extended-spectrum b-lactamases will also limit the choice of antibiotics in certain locales. Thus, local patterns of resistance among common pathogens should be taken into consideration when selecting specific antimicrobial regimens.

Beyond efficacy considerations, the toxicity of a given regimen and its propensity for creating collateral damage will influence antimicrobial selection. In the individual patient, a history of an allergic or other reaction to a specific antibiotic may lead to the selection of an alternative agent. In the local community, overuse of certain antibiotics may lead to collateral damage due to outbreaks of superinfecting or resistant organisms (Paterson 2004). Thus, if a given antimicrobial agent had been implicated, e.g., in a local outbreak of *Clostridium difficile*-associated disease, the use of an alternative agent would be prudent.

Antimicrobial therapy for severe community-acquired IAIs

Patients with community-acquired IAIs who present with severe sepsis or septic shock are at a substantial risk for a poor clinical outcome.

Table 6.1 Recommended antimicrobial agents for patients with community-acquired intra-abdominal infections of mild-to-moderate severity (based on Solomkin et al. 2010).

Single agents	Combination regimens
Cefoxitin Ertapenem Moxifloxacin[a] Ticarcillin/clavulanic acid Tigecycline	Cephazolin, cefuroxime, cefotaxime, or ceftriaxone plus metronidazole Ciprofloxacin[a] or levofloxacin[a] plus metronidazole*
[a]As a result of increased resistance of *E. coli* to fluoroquinolones, local susceptibility profiles should be considered before prescribing these agents.	

Although there are few data suggesting that the microbiology in such patients differs from that of lower-risk patients with community-acquired IAIs, use of inadequate antimicrobial therapy could potentially have much more deleterious consequences. This hypothesis is based on outcome studies of other critically ill patients, e.g., inadequate antimicrobial therapy in patients with ventilator-associated pneumonia has been associated with a twofold increase in mortality (Chastre and Fagon 2002). Moreover, a delay in the administration of appropriate antimicrobial therapy has also been associated with increased mortality in a population of patients presenting with septic shock (Kumar et al. 2006). As a result of this potential for suboptimal outcomes with community-acquired IAIs receiving inadequate antimicrobial therapy, broader-spectrum antimicrobial regimens are recommended for the initial empirical treatment (**Table 6.2**). The planned use of broader-spectrum antimicrobial agents for initial therapy should also have a de-escalation plan to a narrower-spectrum regimen once definitive culture results are available. There is no need to continue a broad-spectrum regimen if more resistant pathogens, such as *Pseudomonas* spp. or enterococci, are not isolated.

Antimicrobial therapy in healthcare-associated IAIs

As a result of changes of the microbial flora that are associated with the healthcare setting, and particularly with prior treatment with antimicrobial agents, resistant pathogens are frequently involved. As with other healthcare-associated infections, resistant microorganisms make empirical antimicrobial choices very difficult.

Antimicrobial therapy for healthcare-associated IAIs needs to be individualized, according to both the patient's history of prior antimicrobial therapy and the resistance patterns of the microbial pathogens in the local environment. The initial empirical regimen should include coverage against a relatively broad range of Gram-negative bacilli and anaerobic organisms. Recommended regimens are similar to those described for treatment of high-severity community-acquired infections. However, empirical treatment regimens for patients with healthcare-associated infections frequently need to be expanded to include additional agents directed against specific Gram-negative pathogens. In addition, the regimen may be broadened to provide coverage of enterococci, resistant Gram-positive cocci, and yeast. Some of these recommendations have been summarized in **Box 6.3**.

When deciding whether or not to utilize additional antimicrobial therapy directed against Gram-negative aerobic pathogens, an assessment needs to be made of the likelihood that the patient will be

> **Box 6.3 Recommended antimicrobial agents for empirical treatment of patients with healthcare-associated intra-abdominal infections (based on Solomkin et al. 2010).**
>
> - Utilize one of the regimens listed in Table 6.2
> - If there is a possibility of significant resistance among the likely Gram-negative pathogens, add a second agent with activity against Gram-negative aerobic bacilli (an aminoglycoside, colistin, a fluoroquinolone, tigecycline), according to local susceptibility profiles
> - Add vancomycin or ampicillin if a cephalosporin or fluoroquinolone-based regimen is being used and the patient has not received extensive prior antimicrobial therapy. If the patient has received extensive prior antimicrobial coverage, add vancomycin to all regimens to provide activity against *Enterococcus faecium*; if there is a high risk or known colonization with vancomycin-resistant *E. faecium*, substitute linezolid
> - Add vancomycin if the patient is colonized with methicillin-resistant *S. aureus* (MRSA) and thought to be at significant risk for an intra-abdominal infection due to this organism
> - Add an echinocandin (anidulafungin, caspofungin, micafungin) if the patient is critically ill and at risk for an infection due to *Candida* spp. Fluconazole should be used in less critically ill patients; an echinocandin or voriconazole can be used in patients infected with non-*C. albicans* spp. resistant to fluconazole

infected with resistant pathogens. This is based in part on knowledge of the frequency with which certain pathogens are encountered in the local environment, as well as their likely resistance patterns. Additional Gram-negative coverage is recommended if more than 10% of the strains of the expected pathogen or pathogens would be resistant to the standard antimicrobial regimen. This approach is analogous to that recommended for the treatment of ventilator-associated pneumonia. Additional agents that might be considered, depending on the types and susceptibilities of local pathogens, include an aminoglycoside, a fluoroquinolone, a glycylcycline, or even the antibiotic colistin if highly resistant strains of *Pseudomonas* or *Acinetobacter* spp. are present locally. The empirical antimicrobial regimen should be narrowed once definitive culture results are available. Continued use of two agents against Gram-negative organisms in an effort to provide synergy is not recommended, and has not been shown to be effective (Cometta et al. 1994, Dupont et al. 2000).

As a result of the frequency with which enterococci are isolated in patients with healthcare-associated IAI, empirical coverage of this microorganism should generally be provided (Sotto et al. 2002, Harbarth and Uckay 2004). In patients with an initial postoperative infection who have not received subsequent courses of antimicrobial therapy, *E. faecalis*, is the usual enterococcal pathogen that will be isolated. Piperacillin/tazobactam and broad-spectrum carbapenems, including imipenem/cilastatin, and doripenem have reasonable activity against this organism. Ampicillin or vancomycin can also be added to a regimen that lacks such anti-enterococcal activity. Patients with healthcare-associated IAIs who have received more extensive antimicrobial therapy are at risk for enterococcal infections due to *E. faecium*. Under these circumstances, vancomycin is the preferred agent for enterococcal coverage, because this organism is generally resistant to penicillins and carbapenems. Increasingly, vancomycin-resistant *E. faecium* is being encountered in patients with

Table 6.2 Recommended antimicrobial agents for patients with community-acquired intra-abdominal infections of high severity (based on Solomkin et al. 2010).

Single agents	Combination regimens
Doripenem Imipenem/cilastatin Meropenem[a] Piperacillin/tazobactam	Ceftazidime[b] or cefepime[a] plus metronidazole Ciprofloxacin[a,b] or levofloxacin[a] plus metronidazole Aztreonam[c] plus metronidazole plus vancomycin

[a] As a result of increased resistance of *E. coli* to fluoroquinolones, local susceptibility profiles should be considered before prescribing these agents.

[b] Addition of ampicillin or vancomycin to the regimen should be considered to provide anti-enterococcal activity. The need for additional anti-enterococcal activity when using meropenem is controversial.

[c] The recommended regimen for patients with a significant allergy to β-lactam antibiotics.

IAIs who have received extensive prior antibiotic therapy. Linezolid, daptomycin, quinupristin–dalfopristin, and tigecycline have activity against this microorganism, and are potential choices (Torres-Viera and Dembry 2004, Eliopoulos 2005). Linezolid is the antibiotic for which most clinical experience has been reported. Empirical use an agent effective against vancomycin-resistant enterococci has not been extensively studied, but could be considered in patients known to be colonized with vancomycin-resistant enterococci or considered to be at very high risk for an infection due to that microorganism.

Staphylococcus aureus is occasionally found as a component of a healthcare-associated IAIs, most commonly with postoperative infections, pancreatic infections, and tertiary peritonitis (Rotstein et al. 1986, Torres-Viera and Dembry 2004). Treatment of IAIs involving staphylococci follows the principles used for treating other staphylococcal infections (Solomkin et al. 2004, Eliopoulos 2005). If methicillin sensitive *S. aureus* is isolated, an anti-staphylococcal penicillin or cephalosporin can be used. For patients with MRSA, vancomycin has generally been used. Linezolid, daptomycin, quinupristin/dalfopristin, and possibly tigecycline are potential alternatives. Very limited experience has been reported regarding the use of any of these agents in IAIs. Empirical therapy directed against MRSA is not generally warranted. However, it might be considered in a patient who has had extensive prior antimicrobial therapy and is known to be colonized with this organism.

Fungal microorganisms, particularly *Candida* spp., are frequently components of healthcare-associated IAIs (Rotstein et al. 1986, Montravers et al. 2004, 2006). Antifungal therapy directed against *Candida* spp. should be used in patients who have a confirmed infection due to this microorganism. Identification of yeasts on the Gram stain of infected peritoneal fluid should also prompt inclusion of antifungal therapy in the empirical regimen selected for these and other higher-risk patients (Bochud et al. 2004). Pre-emptive antifungal therapy in patients who are at high risk for IAIs due to *Candida* spp. also appears to be of benefit (Eggiman et al. 1999, Mazuski 2007).

Antifungal agents that have been evaluated for the treatment of invasive candida infections include amphotericin B and its lipid formulations, the azoles, fluconazole and voriconazole, among others, and the echinocandins, caspofungin, micafungin, and anidulafungin (Bassetti et al. 2006, Spanakis et al. 2006). Fluconazole is the agent most frequently used for treatment of IAIs due to *C. albicans*. However, for critically ill patients, use of an echinocandin has been recommended as first-line therapy instead of fluconazole (Pappas et al. 2004, Reboli et al. 2007). There has been an increased incidence of yeast infections due to non-*C. albicans* spp. in recent years (Maschmeyer 2006), which may apply to patients with healthcare-associated IAIs as well. Some of these non-*C. albicans* spp., particularly *C. glabrata* and *C. krusei*, are resistant to the usual dosages of fluconazole. Use of voriconazole or an echinocandin is an option for treating patients from whom such microorganisms have been isolated.

Duration of antimicrobial therapy

One way with which to avoid resistance and toxicity related to antimicrobial therapy is to limit the duration of that therapy (Raymond et al. 2002, Gleisner et al. 2004, Davey et al. 2005, Dellit et al. 2007). Much of the prolonged use of antimicrobial therapy that occurs in IAIs is likely unnecessary, and may actually lead to a worse outcome (Gleisner et al. 2004, Hedrick et al. 2006).

Patients who do not have a complicated IAIs should not receive prolonged antimicrobial therapy. The primary goal of therapy in such patients is prophylaxis against surgical site infection during the source control procedure. Patients undergoing laparotomy for traumatic or iatrogenic bowel injuries operated on within 12 h of the injury and those undergoing laparotomy for upper gastrointestinal perforations operated on within 24 h should be treated with no more than 24 h of antimicrobial therapy. In addition, patients with non-perforated appendicitis, cholecystitis, bowel obstruction, or bowel infarction, in whom the focus of inflammation or infection has been eliminated by the source control procedure, should receive perioperative antimicrobial therapy for no more than 24 h (Mazuski 2002a).

Shorter courses of antimicrobial therapy are warranted for most complicated IAIs. Limiting the duration of antimicrobial therapy to 3–5 days has been shown to be effective in both retrospective and prospective studies (Andåker et al. 1987, Schein et al. 1994). An alternative approach is to discontinue antimicrobial therapy once the patient has defervesced, has a normalizing white blood cell count, and has had return of gastrointestinal activity (Wilson and Faulkner 1998, Taylor et al. 2000). This approach also leads to decreased utilization of antimicrobial agents without adverse effects on patient outcome.

Some patients with IAIs do not respond optimally to the initial empirical antimicrobial regimen. Patients with persistent signs of infection, such as ongoing fever or leukocytosis, may have an ongoing or recurrent IAI, or an infection at an extra-abdominal site (Lennard et al. 1980, 1982). The recommended approach for these patients is to perform diagnostic imaging or other investigations to localize a source of the abnormal physiological parameters. Prolonged, non-directed antimicrobial therapy, with either the same or different agents, is strongly discouraged.

Patients in whom adequate source control cannot be achieved constitute an exception to the general rule of using short-duration antimicrobial therapy for the treatment of IAI. An example of such a patient is a critically ill individual with tertiary peritonitis, who has ongoing clinical evidence of sepsis. Antimicrobial therapy should most likely be continued for a longer period of time, because early discontinuation of antimicrobial therapy has been associated with increased mortality in such patients (Visser et al. 1998).

■ CLINICAL OUTCOMES

For patients with complicated IAIs, the standard approach of providing physiological resuscitation and support, source control, and appropriate antimicrobial therapy has been associated with a cure rate of around 80% and an overall mortality rate of 2–3% in clinical trials (Mazuski et al. 2002b). However, outcomes are somewhat worse outside a clinical trial setting (Merlino et al. 2001). One statewide survey of patients with complicated IAIs demonstrated an overall mortality rate of 6%, a postoperative abscess rate of 10%, and a reoperation rate of 13% (Mosdell et al. 1991). Outcomes are strongly influenced by the characteristics of the patients and their infections. Mortality due to perforated appendicitis is substantially lower compared with rates observed in patients with other types of complicated IAIs (Wilson and Faulkner 1998, Blomqvist et al. 2001, Anaya and Nathens 2003). In the statewide survey, the mortality rate was 1% among patients with perforated appendicitis, but 13% among patients with infections from another source (Mosdell et al. 1991). The mortality rates of more severely ill patients have been reported to be 17–32% (Mazuski et al. 2002b). Thus, complicated IAIs are still responsible for considerable morbidity and mortality, particularly among patients with a non-appendiceal source of infection, those who have severe sepsis or septic shock, and those who have compromised organ function because of significant pre-existing comorbid conditions. Further research to identify optimal means of treating these patients is warranted.

■ REFERENCES

Adams ML. The medical management of acute appendicitis in a nonsurgical environment: a retrospective case review. *Mil Med* 1990;**155**:345–7.

Akinci D, Akhan O, Ozmen MN, et al. Percutaneous drainage of 300 intraperitoneal abscesses with long-term follow-up. *Cardiovasc Intervent Radiol* 2005;**28**:744–50.

Alamili M, Gögenur I, Rosenberg J. Acute complicated diverticulitis managed by laparoscopic lavage. *Dis Colon Rectum* 2009;**52**:1345–9.

Aldridge KE, Ashcraft D, Cambre K, et al. Multicenter survey of the changing in vitro antimicrobial susceptibilities of clinical isolates of *Bacteroides fragilis* group, *Prevotella*, *Fusobacterium*, *Porphyromonas*, and *Peptostreptococcus* species. *Antimicrob Agents Chemother* 2001;**45**:1238–43.

Al-Omran M, Mamdani MM, McLeod R. Epidemiologic features of acute appendicitis in Ontario, Canada. *Can J Surg* 2003;**46**:263–8.

Altemeier WA, Culbertson WR, Fullen WD, Shook CD. Intra-abdominal abscesses. *Am J Surg* 1973;**125**:70–9.

Alvarado A. A practical score for the early diagnosis of acute appendicitis. *Ann Emerg Med* 1986;**15**:557–64.

Anaya DA, Nathens AB. Risk factors for severe sepsis in secondary peritonitis. *Surg Infect (Larchmt)* 2003;**4**:355–62.

Andåker L, Höjer H, Kihlström E, Lindhagen J. Stratified duration of prophylactic antimicrobial treatment in emergency abdominal surgery. Metronidazole-fosfomycin vs. metronidazole-gentamicin in 381 patients. *Acta Chir Scand* 1987;**153**:185–92.

Andersson RE. Small bowel obstruction after appendicectomy. *Br J Surg* 2001;**88**:1387–91.

Andersson, RE, Petzold MG. Nonsurgical treatment of appendiceal abscess or phlegmon: A systematic review and meta-analysis. *Ann Surg* 2007;**246**:741–8.

Ansaloni L, Catena F, Coccolini F, et al. Surgery versus conservative antibiotic treatment in acute appendicitis: A systematic review and meta-analysis of randomized controlled trials. *Dig Surg* 2011;**28**:210–21.

Arnold RC, Shapiro NI, Jones AE, et al. Multicenter study of early lactate clearance as a determinant of survival in patients with presumed sepsis. *Shock* 2009;**32**:35–9.

Bailey JA, Virgo KS, DiPiro JT, et al. Aminoglycosides for intra-abdominal infection: equal to the challenge? *Surg Infect (Larchmt)* 2002;**3**:315–35.

Bakker J, Coffernils M, Leon M, et al. Blood lactate levels are superior to oxygen-derived variables in predicting outcome in human septic shock. *Chest* 1991;**99**:956–62.

Banks PA, Freeman ML, Practice Parameters Committee of the American College of Gastroenterology. Practice guidelines in acute pancreatitis. *Am J Gastroenterol* 2006;**101**:2379–400.

Bassetti M, Righi E, Tumbarello M, et al. Candida infections in the intensive care unit: Epidemiology, risk factors and therapeutic strategies. *Expert Rev Anti Infect Ther* 2006;**4**:875–85.

Betsch A, Wiskirchen J, Trübenbach J, et al. CT-guided percutaneous drainage of intra-abdominal abscesses: APACHE III score stratification of 1-year results. *Eur Radiol* 2002;**12**:2883–9.

Bilik R, Burnweit C, Shanding B. Is abdominal cavity culture of any value in appendicitis? *Am J Surg* 1998;**175**:267–70.

Blakely ML, Gupta H, Lally KP. Surgical management of necrotizing enterocolitis and isolated intestinal perforation in premature neonates. *Semin Perinatol* 2008;**32**:122–6.

Blomqvist PG, Andersson RE, Granath F, et al. Mortality after appendectomy in Sweden, 1987–1996. *Ann Surg* 2001;**233**:455–60.

Blot S, De Waele JJ. Critical issues in the clinical management of complicated intra-abdominal infections. *Drugs* 2005;**65**:1611–1620.

Bochud PY, Bonten M, Marchetti O, Calandra T. Antimicrobial therapy for patients with severe sepsis and septic shock: an evidence-based review. *Crit Care Med* 2004;**32**:S495–512.

Bone RC, Balk RA, Cerra FB, et al. Definitions for sepsis and organ failure and guidelines for the use of innovative therapies in sepsis. The ACCP/SCCM Consensus Conference Committee. American College of Chest Physicians/Society of Critical Care Medicine. *Chest* 1992;**101**:1644–55.

Bourgaux JF, Defez C, Muller, L, et al. Infectious complications, prognostic factors, and assessment of anti-infectious management of 212 consecutive patients with acute pancreatitis. *Gastroenterol Clin Biol* 2007;**31**:43135.

Brook I. Microbiology of polymicrobial abscesses and implications for therapy. *J Antimicrob Chemother* 2002;**50**:805–10.

Brook I. Microbiology and management of intra-abdominal infections in children. *Pediatrics Int* 2003;**45**:123–9.

Büchler MW, Gloor B, Müller, CA, et al. Acute necrotizing pancreatitis: Treatment strategy according to the status of infection. *Ann Surg* 2000;**232**:619–26.

Buijk SE, Bruining HA. Future directions in the management of tertiary peritonitis. *Intensive Care Med* 2002;**28**:1024–9.

Bundy DG, Byerley JS, Liles EA, et al. Does this child have appendicitis? *JAMA* 2007;**298**:438–51.

Calandra T, Bille J, Schneider R, et al. Clinical significance of Candida isolated from peritoneum in surgical patients. *Lancet* 1989;**ii**:1437–40.

Chastre J, Fagon JY. Ventilator-associated pneumonia. *Am J Respir Crit Care Med* 2002;**165**:867–903.

Cheadle WG, Spain DA. The continuing challenge of intra-abdominal infections. *Am J Surg* 2003;**186**:15S–22S.

Chow JW, Satishchandran V, Snyder TA, et al. In vitro susceptibilities of aerobic and facultative Gram-negative bacilli isolated from patients with intra-abdominal infections worldwide: The 2002 study for monitoring antimicrobial resistance trends (SMART). *Surg Infect (Larchmt)* 2005;**6**:439–48.

Christou NV, Turgeon P, Wassef R, et al. Management of intra-abdominal infections. The case for intraoperative cultures and comprehensive broad-spectrum antibiotic coverage. *Arch Surg* 1996;**131**:1193–201.

Chua K, Frederic Laurent F, Coombs G, et al. Not community-associated methicillin-resistant *Staphylococcus aureus* (CA-MRSA)! A clinician's guide to community MRSA – its evolving antimicrobial resistance and implications for therapy *Clin Infect Dis* 2011;**52**:99–114.

Cometta A, Baumgartner JD, Lew D, et al. Prospective randomized comparison of imipenem monotherapy with imipenem plus netilmicin for treatment of severe infections in nonneutropenic patients. *Antimicrob Agents Chemother* 1994;**38**:1309–13.

Coque TM, Baquero F, Cantón R. Increasing prevalence of ESBL-producing Enterobacteriaceae in Europe. *Euro Surveill* 2008;**13**:19044.

Csendes A, Burdiles P, Maluenda F, et al. Simultaneous bacteriologic assessment of bile from gallbladder and common bile duct in control subjects and patients with gallstones and common duct stones. *Arch Surg* 1996;**131**:389–94.

Cueto J, D'Allemagne B, Vazquez-Frias JA, et al. Morbidity of laparoscopic surgery for complicated appendicitis: an international study. *Surg Endosc* 2006;**20**:717–20.

Davey P, Brown E, Fenelon L Interventions to improve antibiotic prescribing practices for hospital inpatients. *Cochrane Database Syst Rev* 2005;**4**:CD003543.

Dougherty SH. Antimicrobial culture and susceptibility testing has little value for routine management of secondary bacterial peritonitis. *Clin Infect Dis* 1997;**25**(suppl 2):S258–61.

DeLisle S, Perl TM. Vancomycin-resistant enterococci: A road map on how to prevent the emergency and transmission of antimicrobial resistance. *Chest* 2003;**123**:504S–18S.

Dellinger RP, Levy MM, Carlet JM, et al. Surviving Sepsis Campaign: international guidelines for management of severe sepsis and septic shock: 2008. *Crit Care Med* 2008;**36**:296–327.

Dellit TH, Owens RC, McGowan JE Jr, et al. Guidelines for developing an institutional program to enhance antimicrobial stewardship. *Clin Infect Dis* 2007;**44**:159–77.

De Waele JJ, Hoste EA, Blot SI. Blood stream infections of abdominal origin in the intensive care unit: characteristics and determinants of death. *Surg Infect (Larchmt)* 2008;**9**:171–7.

Doria AS, Moineddin R, Kellenberger CJ, et al. US or CT for diagnosis of appendicitis in children and adults? A meta-analysis. *Radiology* 2006;**241**:83–94.

Dupont H. The empiric treatment of nosocomial intra-abdominal infections. *Int J Infect Dis* 2007;**11**:S1–6.

Dupont H, Carbon C, Carlet J, et al. Monotherapy with a broad-spectrum beta-lactam is as effective as its combination with an aminoglycoside in treatment of severe generalized peritonitis: A multicenter randomized controlled trial. *Antimicrob Agents Chemother* 2000;**44**:2028–33.

Edelsberg J, Berger A, Schell S. Economic consequences of failure of initial antibiotic therapy in hospitalized adults with complicated intra-abdominal infections. *Surg Infect (Larchmt)* 2008;**9**:335–47.

Eggiman P, Francioli P, Bille J, et al. Fluconazole prophylaxis prevents intra-abdominal candidiasis in high-risk surgical patients. *Crit Care Med* 1999;**27**:1066–72.

Eliopoulos GM. Antimicrobial agents for treatment of serious infections cause by resistant *Staphylococcus aureus* and enterococci. *Eur J Clin Microbiol Infect Dis* 2005;**24**:826–31.

Eriksson S, Granström L. Randomized controlled trial of appendicectomy versus antibiotic therapy for acute appendicitis. *Br J Surg* 1995;**82**:166–9.

Faber MD, Yee J. Diagnosis and management of enteric disease and abdominal catastrophe in peritoneal dialysis patients with peritonitis. *Adv Chronic Kidney Dis* 2006;**13**:271–9.

Fry DE. Definitive versus temporizing therapy. In Schein M and Marshall JC (eds), *Source Control. A Guide to the Management of Surgical Infections*. Berlin: Springer-Verlag, 2003: 54–8.

Gleisner AL, Argenta R, Pimentel M, et al. Infective complications according to duration of antibiotic treatment in acute abdomen. *Int J Infect Dis* 2004;**8**:155–62.

Goldstein EJC. Intra-abdominal anaerobic infections: Bacteriology and therapeutic potential of newer antimicrobial carbapenem, fluoroquinolone, and desfluoroquinolone therapeutic agents. *Clin Infect Dis* 2002;**35**(suppl 1):S106–11.

Goldstein EJC, Snydman DR. Intra-abdominal infections: Review of the bacteriology, antimicrobial susceptibility and the role of ertapenem in their therapy. *J Antimicrob Chemother* 2004;**53**:ii29–36.

Gupta N, Limbago BM, Patel JB, Kallen AJ. Carbapenem-resistant *Enterobacteriaceae*: Epidemiology and prevention. *Clin Infect Dis* 2011;**53**:60–7.

Hansson J, Körner U, Khorram-Manesh A, et al. Randomized clinical trial of antibiotic therapy versus appendicectomy as primary treatment of acute appendicitis in unselected patients. *Br J Surg* 2009;**96**:473–81.

Harbarth S, Uckay I. Are there patients with peritonitis who require empiric therapy for *Enterococcus*? *Eur J Clin Microbiol Infect Dis* 2004;**23**:73–7.

Harbrecht BG, Franklin GA, Miller FB, et al. Acute appendicitis – not just for the young. *Am J Surg* 2011;**202**:286–90.

Hedrick TL, Evans HL, Smith RL, et al. Can we define the ideal duration of antibiotic therapy? *Surg Infect (Larchmt)* 2006;**7**:419–32.

Hermansson M, Ekedahl A, Ranstam J, Zilling T. Decreasing incidence of peptic ulcer complications after the introduction of the proton pump inhibitors, a study of the Swedish population from 1974–2002. *BMC Gastroenterol* 2009;**9**:25.

Hopkins JA, Lee JCH, Wilson SE. Susceptibility of intra-abdominal isolates at operation: A predictor of postoperative infection. *Am Surg* 1993;**59**:791–6.

Hsueh PR, Hawkey PM. Consensus statement on antimicrobial therapy of intra-abdominal infections in Asia. *Int J Antimicrob Agents* 2007;**30**:129–33.

Jones AE, Shapiro NI, Trzeciak S, et al. Lactate clearance vs central venous oxygen saturation as goals of early sepsis therapy. A randomized clinical trial. *JAMA* 2010;**303**:739–46.

Ko WC, Hsueh PR. Increasing extended-spectrum β-lactamase production and quinolone resistance among Gram-negative bacilli causing intra-abdominal infections in the Asia/Pacific region: Data from the Smart Study 2002–2006. *J Infect* 2009;**59**:95–103.

Kokoska ER, Silen ML, Tracy TF Jr, et al. The impact of intraoperative culture on treatment and outcome in children with perforated appendicitis. *J Pediatr Surg* 1999;**34**:749–53.

Kologlu M, Elker D, Altun H, et al. Validation of MPI and PIA-II in two different group of patients with secondary peritonitis. *Hepatogastroenterology* 2001;**48**:147–51.

Körner, H, Söndenaa, K, Söreide JA, et al. Incidence of acute nonperforated and perforated appendicitis: Age-specific and sex-specific analysis. *World J Surg* 1997;**21**:313–17.

Krobot K, Yin D, Zhang Q, et al. Effect of inappropriate initial empiric antibiotic therapy on outcome of patients with community-acquired intra-abdominal infections requiring surgery. *Eur J Clin Microbiol Infect Dis* 2004;**23**:682–7.

Kumar A, Roberts D, Wood KE, et al. Duration of hypotension before initiation of effective antimicrobial therapy is the critical determinant of survival in human septic shock. *Crit Care Med* 2006;**34**:1589–96.

Lennard ES, Minshew BH, Dellinger EP, Wertz M. Leukocytosis at termination of antibiotic therapy: Its importance for intra-abdominal sepsis. *Arch Surg* 1980;**115**:918–21.

Lennard ES, Dellinger EP, Wertz MJ, Minshew BH. Implications of leukocytosis and fever at conclusion of antibiotic therapy for intra-abdominal sepsis. *Ann Surg* 1982;**195**:19–24.

Liu K, Fogg L. Use of antibiotics alone for treatment of uncomplicated acute appendicitis: A systematic review and meta-analysis. *Surgery* 2011;**150**:673–83.

Livingston EH, Woodward WA, Sarosi, GA, Haley RW. Disconnect between incidence of nonperforated and perforated appendicitis: Implications for pathophysiology and management. *Ann Surg* 2007;**245**:886–92.

Loveday BPT, Mittal A, Phillips A, Windsor JA. Minimally invasive management of pancreatic abscess, pseudocyst, and necrosis: A systematic review of current guidelines. *World J Surg* 2008;**32**:2383–94.

Maher MM, Gervais DA, Kalra MK, et al. The inaccessible or undrainable abscess: how to drain it. *Radiographics* 2004;**24**:717–35.

Malik AA, Bari SU. Conservative management of acute appendicitis. *J Gastrointest Surg* 2009;**13**:966–70.

Marshall, JC, Christou NV, Meakins JL. The gastrointestinal tract. The "undrained abscess" of multiple organ failure. *Ann Surg* 1993;**218**:111–19.

Marshall JC. Intra-abdominal infections. *Microbes Infect* 2004;**6**:1015–25.

Maschmeyer G. The changing epidemiology of invasive fungal infections: New threats. *Int J Antimicrob Agents* 2006;**27**S:S3-S6.

Mason RJ. Surgery for appendicitis: Is it necessary? *Surg Infect (Larchmt)* 2008;**9**:481–8.

Mazuski JE. Antimicrobial treatment for intra-abdominal infections. *Expert Opin Pharmacother* 2007;**8**:2933–45.

Mazuski JE, Sawyer, RG, Nathens AB, et al. The Surgical Infection Society guidelines on antimicrobial therapy for intra-abdominal infections: An executive summary. *Surg Infect (Larchmt)* 2002a;**3**:161–73.

Mazuski JE, Sawyer, RG, Nathens AB, et al. The Surgical Infection Society guidelines on antimicrobial therapy for intra-abdominal infections: evidence for the recommendations. *Surg Infect (Larchmt)* 2002b;**3**:175–233.

Merlino JI, Malangoni MA, Smith CM, Lange RL. Prospective randomized trials affect the outcomes of intraabdominal infection. *Ann Surg* 2001;**233**:859–66.

Montravers P, Gauzit R, Muller C, et al. Emergence of antibiotic-resistant bacteria in cases of peritonitis after intra-abdominal surgery affects the efficacy of empirical antimicrobial therapy. *Clin Infect Dis* 1996;**23**:486–94.

Montravers P, Chalfine A, Gauzit R, et al. Clinical and therapeutic features of nonpostoperative nosocomial intra-abdominal infections. *Ann Surg* 2004;**239**:409–16.

Montravers P, Dupont H, Gauzit R, et al. Candida as a risk factor for mortality in peritonitis. *Crit Care Med* 2006;**34**:646–52.

Mosdell DM, Morris DM, Voltura A, et al. Antibiotic treatment for surgical peritonitis. *Ann Surg* 1991;**214**:543–9.

Mulier S, Penninckx F, Verwaest C, et al. Factors affecting mortality in generalized postoperative peritonitis: Multivariate analysis in 96 patients. *World J Surg* 2003;**27**:379–84.

Nathens AB, Rotstein OD, Marshall JC. Tertiary peritonitis: Clinical features of a complex nosocomial infection. *World J Surg* 1998;**22**:158–63.

Oguntola AS, Adeoti ML, Oyemolade TA. Appendicitis: Trends in incidence, age, sex, and seasonal variations in South-Western Nigeria. *Ann Afr Med* 2010;**9**:213–17.

Pacelli F, Doglietto GB, Alfieri S, et al. Prognosis in intraabdominal infections. *Arch Surg* 1996;**131**:641–5.

Pappas PG, Rex JH, Sobel JD, et al. Guidelines for treatment of candidiasis. *Clin Infect Dis* 2004;**38**:161–89.

Paterson DL. "Collateral damage" from cephalosporin or quinolone antibiotic therapy. *Clin Infect Dis* 2004;**38**(suppl 4):S341–5.

Pfaller MA, Kiekema DJ, Rinaldi MG, et al. Results from the ARTEMIS DISK Global Antifungal Surveillance Study: a 6.5-year analysis of susceptibilities of *Candida* and other yeast species to fluconazole and voriconazole by standardized disk diffusion testing. *J Clin Microbiol* 2005;**43**:5848–59.

Podnos YD, Jimenez JC, Wilson SE. Intra-abdominal sepsis in elderly persons. *Clin Infect Dis* 2002;**35**:62–8.

Raymond DP, Kuehnert MJ, Sawyer RG. Preventing antimicrobial-resistant bacterial infections in surgical patients. *Surg Infect (Larchmt)* 2002;**3**:375–85.

Reboli AC, Rotstein C, Pappas PG, et al. Anidulafungin versus fluconazole for invasive candidiasis. *N Engl J Med* 2007;**356**:2472–82.

Reddy BS, Gatt M, Sowdi R, et al. Gastric colonization predisposes to septic morbidity in surgical patients: A prospective study. *Nutrition* 2008;**24**:632–7.

Rivers E, Nguyen B, Havstad S, et al. Early goal-directed therapy in the treatment of severe sepsis and septic shock. *N Engl J Med* 2001;**345**:1368–77.

Roehrborn A, Thomas L, Potreck O, et al. The microbiology of postoperative peritonitis. *Clin Infect Dis* 2003;**33**:1513–19.

Rotstein OD, Pruett TL, Simmons RL. Microbiologic features and treatment of persistent peritonitis in patients in the intensive care unit. *Can J Surg* 1986;**29**: 247–50.

Sandven P, Giercksky KE, NORGAS Group, Norwegian Yeast Study Group. Yeast colonization in surgical patients with intra-abdominal perforations. *Eur J Clin Microbiol Infect Dis* 2001;**20**:475–81.

Sauerland S, Jaschinski T, Neugebauer EAM. Laparoscopic versus open surgery for suspected appendicitis. *Cochrane Database Syst Rev* 2010;**10**:CD001546.

Savage DC. Microbial ecology of the gastrointestinal tract. *Ann Rev Microbiol* 1977;**31**:107–33.

Schein M. Planned relaparotomies and laparostomy. In: Schein M, Marshall JC (eds), *Source Control. A Guide to the Management of Surgical Infections.* Berlin: Springer-Verlag, 2003: 412–23.

Schein M, Assalia A, Bachus H. Minimal antibiotic therapy after emergency abdominal surgery: A prospective study. *Br J Surg* 1994;**81**:989–91.

Shapiro NI, Howell MD, Talmor D, et al. Serum lactate as a predictor of mortality in emergency department patients with infection. *Ann Emerg Med* 2005;**45**:524–8.

Simillis C, Symeonides P, Shorthouse AJ, Tekkis PP. A meta-analysis comparing conservative treatment versus acute appendectomy for complicated appendicitis (abscess or phlegmon). *Surgery* 2010;**147**:818–29.

Sitges-Serra A, Lopez MJ, Girvent M, et al. Postoperative enterococcal infection after treatment of complicated intra-abdominal sepsis. *Br J Surg* 2002;**89**:361–7.

Snydman DR, Jacobus NV, McDermott LA, et al. Multicenter study of in vitro susceptibility of the *Bacteroides fragilis* group, 1995 to 1996, with comparison of resistance trends from 1990 to 1996. *Antimicrob Agents Chemother* 1999;**43**:2417–22.

Solomkin JS, Hemsell DL, Sweet R, et al. Evaluation of new anti-infective drugs for the treatment of intra-abdominal infections. *Clin Infect Dis* 1992;**15**:S33–42.

Solomkin JS, Mazuski JE, Baron EJ, et al. Guidelines for the selection of anti-infective agents for intra-abdominal infections. *Clin Infect Dis* 2003;**37**:997–1005.

Solomkin JS, Bjornson HS, Cainzos M, et al. A consensus statement on empiric therapy for suspected gram-positive infections in surgical patients. *Am J Surg* 2004;**187**:134–45.

Solomkin JS, Mazuski JE, Bradley JS, et al. Diagnosis and management of complicated intra-abdominal infection in adults and children: Guidelines by the Surgical Infection Society and the Infectious Diseases Society of America. *Surg Infect (Larchmt)* 2010;**11**:79–109.

Sotto A, Lefrant JY, Fabbro-Peray P, et al. Evaluation of antimicrobial therapy management of 120 consecutive patients with secondary peritonitis. *J Antimicrob Chemother* 2002;**50**:569–76.

Spanakis EK, Aperis G, Mylonakis E. New agents for the treatment of fungal infections: Clinical efficacy and gaps in coverage. *Clin Infect Dis* 2006;**43**:1060–8.

Strauss E, Caly WR. Spontaneous bacterial peritonitis: A therapeutic update. *Expert Rev Anti Infect Ther* 2006;**4**:248–60.

Sturkenboom MCJM, Goettsch WG, Picelli G, et al. Inappropriate initial treatment of secondary intra-abdominal infections leads to increased risk of clinical failure and costs. *Br J Clin Pharmacol* 2005;**60**:438–43.

Styrud J, Eriksson S, Nilsson I, et al. Appendectomy versus antibiotic treatment in acute appendicitis. A prospective multicenter randomized controlled trial. *World J Surg* 2006;**30**:1033–7.

Subramanian A, Balentine C, Palacio CH. Outcomes of damage-control celiotomy in elderly nontrauma patients with intra-abdominal catastrophes. *Am J Surg* 2010;**200**:783–9.

Tappenden KA, Deutsch AS. The physiological relevance of the intestinal microbiota – Contributions to human health. *J Am Coll Nutr* 2007;**26**:679S–83S.

Taylor E, Dev V, Shah D, et al. Complicated appendicitis: Is there a minimum intravenous antibiotic requirement? A prospective randomized trial. *Am Surg* 2000;**66**:887–90.

Teppler H, McCarroll K, Gesser RM, Woods GL. Surgical infections with *Enterococcus*: Outcome in patients treated with ertapenem versus piperacillin-tazobactam. *Surg Infect (Larchmt)* 2002;**3**:337–49.

Theisen J, Bartels H, Weiss W, et al. Current concepts of percutaneous abscess drainage in postoperative retention. *J Gastrointest Surg* 2005;**9**:280–3.

Torres-Viera C, Dembry LM. Approaches to vancomycin-resistant enterococci. *Curr Opin Infect Dis* 2004;**17**:541–7.

Trick WE, Fridkin SK, Edwards JR, et al. Secular trend of hospital-acquired candidemia among intensive care unit patients in the United States during 1989–1999. *Clin Infect Dis* 2002;**35**:627–30.

Urban BA, Fishman EK. Targeted helical CT of the acute abdomen: Appendicitis, diverticulitis, and small bowel obstruction. *Semin Ultrasound CT MR* 2000;**21**:20–39.

Van Ruler O, Mahler CW, Boer KR, et al. Comparison of on-demand vs planned relaparotomy strategy in patients with severe peritonitis. A randomized trial. *JAMA* 2007;**298**:865–73.

Varadhan KK, Humes DJ, Neal KR, Lobo DN. Antibiotic therapy versus appendectomy for acute appendicitis: A meta-analysis. *World J Surg* 2010;**34**:199–209.

Verrall, R. The *Streptococcus milleri* group. *Infect Control* 1986;**11**:558–60.

Visser MR, Bosscha K, Olsman J, et al. Predictors of recurrence of fulminant bacterial peritonitis after discontinuation of antibiotics in open management of the abdomen. *Eur J Surg* 1998;**164**:825–9.

Wacha H, Hau T, Dittmer R, et al. Risk factors associated with intra-abdominal infections: A prospective multicenter study. *Langenbeck's Arch Surg* 1999;**384**:24–32.

Wagner JM, McKinney WP, Carpenter JL. Does this patient have appendicitis? *JAMA* 1996;**276**:1589–94.

Waibel BH, Rotondo MR. Damage control in trauma and abdominal sepsis. *Crit Care Med* 2010;**38**(suppl):S421–30.

Waites KB, Duffy LB, Dowzicky MJ. Antimicrobial susceptibility among pathogens collected from hospitalized patients in the United States and in vitro activity of tigecycline, a new glycylcycline antimicrobial. *Antimicrob Agents Chemother* 2006;**50**:3479–84.

Wang YR, Richter JE, Dempsey DT. Trends and outcomes of hospitalizations for peptic ulcer disease in the United States, 1993 to 2006. *Ann Surg* 2010;**251**:51–8.

Wilson SE, Faulkner K. Impact of anatomical site on bacteriological and clinical outcome in the management of intra-abdominal infections. Am Surg 1998;**64**:402– 7.

Wong PF, Gilliam AD, Kumar S, et al. Antibiotic regimens for secondary peritonitis of gastrointestinal origin in adults. *Cochrane Database Syst Rev* 2005;**2**:CD004539.

Yoshida M, Takada T, Kawarada Y, et al. Antimicrobial therapy for acute cholecystitis: Tokyo Guidelines. *J Hepatobiliary Pancreat Surg* 2007;**14**:83–90.

Chapter 7 Perirectal abscesses and pilonidal disease

Susan Galandiuk

Compared with other surgical infections discussed in this book, many of which are potentially fatal and complex in their management, the etiology of primary and recurrent perirectal abscesses and pilonidal disease is often overlooked and their treatment delegated to the most junior personnel. Although these infections are infrequently fatal, considerable morbidity can attend those perineal infections that are not managed in a prompt and appropriate fashion.

PERIRECTAL ABSCESSES

The cryptoglandular origin of abscess formation is generally accepted, and infected anal glands have been demonstrated (Lockhart-Mummery 1929, Parks 1961). Anal glands extend from anal crypts through the lower half of the internal anal sphincter. An infection arising in these crypts and glandular infections leads to an infection in the intersphincteric plane where many glands terminate. Most anorectal abscesses are due to infections within this intersphincteric space. Persistence of anal gland epithelium would result in the internal opening remaining patent, with prevention of healing. One may consider the pelvic floor as a cone within a cone; the inner cone consists of the rectum and internal sphincter and the outer cone (in caudal to cranial order) of the external anal sphincter, puborectalis muscle, and levator ani muscle. An infection within the intersphincteric plane between these two cones can extend: (1) distally between the internal and external anal sphincter muscles – *perianal abscess*, (2) through the external anal sphincter muscle as well – *ischiorectal abscess*, (3) proximally between the internal and external sphincter muscles – *intersphincteric abscess*, or (4) above the levator ani muscle – *supralevator abscess*, or (5) perforate through the internal sphincter again, to lie beneath the rectal mucosa – *submucosal abscess*.

Perirectal and ischiorectal abscesses are the most frequent types, followed by the less common intersphincteric and supralevator abscesses (McElwain et al. 1975, Read and Abcarian 1979, Ramanujam et al. 1984). Factors involved in the cause of perirectal abscesses are diarrhea, trauma, hard stool, or foreign body), tissue injury (i.e., fissure), Crohn disease, immunocompromised host, perforating carcinoma, hidradenitis suppurativa, tuberculosis (TB), and pelvic infections such as diverticulitis or appendicitis (Gordon 2007).

Figure 7.1a demonstrates the sites of these various types of perirectal abscesses, and **Figure 7.1b** the location of fistulas. Perirectal abscesses tend to occur more frequently in males than in females (Goligher 1984, Ramanujam et al. 1984). Diagnosis of common perianal abscesses is usually straightforward and based on clinical findings and symptoms, including constant pain aggravated by defecation and various types of Valsalva maneuvers such as coughing and sneezing, and occasionally by fever. An erythematous, tender swelling in the perianal area most frequently occurs with perianal abscesses, and more diffuse swelling with ischiorectal abscesses. The most common symptoms of perirectal abscess are pain (98%), swelling (50%), and bleeding per rectum (16%), followed by other symptoms such as purulent anal discharge, diarrhea, and fever (Vasilevsky and Gordon 1984). In patients for whom the diagnosis is unclear, needle aspiration may confirm the presence of pus, or endorectal ultrasonography may confirm and map out the extent of perianal disease (Law et al. 1989). Differential diagnosis includes periurethral abscesses in the male, or Bartholin gland abscesses in the female. Tubercular abscesses are usually characterized by less viscous pus than conventional abscesses and may be associated with known pulmonary TB. Other differential diagnoses include hidradenitis suppurativa, sebaceous cysts, actinomycosis, fissure *in ano*, pilonidal sinuses, and folliculitis of the

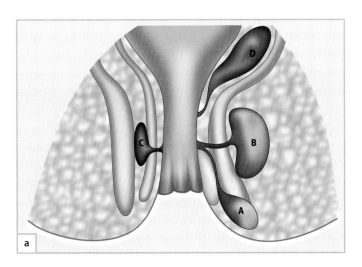
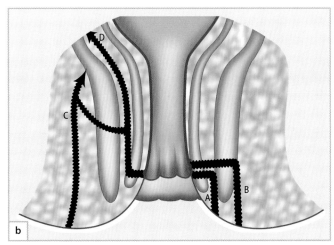

Figure 7.1 (a) Types of perirectal abscesses: (A) Perianal, (B) ischiorectal, (C) intersphincteric, and (D) supralevator. **(b) Types of fistulas:** (A) Intersphincteric, (B) transsphincteric, (C) extrasphincteric, and (D) suprasphincteric.

perianal skin. A pelvic abscess due to intra-abdominal disease may present in the perineal area with fever and a palpable pelvic mass on digital rectal or vaginal examination.

Treatment

Parenteral or oral antibiotics do not have a place in the treatment of perirectal abscesses, except in the following circumstances:

- The presence of a prosthesis, such as a hip prosthesis, pacemaker, or cardiac valve replacement
- Immunocompromised patients such as transplant recipients, those with diabetes, human immunodeficiency virus (HIV) positivity, or acquired immune deficiency syndrome (AIDS), and granulocytopenic patients such as those with leukemia or after aggressive cancer chemotherapy
- As a temporizing measure if immediate surgical drainage is not possible due to unavailability of a surgeon, or a patient is anticoagulated or in extremely poor general medical condition.
- Significant cellulitis or an unusual degree of infection, such as a massive pelvic/perianal infection with suspicion of the presence of gas-forming organisms
- When systemic antibiotics are used, large doses should be given and terminated promptly to avoid meticillin-resistant *Staphylococcus aureus* and *Clostridium difficile* superinfections.

Digital rectal examination at the level of the dentate line for signs of induration is usually the most accurate way of identifying an internal fistula opening if one is present, and is superior to visual inspection with a rigid sigmoidoscope or anoscope. Rigid sigmoidoscopy does, however, permit visual inspection of the lower rectum for signs of rectal Crohn disease, specific proctitis such as can occur in HIV-positive and AIDS patients, as well as other pathology such as perforating carcinomas.

Perianal abscesses can usually be drained in the office under local anesthesia. This author prefers to use 1% lidocaine with 1:200 000 epinephrine. Ischiorectal abscesses are often too deep to drain without general or regional anesthesia. This is also true of higher abscesses or abscesses in the postanal space. In patients in whom the area is too tender for an adequate examination, or in patients in whom no physical abnormality can be detected despite significant symptoms or perirectal pain with or without pyrexia, an examination under anesthesia is warranted. Two important considerations in treating perirectal abscesses are to provide a large enough opening in the skin to prevent closure and re-accumulation of pus. Although one does want to ensure adequate drainage, excessive manipulation to break up loculations can result in trauma to the anal canal innervation. If an internal fistula opening is identified, and the surgeon treating the abscess is knowledgeable, a primary fistulotomy can be performed. A recent Cochrane review on this topic identified 6 trials involving 479 patients in which incision and drainage of a perianal abscess alone was compared with incision and drainage with treatment of the fistula (Malik et al. 2010). There was a significant reduction in abscess recurrence, persistent abscess or fistula, and repeat surgery in the latter group (relative risk = 0.13, 95% confidence interval 0.07–0.24).

Due to edema and the friable nature of tissue in the presence of infection, a false passage can easily be made, and therefore fistulotomy should be undertaken *only* if the internal opening and fistula are very obvious. The author prefers to drain abscesses by making a cruciate incision over the abscess and excising the "corners" to provide for a large cutaneous opening for drainage. This large opening prevents premature primary closure and eliminates the need for packing of the wound (**Figure 7.2**). Radial counter incisions should be used liberally

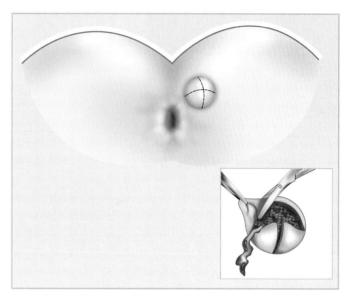

Figure 7.2 Perirectal abscess drainage: Cruciate incision with excision of "corners" allows for adequate drainage without the need for packing.

if a large abscess is present, and large Penrose drains can be placed through these counter-incisions to keep the skin edges open and ensure adequate drainage. Perioperative antibiotics are unnecessary before anorectal procedures, except in the circumstances outlined above. The author performs drainage, whether in the office or in the operating room, with nearly all patients in a prone jack-knife position rather than in a lithotomy position. This gives the best exposure to the area and permits the most careful examination. Pregnant women and those unable to be positioned in this manner can be placed in a left or right lateral or lithotomy position.

RECURRENT ABSCESSES AND FISTULAS

Unless there is an unusual appearance to the abscess, or unusual appearance or consistency of the pus, the author often does not obtain cultures. The presence of enteric organisms when culturing perirectal abscesses does not indicate the presence of a fistula. When initially treated for perirectal abscess, the patient should be informed that the abscess may recur. If it recurs, then a fistula is probably present, and will require definitive surgery. Fistulas represent a chronic anorectal disease, and recurring anorectal abscesses are an acute expression of the presence of a fistula (Gordon 2007). Recurrent abscesses occur when persistent fistular tracts are overlooked, abscesses are incompletely or only partially drained, or there is inflammation of extra-anal origin such as with hidradenitis suppurativa or pilonidal disease. Three-quarters of patients with recurrent perirectal abscesses have persistent fistula(s), with a third of these having had previous surgery (Chrabot et al. 1983). Of these patients with previous drainage, two-thirds have an undiagnosed fistula, and a third a missed fistula component. The incidence of a persistent fistula after initial abscess drainage varies from 35 to 95% in various series (Killingback 1988). In looking for the internal fistula opening associated with a perirectal abscess, the Goodsall rule applies (**Figure 7.3**). For abscesses or external fistula openings on the posterior half of the anal circumference, the internal opening is likely to be in the posterior midline, with a curved fistula tract, whereas, for those abscesses and external fistula

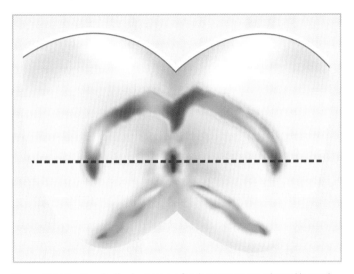

Figure 7.3 The Goodsall rule: Anterior fistula tracts are straight and located radial to the external opening, and posterior fistula tracts are curved and with internal opening at the posterior midline.

openings on the anterior half of the anal circumference, the internal opening will be located on the external opening with a linear fistula tract. One exception to this is the horseshoe abscess or fistula, which is discussed later. Anterior abscesses may be extensions originating from an internal fistula opening in the posterior midline. Although the definitive treatment of fistulas is beyond the scope of this chapter, several important points are pertinent to their management:

- One should err on the side of conservatism.
- As the puborectalis muscle is a sling extending from the symphysis and surrounding the rectum posteriorly and laterally, there is no puborectalis anteriorly and therefore less muscle mass. More caution and conservatism should therefore be exercised when treating anterior fistulas.
- Primary fistulotomy should not be performed when the involved part of the anal sphincter is more than 1 cm wide or thick. In these cases, a "delayed" fistulotomy is performed using a "seton." This seton may be a no. 2 silk suture, or the author's preference, a vessel loop or a 3/8 inch Penrose drain. The seton is passed through the fistula tract and tied tightly, or tied using silk suture when the Penrose drain is used. This results in local ischemia of the involved anal sphincter with subsequent necrosis. Two weeks later when the patient is seen in the office, the seton, now loose, is again tightened. This tightening does cause significant discomfort, and oral pain medications are routinely prescribed. This same process is repeated until the sphincter muscle has been divided and the seton has fallen out. In slowly dividing the muscle in this manner, the seton causes a foreign body reaction and scarring, which in turn results in the ends of the divided sphincter muscle being scarred or fixed in place with maintenance of good continence. This differs from the "snapping apart" of the sphincter like an elastic band, which occurs if the muscle is divided primarily, and could result in impaired continence.

Most primary fistula openings are posterior or anterior in the anal canal. There is a higher density of anal crypts in the posterior half of the anus (Marti 1990). Lateral location and increased number of fistula openings are related to increasing fistula complexity. Sigmoidoscopy can differentiate between anal canal and rectal fistula openings. In 355 patients undergoing abscess drainage, an internal fistula opening was identified in a third, whereas, in another study of 232 patients, fistulas developed in two-thirds (Scoma et al. 1974, Ramanujam et al. 1984).

Fistulography may be useful in patients with suspected complex fistulas and those with fistulas with high or supralevator extensions, and also in patients with recurrent fistulas. However, routine fistulography is generally not helpful (Kuijpers and Schulpen 1985).

Injection of hydrogen peroxide into external fistula openings may be helpful in demonstrating internal fistula openings. Methylene blue causes significant discoloration of adjacent tissue and is therefore less useful.

■ Special considerations

Although drainage of perianal and ischiorectal abscesses is relatively straightforward, other types of abscesses may require special treatment.

Intersphincteric abscesses

Intersphincteric abscesses are an important cause of persistent undiagnosed anal pain, which is often aggravated by defecation. Swelling may not occur with this type of abscess, and there may be no external sign of infection. Abscesses may drain spontaneously before the patient is seen, and examination under anesthesia may be required before a diagnosis can be made. All patients with an intersphincteric abscess have a fistula (Chrabot et al. 1983).

Submucosal abscess

A high intermuscular or submucosal abscess is a variant of an intersphincteric abscess. It may rupture directly into the rectum. Transrectal unroofing of the abscess is usually sufficient.

Supralevator abscess

Before definitive treatment of a supralevator abscess, one must first determine the origin of the fistula, and whether it represents an upward extension of an intersphincteric abscess, an ischiorectal abscess, or an extension of pelvic inflammation such as Crohn disease, diverticulitis, or appendicitis.

- If the abscess is secondary to upward extension of an intersphincteric abscess, it should be drained into the rectum by dividing the involved internal sphincter (Gordon 2007). Drainage through the ischiorectal space should be avoided because this will convert the process into a supralevator fistula.
- If the abscess has occurred as an extension of an ischiorectal abscess, it should be drained through the ischiorectal space, because drainage through the rectum would create an extrasphincteric fistula (Gordon 2007).
- With abscesses originating from pelvic sources, drainage can be achieved transrectally, through the ischiorectal space or through the abdominal wall (i.e., CT-guided drainage). If there is an opening in the levator muscle through which pus is draining, it can be widened to facilitate drainage, and a drain placed to ensure adequate drainage. Treatment of the pelvic source of the abscess is required in nearly all patients.

Horseshoe abscess

The tethering effect of the anococcygeal ligament may prevent posterior infections or abscesses (postanal space abscesses) from posterior extension. These infections may extend anteriorly and laterally to either or both sides of the perianal area to form a "horseshoe" abscess. This is explained by the fact that purulence generally spreads along the path of least resistance. Knowledge of this type of extension of posterior infections is essential for proper treatment. Horseshoe abscesses can occur at three levels: Intersphincteric, ischiorectal, and supralevator, of which the second is the most common.

Posterior drainage should be performed, possibly with delayed fistulotomy and counter-incisions for anterolateral extensions (Hanley 1965) (**Figure 7.4**).

Postoperative care

Wounds from drained abscesses heal by secondary intention, which generally proceeds over 2–3 weeks. Sitz baths taken three to four times daily for 10–15 min in very warm water will ease incisional discomfort as well as maintain proper perianal hygiene. Patients are also instructed to take a laxative such as milk of magnesia twice daily until they have their first bowel movement after the drainage procedure. This counteracts both the constipation secondary to opiate pain medications and that due to apprehension about having a bowel movement after anorectal surgery. Patients are also advised to take a psyllium or methylcellulose product to soften the consistency of their bowel movements to decrease both pain and potential bleeding. Patients are seen 1 week after abscess drainage, and then biweekly until the wound has closed. If exuberant granulation tissue is present, topical treatment with silver nitrate sticks may speed healing.

Massive perineal infection and soft-tissue necrosis

Crepitation or necrosis of the overlying skin with or without systemic sepsis may be a sign of infection with a gas-forming organism. Many fatal perianal infections have been reported (Abcarian et al. 1983, Di Falco et al. 1986, Morpurgo et al. 2001). Delay in diagnosis, inadequate initial treatment, and the presence of associated diseases contribute to the morbidity and mortality after massive soft-tissue sepsis in the perianal area. Extensive infection of this type occurs in <1% of patients with anorectal infections (Morpurgo et al. 2001). Conditions frequently associated with extensive soft-tissue sepsis and necrosis include diabetes mellitus, blood dyscrasias, organic heart disease, chronic renal failure, hemorrhoids, previous abscesses or fistulas, and anal trauma (Abcarian et al. 1983). Symptoms that

may herald such massive infection include tachycardia, fever, hypotension, and crepitus or necrosis of the overlying skin (**Figure 7.5a**). Severe pain is typically the first symptom. In some patients, soft-tissue gas can also be seen on conventional radiographs. Treatment of choice in these patients is prompt drainage and debridement (**Figure 7.5b**) and proper systemic antibiotics. Radical debridement and drainage must be performed as soon as possible, especially in the presence of gas-forming organisms. Appropriate systemic antibiotic treatment is essential. In some reports, *Escherichia coli* is the most frequently cultured organism, whereas others report predominantly *Clostridium* spp. (Morpurgo et al. 2001). These infections may spread from the supralevator space to the pre-peritoneal space, or alternatively extend to the perirectal soft tissue with necrosis of skin, subcutaneous tissue, or muscle. As the testicles receive their blood supply from the spermatic vessels, they are not usually necrotic and can be banked in an abdominal wall or thigh "pocket" if surrounding tissue is debrided. The mortality rate for this type of infection can be as high as 40%. Repeated examination and debridement as necessary are important.

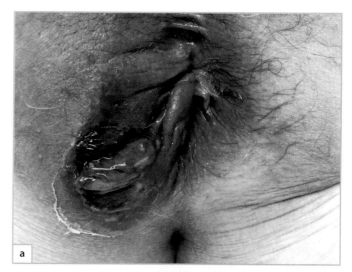

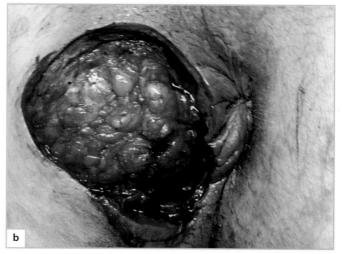

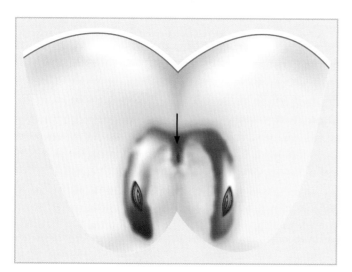

Figure 7.4 Technique of counter-incision for horseshoe abscess, with or without simultaneous treatment of posterior internal fistula opening (arrow).

Figure 7.5 Perirectal abscess with necrotizing infection in a patient with type 1 diabetes. (a) Preoperatively and (b) after wide excision.

Crohn disease

If unusual disease is encountered in terms of the number of abscesses present, extent of the abscess(es), or unusual location, then skin margins or granulation tissue or both should be sent for histological examination to see whether there is evidence of Crohn disease or any other unusual pathology. Perirectal abscesses in patients with Crohn disease may be more difficult diagnoses than in other patients. Many abscesses in these patients have already drained spontaneously at the time of first presentation, and present as fistulas. Complex fistulas with atypical location of the external fistula opening are more common in this group of patients. Although abscesses and fistulas in patients with Crohn disease may have a cryptoglandular origin, they more commonly originate from perforated fissures or ulcers that are visible by proctoscopy. Anal stricture secondary to Crohn disease may also complicate diagnosis of this condition (Galandiuk et al. 2005). There is a tendency for the wounds of patients with Crohn disease to heal poorly. Metronidazole may be especially helpful in these patients because of its immmunosuppressive effect. In some patients, diagnosis may be aided by the use of endorectal ultrasonography (Law et al. 1989). Some of these patients may ultimately require proctectomy for their disease. Abscesses should be drained, but great caution exercised in treating fistulas.

Leukemic and granulocytopenic patients

Perianal sepsis may be fatal in patients with leukemia and is treated differently from that in "normal" patients. In severely granulocytopenic patients, pus may not form and there may be diffuse infiltration, and induration without fluctuation. In such immunocompromised patients, digital or sigmoidoscopic manipulation may lead to bacteremia and should be avoided. These patients should be treated aggressively with intravenous antibiotics. Sitz baths and analgesics should be used accordingly. Perianal infections in patients with leukemia are associated with a 45–78% mortality rate (Barnes et al. 1984). Although there is controversy over whether to aggressively perform drainage in these patients, or to treat them only with intravenous antibiotics, one study suggested that fewer postoperative complications occurred in these patients if the granulocyte count was >1000/mm^3 (Barnes et al. 1984, Shaked et al. 1986, Carlson et al. 1988). Candidates most suitable for surgical treatment are leukemia patients in remission and those with chronic forms of leukemia. Surgery should be reserved for those who do not respond to conservative therapy and in whom there is palpable fluctuance (North et al. 1996). Attention should also be paid to the platelet count, and transfusions given as needed should surgery be necessary.

HIV-positive and AIDS patients

HIV-positive and AIDS patients may also present with perirectal abscess or sepsis. In one study, the frequency of anorectal symptoms was 32% in HIV-positive patients, 43% in HIV-symptomatic patients, and 25% in AIDS patients (Miles et al. 1990). In that study, the incidence of hospital admission due to anorectal disease was 14 times higher in HIV-positive homosexual and bisexual men than in the general male population. In one report, 80% of perianal wounds in HIV-symptomatic patients did not heal within 30 days postoperatively, with a 16% rate of major complications (Wexner et al. 1986). In that series, perirectal abscess was present in 16 of 51 HIV-positive patients requiring anorectal surgery. Condylomata acuminata are often present and can even spread to the healing abscess drainage site. These patients may also have diarrhea from colitis due to cytomegalovirus or other infectious pathogens, which may further impair wound healing. Due to the high rate of non-healing of these wounds, conservatism is advised in dealing with these patients. A patient with a CD4 lymphocyte count <200 or a clinical AIDS patient has higher morbidity rates than those who are HIV positive but under control (Moenning et al. 1991). In the current era of highly active antiretroviral therapy (HAART), most HIV-positive individuals have low viral loads and normal wound healing (Horberg et al. 2006, Nadal et al. 2008). They can largely be treated without special considerations other than contact precautions.

PILONIDAL ABSCESS

Pilonidal disease is a relatively simple yet frequently frustrating problem that is characterized by its likelihood to recur. It most frequently occurs in young men who are hirsute, but can also occur in women. There are three different types of buttock contour: those individuals who have a relatively deep buttock cleft and individuals with a relatively sloping buttock cleft – more common among women; and the intermediate type (Nivatvongs et al. 1983). Pilonidal disease is more common among the first type, where there is more friction between the buttocks during walking and daily activities, and hair in this area can be driven back down the hair follicle and result in an abscess or infected cyst within the hair follicle itself. Examination of individuals with pilonidal disease will usually reveal the presence of "pilonidal pits," a frequent diagnostic sign (**Figure 7.6**).

Traditionally, treatments for pilonidal disease have involved either local office procedures designed to temporize by draining infected fluid collections, or more definitive treatments in the operating room aimed at complete excision of the infection. The latter can be divided into procedures in which the wound is left open for closure by secondary intention, or closed primarily. Procedures in which the wound is closed primarily are further divided into those with closure in the midline and those closed off midline. In all cases of operative excision, complete removal of the infected material with excision of infected collections, which often extend down to the presacral fascia, is of paramount importance. Excision and allowing these wounds to

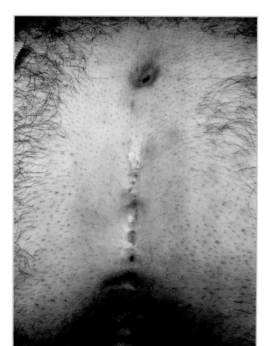

Figure 7.6 Chronic pilonidal abscess. Note the multiple draining pilonidal pits in the natal cleft and hirsute nature of the patient.

close secondarily or "marsupializing" them (i.e., suturing the edges of the wound down to the fascia and allowing secondary closure) is a very slow process. As a result of the same friction on the buttock crease, as mentioned earlier, while walking or doing normal daily activities, these wounds are notoriously hard to heal. In addition, the posterior location of the wounds means that it is always difficult for patients to care for it themselves, often leading patients to enlist the aid of a family member or nursing help to help with weekly shaving or depilation of hair and dressing changes. Simple sitz baths with an antibacterial soap may be helpful. Negative pressure dressings have also been used to help hasten wound healing albeit at significant cost. Despite the longer time to heal and need to do dressing changes, a recent Cochrane study did show that open healing reduces the risk of recurrence by 35% when compared with any closed method (Al-Khamis et al. 2010). Primary incision and closure of pilonidal abscesses with midline incisions have been associated with a significant surgical site infection rate and subsequent healing by secondary intention.

High surgical site infection rates with primary closure has led to the development of alternative approaches using an "off-midline" incision. One approach that has led to reports of the highest degree of healing has been the concept of excision of the contributing hair follicles and lateral placement of the incision, as advocated by Bascom (1983) (**Figure 7.7**). In that early report of 161 patients with a mean 3.5-year follow-up, his mean time to healing was 3 weeks, with 17% of patients returning with complaints of drainage of recurrent disease requiring intervention. With this technique, an incision is made just lateral to the midline, and the incision is angled downward toward the midline where the infected abscess is excised, including excision of the pilonidal pits, which through a modification can easily be excised using a skin-punch biopsy. The pits can then be closed primarily, as is the lateral incision. If patients come with a primarily infected pilonidal cyst, lateral drainage in the office also permits a future lateral excision and facilitates the delayed definitive procedure. There are numerous variations for treating chronic pilonidal sinus that are beyond the scope of this chapter. Suffice it to say that the aforementioned Cochrane review (Al-Khamis et al. 2010) provides evidence that midline compared with "off-midline" procedures are associated with higher rates of surgical site infection (relative risk = 3.72, 95% confidence interval 1.86–7.42) as well as higher recurrence rates (Peto odds ratio 4.54, 95% confidence interval 2.30–8.96).

Regardless of which way the pilonidal disease is approached, frequent office follow-up is required to insure that the wound stays hair free. As this often occurs in hirsute individuals, failure to keep the vicinity of the wound free of hair can lead to a prompt persistence or recurrence of the problem, as this is the source of the problem in the first place. Hair growing into the wound also contributes to non-healing.

In cases in which patients have had multiple prior procedures or there are persistent wounds, flap procedures may be desirable. The goal of these procedures is to provide additional soft-tissue coverage to the wound while also "obliterating" or flattening the contour and "indentation" of the buttock cleft. Numerous flap procedures have been proposed, including a rhomboid flap (Limberg flap), Z-plasty, and others (Mentes et al. 2008, Ates et al. 2011). The rhomboid flap is a relatively simple procedure that provides for excision of the wound with a minimal tissue rotation (**Figure 7.8**). Because of the vascularity of these wounds, I favor placement of a suction drain for a short time if such procedures are performed and especially in obese patients.

After surgery for pilonidal disease, recurrence rates of 7% and higher are observed (Al-Khamis et al. 20101). Flap procedures are generally *not* performed for initial treatment of pilonidal disease and, without proper follow-up, such procedures can be associated with intrinsic wound healing complications.

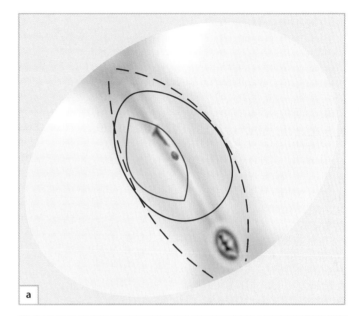

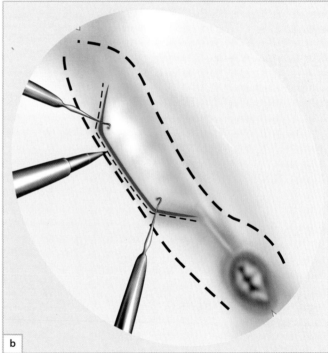

Figure 7.7 **(a) The ellipse of skin to be removed is marked in red.** The area to be mobilized as a full-thickness skin flap is outlined in blue. (With permission from Bascom and Bascom (2002).) (b) Fit of the flap from the right is checked before the flap from the left is cut away. Marking is designed for a cleft floor that is shallower and less tense and for a suture line near the surface. (Redrawn with permission from Bascom and Bascom 2002; © 2002, American Medical Association. All rights reserved.)

▪ CONCLUSIONS

Treatment of perirectal abscesses is based on prompt drainage and recognition. An abscess is the acute form and a fistula is the chronic form of anorectal infection. Sound knowledge of pelvic floor anatomy should allow the clinician to identify and properly treat abscesses in this area. Although they can be confused by aberrant locations, pilonidal infections are quite different from perirectal abscesses and fistulas.

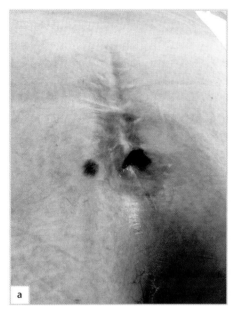
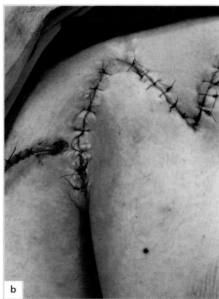
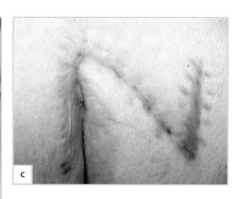

Figure 7.8 (a) Chronic pilonidal abscess after midline incision in 17-year-old girl. Chronic drainage kept her from attending school for over 1 year. (b) Chronic abscess excised and treated by Limberg (rhomboid flap) with delayed healing of left suture line 4 months postoperatively. (c) Healed flap 6 months postoperatively

■ REFERENCES

Abcarian H, Eftaiha M. Floating free-standing anus: A complication of massive anorectal infection. *Dis Colon Rectum* 1983;**26**:516–21.

Al-Khamis A, McCallum I, King PM, Bruce J. Healing by primary versus secondary intention after surgical treatment for pilonidal sinus. *Cochrane Database Syst Rev* 2010;(**1**):CD006213.

Ates M, Dirican A, Sarac M, Aslan A, Colak C. Short and long-term results of the Karydakis flap versus the Limberg flap for treating pilonidal sinus disease: a prospective randomized study. *Am J Surg* 2011;**202**:568–73.

Barnes SG, Sattler FR, Ballard JO. Perirectal infections in acute leukemia: improved survival after incision and debridement. *Ann Intern Med* 1984;**100**: 515–18.

Bascom J. Pilonidal disease: long-term results of follicle removal. *Dis Colon Rectum* 1983;**26**:800–7.

Bascom J, Bascom T. Failed pilonidal surgery: new paradigm and new operation leading to cures. *Arch Surg* 2002;**137**:1146–50

Carlson GW, Ferguson CM, Amerson JR. Perianal infections in acute leukemia: second place winner. Conrad-Jobst Award. *Am Surg* 1988;**54**: 693–5.

Chrabot CM, Prasad MI, Abcarian H. Recurrent anorectal abscesses. *Dis Colon Rectum* 1983;**26**:105–8.

Di Falco G, Guccione C, D'Annibale A, et al. Fournier's gangrene following a perianal abscess. *Dis Colon Rectum* 1986;**29**:582–5.

Galandiuk S, Kimberling J, Al-Mishlab TG, Stromberg AJ. Perianal Crohn disease: predictors of need for permanent diversion. *Ann Surg* 2005;**241**:796–801.

Goligher J, Duthie H, Nixon H. Anorectal abscess. In: Goligher JC (ed), *Surgery of the Anus, Rectum and Colon*, 5th edn. London: Baillière Tindall, 1984: 167–77.

Gordon PH. Anorectal abscesses and fistula-in-ano. In: Gordon PH, Nivatvongs S (eds), *Principles and Practice of Surgery of the Colon, Rectum and Anus*, 3rd edn. New York: Informa Healthcare USA, 2007: 192–230.

Hanley PH. Conservative surgical correction of horseshoe abscess and fistula. *Dis Colon Rectum* 1965;**8**:364–8.

Horberg MA, Hurley LB, Klein DB, et al. Surgical outcomes in human immunodeficiency virus-infected patients in the era of highly active antiretroviral therapy. *Arch Surg* 2006;**141**:1238–45.

Killingback M. Anal fissure and fistula with special reference to high fistula. In: Decosse JJ, Todd IP (eds), *Anorectal Surgery*. London: Churchill Livingstone, 1988: 56–92.

Kuijpers HC, Schulpen T. Fistulography for fistula-in-ano. Is it useful? *Dis Colon Rectum* 1985;**28**:103–4.

Law PJ, Talbot RW, Bartram CI, Northover JM. Anal endosonography in the evaluation of perianal sepsis and fistula in ano. *Br J Surg* 1989;**76**:752–5.

Lockhart-Mummery JP. Discussion on fistula-in-ano. *Proc R Soc Med* 1929;**22**:1331–58.

McElwain JW, MacLean MD, Alexander RM, et al. Anorectal problems: Experience with primary fistulectomy for anorectal abscess, a report of 1000 cases. *Dis Colon Rectum* 1975;**18**: 646–9.

Malik AI, Nelson RL, Tou S. Incision and drainage of perianal abscess with or without treatment of anal fistula (Review). *Cochrane Database Syst Rev* 2010;(**7**):CD006827.

Marti MC. Anorectal abscesses and fistulas. In: Marti MC, Givel JC (eds), *Surgery of Anorectal Diseases*. Berlin: Springer, 1990: 84–98.

Mentes O, Bagci M, Bilgin T, Ozgul O, Ozdemir M. Limberg flap procedure for pilonidal sinus disease: results of 353 patients. *Langenbeck's Arch Surg* 2008;**393**:185–9.

Miles AJG, Mellor CH, Gazzard B, et al. Surgical management of anorectal disease in HIV-positive homosexuals. *Br J Surg* 1990;**77**: 869–71.

Moenning S, Huber P, Simonton C, et al. Prediction of morbidity by T4 lymphocyte count in the HIV positive or AIDS anorectal outpatient. *Dis Colon Rectum* 1991;**34**:17.

Morpurgo E, Galandiuk S. Fournier's gangrene. *Surg Clin North Am* 2001;**82**:1213–24.

Nadal SR, Manzione CR, Couto Horta SH. Comparison of perianal diseases in HIV-positive patients during periods before and after protease inhibitors use. What changed in the 21st century? *Dis Colon Rect* 2008;**51**:1491–4.

Nivatvongs S, Fang DT, Kennedy HL. The shape of the buttocks: a useful guide for selection of anesthesia and patient position in anorectal surgery. *Dis Colon Rect* 1983;**26**: 85–6.

North JH Jr, Weber TK, Rodriguez-Bigas MA, Meropol NJ, Petrelli NJ. The management of infectious and noninfectious anorectal complications in patients with leukemia. *J Am Coll Surg* 1996;**183**:322–8.

Parks AG. Pathogenesis and treatment of fistula-in-ano. *BMJ* 1961;**i**:463–9.

Ramanujam PS, Prasad MI, Abcarian H, Tan AB. Perianal abscesses and fistulas: a study of 1023 patients. *Dis Colon Rectum* 1984;**27**:593–7.

Read DR, Abcarian H. A prospective survey of 474 patients with anorectal abscess. *Dis Colon Rectum* 1979;**22**: 566–8.

Scoma JA, Salvati EP, Rubin RJ. Incidence of fistulas subsequent to anal abscesses. *Dis Colon Rectum* 1974;**17**: 357–9.

Shaked AA, Shinar E, Freund H. Managing the granulocytopenic patient with acute perianal inflammatory disease. *Am J Surg* 1986;**152**:510–12.

Vasilevsky CA, Gordon PA. The incidence of recurrent abscess or fistula-in-ano following anorectal suppuration. *Dis Colon Rectum* 1984;**27**:126–30.

Wexner SD, Smithy WB, Milsom JW, et al. The surgical management of anorectal diseases in AIDS and pre-AIDS patients. *Dis Colon Rectum* 1986;**29**:719–23.

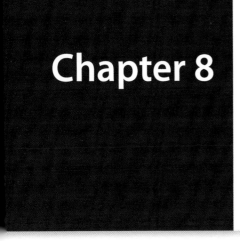

Chapter 8

Hospital-acquired and ventilator-associated pneumonia

Philip S. Barie

Hospital-acquired pneumonia (HAP) occurs by definition more than 48 h after hospitalization, and is commonplace among surgical patients. Most cases of HAP develop during mechanical ventilation, and are thus termed "ventilator-associated pneumonia" (VAP), which comprises nearly a third of all intensive care unit (ICU) infections (Chastre and Fagon 2002, Rello et al. 2002) (**Figure 8.1**). The incidence of VAP varies markedly in published reports, depending on the diagnostic criteria used. Clinical criteria alone (e.g., those of the US Centers for Disease Control and Prevention [CDC], which do not require the identification of a pathogen) overestimate the incidence of VAP compared with either microbiological or histological data (Meduri et al. 1994, Fagon et al. 2000). In a systematic review of 89 studies in which the incidence of VAP was reported among mechanically ventilated patients, the authors reported a pooled incidence of VAP of 22.8% (95% confidence interval [CI] (18.8–26.9%) despite substantial heterogeneity of diagnostic criteria (Safdar et al. 2005). However, the incidence of VAP may be decreasing, although it remains higher in surgical units compared with medical units, and especially so in trauma, burn, and neurosurgical patients. The National Nosocomial Infection Surveillance (NNIS) system reported for 1992–2000 that VAP occurred at a rate of 7.5 cases/1000 ventilator days in medical ICUs and 13.6/1000 ventilator days in surgical ICUs (NNIS 2000). By contrast, NNIS data inclusive of 1992–2004 indicate the rates of VAP to be 3.7 cases/1000 ventilator days in medical ICUs and 8.6/1000 ventilator days in surgical ICUs (Table 8.1) (NNIS 2004). Data from 2006–2008 from the National Healthcare Safety Network (NHSN), the CDC's successor program to NNIS, suggest a further decrease, the rates of VAP being 2.2 cases/1000 ventilator days in medical ICUs and 3.8/1000 ventilator days in surgical ICUs (**Table 8.1**) (Edwards et al. 2009). However, the number of reporting hospitals is much larger in NHSN compared with NNIS.

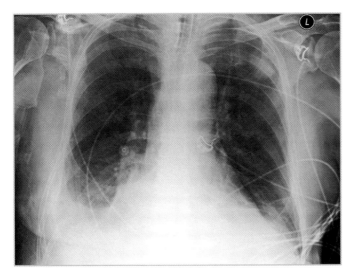

Figure 8,1 A ventilator-associated pneumonia in the right lower lobe in an 87 year old trauma patient. Bronchoalveolar lavage documented methicillin-sensitive *Staphylococcus aureus* which responded to appropriate antibiotic therapy. The patient had an incidental left upper lobe lung lesion identified.

RISK FACTORS

Risk factors for VAP are summarized in **Box 8.1**. Perhaps most important is airway intubation itself, the use of which appears to have decreased only modestly in surgical units despite the availability of techniques for non-invasive positive pressure ventilation (NIPPV) (see Table 8.1). The incidence of VAP varies with the duration of

Table 8.1 Rates of healthcare-associated pneumonia among various intensive care unit (ICU) types

| ICU type | TT use | | VAP rate | Mean/Median |
	1992–2004	2006–2008	1992–2004	2006–2008
Medical	0.46	0.48	4.9/3.7	2.4/2.2
Pediatric	0.39	0.42	2.9/2.3	1.8/0.7
Surgical	0.44	0.39	9.3/8.3	4.9/3.8
Cardiovascular	0.43	0.39	7.2/6.3	3.9/2.6
Neurosurgical	0.39	0.36	11.2/6.2	5.3/4.0
Trauma	0.56	0.57	15.2/11.4	8.1/5.2

Based on data from National Nosocomial Infections Surveillance (NNIS) System Report (2004) and Edwards et al. (2009). Data available at www.cdc.gov.

TT use, number of days of indwelling endotracheal tube or tracheostomy/1000 patient days in ICU; VAP, ventilator-associated pneumonia

Infection rates are indexed per 1000 patient-days.

Box 8.1 Risk factors for ventilator-associated pneumonia.

- Age ≥60 years
- Acute respiratory distress syndrome
- Chronic obstructive pulmonary disease or other underlying pulmonary disease
- Coma or impaired consciousness
- Serum albumin <2.2 g/dl
- Burns, trauma
- Blood transfusion
- Organ failure
- Supine position
- Large-volume gastric aspiration
- Sinusitis
- Immunosuppression

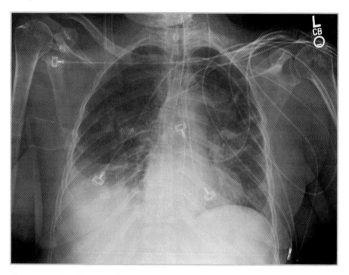

Figure 8.2 A left upper lobe *Pseudomonas aeruginosa* pneumonia confirmed by bronchoalveolar lavage. The right subpulmonic effusion is identified and has been contributed to by this patients extensive abdominal malignancy.

mechanical ventilation (MV), increasing at a rate of 3% per day over the first 5 days, 2% per day over days 5–10, and 1% per day after that (Cook et al. 1998a). The risk of HAP increases 6- to 20-fold in mechanically ventilated patients (Celis et al. 1988, Torres et al. 1990, Chastre and Fagon 2002); patients with respiratory failure managed with NIPPV have a lower incidence of pneumonia (Brochard et al. 1995, Antonelli et al. 1998, Hilbert et al. 2001). VAP is especially common in patients with the acute respiratory distress syndrome (ARDS), owing to prolonged MV and devastated local airway host defenses (Chastre et al. 1998, Markowicz et al. 2000).

Whether VAP is an independent risk factor for mortality is controversial (Barie 2000). Most recent series have reported a crude mortality rate in patients with VAP of 9–27% (CDC 2000, Rello et al. 2002, Kollef 2006), although rates can exceed 75% in high-risk patients infected with multidrug-resistant (MDR) organisms (Craven et al. 1986, Chastre et al. 1998). Attribution of mortality in patients with VAP has been problematic because they are systemically more ill compared with non-VAP patients. Several authors have addressed this issue with a matched cohort study design. Heyland et al. (1999) matched 177 patients who developed VAP to controls by age, admission diagnosis, location before the ICU, and admission Acute Physiology and Chronic Health Evaluation (APACHE) II score. Patients with VAP had a longer ICU length of stay (LOS), but no increase in mortality (23.7% vs 17.7%, *p* = 0.19). Furthermore, attributable mortality was highest for patients infected with high-risk MDR organisms, defined as meticillin-resistant *Staphylococcus aureus* (MRSA), *Pseudomonas aeruginosa, Acinetobacter baumannii*, and *Stenotrophomonas maltophilia* (**Figure 8.2**). However, appropriate initial empirical therapy may mitigate adverse outcomes (Kollef et al. 2000). Hugonnet et al. (2004) matched patients with and without VAP by age, severity of illness, and duration of MV before the development of VAP. Compared with non-VAP patients, patients with VAP had an increased ICU LOS, prolonged duration of MV, and higher ICU cost, but not mortality (32.0% vs 24.7%, *p* = 0.26). However, when these and other matched-cohort studies were pooled by meta-analysis, patients with VAP were more than twice as likely to die compared with those without VAP (odds ratio [OR] 2.03, 95% CI 1.16–3.56, *p* = 0.03), and incurred both a longer ICU LOS and a mean increased ICU cost of $10 019 (Safdar et al. 2005).

Using a competing risk survival analysis, treating ICU discharge as a competing risk for ICU mortality, in a marginal structural modeling approach to adjust for time-varying confounding by disease severity, Bekaert et al. (2011) studied 685/4479 (15.3%) patients from the longitudinal prospective (1997–2008) French multicenter outcome database, who acquired at least one episode of VAP. Patients were included if they stayed in the ICU for at least 2 days and received MV within 48 h of ICU admission. It was estimated that 4.4% (95% CI, 1.6–7.0%) of the deaths in the ICU by day 30 and 5.9% (95% CI 2.5–9.1%) by day 60 were attributable to VAP. With an observed ICU mortality rate of 23.3% on day 30 and 25.6% on day 60, the ICU mortality rate attributable to VAP was about 1% by day 30 and 1.5% by day 60.

Noting that the attributable ICU mortality of VAP may be modest, Tseng et al. (2012) examined risk factors associated independently with mortality from VAP in a study of 163 patients. Variables examined were the Sequential Organ Failure Assessment (SOFA) score, APACHE-II scores, oxygenation index, underlying comorbidities (Charlson Comorbidity Index), septic shock status, tracheostomy status, and microbiology. Of 163 patients 92 survived. Multivariable logistic regression analysis identified that a pre-existing Charlson Comorbidity Index score (*p* = 0.011), initial oxygenation index (*p* = 0.025), SOFA score (*p* = 0.043), VAP caused by *Acinetobacter baumannii* (*p* = 0.030), and infection with MDR pathogens (*p* = 0.003) were independent risk factors for hospital mortality in patients with VAP. However, the small number of deaths decreases the statistical power, variables related to antibiotic choice, timing, and duration were not examined, and it is unclear how many surgical patients comprised the study population.

■ PATHOGENESIS

Both impaired host immunity and displacement of normal oropharyngeal flora by pathogens predispose the critically ill, mechanically ventilated patient to VAP. Normal non-specific host defenses, such as the epiglottis, vocal cords, cough reflex, and ciliated epithelium and mucus of the upper airways, are either bypassed or rendered ineffective by airway intubation. Bacteria gain access to the lower respiratory tract via aspiration through the endotracheal tube (where they may establish colonies impervious to the effects of antibiotics in the glycocalyx biofilm that coats the lumen of artificial airway devices) (Wilson et al. 2012), migration around it (particularly if cuff inflation pressure is not maintained) (Zolfaghari and Wyncoll 2011, Ramirez et al. 2012), or, in rare instances, hematogenous spread from bloodstream infections (usually when the host is neutropenic) (Fujitani et al. 2011). Displacement of normal flora by pathogens is also necessary for the development of VAP (Johanson et al. 1969, 1972, Bonten et al. 1996). Both the facial sinuses and stomach may serve as potential pathogen reservoirs, but measures to minimize passage of pathogens from these sources into the lower airways have provided mixed results.

Due to indiscriminant use of broad-spectrum antibiotics, MDR pathogens are implicated increasingly in VAP (Garnacho-Montero 2003, Neuhauser et al. 2003, Hidron et al. 2008, Kallen et al. 2010). Recently (2006–7), the most common pathogens isolated from patients with VAP have been *S. aureus* (24%, most of which are MRSA), *Pseudomonas* spp. (16%, of which about 40% are MDR), *Enterobacter* spp. (8%), *Actnetobacter* spp. (8%; half are MDR), *Klebsiella* spp. (7%, of which about 15% are MDR), and *Escherichia coli* (5%) (Hidron et al. 2008, Kallen et al. 2010). Infection with MRSA is particularly common in patients with diabetes mellitus and after traumatic brain injury (Lowy 1998, Fridkin 2001, Fry and Barie 2011). *P. aeruginosa*, the most common Gram-negative pathogen in VAP, is increasingly common with an MDR phenotype, especially to fluoroquinolones (Neuheuser et al. 2003, Scheld 2003) third-generation cephalosporins (NNIS 2003), and increasingly to carbapenems (Apisarnthanarak and Mundy 2010).

Anaerobic bacteria are isolated infrequently from patients with VAP, although this finding may represent an inability to culture these organisms effectively from the oxygen-enriched environment of the mechanically ventilated airway (Marik and Careau 1999). Although isolation of fungi such as *Candida* spp. and *Aspergillus fumigatus* from endotracheal aspirates is common, it nearly always represents colonization of the immunocompetent host (Loo et al. 1996, El-Ebiary et al. 1997), with *Candida* spp. estimated to cause VAP in only about 2% of cases (Hidron et al. 2008). However, when fungi are isolated from two or more normally sterile sites (e.g., urine and lower respiratory tract) in an immunocompromised patient, systemic antifungal therapy should be considered (Pappas et al. 2009).

■ PREVENTION

It has been estimated that up to 55% of cases of VAP may be preventable using current evidence-based tactics (Umscheid et al. 2011). Prevention of VAP requires a thorough understanding of modifiable risk factors. Strict infection control, including hand hygiene with alcohol-based hand disinfectants, gowning, and gloving, minimizes person-to-person transmission of pathogens and is paramount to deterring all ICU infections (Pittet et al. 2000, Girou et al. 2002). Prevention of VAP begins with minimization of endotracheal intubation and the duration of MV. Non-invasive PPV should always be considered instead of intubation, because there is a lower incidence of VAP (Brochard et al. 1995, Antonelli et al. 1998, Hilbert et al. 2001, Girou et al. 2003). Evidence-based strategies to decrease the duration of MV include daily interruption of sedation (Kress et al. 2000), standardized weaning protocols (Rice et al. 2012), and adequate ICU staffing (Marelich et al. 2000).

Technological improvements in endotracheal tube design may decrease the risk of VAP. Improved design of the balloon cuff, to decrease longitudinal folding of standard high-volume, low-pressure polyvinyl chloride cuffs, through which aspirated secretions may gain access to the lower airway, by improving the seal between cuff and mucosa may decrease the risk of VAP from the microaspirations that are ubiquitous in the ICU (Nseir et al. 2011, Zolfaghari and Wyncoll 2011). Coating the endotracheal tube with an antibacterial silver alloy was successful in decreasing the incidence of VAP and delaying its onset in a randomized trial (Kollef et al. 2008). If endotracheal intubation is required, orotracheal intubation may decrease the risk of developing VAP compared with the nasotracheal route. Holzapfel et al. (1993) found that the incidence of VAP in patients who were randomized to orotracheal intubation was only half that of patients intubated nasotracheally (6% vs 11%). Considering this and the association between nasotracheal intubation and the development of nosocomial sinusitis (Rouby et al. 1994), orotracheal intubation is preferred.

Once intubation has occurred, most standard preventive measures against VAP aim to decrease the risk of aspiration (Pieracci and Barie 2007, Ramirez et al. 2012). Evidence indicates that semirecumbent positioning (30–45° head-up) is protective, compared with supine positioning, especially during enteral feeding (Torres et al. 1992, Orozco-Levy et al. 1995, Draculovic et al. 1999). Both maintenance of endotracheal cuff pressure >20 cmH$_2$O (Cook et al. 1998b, Nseir et al. 2011), and continuous aspiration of subglottic secretions achieved through the use of an endotracheal tube equipped with an additional lumen above the balloon, reduce the incidence of VAP. In a systematic review of 13 randomized trials (2442 patients), 12 reported a reduction in VAP rates associated with subglottic secretion drainage arm; by meta-analysis, the hazard ratio for VAP was 0.55 (95% CI, 0.46–0.66; p <0.00001). The use of subglottic secretion drainage was also associated with reduced ICU LOS, decreased duration of MV, and increased time to first episode of VAP. There was no effect on mortality (Muscedere et al. 2011).

Compared with postpyloric feeding, intragastric feeding results in more episodes of both gastroesophageal reflux and aspiration (Torres et al. 1992). However, randomized controlled trials (RCTs) comparing rates of VAP have produced variable results (Orozco-Levy et al. 1995, Draculovic et al. 1999). Heyland et al. (2001) performed a meta-analysis of 11 RCTs and reported a relative risk (RR) of 0.77 (95% CI 0.60–1.00, p = 0.05) for VAP with postpyloric compared with gastric feedings. Based on these data, most expert recommendations do not differentiate between gastric and postpyloric feeding (Kearns et al. 2000, Montejo et al. 2000, Heyland et al. 2001). Pro-motility agents such as erythromycin may facilitate safe intragastric feeding should this route be used (Berne et al. 2002). The timing of onset of enteral feedings may also influence the risk of developing VAP. Initiation of enteral feeding on day 1 compared with day 5 resulted in significantly more episodes of VAP (49.3% vs 30.7%, p = 0.02) and a longer ICU LOS in one prospective trial of 150 patients (Ibrahim et al. 2002). More recently, Shorr et al. (2004) reported that enteral nutrition begun ≤48 h after the initiation of MV was independently associated with the development of VAP (odds ratio [OR] 2.65, 95% CI 1.93–3.63, p <0.0001).

Pharmacological strategies intended to minimize the risk of aspiration of pathogenic bacteria include selective decontamination of the digestive tract (SDD) with either topical or systemic antibiotics or antiseptics, and minimization of prophylaxis against stress ulcer. Myriad clinical trials have addressed SDD which, on balance, show a significant decrease in the incidence of VAP (Reed 2011). However, enthusiasm for use of SDD has been limited by questionable study methodology (van Nieuwenhoven et al. 2001), use of narrow patient subsets from ICUs in which MDR pathogens were rare (de Smet et al. 2012), and an increased number of infections caused by MDR pathogens observed after SSD (Misset et al. 1994, Lingnau et al. 1998). For these reasons, SDD is currently not used widely for the routine prevention of VAP.

Alternatively, oropharyngeal decontamination can be accomplished with a topical antiseptic, such as chlorhexidine. A systematic review and meta-analysis of 14 studies (2481 patients), 12 of which investigated the effect of chlorhexidine (2341 patients) and 2 that evaluated povidone–iodine (140 patients), found that antiseptic use resulted in a significant reduction in the risk of VAP (RR 0.67; 95% CI 0.50–0.88; $p = 0.004$). Chlorhexidine application was effective (RR 0.72; 95% CI 0.55–0.94; $p = 0.02$), whereas the analysis of povidone–iodine was underpowered. Favorable effects were more pronounced in subgroup analyses for 2% chlorhexidine (RR 0.53, 95% CI 0.31–0.91), and in cardiothoracic surgical studies (RR 0.41, 95% CI 0.17–0.98) (Labeau et al. 2011).

Prophylaxis of stress-related gastric mucosal hemorrhage is a known risk factor for the development of VAP (Bonten et al. 1996, 1997a); its use should be reserved for patients at high risk for hemorrhage (e.g., prolonged MV, intracranial hemorrhage, coagulopathy, glucocorticoid therapy). RCTs comparing histamine H_2-receptor antagonists, sucralfate, and antacids have yielded conflicting results (Bonten et al. 1994, 1995, Cook et al. 1998c); no agent is preferred for prophylaxis based solely on efficacy for prevention of VAP.

Ample data document the relationship between blood transfusion and infection risk in surgical (Ottino et al. 1987, Braga et al. 1992), trauma (Claridge et al. 2002, Hill et al. 2003, Robinson et al. 2005), and critically ill patients (Taylor et al. 2002). Shorr et al. (2004) found red blood cell transfusion to be independently associated with the development of VAP (OR 1.89, 95% CI 1.33–2.68, $p = 0.0004$). Earley et al. (2006) documented a decreased incidence of VAP in a surgical ICU after implementation of an anemia management protocol. After implementation of the protocol, fewer blood transfusions were administered despite equivalent outcomes, and the incidence of VAP decreased from 8.1% to 0.8% ($p = 0.002$).

Several antibiotic administration strategies, including "de-escalation" and antibiotic rotation or "cycling," have been suggested to prevent VAP caused by MDR pathogens. De-escalation refers to the process of tailoring empirical broad-spectrum antimicrobial coverage to specific pathogens once microbiologic data from lower respiratory tract samples become available. Discontinuation of unnecessary antibiotics at this point curtails not only the emergence of MDR organisms, but also the risk of drug toxicity. Antibiotic cycling offers the potential for antibiotic classes to be used on a scheduled basis to preserve overall activity against predominant pathogens (Fridkin and Gaynes 1999, Carlet et al. 2004). Several prospective trials have documented improved microbial ecology (Barie et al. 2005, Dortch et al. 2011), decreased incidence of VAP (Kollef et al. 1997, Gruson et al. 2003), improved initial adequacy of therapy (Kollef et al. 2000), and decreased mortality (Raymond et al. 2001) after the implementation of scheduled antibiotic rotation. However, these studies have been limited by the use of historical controls, and thus possible confounding by other changes in care. Other data have challenged the efficacy of antibiotic cycling (van Loon et al. 2005). Pending further research, cycling of antibiotics may be considered if multiple classes of antibiotics are cycled frequently together with other tactics to prevent the emergence of MDR pathogens (Kollef et al. 2006).

Education of staff concerning modifiable risk factors may be cost-effective in preventing VAP. Zazk et al. (2002) demonstrated that an education program administered to respiratory care practitioners and intensive care nurses which highlighted correct practices for the prevention of VAP resulted in a significantly decreased incidence of VAP and increased cost savings.

Tracheostomy

Timing of tracheostomy remains controversial. Proponents argue that patient comfort and pulmonary toilet are improved, the risk of glottic injury and post-extubation swallowing dysfunction is decreased

(Bordon et al. 2011), and the incidence of VAP is lower. Wang et al. (2011) conducted a meta-analysis, the objective of which was to review systematically and synthesize all randomized trials to compare important outcomes in mechanically ventilated, critically ill patients who received an "early" (e.g., ≤7 days of translaryngeal intubation) or "late" tracheostomy (any time thereafter). Seven trials (1044 patients) were analyzed. Early tracheostomy for critically ill patients did not reduce short-term mortality (RR 0.86, 95% CI 0.65–1.13), long-term mortality (RR 0.84, 95% CI 0.68–1.04), or the incidence of VAP (RR 0.94, 95% CI 0.77–1.15) The timing of tracheostomy was not associated with a reduced duration of MV (weighted mean difference [WMD] -3.90 days, 95% CI -9.71 to 1.91) or sedation (WMD -7.09 days, 95% CI, -14.64 to 0.45), a shorter stay in the ICU (WMD -6.93 days, 95% CI -16.50 to 2.63) or hospital (WMD 1.45 days, 95% CI -5.31 to 8.22), or more complications (RR 0.94, 95% CI 0.66–1.34).

■ DIAGNOSIS

The goals in diagnosing VAP are to determine whether the patient has pneumonia, and the etiological pathogen. Poor specificity is particularly problematic in the diagnosis of VAP because it not only exposes individual patients to unnecessary risk from overtreatment with antibiotics, but also increases selection pressure and thus the emergence of MDR bacteria within the ICU (Neuhauser et al. 2003, Niederman 2003, Pieracci and Barie 2007). Conversely, inadequate initial therapy in patients with VAP (poor sensitivity) has been associated consistently with increased mortality that cannot be reduced by subsequent changes in antibiotics (Alvarez-Lerma 1996). The diagnosis of VAP should be considered in the presence of one or more of the following: Fever, leukocytosis or leukopenia, purulent sputum, hypoxemia, or a new or evolving infiltrate viewed on chest radiograph. However, several non-infectious respiratory disease processes may mimic these signs, such as congestive heart failure, atelectasis, pulmonary thromboembolism, pulmonary hemorrhage, and ARDS (Rangel-Frausto 1995, Barie et al. 2005), making clinical criteria alone nonspecific (**Figure 8.3**). Fabregas et al. (1999) found the presence of a new infiltrate on chest radiograph, along with two of the three aforementioned clinical criteria, to be 69% sensitive and 75% specific for the diagnosis of VAP when compared with postmortem histology. Several subsequent reports have confirmed the low specificity of clinical acumen in the diagnosis of VAP (Baughman 2003, Mabie and Wunderink 2003), and clinically diagnosed VAP is confirmed microbiologically in fewer than 50% of cases (Rodriguez de Castro et al. 1996, Fagon et al. 2000).

Pugin et al. (1991) standardized clinical, radiographic, and microbiological criteria into the Clinical Pulmonary Infection Score (CPIS). Temperature, leukocyte count, chest radiograph infiltrates, the appearance and volume of tracheal secretions, $PaO_2{:}FiO_2$ (ratio of partial arterial O_2 pressure to fraction of inspired O_2), and culture and Gram stain of tracheal aspirate (0–2 points each) yield a maximum CPIS score of 12 points; a score of >6 points indicates a high probability of VAP. Despite favorable test performance of the CPIS in its initial description, and its subsequent modification to include radiological progression of pulmonary infiltrates (Singh et al. 2000), the specificity of CPIS is no better than clinical acumen alone when compared with lower respiratory tract cultures obtained via bronchoscopic brochoalveolar lavage (BAL) or protected specimen brush (PSB) (Fartoukh et al. 2003, Luyt et al. 2004, Veinstein et al. 2006). Croce et al. (2006) have argued that the CPIS has no probative value for trauma patients. The NNIS diagnostic criteria for nosocomial pneumonia (CDC 2012), which include similar combinations of clinical and radiographic parameters, perform equivalently to the CPIS when compared with quantitative

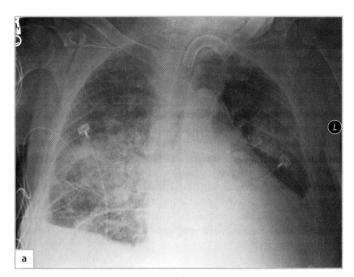

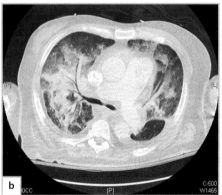

Figure 8.3 (a) An aggressive *Enterobacter* spp bilateral pneumonia. (b) A chest CT scan of the patient in (a), identifying the severe compromise of ventilating units within the lung.

lower respiratory tract cultures (Miller et al. 2006). Incorporation of Gram stain results into the CPIS improves specificity only marginally (Fartoukh et al. 2003). However, the negative predictive value of a negative Gram stain in a clinically stable patient approaches 100% (Blot et al. 2000).

As a result of the low specificity of clinical signs, radiographic criteria, and microscopic examination of lower respiratory tract samples, culture of lower respiratory tract samples before any manipulation of antibiotics is mandatory for workup of a suspected VAP to minimize false-negative results. Two questions are debated: The method of specimen collection (invasive vs non-invasive), and the method of specimen analysis (semi-quantitative vs quantitative). Non-invasive techniques include sampling of the lower respiratory tract via endotracheal aspirate (EA), blinded plugged telescoping catheter (PTC), blinded PSB, and mini-BAL. EAs are less specific due to both an increased likelihood of contamination by oropharyngeal flora (indicated by the presence of squamous epithelial cells on Gram stain) and an increased likelihood that the presence of organisms indicates colonization rather than infection.

Invasive techniques (BAL or PSB) collect lower respiratory tract samples usually by fiberoptic bronchoscopy, but non-bronchoscopic "blind" techniques have been described. The main theoretical advantage of bronchoscopy is direct visualization of the airways. However, invasive techniques are more expensive and resource intensive than their non-invasive counterparts, and may not be readily available. Although bronchoscopy is generally well tolerated, a reduction in SaO_2 (arterial O_2 saturation) may be observed for up to 24 h afterward, possibly related to alveolar flooding caused by residual lavage fluid.

However, this transient desaturation is of unclear importance, not having been correlated with poorer outcomes (Torres and Mustafa 2000).

Irrespective of collection method, respiratory tract cultures may be analyzed using either semiquantitative or quantitative microbiology. The crucial issue is distinction of colonization from infection (Niederman 1990). Whereas semiquantitative microbiology reports growth in terms of ordinal categories (e.g., light, moderate, or heavy), quantitative microbiology reports growth in number of colony-forming units (CFU)/ml of aliquot. In the latter case, a threshold value is selected to distinguish colonization from infection. Commonly used thresholds are 10^3 CFU/ml for PSB, 10^4 CFU/ml for BAL, and 10^5 CFU/ml for EA, lowered by one order of magnitude if antibiotics have been changed recently or started before sample acquisition (American Thoracic Society 2005).

Endotracheal aspirates possess inferior specificity when compared with both blinded PTC (Vidaur et al. 2005) and bronchoscopic BAL or PSB (Sanchez-Nieto et al. 1998, Wu et al. 2002, Elatrous et al. 2004, Brun-Buisson et al. 2005). Two systematic reviews, one of bronchoscopic BAL (Torres and Mustafa 2000) and one of blinded invasive techniques (Campbell 2000), reported similar test characteristics for the two techniques. However, methodological variability is widespread. Of 23 studies 16 (70%) in the former review used histology as a reference standard, compared with only 4 of 15 studies (27%) analyzed in the latter review. Furthermore, the remainder of studies analyzed in the review of blinded invasive techniques used either bronchoscopic BAL or PSB as the reference category. Both reviews reported substantial interstudy variability in sampling technique as well as threshold values. A recent study reported that, compared with a reference standard of bronchoscopic BAL (threshold 10^4 CFU/ml), blinded PTC was 77% sensitive and 94% specific (Sanchez-Nieto et al. 1998). Thus, despite the limitations, it is likely that bronchoscopic techniques are more specific than blinded techniques, and that either technique is superior to EA.

Evidence-based recommendations for the diagnosis of VAP have been difficult to formulate because trials have compared various permutations of collection and analytical methodology, threshold values, and reference categories. The largest randomized trial of this type compared an invasive, quantitative approach with a non-invasive, semiquantitative approach (Fagon et al. 2000). A total of 413 patients suspected of having VAP were randomized to evaluation with either bronchoscopic BAL or PSB with quantitative cultures, or "clinical" management consisting of semiquantitative analysis of EAs. Antibiotic therapy was discontinued in clinically stable patients with negative culture results, regardless of the study arm. Compared with the clinical strategy, patients in the invasive group demonstrated decreased 14-day mortality rates (16% vs 25%, $p = 0.02$), less antibiotic use (11.9 vs 7.7 antibiotic-free days), decreased sepsis-related organ failure, and decreased 28-day mortality after adjustment for severity of illness. The clinical strategy also resulted in more and broader-spectrum antibiotic therapy compared with the invasive strategy, and increased emergence of fungi. It is unclear whether these improved outcomes resulted from the use of an invasive versus a non-invasive sputum collection strategy, or a quantitative versus a semiquantitative analysis strategy.

Two randomized trials have compared outcomes of patients with suspected VAP managed with an invasive versus a non-invasive approach when both samples were cultured quantitatively. Sanchez-Nieto et al. (1998) randomized 51 patients with suspected VAP to EA versus bronchoscopic BAL or PSB. Initial antibiotic therapy was modified in a significantly higher percentage of patients with invasive compared with non-invasive approaches (42% vs 16%, $p < 0.05$), but there was no difference in severity-adjusted mortality, ICU LOS, or duration of

MV. Ruiz et al. (2002) randomized 76 patients with suspected VAP to EA versus bronchoscopic BAL or PSB, and found no difference in incidence of antibiotic modification, duration of MV, ICU LOS, or crude or adjusted mortality. In both studies, antibiotics were continued in all patients with negative cultures.

Shorr et al. (2005) performed a meta-analysis of the aforementioned trials comparing EA (either quantitative or semiquantitative) with bronchoscopic quantitative cultures. There was no survival advantage to the invasive approach, but patients diagnosed invasively were more likely to undergo changes in antimicrobial regimen.

Samples obtained via bronchoscopic BAL or PSB and then analyzed quantitatively have the highest specificity in diagnosing VAP. Reported outcomes in patients managed with an invasive versus a "clinical" strategy are conflicting. Several trials demonstrate that patients so managed are also more likely to undergo antibiotic changes. Trials rebutting the use of the invasive/quantitative strategy are limited because patients with negative cultures continued to receive antibiotics, which negates the putative benefit (the ability to discontinue antimicrobial therapy). This last point is important because the value of invasive, quantitative specimens lies not with the decision to initiate therapy (these cultures will not become available for 48–72 h), but rather with either de-escalation or discontinuation of antibiotic therapy when appropriate.

Ventilator-associated tracheobronchitis

A controversial new entity, ventilator-associated tracheobronchitis (VAT) has been described (Craven and Hjalmarson 2011). Progression of colonization to VAT and, in some patients, to VAP is related to the quantity, types, and virulence of invading bacteria versus containment by host defenses. Diagnostic criteria for VAT and VAP overlap in terms of clinical signs and symptoms, and they share similar microbiological criteria when endotracheal sputum aspirate samples are used. In addition, the diagnosis of VAP requires a new, persistent radiographic infiltrate, which may be difficult to assess in critically ill patients, as well as a positive bacterial culture of an EA or BAL specimen. The weak link in the diagnosis of VAT (and VAP) is arguably the requirement for no new or changing radiographic infiltrate for VAT. Multiple studies have documented the inaccuracy of routine radiographic interpretation (Wunderink 2000). At least 30% of infiltrates in the lower lobes found by chest computed tomography (CT) are missed by portable supine chest radiographs. Conversely, multiple other causes of new or changing radiographic infiltrates may cause the misdiagnosis of VAT as VAP, or sterile inflammation as infection.

Contention has arisen because of mandated public reporting of hospital-acquired infections and the potential that VAP will be added to the list of infections reported as a quality standard to measure hospital safety (Wunderink 2011). Reports from multiple hospitals of VAP rates of zero for prolonged periods may be achievable by greater attention to prevention tactics, but are inherently dubious. Aside from the fact that VAP rates that are very low or zero or are not well documented, said low rates have not been associated with corresponding decreases in antibiotic use or mortality. Is the reporting system being manipulated to avoid the diagnosis of VAP, while continuing to treat patients using antibiotics suitable for VAP?

Dallas et al. (2011) examined the questions of the veracity and importance of VAT in a small epidemiological study of 28 patients with VAT and 83 with VAP (incidence, 1.4% and 4.0%, respectively). Although VAP was more common in surgical than medical ICU patients (5.3% vs 2.3%, p <0.001), as expected, the occurrence of VAT was similar (1.3% vs 1.5%, p = 0.845). Progression of VAT to VAP was

observed in nine patients (32.1%) despite antibiotic therapy. There was no difference in hospital mortality rates between patients with VAP and VAT (19.3% vs 21.4%, p = 0.789). The VAT entity always prolonged the duration of MV. The pathogens associated with VAT were often MDR, including MRSA, *P. aeruginosa*, and other non-fermenting Gram-negative bacteria, but the *Enterobacteriaceae* were significantly less likely to cause VAT than VAP. Dallas et al. also documented that the prevalence of VAT is much less frequent than that of VAP (3.2/1000 vs 9.4/1000 ventilator days).

Despite VAT likely being a real entity, possibly being an intermediate step between colonization and VAP, every aspect of its diagnosis is problematic. Diagnostic criteria are all of the standard criteria for VAP except the criterion of radiographic infiltrate. The outcome for VAT may be increased tracheal secretions; alternatively, worsening oxygenation is less likely to occur with VAT, which may help distinguish it from VAP.

Systemic antibiotics have an unclear benefit in VAT. They do appear to be a risk factor for the development of VAT. Lack of antibiotic treatment of VAT is associated with an increased risk of subsequent VAP and prolonged MV, but systemic antibiotics do not appear to prevent progression consistently. Aerosolized antibiotics might be the ideal treatment of VAT, but data are lacking.

TREATMENT

Neither the decision to treat nor the choice of agent involves interpretation of lower respiratory tract cultures, which do not become available for 48–72 h. Rather, the treatment decision is based on clinical suspicion and Gram stain. Choice of agent is based on both individual patient risk factors for infection with MDR organisms and data from institutional (ideally unit specific) antibiograms (Barie 2012). Most data indicate that antimicrobial therapy may be withheld safely if (1) a Gram-stained lower respiratory tract sample reveals no organisms and (2) the patient does not have severe sepsis (Croce et al. 1995, Ibrahim et al. 2001, Iregui et al. 2002, Kollef et al. 2005). Clinical signs of infection along with a negative Gram stain suggest either an extrapulmonary source of infection or sterile inflammation (e.g., intracranial hemorrhage) (Barie et al. 2005). It is crucial when treating VAP to administer "adequate therapy," meaning at least one antimicrobial agent to which the pathogen is sensitive, in the correct dose, via the correct route of administration, and in a timely manner. A second crucial aspect of VAP therapy involves serial re-evaluation and interpretation of initial microbiology so that: (1) Therapy may be discontinued if no organism is isolated and the patient has not deteriorated clinically; (2) therapy is de-escalated to treat only the specific etiological pathogen; and (3) an endpoint of therapy may be identified and adhered to in prospect.

There are ample data detailing the increased mortality associated with inadequate initial antimicrobial therapy in patients with VAP. Iregui et al. (2002) showed that delayed therapy (defined as initial antibiotic treatment administered ≥24 h after meeting diagnostic criteria for VAP) was independently associated with hospital mortality (OR 7.68, 95% CI 4.50–13.09, p <0.001). The mean difference in time to antibiotic administration between groups was 16 h. Similarly, Kollef et al. (2000) reported that inadequate initial antimicrobial therapy was an independent risk factor for ICU mortality in patients with Gram-negative infections (OR 4.22, 95% CI 3.57–4.98, p <0.001). Alvarez-Lerma et al. (1996) demonstrated that attributable mortality from VAP was significantly lower among patients receiving initial appropriate antibiotic treatment compared with receipt of inappropriate treatment (16.2% vs 24.7%; p = 0.03). The essential nature of appropriate initial therapy is underscored by the fact that Alvarez-Lerma et al. demonstrated that switching to appropriate therapy once culture results became available did not ameliorate the excess mortality associated with inadequate initial therapy.

Choice of initial antimicrobial therapy depends on patient risk factors for MDR pathogens (**Box 8.2**) and local microbiological data that may be obtained from the unit-specific antibiogram. Having a current and frequently updated antibiogram increases the likelihood that appropriate initial antibiotic treatment will be prescribed (Rello et al. 1999, Gruson et al. 2000, Ibrahim et al. 2001). In general, therapy for patients at risk for infection with an MDR organism should provide coverage against MRSA, *P. aeruginosa*, and extended-spectrum b-lactamase-producing Klebsiella spp. and *Escherichia coli*. This will likely require at least two drugs, one effective against MRSA (e.g., vancomycin or linezolid) and one effective against MDR Gram-negative bacilli, particularly *Pseudomonas* spp. (e.g., meropenem). Empirical therapy against *A. baumannii* may be indicated, depending on the patient and the microbial ecology of the unit. Patients with early onset VAP (occurring <5 days after intubation) and none of the aforementioned risk factors may be candidates for narrower-spectrum therapy. Trauma patients, who tend to develop VAP sooner than critically ill surgical patients, may also be candidates for narrower-spectrum therapy of earlier episodes of VAP (Becher et al. 2011).

Box 8.2 Risk factors for ventilator-associated pneumonia (VAP) with multidrug-resistant organisms.

- Late-onset VAP (occurring ≥5 days after intubation)
- Antibiotics within previous 90 days
- Hospitalization within previous 90 days
- Current hospitalization >5 days
- Admission from a long-term care/hemodialysis facility
- High frequency of antibiotic resistance in the community
- Immunosuppressive disease or therapy

Antimicrobial therapy for VAP should be administered initially via the intravenous (IV) route. Enteral therapy may be considered if patients demonstrate an adequate response to IV therapy, gastrointestinal function is normal, and the antibiotics used possess high bioavailability when administered orally or enterally. Linezolid and fluoroquinolones have oral bioavailability adequate to the task (Paladino 1995). Aerosolized antibiotics are theoretically attractive to optimize pulmonary antibiotic concentrations. Limited data suggest that addition of aerosolized aminoglycosides or colistin to intravenous therapy may improve response rates in patients with MDR organisms or refractory pneumonia. Adverse events can occur, especially with colistin. Aerosolized antibiotics administered by conventional nebulizer therapy may not achieve standardized droplet size or complete dispersal within the lower airways, to ensure tolerability and good drug delivery, so further research into the use and delivery of aerosolized antibiotics is needed (Wood 2011, Arnold et al. 2012, Florescu et al. 2012).

Inadequate dosing of antibiotics leads to the emergence of MDR bacteria and is associated with poorer outcomes in VAP (Guillermot et al. 1998). Appropriate initial dosing of vancomycin (15 mg/kg every 12 h) and aminoglycosides (gentamicin or tobramycin 7 mg/kg once daily; amikacin 20 mg/kg once daily) is necessary to achieve high peak: MIC (minimum inhibitory concentration) to optimize bacterial killing; although single daily dose aminoglycoside therapy has not been associated with increased toxicity, the higher doses of vancomycin necessary to achieve recommended trough concentrations of 1–20 µg/ml have been associated with an increased risk of nephrotoxicity (Cano et al. 2012). Increasing resistance to fluoroquinolones (levofloxacin 750 mg/day, ciprofloxacin 400 mg every 8 h) makes their empirical use increasingly dubious (Neuhauser et al. 2003, Nseir et al. 2005).

Certain points regarding specific antibiotics warrant further discussion. Most notably, linezolid has emerged as an effective alternative therapy for VAP caused by Gram-positive bacteria, and MRSA in particular. Linezolid is theoretically appealing for the treatment of VAP because achievable concentrations in bronchial secretions exceed those in serum, dose adjustment is not needed for renal insufficiency, and enteral administration has equivalent bioavailability. However, a meta-analysis of linezolid versus glycopeptide (vancomycin or teicoplanin) for the treatment of nosocomial pneumonia suggests equivalent efficacy and, perhaps surprisingly, more adverse events with linezolid therapy (Kalil et al. 2010). Nine trials (vancomycin [n = 7], teicoplanin [n = 2]) were included (2329 patients). The RR for clinical cure was 1.01 (95% CI, 0.93–1.10; p = 0.83), and for microbiological eradication, 1.10 (95% CI 0.98–1.22, p = 0.10). Subgroup analysis for MRSA yielded an RR for microbiological eradication of 1.10 (95% CI 0.87–1.38, p = 0.44). Comparing linezolid only with vancomycin, the RR for clinical cure was 1.00 (95% CI 0.90–1.12), for microbiological eradication 1.07 (95% CI 0.90–1.26, p = 0.45), and for MRSA 1.05 (95% CI 0.82–1.33, p = 0.71). No differences were observed for all-cause mortality (RR 0.95, 95% CI 0.76–1.18, p = 0.63) or acute kidney injury (RR 0.89, 95% CI 0.56–1.43, p = 0.64), but risks of thrombocytopenia (RR 1.93, 95% CI 1.30–2.87, p = 0.001) and gastrointestinal events (RR 2.02. 95% CI 1.10–3.70, p = 0.02) were higher with linezolid.

Abundant data document the association between prior fluoroquinolone use and the emergence of VAP caused by MDR pathogens, particularly MRSA and Pseudomonas spp. (Trouillet et al. 2002, Nseir et al. 2005) (**Figure 8.4**). Fluoroquinolone use in the treatment of VAP should therefore be judicious, probably not for empirical use, but rather part of a program of de-escalation based on institutional antibiograms that are updated frequently. Whereas multidrug therapy against MRSA and *P. aeruginosa* is necessary to achieve adequate initial empirical coverage in patients with suspected VAP until culture results become available, combination therapy directed against a specific pathogen (e.g., "double-coverage" of *Pseudomonas* spp., meaning three antibiotics initially) is controversial. Proponents (usually of a b-lactam agent plus an aminoglycoside) argue that the high risk of an MDR Gram-negative bacillus as the etiological agent requires two drugs to maximize the possibility that at least one will provide coverage. Detractors point to a lack of evidence of benefit, increased risk of toxicity, and possibly increased mortality (Kett et al. 2011). Neither in vitro nor in vivo synergy of such Gram-negative combination therapy has been demonstrated consistently (Hilf et al. 1989, Fowler et al. 2003). A meta-analysis of all trials of b-lactam monotherapy versus b-lactam–aminoglycoside combination therapy for immunocompetent patients with sepsis, including 64 trials and 7586 patients, found no difference in either mortality (RR 0.90, 95% CI 0.77–1.06) or the development of resistance (Paul et al. 2004). In fact, clinical failure was more common with combination therapy, as was acute kidney injury.

After initiation of adequate antimicrobial therapy for suspected VAP, results of lower respiratory tract cultures may reveal: (1) No growth or insignificant growth (below the predetermined threshold value); (2) meaningful (above threshold) growth of a pathogen sensitive to a narrow-spectrum agent; or (3) growth of a pathogen sensitive only to a broad-spectrum agent. Regarding the first scenario, data indicate that antimicrobial therapy may be discontinued safely as long as the patient has not deteriorated clinically (Croce et al. 1995, Bonten et al. 1997b, Kollef et al. 2005, Shorr et al. 2005). In the second scenario, therapy is de-escalated to a narrow-spectrum agent with activity against the pathogen isolated (Eachempati et al. 2009, Niederman et al. 2011). In the last scenario, the initial broad-spectrum

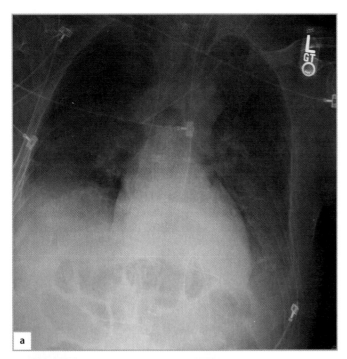

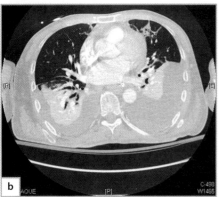

Figure 8.4 (a) A bilateral multidrug resistance *Pseudomonas aeruginosa* pneumonia following subtotal gastrectomy. (b) The bilateral effusions in association with the pneumonia. The left-sided effusion proved to be an empyema treated with chest tube drainage.

agent to which the pathogen is susceptible is continued. The goal of adequate empirical therapy is to initiate a combination of antibiotics likely to cover all possible etiological pathogens, followed by tailored therapy if possible. The ideal treatment of suspected VAP thus involves an initial period of perfect sensitivity followed by a period of perfect specificity, once microbiology results are available. In this fashion, no patient with VAP is untreated, and no patient without VAP is treated after microbiological data are available.

Once pathogen-specific therapy has been initiated, its duration must be determined such that prolonged and unnecessary periods of antibiotic administration are avoided. Resolution of clinical and radiographic parameters typically lags behind the eradication of infection (Luna et al. 2003). Vidaur et al. (2005) found that improved oxygenation and normalization of temperature occurred within 3 days in VAP patients without ARDS. Dennesen et al. (2001) observed a clinical response to therapy of VAP, defined as normalization of temperature, white blood cell count, SaO_2, and quality of tracheal aspirates, within 6 days of therapy.

A randomized, multicenter trial of 401 patients with microbiologically confirmed VAP assigned participants to receive either 8 or 15 days of antibiotic therapy (Chastre et al. 2002). All patients received adequate initial therapy after invasive/quantitative specimen collec-

tion and analysis, and patients whose therapy ended at 8 days were stable clinically at that time. Patients treated for 8 days had equivalent mortality, ICU LOS, duration of MV, and recurrence of infection despite significantly more antibiotic-free days. Recurrent infections were less likely to be caused by MDR pathogens in patients treated for 8 days. However, patients with VAP caused by non-fermenting Gram-negative bacilli (NFGNB, e.g., *P. aeruginosa*, *A. baumannii*, *S. maltophilia*) were more likely to develop recurrent pneumonia if treated for 8 days only. Thus, an 8-day course of initially appropriate antimicrobial therapy appears safe and effective provided that the patient has not deteriorated, especially if the pathogen is not an NFGNB. A recent meta-analysis supports this conclusion (Pugh et al. 2011). Eight studies (1703 patients) were included; few patients with a high probability of HAP were not on MV. For patients with VAP, a short (7.8-day) course of antibiotics compared with a prolonged (10- to 15-day) course increased 28-day antibiotic-free days (OR 4.02, 95% CI 2.26–5.78) and reduced the recurrence of VAP due to MDR organisms (OR 0.44, 95% CI 0.21–0.95), without affecting other outcomes adversely. However, for cases of VAP due to NFGNB, recurrence was greater after short-course therapy (OR 2.18, 95% CI 1.14–4.16). In three studies, discontinuation guided by the serum procalcitonin concentration led to a reduction in duration of therapy and increased 28-day antibiotic-free days (mean difference [MD] 2.80, 95% CI 1.39–4.21) without affecting other outcomes.

In select patients, a shorter course of therapy may be effective for the treatment of VAP. Singh et al. (2000) randomized patients with suspected VAP and a CPIS score ≤6 points to receive either standard therapy (physician discretion) versus ciprofloxacin monotherapy, with re-evaluation at day 3 and discontinuation of antibiotics if the CPIS remained ≤6. If the CPIS remained ≤6 at the 3-day evaluation point, antibiotics were continued in 96% (24/25) of patients in the standard therapy group, but in none of the patients in the experimental therapy group (p = 0.0001). Mortality and ICU LOS did not differ despite a shorter duration (p = 0.0001); cost of antimicrobial therapy was decreased (p = 0.003) in the experimental arm.

Patients treated for VAP who do not improve clinically after appropriate antimicrobial therapy pose a dilemma. Inadequate therapy, misdiagnosis, or a pneumonia-related complication (e.g., empyema or lung abscess) must all be considered. A diagnostic evaluation should be repeated, including quantitative cultures of the lower respiratory tract (using a lower diagnostic threshold given recent antibiotic exposure), and consideration of broadened coverage until new data become available.

The literature suggests a discrepancy between the principles of care discussed herein and contemporary clinical practice. Rello et al. (1997) reported that, in a cohort of 113 patients with VAP, nearly 25% received inadequate initial therapy. In a second cohort study of 398 ICU patients with suspected VAP from 20 ICUs throughout the USA, Kollef et al. (2006) documented more than 100 different antibiotic regimens prescribed as initial therapy of VAP. Furthermore, the mean duration of therapy was 11.8 ± 5.9 days, and in 61.6% of cases there was neither escalation nor de-escalation. The use of standardized treatment protocols can improve substantially the likelihood that adequate therapy is delivered for an appropriate duration. Ibrahim et al. (2001) compared outcomes before and after implementation of a VAP treatment protocol that involved standardized, broad-spectrum initial coverage, with termination after 7 days of absent persistent signs of active infection. The proportions of patients who received inadequate initial therapy and therapy of inappropriate duration were significantly lower in the protocol arm. Several additional studies have confirmed the effectiveness of protocol-driven therapy (Evans et al. 1998, Micek et al. 2004).

REFERENCES

Alvarez-Lerma F. Modification of empiric antibiotic treatment in patients with pneumonia acquired in the intensive care unit: ICU-Acquired Pneumonia Study Group. *Intensive Care Med* 1996;**22**:387–94.

American Thoracic Society: Guidelines for the management of adults with hospital-acquired, ventilator-associated, and healthcare-associated pneumonia. *Am J Respir Crit Care Med* 2005;**171**:388–416.

Antonelli M, Conti G, Rocco M, et al. A comparison of noninvasive positive pressure ventilation and conventional mechanical ventilation in patients with acute respiratory failure. *N Engl J Med* 1998;**339**:429–35.

Apisarnthanarak A, Mundy LM. Use of high-dose 4-hour infusion of doripenem, in combination with fosfomycin, for treatment of carbapenem-resistant *Pseudomonas aeruginosa* pneumonia. *Clin Infect Dis* 2010;**51**:1352–4.

Arnold HM, Sawyer AM, Kollef MH. Use of adjunctive aerosolized antimicrobial therapy in the treatment of *Pseudomonas aeruginosa* and *Acinetobacter baumannii* ventilator-associated pneumonia. *Respir Care* 2012;**40**:186–92.

Barie PS. Importance, morbidity, and mortality of pneumonia in the surgical intensive care unit. *Am J Surg* 2000;**197**:S2–7.

Barie PS. Multidrug-resistant organisms and antibiotic management. *Surg Clin North Am* 2012;**92**:345–91.

Barie PS, Hydo LJ, Shou J, et al. Influence of antibiotic therapy on mortality of critical surgical illness caused or complicated by infection. *Surg Infect (Larchmt)* 2005;**6**:41–54.

Baughman RP. Diagnosis of ventilator-associated pneumonia. *Curr Opin Crit Care* 2003;**95**:397–402.

Becher RD, Hoth JJ, Neff LP, et al. Multidrug-resistant pathogens and pneumonia: comparing the trauma and surgical intensive care units. *Surg Infect (Larchmt)* 2011;**12**:267–72.

Bekaert M, Timsit JF, Vansteelandt S, et al.; Outcomerea Study Group. Attributable mortality of ventilator-associated pneumonia: a reappraisal using causal analysis. *Am J Respir Crit Care Med* 2011;**184**:1133–9.

Berne JD, Norwood SH, McAuley CE, et al. Erythromycin reduces delayed gastric emptying in critically ill trauma patients: a randomized, controlled trial. *J Trauma* 2002;**53**:422–5.

Blot FB, Raynard B, Chachaty E, et al. Value of gram stain examination of lower respiratory tract secretions for early diagnosis of nosocomial pneumonia. *Am J Respir Crit Care Med* 2000;**162**:1731–7.

Bonten MJM, Gaillard CA, van Tiel FH, et al. The stomach is not a source for colonization of the upper respiratory tract and pneumonia in ICU patients. *Chest* 1994;**105**:878–84.

Bonten MJ, Gaillard CA, van der Geest S, et al. The role of intragastric acidity and stress ulcer prophylaxis on colonization and infection in mechanically ventilated ICU patients: A stratified, randomized, double-blind study of sucralfate versus antacids. *Am J Respir Crit Care Med* 1995;**152**:1825–34.

Bonten MJ, Bergmans DC, Ambergen AW, et al. Risk factors for pneumonia, and colonization of respiratory tract and stomach in mechanically ventilated ICU patients. *Am J Respir Crit Care Med* 1996;**154**:1339–46.

Bonten MJ, Gaillard CA, de Leeuw PW, Stobberingh EE. Role of colonization of the upper intestinal tract in the pathogenesis of ventilator-associated pneumonia. *Clin Infect Dis* 1997a;**24**:309–19.

Bonten MJ, Bergmans DC, Stobberingh EE, et al. Implementation of bronchoscopic techniques in the diagnosis of ventilator-associated pneumonia to reduce antibiotic use. *Am J Respir Crit Care Med* 1997b;**156**:1820–4.

Bordon A, Bokhari R, Sperry J, et al. Swallowing dysfunction after prolonged intubation: analysis of risk factors in trauma patients. *Am J Surg* 2011;**202**:679–82.

Braga M, Vignali A, Radaelli G, et al. Association between perioperative blood transfusion and postoperative infection in patients having elective operations for gastrointestinal cancer. *Eur J Surg* 1992;**158**:531–6.

Brochard L, Mancebo J, Wysocki M, et al. Noninvasive ventilation for acute exacerbations of chronic obstructive pulmonary disease. *N Engl J Med* 1995;**333**:817–22.

Brun-Buisson C, Fartoukh M, Lechapt E, et al. Contribution of blinded, protected quantitative specimens to the diagnostic and therapeutic management of ventilator-associated pneumonia. *Chest* 2005;**128**:533–44.

Campbell GD. Blinded invasive diagnostic procedures in ventilator-associated pneumonia. *Chest* 2000;**117**:207S-11S.

Cano EL, Haque NZ, Welch VL, et al. Improving Medicine through Pathway Assessment of Critical Therapy of Hospital-Acquired Pneumonia (IMPACT-HAP) Study Group. Incidence of nephrotoxicity and association with vancomycin use in intensive care unit patients with pneumonia: Retrospective analysis of the IMPACT-HAP Database. *Clin Ther* 2012;**34**:149–57.

Carlet J, Ben Ali A, Chalfine A. Epidemiology and control of antibiotic resistance in the intensive care unit. *Curr Opin Infect Dis* 2004;**17**:309–16.

Celis R, Torres A, Gatell JM, et al. Nosocomial pneumonia: A multivariate analysis of risk and prognosis. *Chest* 1998;**93**:318–24.

Centers for Disease Control and Prevention. Monitoring hospital acquired infections to promote patient safety: United States, 1990–1999. *MMWR* 2000;**49**:149–53.

Centers for Disease Control and Prevention. Definitions for health care-associated infections. www.cdc.gov/ncidod/dhqp/nnis.html. Accessed April 15, 2012.

Chastre J, Fagon J-Y. Ventilator-associated pneumonia. *Am J Respir Crit Care Med* 2002;**165**:867–903.

Chastre J, Trouillet JL, Vuagnat A, et al. Nosocomial pneumonia in patients with acute respiratory distress syndrome. *Am J Respir Crit Care Med* 1998;**157**:1165–72.

Chastre J, Wolff M, Fagon JY, et al. Comparison of 8 vs. 15 days of antibiotic therapy for ventilator-associated pneumonia in adults: A randomized trial. *JAMA* 2002;**290**:2588–98.

Claridge JA, Sawyer RG, Schulman AM, et al. Blood transfusions correlate with infections in trauma patients in a dose-dependent manner. *Am Surg* 2002;**68**:566–72.

Cook DJ, Walter SD, Cook RJ, et al. Incidence and risk factors for ventilator-associated pneumonia in critically ill patients. *Ann Intern Med* 1998a;**129**:433–40.

Cook D, De Jonghe B, Brochard L, Brun-Buisson C. Influence of airway management on ventilator-associated pneumonia: Evidence from randomized trials. *JAMA* 1998b;**279**:781–7.

Cook D, Guyatt G, Marshall J, et al. A comparison of sucralfate and ranitidine for the prevention of upper gastrointestinal bleeding in patients requiring mechanical ventilation. *N Engl J Med* 1998c;**338**:791–7.

Craven DE, Hjalmarson KI. Ventilator-associated tracheobronchitis and pneumonia: Thinking outside the box. *Clin Infect Dis* 2010;**51**(suppl 1):S59–66. Erratum in: *Clin Infect Dis* 2010;**51**:1114.

Craven DE, Kunches LM, Kilinsky V, et al. Risk factors for pneumonia and fatality in patients receiving continuous mechanical ventilation. *Am Rev Respir Dis* 1986;**133**:792–6.

Croce MA, Fabian TC, Schurr MJ, et al. Using bronchoalveolar lavage to distinguish nosocomial pneumonia from systemic inflammatory response syndrome: a prospective analysis. *J Trauma* 1995;**39**:1134–9.

Croce MA, Swanson JM, Magnotti LJ, et al. The futility of the clinical pulmonary infection score in trauma patients. *J Trauma* 2006;**60**:523–7.

Dallas J, Skrupky L, Abebe N, et al. Ventilator-associated tracheobronchitis in a mixed surgical and medical ICU population. *Chest* 2011;**139**:513–18.

Dennesen PJ, van der Ven AJ, Kessels AG, et al. Resolution of infectious parameters after antimicrobial therapy in patients with ventilator-associated pneumonia. *Am J Respir Crit Care Med* 2001;**163**:1371–5.

de Smet AM, Bonten MJ, Kluytmans JA. For whom should we use selective decontamination of the digestive tract? *Curr Opin Infect Dis* 2012;**25**:211–17.

Drakulovic MB, Torres A, Bauer TT, et al. Supine body position as a risk factor for nosocomial pneumonia in mechanically ventilated patients: A randomised trial. *Lancet* 1999;**354**:1851–8.

Dortch MJ, Fleming SB, Kauffmann RM, et al. Infection reduction strategies including antibiotic stewardship protocols in surgical and trauma intensive care units are associated with reduced resistant gram-negative healthcare-associated infections. *Surg Infect (Larchmt)* 2011;**12**:15–25.

Eachempati SR, Hydo LJ, Shou J, Barie PS. Does de-escalation of antibiotic therapy for ventilator-associated pneumonia affect the likelihood of recurrent pneumonia or mortality in critically ill surgical patients? *J Trauma* 2009;**66**:1343–8.

Earley AS, Gracias VH, Haut E, et al. Anemia management program reduces transfusion volumes, incidence of ventilator-associated pneumonia, and cost in trauma patients. *J Trauma* 2006;**61**:1–7.

Edwards JR, Peterson KD, Mu Y, et al. National Healthcare Safety Network (NHSN) report: Data summary for 2006 through 2008, issued December 2009. *Am J Infect Control* 2009;**37**:783–805.

Elatrous S, Boukef R, Besbes LO, et al. Diagnosis of ventilator-associated pneumonia: Agreement between quantitative cultures of endotracheal aspiration and plugged telescoping catheter. *Intensive Care Med* 2004;**30**:853–858.

El-Ebiary M, Torres A, Fabregas N, et al. Significance of the isolation of Candida species from respiratory samples in critically ill, non-neutropenic patients. *Am J Respir Crit Care Med* 1997;**156**:583–90.

Evans RS, Pestotnik SL, Classen DC, et al. A computer-assisted management program for antibiotics and other anti-infective agents. *N Engl J Med* 1998;**338**:232–8.

Fabregas N, Ewig S, Torres A, et al. Clinical diagnosis of ventilatory associated pneumonia revisited: comparative value using immediate post-mortem lung biopsies. *Thorax* 1999;**54**:867–73.

Fagon JY, Chastre J, Wolff M, et al. Invasive and noninvasive strategies for management of suspected ventilator-associated pneumonia. A randomized trial. *Ann Intern Med* 2000;**132**:621–30.

Fartoukh M, Maitre B, Honore S, et al. Diagnosing pneumonia during mechanical ventilation: the clinical pulmonary infection score revisited. *Am J Respir Crit Care Med* 2003;**168**:173–9.

Florescu DF, Qiu F, McCartan MA, et al. What is the efficacy and safety of colistin for the treatment of ventilator-associated pneumonia? A systematic review and meta-regression. *Clin Infect Dis* 2012;**54**:670–80.

Fowler RA, Flavin KE, Barr J, et al. Variability in antibiotic prescribing patterns and outcomes in patients with clinically suspected ventilator-associated pneumonia. *Chest* 2003;**123**:835–44

Fridkin SK. Increasing prevalence of antimicrobial resistance in intensive care units. *Crit Care Med* 2001;**29**:64–8.

Fridkin SK, Gaynes RP. Antimicrobial resistance in intensive care units. *Clin Chest Med* 1999;**20**:303–16

Fry DE, Barie PS. The changing face of *Staphylococcus aureus*: A continuing surgical challenge. *Surg Infect (Larchmt)* 2011;**12**:191–203.

Fujitani S, Sun HY, Yu VL, Weingarten JA. Pneumonia due to *Pseudomonas aeruginosa*: Part I: Epidemiology, clinical diagnosis, and source. *Chest* 2011;**139**:909–19.

Garnacho-Montero J, Ortiz-Leyba C, Jimenez-Jimenez FJ, et al. Treatment of multidrug-resistant Acinetobacter baumannii ventilator-associated pneumonia (VAP) with intravenous colistin: A comparison with imipenem-susceptible VAP. *Clin Infect Dis* 2003;**36**:1111–18.

Girou E, Loyeau S, Legrand P, et al. Efficacy of hand rubbing with alcohol based solution versus standard hand washing with antiseptic soap: Randomized clinical trial. *BMJ* 2002;**325**:362–6.

Girou E, Brun-Buisson C, Taille S, et al. Secular trends in nosocomial infections and mortality associated with noninvasive ventilation in patients with exacerbations of COPD and pulmonary edema. *JAMA* 2003;**290**:2985–91.

Gruson D, Hilbert G, Vargas F, et al. Rotation and restricted use of antibiotics in a medical intensive care unit: impact on the incidence of ventilator-associated pneumonia caused by antibiotic resistant gram-negative bacteria. *Am J Respir Crit Care Med* 2000;**162**: 837–43.

Gruson D, Hilbert G, Vargas F, et al. Strategy of antibiotic rotation: Long term effect on incidence and susceptibilities of gram-negative bacilli responsible for ventilator-associated pneumonia. *Crit Care Med* 2003;**31**:1908–14.

Guillemot D, Carbon C, Balkau B, et al. Low dosage and long treatment duration of β-lactam: Risk factors for carriage of penicillin-resistant *Streptococcus pneumoniae*. *JAMA* 1998;**279**:365–70.

Heyland DK, Cook DJ, Griffith L, et al. The attributable morbidity and mortality of ventilator-associated pneumonia in the critically ill patient. *Am J Respir Crit Care Med* 1999;**159**:1249–56.

Heyland DK, Drover J, MacDonald S, et al. Effect of postpyloric feeding on gastroesophageal regurgitation and pulmonary microaspiration: Results of a randomized controlled trial. *Crit Care Med* 2001;**29**:1495–501.

Hidron AI, Edwards JR, Patel J, et al; National Healthcare Safety Network Team; Participating National Healthcare Safety Network Facilities. NHSN annual update: Antimicrobial-resistant pathogens associated with healthcare-associated infections: annual summary of data reported to the National Healthcare Safety Network at the Centers for Disease Control and Prevention, 2006–2007. *Infect Control Hosp Epidemiol* 2008;**29**:996–1011. Erratum in: *Infect Control Hosp Epidemiol* 2009;**30**:107.

Hilbert G, Gruson D, Vargas F, et al. Noninvasive ventilation in immunosuppressed patients with pulmonary infiltrates, fever, and acute respiratory failure. *N Engl J Med* 2001;**344**:817–22.

Hilf M, Yu VL, Sharp J, et al. Antibiotic therapy for Pseudomonas aeruginosa bacteremia: Outcome correlations in a prospective study of 200 patients. *Am J Med* 1989;**87**:540–6.

Hill GE, Frawley WH, Griffith KE, et al. Allogeneic blood transfusion increases the risk of postoperative bacterial infection: a meta-analysis. *J Trauma* 2003;**54**:908–914.

Holzapfel L, Chevret S, Madinier G, et al. Influence of long-term oro-or nasotracheal intubation on nosocomial maxillary sinusitis and pneumonia: Results of a prospective, randomized trial. *Crit Care Med* 1993;**21**:1132–8.

Hugonnet S, Eggiman P, Borst F, et al. Impact of ventilator-associated pneumonia on resource utilization and patient outcome. *Infect Control Hosp Epidemiol* 2004;**25**:1090–6.

Ibrahim EH, Ward S, Sherman G, et al. Experience with a clinical guideline for the treatment of ventilator associated pneumonia. *Crit Care Med* 2001;**29**:1109115.

Ibrahim EH, Mehringer L, Prentice D, et al. Early versus late enteral feeding of mechanically ventilated patients:results of a clinical trial. *JPEN* 2002;**26**:174–81.

Iregui M, Ward S, Sherman G, et al. Clinical importance of delays in the initiation of appropriate antibiotic treatment for ventilator-associated pneumonia. *Chest* 2002;**122**:262–8.

Johanson WG, Pierce AK, Sanford JP. Changing pharyngeal bacterial flora of hospitalized patients: Emergence of gram negative bacilli. *N Engl J Med* 1969;**281**:1137–40.

Johanson WG, Pierce AK, Sanford JP, et al. Nosocomial respiratory infections with gram-negative bacilli: The significance of colonization of the respiratory tract. *Ann Intern Med* 1972;**77**:701–6.

Kalil AC, Murthy MH, Hermsen ED, et al. Linezolid versus vancomycin or teicoplanin for nosocomial pneumonia: a systematic review and meta-analysis. *Crit Care Med* 2010;**38**:1802–8.

Kallen AJ, Hidron AI, Patel J, Srinivasan A. Multidrug resistance among gram-negative pathogens that caused healthcare-associated infections reported to the National Healthcare Safety Network, 2006–2008. *Infect Control Hosp Epidemiol* 2010;**31**:528–31.

Kearns PJ, Chin D, Mueller L, et al. The incidence of ventilator-associated pneumonia and success in nutrient delivery with gastric versus small intestinal feeding: A randomized clinical trial. *Crit Care Med* 2000;**28**:1742–6.

Kett DH, Cano E, Quartin AA, et al., Improving Medicine through Pathway Assessment of Critical Therapy of Hospital-Acquired Pneumonia (IMPACT-HAP) Investigators. Implementation of guidelines for management of possible multidrug-resistant pneumonia in intensive care: An observational, multicentre cohort study. *Lancet Infect Dis* 2011;**11**:181–9.

Kress J, Pohlman A, O'Connor M, Hall J. Daily interruption of sedative infusions in critically ill patients undergoing mechanical ventilation. *N Engl J Med* 2000;**342**:1471–7.

Kollef MH. Is antibiotic cycling the answer to preventing the mergence of bacterial resistance in the intensive care unit? *Clin Infect Dis* 2006;**43**: S82–8.

Kollef MH, Vlasnik J, Sharpless L, et al. Scheduled rotation of antibiotic classes: A strategy to decrease the incidence of ventilator-associated pneumonia due to antibiotic-resistant gram-negative bacteria. *Am J Respir Crit Care Med* 1997;**156**:1040–8.

Kollef MH, Ward S, Sherman G, et al. Inadequate treatment of nosocomial infections is associated with certain empiric antibiotic choices. *Crit Care Med* 2000;**28**:3456–64.

Kollef MH, Kollef KE. Antibiotic utilization and outcomes for patients with clinically suspected VAP and negative quantitative BAL cultures results. *Chest* 2005;**128**:2706–13.

Kollef MH, Morrow LE, Niederman MS, et al. Clinical characteristics and treatment patterns among patients with ventilator-associated pneumonia. *Chest* 2006;**129**:1210–18.

Kollef MH, Afessa B, Anzueto A, et al., NASCENT Investigation Group. Silver-coated endotracheal tubes and incidence of ventilator-associated pneumonia: the NASCENT randomized trial. *JAMA* 2008;**300**:805–13.

Labeau SO, Van de Vyver K, Brusselaers N, et al. Prevention of ventilator-associated pneumonia with oral antiseptics: a systematic review and meta-analysis. *Lancet Infect Dis* 2011;**11**:845–4.

Lingnau W, Berger J, Javorsky F, et al. Changing bacterial ecology during a five year period of selective intestinal decontamination. *J Hosp Infect* 1998;**39**:195–206.

Loo VG, Bertrand C, Dixon C, et al. Control of construction-associated nosocomial aspergillosis in an antiquated hematology unit. *Infect Control Hosp Epidemiol* 1996;**17**:360–4.

Lowy FD. Staphylococcus infections. *N Engl J Med* 1998;**320**:520–32.

Luna CM, Blanzaco D, Niederman MS, et al. Resolution of ventilator-associated pneumonia: Prospective evaluation of the clinical pulmonary infection score as an early clinical predictor of outcome. *Crit Care Med* 2003;**31**:676–82.

Luyt CE, Chastre J, Fagon J, et al. Value of the clinical pulmonary infection score for the identification and management of ventilator-associated pneumonia. *Intensive Care Med* 2004;**30**:844–52.

Mabie M, Wunderink RG. Use and limitations of clinical and radiologic diagnosis of pneumonia. *Semin Respir Infect* 2003;**18**:72–9.

Marelich GP, Murin S, Battistella F, et al. Protocol weaning of mechanical ventilation in medical and surgical patients by respiratory care practitioners and nurses: effect on weaning time and incidence of ventilator-associated pneumonia. *Chest* 2000;**118**:459–67.

Marik PE, Careau P. The role of anaerobes in patients with ventilator-associated pneumonia and aspiration pneumonia: A prospective study. *Chest* 1999;**115**:178–83.

Markowicz P, Wolff M, Djedaini K, et al. Multicenter prospective study of ventilator-associated pneumonia during acute respiratory distress syndrome. Incidence, prognosis, and risk factors. ARDS Study Group. *Am J Respir Crit Care Med* 2002;**161**:1942–8.

Meduri GU, Mauldin GL, Wunderink RG, et al. Causes of fever and pulmonary densities in patients with clinical manifestations of ventilator-associated pneumonia. *Chest* 1994;**106**:221–35.

Micek ST, Ward S, Fraser V, Kollef M. A randomized controlled trial of an antibiotic discontinuation policy for clinically suspected ventilator-associated pneumonia. *Chest* 2004;**125**:1791–9.

Miller PR, Johnson JC, III, Karchmer T, et al. National nosocomial infection surveillance system: From benchmark to bedside in trauma patients. *J Trauma* 2006;**60**:98–103.

Misset B, Kitzis MD, Conscience G, et al. Mechanisms of failure to decontaminate the gut with polymixin E, gentamycin and amphotericin B in patients in intensive care. *Eur J Clin Microbiol Infect Dis* 1994;**13**:165–70.

Montejo JC, Grau T, Acosta J, et al. Multicenter, prospective, randomized, single-blind study comparing the efficacy and gastrointestinal complications of early jejunal feeding with early gastric feeding in critically ill patients. *Crit Care Med* 2000;**30**:796–800.

Muscedere J, Rewa O, McKechnie K, et al. Subglottic secretion drainage for the prevention of ventilator-associated pneumonia: a systematic review and meta-analysis. *Crit Care Med* 2011;**39**:1985–91.

National Nosocomial Infections Surveillance (NNIS) system report: Data summary from January 1992–April 2000, issued June 2000. *Am J Infect Control* 2000;**28**:429–48.

National Nosocomial Infections Surveillance (NNIS) System Report, data summary from January 1992 through June 2003, issued August 2003. *Am J Infect Control* 2003;**31**:481–98.

National Nosocomial Infections Surveillance (NNIS) System Report, data summary from January 1992 to June 2004, issued October 2004. *Am J Infect Control* 2004;**32**:470–85.

Neuhauser MM, Weinstein RA, Rydman R, et al. Antibiotic resistance among Gram-negative bacilli in US intensive care units: implications for fluoroquinolone use. *JAMA* 2003;**289**:885–8.

Niederman MS. Gram-negative colonization of the respiratory tract: Pathogenesis and clinical consequences. *Semin Respir Infect* 1990;**5**:173–84.

Niederman MS. Appropriate use of antimicrobial agents: Challenges and strategies for improvement. *Crit Care Med* 2003;**31**:608–16.

Niederman MS, Soulountsi V. De-escalation therapy: Is it valuable for the management of ventilator-associated pneumonia? *Clin Chest Med* 2011;**32**:517–34.

Nsier S, Pompeo C, Soubrier S, et al. First-generation fluoroquinolone use and subsequent emergence of multiple drug-resistant bacteria in the intensive care unit. *Crit Care Med* 2005;**33**:283–9.

Nseir S, Zerimech F, Jaillette E, et al. Microaspiration in intubated critically ill patients: Diagnosis and prevention. *Infect Disord Drug Targets* 2011;**11**:413–23.

Orozco-Levi M, Torres A, Ferrer M, et al. Semirecumbent position protects from pulmonary aspiration but not completely from gastroesophageal reflux in mechanically ventilated patients. *Am J Respir Crit Care Med* 1995;**152**:1387–90.

Ottino G, De Paulis R, Pansini S, et al. Major sternal wound infection after open heart surgery: A multivariate analysis of risk factors in 2,579 consecutive procedures. *Ann Thorac Surg* 1987;**44**:173–9.

Paladino JA. Pharmacoeconomic comparison of sequential IV/oral ciprofloxacin versus ceftazidime in the treatment of nosocomial pneumonia. *Can J Hosp Pharm* 1995;**48**:276–83.

Pappas PG, Kauffman CA, Andes D, et al., Infectious Diseases Society of America. Clinical practice guidelines for the management of candidiasis: 2009 update by the Infectious Diseases Society of America. *Clin Infect Dis* 2009;**48**:503–35.

Paul M, Benuri-Silibiger I, Soares-Weiser K, Leibovici L. Beta-lactam monotherapy versus beta-lactam-aminoglycoside combination therapy for sepsis in immunocompetent patients: Systematic review and meta-analysis of randomized trials. *BMJ* 2004;**328**:328–668.

Pieracci FM, Barie PS. Strategies in the prevention and management of ventilator-associated pneumonia. *Am Surg* 2007;**73**:419–32.

Pittet D, Hugonnet S, Harbarth S, et al. Effectiveness of a hospital-wide programme to improve compliance with hand hygiene. *Lancet* 2000;**356**:1307–12.

Pugh R, Grant C, Cooke RP, Dempsey G. Short-course versus prolonged-course antibiotic therapy for hospital-acquired pneumonia in critically ill adults. *Cochrane Database Syst Rev* 2011;**10**:CD007577.

Pugin J, Auckenthaler R, Mili N, et al. Diagnosis of ventilator-associated pneumonia by bacteriologic analysis of bronchoscopic and nonbronchoscopic "blind" bronchoalveloar lavage fluid. *Am Rev Respir Dis* 1991;**143**:1121–9.

Ramirez P, Bassi GL, Torres A. Measures to prevent nosocomial infections during mechanical ventilation. *Curr Opin Crit Care* 2012;**18**:86–92.

Rangel-Frausto MS, Pittet D, Costigan M, et al. The natural history of the systemic inflammatory response syndrome (SIRS). A prospective study. *JAMA* 1995;**273**:117–23.

Raymond DP, Pelletier SJ, Crabtree TD, et al. Impact of a rotating empiric antibiotic schedule on infectious mortality in an intensive care unit. *Crit Care Med* 2001;**29**:1101–8.

Reed RL. Prevention of hospital-acquired infections by selective digestive decontamination. *Surg Infect (Larchmt)* 2011;**12**:221–9.

Rello J, Gallego M, Mariscal D, et al. et al. The value of routine microbial investigation in ventilator-associated pneumonia. *Am J Respir Crit Care Med* 1997;**156**:196–200.

Rello J, Sa-Borges M, Correa H, et al. Variations in etiology of ventilator-associated pneumonia across four treatment Sites. Implications for antimicrobial prescribing practices. *Am J Respir Crit Care Med* 1999;**160**:608–13.

Rello J, Ollendorf DA, Oster G, et al. Epidemiology and outcomes of ventilator-associated pneumonia in a large US database. *Chest* 2002;**122**:2115–21.

Rice TW, Morris S, Tortella BJ, et al. Deviations from evidence-based clinical management guidelines increase mortality in critically injured trauma patients. *Crit Care Med* 2012;**40**:778–86.

Robinson WP 3rd, Ahn J, Stiffler A, et al. Blood transfusion is an independent predictor of increased mortality in nonoperatively managed blunt hepatic and splenic injuries. *J Trauma* 2005;**58**:437–44.

Rodriguez de Castro F, Sole-Violan J, Aranda Leon A, et al. Do quantitative cultures of protected brush specimens modify the initial empirical therapy in ventilated patients with suspected pneumonia? *Eur Respir J* 1996;**9**:37–41.

Rouby JJ, Laurent P, Gosnach M, et al. Risk factors and clinical relevance of nosocomial maxillary sinusitis in the critically ill. *Am J Respir Crit Care Med* 1994;**150**:776–83.

Ruiz M, Torres A, Ewig S, et al. Noninvasive versus invasive microbial investigation in ventilator-associated pneumonia: evaluation of outcome. *Am J Respir Crit Care Med* 2002;**162**:119–25.

Safdar N, Dezfulian C, Collard HR, Saint S. Clinical and economic consequences of ventilator-associated pneumonia: A systematic review. *Crit Care Med* 2005;**33**:2184–93.

Sanchez-Nieto JM, Torres A, Garcia-Cordoba F, et al. Impact of invasive and noninvasive quantitative culture sampling on outcome of ventilator-associated pneumonia. *Am J Respir Crit Care Med* 1998;**157**:371–6.

Scheld WM. Maintaining fluoroquinolone class efficacy: Review of influencing factors. *Emerg Infect Dis* 2003;**9**:1–9.

Shorr AF, Duh MS, Kelly KM, Kollef MH. Red blood cell transfusion and ventilator-associated pneumonia: a potential link? *Crit Care Med* 2004;**32**:666–74.

Shorr AF, Sherner JH, Jackson WL, Kollef MH. Invasive approaches to the diagnosis of ventilator-associated pneumonia: A meta-analysis. *Crit Care Med* 2005;**33**:46–53.

Singh N, Rogers P, Atwood CW, et al. Short-course empiric antibiotic therapy for patients with pulmonary infiltrates in the intensive care unit. *Am J Respir Crit Care Med* 2000;**162**:505–11.

Souweine B, Veber B, Bedos JP, et al. Diagnostic accuracy of protected specimen brush and bronchioalveolar lavage in nosocomial pneumonia: Impact of previous antimicrobial treatment. *Crit Care Med* 1998;**26**:236–44.

Taylor RW, Manganaro L, O'Brien J, et al. Impact of allogenic packed red blood cell transfusion on nosocomial infection rates in the critically ill patient. *Crit Care Med* 2002;**30**:2249–54.

Torres A, Mustafa E. Bronchoscopic BAL in the diagnosis of ventilator-associated pneumonia. *Chest* 2000;**117**:198–202.

Torres A, Aznar R, Gatell JM, et al. Incidence, risk, and prognosis factors of nosocomial pneumonia in mechanically ventilated patients. *Am Rev Respir Dis* 1990;**142**:523–8.

Torres A, Serra-Batlles J, Ros E, et al. Pulmonary aspiration of gastric contents in patients receiving mechanical ventilation: The effect of body position. *Ann Intern Med* 1992;**116**:540–3.

Trouillet J, Vuagnat A, Combes A, et al. *Pseudomonas aeruginosa* ventilator-associated pneumonia: Comparison of episodes due to piperacillin-resistant versus piperacillin-susceptible organisms . *Clin Infect Dis* 2002;**34**:1047–54.

Tseng CC, Liu SF, Wang CC, et al. Impact of clinical severity index, infective pathogens, and initial empiric antibiotic use on hospital mortality in patients with ventilator-associated pneumonia. *Am J Infect Control* 2012;Jan 11. **40**:648–52.

Umscheid CA, Mitchell MD, Doshi JA, et al. Estimating the proportion of healthcare-associated infections that are reasonably preventable and the related mortality and costs. *Infect Control Hosp Epidemiol* 2011;**32**: 101–14.

van Loon HJ, Vriens MR, Fluit AC, et al. Antibiotic rotation and development of Gram-negative antibiotic resistance. *Am J Respir Crit Care Med* 2005;**171**:480–7.

van Nieuwenhoven CA, Buskens E, van Tiel FH, Bonten MJ. Relationship between methodological trial quality and the effects of selective digestive decontamination on pneumonia and mortality in critically ill patients. *JAMA* 2001;**286**:335–40.

Veinstein A, Brun-Buisson C, Derrode N, et al. Validation of an algorithm based on direct examination of specimens in suspected ventilator-associated pneumonia. *Intensive Care Med* 2006;**32**:676–83.

Vidaur L, Gualis B, Rodríguez A, et al. Clinical resolution in patients with suspicion of VAP: A cohort study comparing patients with and without ARDS. *Crit Care Med* 2005;**33**:1248–53.

Wang F, Wu Y, Bo L, et al. The timing of tracheotomy in critically ill patients undergoing mechanical ventilation: a systematic review and meta-analysis of randomized controlled trials. *Chest* 2011;**140**:1456–65.

Wilson A, Gray D, Karakiozis J, Thomas J. Advanced endotracheal tube biofilm stage, not duration of intubation, is related to pneumonia. *J Trauma Acute Care Surg* 2012;**72**:916–23.

Wood GC. Aerosolized antibiotics for treating hospital-acquired and ventilator-associated pneumonia. *Expert Rev Anti Infect Ther* 2011;**9**:993–1000.

Wu CL, Yang DI, Wang NY, et al. Quantitative culture of endotracheal aspirates in the diagnosis of ventilator associated pneumonia in patients with treatment failure. *Chest* 2002;**122**:662–8.

Wunderink RG. Radiologic diagnosis of ventilator-associated pneumonia. *Chest* 2000;**117**(4 suppl 2):188S–90S.

Wunderink RG. Ventilator-associated tracheobronchitis: public-reporting scam or important clinical infection? *Chest* 2011;**139**:485–8.

Zazk JE, Garrison T, Trovillion E, et al. Effect of an education program aimed at reducing the occurrence of ventilator-associated pneumonia. *Crit Care Med* 2002;**30**:2407–12.

Zolfaghari PS, Wyncoll DL. The tracheal tube: Gateway to ventilator-associated pneumonia. *Crit Care* 2011;**15**:310.

Chapter 9 Postoperative urinary tract infections

Jeffrey A. Claridge, Joseph F. Golob

■ DEFINITION AND DIAGNOSIS

Urinary tract infections (UTIs) include those infections of the lower urinary tract (cystitis) and the upper urinary tract (pyelonephritis). Most UTIs are considered uncomplicated because they occur spontaneously without previous urinary tract instrumentation. However, within the surgical population, virtually all UTIs are of the complicated (urinary catheter in place and/or functional/anatomical urinary tract abnormality) and healthcare-associated variety due to urological instrumentation and/or indwelling urinary catheter placement (Klevens et al. 2007).

The Centers for Disease Control and Prevention (CDC) have very specific definitions of UTIs. The CDC divides UTIs into three categories: Symptomatic UTIs, asymptomatic UTIs, and other UTIs. The symptomatic and asymptomatic categories include definitions with and without an indwelling urinary catheter. If a urinary catheter is present at the time of urine collection, or was collected within 48 h of catheter removal, the infection is called a catheter-associated urinary tract infection (CAUTI). The definitions, evaluation, and diagnosis of CAUTI are detailed in **Figure 9.1**.

The definitions by the CDC use a variety of signs and symptoms. In a symptomatic UTI, the patient may complain of urgency, frequency, dysuria, or abdominal pain. On physical exam, patients may demonstrate suprapubic tenderness and/or costovertebral tenderness. Signs of both symptomatic and asymptomatic UTIs include: Fever (>38°C), positive urinalysis for leukocyte esterase and/or nitrite, pyuria (≥10 white blood cells/mm^3 of unspun urine or ≥3 white blood cells/high power field in spun urine), and a positive urine culture of ≥10^5 colony-forming units (CFU)/ml.

Obtaining urinalysis and urine cultures are ideally done before starting any antibiotics in patients for whom there is concern about a UTI. If possible, the indwelling urinary catheter should be removed and a clean-catch midstream urine sample obtained because it is more difficult to distinguish true pathogens from colonizing organisms in catheterized patients. If the catheter must be maintained, the urine sample should be removed from the port within the catheter tubing and not the urine bag. If there is no tubing port, the last resort is to remove the closed drainage system and obtain the sample directly from the urinary catheter. However, there are some data that this technique

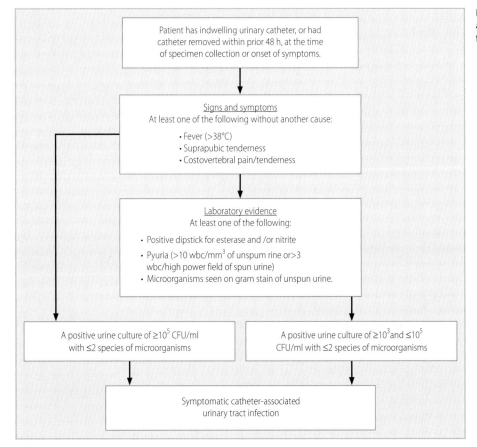

Figure 9.1 Identification of the catheter-associated urinary tract infection. (From Centers for Disease Control and Prevention 2012.)

Patient has indwelling urinary catheter, or had catheter removed within prior 48 h, at the time of specimen collection or onset of symptoms.

Signs and symptoms
At least one of the following without another cause:

- Fever (>38°C)
- Suprapubic tenderness
- Costovertebral pain/tenderness

Laboratory evidence
At least one of the following:

- Positive dipstick for esterase and /or nitrite
- Pyuria (>10 wbc/mm^3 of unspun rine or>3 wbc/high power field of spun urine)
- Microorganisms seen on gram stain of unspun urine.

A positive urine culture of ≥10^5 CFU/ml with ≤2 species of microorganisms

A positive urine culture of ≥10^3 and ≤10^5 CFU/ml with ≤2 species of microorganisms

Symptomatic catheter-associated urinary tract infection

may increase the risk of introducing pathogens into the urinary tract (Gould et al. 2010).

Unfortunately, there are limited data to support when to obtain urinalysis and urine cultures in the surgical patient population. Even in the setting of fever and/or leukocytosis, it may not be prudent to obtain a urine specimen, especially from catheterized patients. Pyuria and bacteriuria ($\geq 10^2$ CFU/ml) are frequent in the catheterized patient and may or may not signify an infection that needs to be treated (Tambyah and Maki 2000). Data from our institution demonstrated that, in 510 critically ill trauma patients, fever, leukocytosis, or both did not predict a UTI (Golob et al. 2008). Some continue to advocate evaluation of the urinary tract when patients develop fever, or otherwise unexplained systemic manifestations compatible with infection, including malaise, altered mental status, hypotension, or metabolic acidosis (Fekete 2011). However, data do not support obtaining routine surveillance urine cultures in patients who are asymptomatic with long-term indwelling urinary catheters, such as spinal cord-injured patients (Nicolle 2005). Screening with routine urinalysis is appropriate only for pregnant women and patients undergoing urological procedures in which mucosal bleeding is anticipated, because these asymptomatic patients benefit from treatment to minimize risk of bacteriuria (Nicolle 2005, Lin et al. 2008).

■ EPIDEMIOLOGY

CAUTIs account for more than 40% of all nosocomial infections and are the leading cause of secondary nosocomial bacteremias (Stamm 1991, Warren 2001). It has been shown that approximately 20% of hospital-acquired bacteremias arise from the urinary tract (urosepsis). Of these bacteremias, approximately 10% result in sepsis, multiorgan dysfunction, and eventual death (Gould et al. 2009). In 1992, CAUTIs were responsible for approximately 900 000 additional hospital-days per year and contribute to more than 7000 deaths annually. UTIs increase healthcare costs by up to $500 million per year (Hashmi et al. 2003).

According to the National Healthcare Safety Network (NHSN), general surgery and trauma patients, especially those treated in the intensive care unit (ICU), have some of the highest rates of both indwelling urinary catheter usage and CAUTIs. The NHSN is a CDC organization that collects data from a collaboration of hospitals regarding patient safety issues. Included in this data collection are urinary catheter usage and CAUTIs for both surgical and medical patient populations. The NHSN reports usage of indwelling urinary catheters as: Number of urinary catheter-days/number of patient-days. CAUTIs are reported by normalizing the data to 1000 urinary catheter-days through the following calculation:

[Number of CAUTIs/Number of urinary catheter-days] × 1000.

Table 9.1 contains data from the 2009 NHSN report regarding urinary catheter usage and CAUTIs in specific patient populations.

ICU surgical and trauma patients have a urinary catheter usage of 0.79 and 0.83, respectively. Not surprising, these patient populations have some of the highest CAUTI rates. The CAUTI rate in ICU surgical patients is 2.6 CAUTIs per 1000 urinary catheter-days and in ICU trauma patients it is 3.4 CAUTIs/1000 urinary catheter-days. This is in comparison to a medical ICU rate of 2.3 CAUTIs/1000 urinary catheter-days. The highest rates of CAUTI are in burn and neurosurgical ICU patients (4.4 CAUTIs/1000 urinary catheter-days) despite burn units having the lowest ICU rate of catheter usage (0.54) (Dudeck et al. 2009).

Table 9.1 NHSN urinary catheter usage and associated CAUTIs (catheter-associated urinary tract infections).

NHSN urinary catheter usage per patient-days	
Surgical ICU	0.79
Trauma ICU	0.83
Neurosurgical ICU	0.77
Medical ICU (teaching hospital)	0.74
Burn ICU	0.56
Urology – ward	0.21
Gynecology – ward	0.20
Surgical – ward	0.23
Orthopedics – ward	0.28
NHSN CAUTIs per 1000 urinary catheter-days	
Surgical ICU	2.6
Trauma ICU	3.4
Neurosurgical ICU	4.4
Medical ICU (teaching hospital)	2.3
Burn ICU	4.4
Urology – ward	1.2
Gynecology – ward	1.0
Surgical – ward	1.8
Orthopedics – ward	1.6

ICU, intensive care unit; NHSN, National Healthcare Safety Network.

■ PATHOPHYSIOLOGY

The major risk factor for bacteriuria and UTIs in the surgical patient is an indwelling urinary catheter. The risk of UTI is directly proportional to the duration the urinary catheter is in place. The daily incidence of UTI in the presence of an indwelling catheter is up to 5% per day. After 1 week of catheterization, 25% of patients will have bacteriuria or candiduria. However, only 10–25% of these patients will go on to meet the CDC definition of UTIs (Stark and Maki 1984, Tambyah and Maki 2000, Maki and Tambyah 2001).

Other important UTI risk factors in a surgical population include patients with other infectious sites, prolonged hospital stay, diabetes, malnutrition, female sex, and ureteral stent placement (Kunin and McCormack 1966, Platt et al. 1986, Wald et al. 2008, Marchaim 2011). There is also less rigorous data to support older age, disconnection of the closed drainage system, renal impairment, insertion of the catheter outside the operating room, and a lower professional training of the person inserting the catheter as risk factors for UTIs (Gould et al. 2010).

The microbiology of uncomplicated cystitis and pyelonephritis consists mainly of *Escherichia coli* (75–95%), *Proteus mirabilis*, *Klebsiella pneumoniae*, and *Staphylococcus saprophyticus* (Echols et al. 1999, Czaja et al. 2007). Surgical patients with a CAUTI tend to grow the same bacteria with the addition of *Pseudomonas*, *Serratia*, and *Providencia* spp., as well as various enterococci, staphylococci, and fungi (Hooton 2011). The broader bacterial flora seen in patients with complicated UTIs result from the presence of underlying chronic comorbid conditions, longer hospital courses, multiple different antibiotic drug therapies during hospital admission, and frequent manipulations and contact with healthcare workers whose hands can become vehicles of bacterial transfer (Marchaim 2011).

These bacteria that cause UTIs are often chronic colonizers of the gut and perineum and subsequently invade the urinary system. The presence of an indwelling urinary catheter creates an easy path for the bacteria to follow. Bacterial adhesion onto the urinary catheter and subsequently the urothelial cells has been suggested to be the single most important bacterial virulence factor in causing CAUTIs (Richards et al. 1999, Meyrier 2011).

The two most common UTI microbes, *E. coli* and *P. mirabilis*, have flagella and fimbriae as virulence factors that facilitate migration into the urinary bladder from the pericatheter space within the urethra. The flagella allow the organisms to be mobile, exit the fecal reservoir, and migrate up the biofilm of the indwelling urinary catheter. Once in the bladder, the fimbriae adhesion systems have an overall positive electrical charge and promote adhesion to the negatively charged uroepithelial cell membrane via hydrophobicity. Once this adhesion occurs, the bacteria can than cause cystitis and continue to spread into the upper urinary tract causing pyelonephritis (Mulvey 2002, Oelschlaeger et al. 2002).

In addition to bacteria, fungi can also colonize and infect the urinary tract. Although *Aspergillus*, *Fusarium*, *Trichosporon*, and *Mucor* spp., and cryptococci have been implicated in UTIs, *Candida albicans* and other *Candida* spp. are the most common pathogens. The National Nosocomial Infections Surveillance System (now the NHSN) reported that candida UTIs increased from 22% for the period 1986–1989 to nearly 40% in 1992–1997 (Richards et al. 1999). It is unclear from the data if this candiduria was an actual infection or colonization. A large prospective study identified several risk factors for fungiuria with the top three being: Prior antibiotic therapy (90%), indwelling urinary catheter (83%), and diabetes (39%) (Kauffman et al. 2000).

Differentiation between infection and colonization in fungiuria can be difficult. Most cases of candiduria are asymptomatic and most likely represent colonization. Infected patients may or may not display the typical UTI symptoms such as dysuria, frequency, and suprapubic pain. Pyuria, presence of pseudohyphae, or the number of colonies growing in culture do not help distinguish colonization (Kauffman et al. 2000). Evaluation of the entire clinical picture needs to occur in order to diagnosis and treat a candida UTI.

■ TREATMENT

The single best way to treat a CAUTI is to remove the indwelling urinary catheter. This method alone has been shown in two-thirds of patients with bacteriuria to assist in clearing the bacteria within 1 week (Hartstein et al. 1981). If the patient is showing systemic signs of a possible UTI, and the appropriate microbiological studies have been obtained (urinalysis and urine culture), empirical antibiotics can be initiated pending the culture results. Choosing the empirical antibiotic should be based on normal UTI flora, previous culture results, and/or the hospital's antibiogram. The typical UTI profile of Gram-negative bacilli may be treated with a third-generation cephalosporin or a fluoroquinolone. If *Pseudomonas* spp. is suspected, treatment with fluoroquinolone alone or a penicillin in combination with an aminoglycoside can be utilized. When expanded-spectrum b-lactamase producing Gram-negative pathogens are encountered, a carbapenem choice may be desirable. If Gram-positive cocci are seen on Gram stain, they may represent enterococci or staphylococci, and vancomycin should be started. Once culture and susceptibility results are available, the antibiotics should be tailored to treat the specific organism.

The duration of treatment remains unclear, especially in patients with a CAUTI. In normal hosts with an uncomplicated UTI, 3 days of treatment with a penicillin derivative, trimethoprin sulfa, fluoroquinolone, or nitrofurantoin is adequate. If the host is compromised (chronic steroids, diabetes, lupus, cirrhosis, or multiple myeloma) then 5 days of antibiotics should be used (Cunha 2007). It has been suggested that in patients with a urinary catheter, the catheter should be changed and treatment for 10–14 days is usually adequate (Trautner and Darouiche 2004). Unfortunately, even with an extended duration of antibiotics, there is a high relapse rate if the indwelling urinary catheter is left in place (Stamm 1991).

Asymptomatic candiduria rarely requires antifungal treatment unless it occurs in the setting of neutropenia or urinary tract surgery. Symptomatic candiduria should always be treated. Treatment should be tailored to the *Candida* spp., and according to whether ascending or disseminated infection is present. Changing the urinary catheter and a 14-day course of an appropriate antifungal should be utilized. If amphotericin B is required, the non-lipid formulation should be used because the lipid formulation does not penetrate into the kidney to achieve high concentrations in the bladder. Amphotericin B bladder irrigations can be used to clear fungiuria, but should not be used as sole treatment.

■ PREVENTION

The single best UTI prevention strategy is to avoid inserting unnecessary urinary catheters and to remove any unneeded ones. There has been substantial research on other methods to prevent CAUTIs such as utilization of external drainage systems in male patients, intermittent catheterization versus indwelling catheters, drug-impregnated catheters, preconnected closed catheters versus standard catheters, systemic antimicrobial prophylaxis, topical antimicrobials, and bladder irrigations.

In male patients without urinary tract obstruction and/or urinary retention, there is some evidence to suggest that use of an external condom catheter over an indwelling catheter will decrease the risk of a UTI, bacteriuria, and death (Gould et al. 2010). Likewise, intermittent catheterization is associated with lower rates of bacteriuria and symptomatic UTIs in patients requiring long-term indwelling catheters such as spinal cord-injured patients (Weld and Dmochowski 2000). However, there are no data to demonstrate that intermittent catheterization is superior to indwelling urinary catheters in critically ill surgical/trauma patients.

There continues to be mixed results on the utilization of silver-coated catheters and nitrofurazone-impregnated catheters. Both the silver-coated and nitrofurazone catheters seem to be effective if duration of use was less than 7 days. After 1 week of use, there was no difference in UTI rates between these special catheters and a standard latex catheter, questioning the cost–benefit ratio for these special catheters (Gould et al. 2010).

Since 1966, the utilization of closed urinary drainage systems have been the standard of care after a study published by Kunin showed a dramatic decrease in UTIs (Kunin and McCormack 1966). More recent data demonstrated that disconnecting the drainage system increases the risk of bacteriuria. Therefore, the CDC recommends the use of a closed urinary drainage system (category IB) with consideration of the presealed catheter tubing junctions (category II) (Gould et al. 2009).

To date, there is no evidence to suggest that systemic antibiotic prophylaxis against UTIs is beneficial in patients with either short- or long-term indwelling urinary catheter usage (Neil-Weise 2005). Topical antimicrobial agents such as methenamine do not prevent CAUTIs and may actually increase the risk due to more frequent catheter manipulations (Warren 2001). Soaking catheters in an anti-infective solution, placement of anti-infection solution into drainage bag, or continuous bladder irrigations have not been shown to decease the risk of CAUTIs (Warren et al. 1978, Maki and Tambyah 2001, Warren 2001).

When placing a urinary catheter, sterile aseptic technique should be employed by a health professional familiar with the technique of inserting the catheter appropriately. The person inserting the catheter should wash his or her hands and use sterile gloves, sterile drapes, and an antiseptic solution to clean the urethral orifice. Once in place, a closed drainage system should be used and manipulations to the catheter should be avoided. The collection tubing and bag should always be located below the patient. Finally, prompt removal of unnecessary catheters is key to avoiding CAUTIs.

CONCLUSION

This chapter has presented the contemporary view of the diagnosis, prevention, and management of CAUTIs in the surgical patient. The standard practice methods for prevention and the antibiotic therapy for these infections are well understood. Concern about these complications is best reflected in the current policy of the US Medicare program, which refuses to pay supplemental costs to hospitals for patient care when a CAUTI has occurred. CAUTIs and certain other hospital-acquired infections (e.g., intravascular catheter infections) have been labeled "never events" by healthcare policy, the rationale being that these complications are totally preventable and should "never" occur. However, anyone who has cared for critically ill patients with ongoing and necessary urinary bladder catheterization knows that these infections will occur in the most capable practices. Risk models can be formulated (Fry et al. 2010) to identify the clinical profile of the patient who is likely to develop a CAUTI.

An issue that obscures analytical methods for prevention and treatment of CAUTIs is the criterion for establishment of this diagnosis. Although Claridge and Golob (Golob et al. 2008) have used the conventional definitions that are employed in the diagnosis of a CAUTI, the diagnosis of a CAUTI requires additional investigation and assessment. The sacred threshold of 10^5 organisms/ml of urinary sample is considered the standard for the diagnosis, but from whence was that derived? The classic research that defined the 10^5 microbes/ml threshold was by Kass (1957). This was done by studying uncomplicated community-acquired, not catheter-associated, UTIs. This threshold of bacterial presence in the sampled urine has been generally extrapolated to apply in CAUTIs. With the indwelling foreign body within the urethra as a direct conduit to the external perineal surface of critically ill patients, it is logical to assume that the catheter will have colonization. With binding and division of bacteria on the surface of the foreign body, and the development of biofilms that compromise efficient elimination of colonization, it may be that urine specimens derived from the densely colonized catheter or from the urethra after removal of the catheter have colony counts that do not accurately reflect invasive infection. False-positive urinary cultures leads to excessive rates of CAUTI being identified and certainly excessive antibiotic administration.

If false-positive cases are identified and reported, this actually dilutes the impact of truly invasive CAUTIs. Laupland et al. (2005) and Clec'h et al. (2007) concluded that a CAUTI was not an independent variable in contributing to hospital deaths. Tambyah et al. (2002) found attributable costs of only $589 per patient for 235 patients with a CAUTI based on positive cultures. In a multi-hospital study of hospital-acquired infections, Anderson et al. (2007) noted attributable costs of $25 000 for each ventilator-associated pneumonia and >$10 000 for each surgical site infection, but only $758 for each CAUTI. If colonization of the urinary tract is counted as a CAUTI, then the denominator of population analyses is distorted and the cost-effectiveness of interventions will be equally distorted.

The true diagnosis of a CAUTI must be refined. Perhaps the measurement of leukocyte esterase, nitrites, or other objective biomarkers of a UTI will supplement the quantitative microbial culture. There is no question that a CAUTI can be a severe event in the recovery of surgical patients. Effective preventive strategies and cost-effective treatment require that the diagnosis must be accurate.

REFERENCES

Anderson DJ, Kirkland KB, Kaye KS, et al. Underresourced hospital infection control and prevention programs: penny wise and pound foolish? *Infect Control Hosp Epidemiol* 2007;**28**:767–73.

Centers for Disease Control and Prevention. Cath*eter-associated urinary tract infection (CAUTI) event*. Available at: www.cdc.gov\nhsn\pdfs\pscmanual\7pscCAUTIcurrent.pdf (accessed February 26, 2012).

Clec'h C, Schwebel C, Français M, et al. Does catheter-associated urinary tract infection increase mortality in critically ill patients? *Infect Control Hosp Epidemiol* 2007;**28**:1367–73.

Cunha B. *Antibiotic Essentials*, 6th edn. Royal Oak, MI: Physician Press, 2007.

Czaja CA, Scholes D, Hooton TM, et al. Population-based epidemiologic analysis of acute pyelonephritis. *Clin Infect Dis* 2007;**45**:273–80.

Dudeck MA Horan TC, Peterson KD, et al. *National Healthcare Safety Network (NHSN) Report, Data Summary for 2009, Device-associated Module*. 2009. Available at: www.cdc.gov/nhsn/PDFs/datastat/2010NHSNReport.pdf (accessed June 25, 2012

Echols RM, Tosiello RL, Haverstock DC, et al. Demographic, clinical, and treatment parameters influencing the outcome of acute cystitis. *Clin Infect Dis* 1999;**29**:113–19.

Fekete T. Urinary tract infections associated with urethral catheters. 2011. Available at: www.uptodate.com.

Fry DE, Pine M, Jones BL, Meimban RJ. Patient characteristics and the occurrence of never events. *Arch Surg* 2010;**145**:148–51.

Golob JF Jr, Claridge JA, Sando MJ, et al. Fever and leukocytosis in critically ill trauma patients: it's not the urine. *Surg Infect* 2008;**9**:49–56.

Gould FK, Brindle R, Chadwick PR, et al. Guidelines (2008) for the prophylaxis and treatment of methicillin-resistant Staphylococcus aureus (MRSA) infections in the United Kingdom. *J Antimicrob Chemother* 2009;**63**:849–61.

Gould CV, Umscheid CA, Agarwal RK, Kuntz G, Pegues DA. Guideline for prevention of catheter-associated urinary tract infection 2009. *Infect Control Hosp Epidemiol* 2010;**31**:319–26.

Hartstein AI, Garber SB, Ward TT, et al. Nosocomial urinary tract infection: a prospective evaluation of 108 catheterized patients. *Infect Control* 1981;**2**:380–6.

Hashmi S, Kelly E, Rogers SO, et al. Urinary tract infection in surgical patients. *Am J S* 2003;**186**:53–6.

Hooton T. *Acute complicated cysitis and pylonephritis*, 2011. Available at: www.uptodate.com (accessed May 15, 2012).

Kass EH. Bacteruria and the diagnosis of infection of the urinary tract. *Arch Intern Med* 1957;**100**:709–14.

Kauffman CA, Vazquez JA, Sobel JD, et al. Prospective multicenter surveillance study of funguria in hospitalized patients. The National Institute for Allergy and Infectious Diseases (NIAID) Mycoses Study Group. *Clin Infect Dis* 2000;**30**:14–18.

Klevens RM, Edwards JR, Richards CL Jr, et al. Estimating health care-associated infections and deaths in U.S. hospitals, 2002. *Public Health Rep* 2007;**122**:160–6.

Kunin CM, McCormack RC. Prevention of catheter-induced urinary-tract infections by sterile closed drainage. *N Engl J Med* 1966;**274**:1155–61.

Laupland KB, Bagshaw SM, Gregson DB, et al. Intensive care unit-acquired urinary tract infections in a regional critical care system. *Crit Care* 2005;**9**:R60–5.

Lin K, Fajardo K, Force USPST. Screening for asymptomatic bacteriuria in adults: evidence for the U.S. Preventive Services Task Force reaffirmation recommendation statement. *Ann Intern Med* 2008;**149**:W20–4.

Maki DG, Tambyah PA. Engineering out the risk for infection with urinary catheters. *Emerging Infect Dis* 2001;**7**:342–7.

Marchaim DKK. *Infection in the intensive care unit*, 2011. Available at: www.uptodate.com (accessed May 15, 2012).

Meyrier A. *Bacterial adherehnce and other virulence facture for urinary tract infection*, 2011. Available at: www.uptodate.com (accessed May 15, 2012).

Mulvey MA. Adhesion and entry of uropathogenic *Escherichia coli*. *Cell Microbiol* 2002;**4**:257–271.

Neil-Weise B. Antibiotic policies for short-term catheter bladder drainage in adults. *Cochrane Database Syst Rev* 2005.

Nicolle LE. Infectious Diseases Society of America guidelines for the diagnosis and treatment of asymptomatic bacteriuria in adults. *Clin Infect Dis* 2005;**40**:643.

Oelschlaeger TA, Dobrindt U, Hacker J. Virulence factors of uropathogens. *Curr Opin Urol* 2002;**12**:33–8.

Paradisi F, Corti G, Mangani V. Urosepsis in the critical care unit. *Crit Care Clinics* 1998;**14**:165–80.

Platt R, Polk BF, Murdock B, et al. Risk factors for nosocomial urinary tract infection. *Am J Epidemiol* 1986;**124**:977–85.

Richards MJ, Edwards JR, Culver DH, et al. Nosocomial infections in medical intensive care units in the United States. National Nosocomial Infections Surveillance System. *Crit Care Med* 1999;**27**:887–92.

Stamm WE. Catheter-associated urinary tract infections: epidemiology, pathogenesis, and prevention. *Am J Med* 1991;**91**:65S–71S.

Stark RP, Maki DG. Bacteriuria in the catheterized patient. What quantitative level of bacteriuria is relevant? *N Engl J Med* 1984;**311**:560–4.

Tambyah PA, Knasinski V, Maki DG. The direct costs of nosocomial catheter-associated urinary tract infection in the era of managed care. *Infect Control Hosp Epidemiol* 2002;**23**:27–31.

Tambyah PA, Maki DG. Catheter-associated urinary tract infection is rarely symptomatic: a prospective study of 1,497 catheterized patients. *Arch Intern Med* 2000;**160**:678–82.

Trautner BW, Darouiche RO. Role of biofilm in catheter-associated urinary tract infection. *Am J Infect Control* 2004;**32**:177–83.

Wald HL, Ma A, Bratzler DW, et al. Indwelling urinary catheter use in the postoperative period: analysis of the national surgical infection prevention project data. *Arch Surg* 2008;**143**:551–7.

Weld KJ, Dmochowski RR. Effect of bladder management on urological complications in spinal cord injured patients. *Journal of Urology* 2000;**163**:768–72.

Warren JW, Platt R, Thomas RJ, et al. Antibiotic irrigation and catheter-associated urinary-tract infections. *N Engl J Med* 1978;**299**:570–3.

Warren JW. Catheter-associated urinary tract infections. *Int J Antimicrob Agents* 2001;**17**:299–303.

Chapter 10 — Catheter-related bloodstream infections

William P. Schecter

INTRODUCTION

In 1656, Christopher Wren, the genius who designed St Paul's Cathedral in London, injected opium drops intravenously into dogs using a quill and bladder as the first intravascular device. However, major advances in intravenous therapy did not occur until the twentieth century. Before the Second World War, metal needles were the prime method of access to the vascular system.

Rudimentary flexible plastic catheters were first inserted by venous cut-down in 1945. In 1950, the "Rochester" plastic intravenous catheter was introduced into clinical practice (Rosenthal et al. 2006). In the 1960s percutaneous plastic catheters were developed for central venous access, which quickly became routine hemodynamic monitors and access ports for intravenous alimentation. In the 1970s both implantable ports and the Broviac catheter for long-term vascular access were introduced. The explosion of intravenous therapy in the latter decades of the twentieth century was associated with a concomitant epidemic of catheter-related bloodstream infections (CRBSIs).

EPIDEMIOLOGY

US intensive care patients experience 15 million days of central venous catheter (CVC) exposure each year (Mermel et al. 2003); 80 000 CRBSIs occur in intensive care units (ICUs) each year (Mermel et al. 2003) giving an incidence rate of 0.0053 CRBSIs/day of CVC exposure in the ICU. The extent of hospital-acquired CRBSIs, however, is much greater. If we include CRBSIs associated with peripheral intravenous, arterial catheters, and vascular catheters connected to other medical devices, an estimated 250 000 cases occur in the USA each year. These infections are responsible for increased hospital length of stay and cost of care estimated to be $2.3 billion per year (Dimick et al. 2001, Renaud and Brun-Buisson 2001, Blot et al. 2005, Warren et al. 2006a). CRBSIs are associated with 28 000 deaths per year (O'Grady et al. 2011). The risk of CRBSIs is even greater in the developing world (Rosenthal et al. 2006).

It is important to differentiate local infection from catheter colonization and bloodstream infection when considering CRBSIs. Local infection refers to the presence of purulence at the catheter insertion site. Catheter colonization is defined as growth >15 colony-forming units (CFU) using the semiquantitative roll-plate culture technique (Pronovost 2008). A CRBSI is defined as a positive blood culture with clinical and microbiological evidence pointing to the catheter as the source of the infection. This evidence may include comparison of cultured blood drawn from a peripheral vein with blood drawn through the catheter (Pronovost et al. 2006).

PATHOPHYSIOLOGY

There are four recognized causes of CRBSI:

1. A direct route is created alongside the barrel of the catheter, which permits skin bacteria to proliferate distally and results in infection of the catheter tip and bacteremia (Maki et al. 1977, Renaud and Brun-Buisson 2001, Safdar and Maki 2004). Catheters placed through moist contaminated areas such as the groin or burn eschar are associated with an increased risk for bacteremia (Robinson et al. 1995, Goetz et al. 1998, Merrer et al. 2001). Repeated venopuncture at one site increases the risk of local skin infection once successful venous catheterization has been achieved, increasing the risk of CRBSI.

2. Catheters constructed with materials having irregular surfaces have an increased risk of infection because of increased adherence by organisms such as *Staphylococcus epidermidis* and *Candida albicans* (Stillman et al. 1977, Hawser and Douglas 1994). The patient forms a protein sheath around the catheter consisting of fibrin and fibronectin (Mehall et al. 2002). Certain organisms such as *Staphylococcus aureus* can adhere to these proteins by producing clumping factors (ClfA and ClfB) (Herrmann et al. 1991, McDevitt et al. 1995, Ni Eidhin et al. 1998, Mehall et al. 2002). Other organisms such as coagulase-negative staphylococci (von Eiff et al. 2002, Mack et al. 2007), *Pseudomonas aeruginosa* (Murga et al. 2001), and *Candida* spp. (Douglas 2003) produce an extracellular polymeric substance (EPS) composed primarily of exopolysaccharide, which forms a biofilm layer that can bind antimicrobials before contact with the cell wall and neutralize polymorphonucleocytes (Farber et al. 1990, Donlan 2000, von Eiff et al. 2002). Repeated puncture of a vascular conduit created as vascular access for hemodialysis increases the risk for mycotic pseudoaneurysm formation. The risk and consequences are greater with a prosthetic conduit compared with an arteriovenous fistula or autogenous conduit (National Kidney Foundation 2001).

3. The catheter or intravenous extension tubing can be contaminated by the hands of healthcare workers (HCW), contaminated fluids, or contaminated devices (e.g. pressure transducers) (Raad et al. 1993, Dobbins et al. 2002). Contamination of infusion solutions is a possible but infrequent cause of CRBSIs (Raad et al. 2001).

4. Catheters can occasionally be infected by circulating organisms from a remote site of infection (Annaissie et al. 1995). The risk of infection by this mechanism increases if the indwelling catheter directly injures the endothelium and causes local thrombosis or chemical phlebitis. Intravascular thrombus creates a scaffolding for seeding by circulating organisms.

MICROBIOLOGY

The most common organisms associated with CRBSIs are coagulase-negative staphylococci, *S. aureus*, enterococci and *Candida* spp. (Wisplinghoff et al. 2004). Gram-negative bacilli account for 19–21% of all CRBSIs (**Table 10.1**) (Wisplinghoff et al. 2004, Gaynes and Edwards 2005). Many organisms causing hospital-acquired infections, including *Klebsiella pneumoniae*, *Escherichia coli*, *Pseudomonas aeruginosa*, and *Candida* spp., are now resistant to previously effective antibiotics (Gaynes and Edwards 2005, Lipitz-Snydermanet et al. 2011).

Table 10.1 Categories of recommendations.

Category IA	Strongly recommended for implementation and strongly supported by well-designed experimental, clinical, or epidemiological studies
Category IB	Strongly recommended for implementation and supported by some experimental, clinical, or epidemiological studies and a strong theoretical rationale; or an accepted practice (e.g., aseptic technique) supported by limited evidence
Category IC	Required by state or federal regulations, rules, or standards
Category II	Suggested for implementation and supported by suggestive clinical or epidemiological studies or a theoretical rationale
Unresolved issue	Represents an unresolved issue for which evidence is insufficient or no consensus regarding efficacy exists

However, meticillin-resistant *S. aureus* (MRSA) is a particularly important pathogen that plays a major role in central line-associated bloodstream infection (CLABSIs) (Gaynes and Edwards 2005, Lipitz-Snyderman et al. 2011).

The special problem of MRSA CRBSIs

S. aureus CRBSI (SACRBSI) is a special problem because of its tendency to cause deep infections at multiple metastatic sites remote from the initial source of the infection. Locating the occult source of infection is particularly challenging; it is often never identified even after an extensive evaluation. The mortality rate for MRSA bacteremia is higher than for meticillin-susceptible *S. aureus* (MSSA) (Cosgrove et al. 2003). Endocarditis may be a complicating event from SACRBSIs. This risk of endocarditis is increased by a permanent intracardiac device, hemo-dialysis dependency, spinal infection, and non-vertebral osteomyelitis (Kaasch et al. 2011). All patients with a SACRBSI should be evaluated by echocardiography. Transesophageal echo (TEE) is the diagnostic tool of choice because of increased sensitivity compared with trans-thoracic echo (TTE). All patients with a positive blood culture should receive a follow-up blood culture within 48 h of the initiation of drug therapy regardless of their clinical response to exclude prolonged bacteremia. The decision to use empirical antibiotic therapy for a presumed MRSA CRBSI before blood culture data should be based on clinical suspicion and knowledge of the prevalence of MRSA in one's particular hospital microbial flora.

Reduction of CRBSIs in the ICU: The Keystone Project

A prospective cohort study of surgical ICU patients demonstrated near elimination of CRBSIs by adherence to evidence-based guidelines (Berenholtz et al. 2004). Five interventions, with the strongest evidence and the lowest barriers to implementation, were chosen: Handwashing, use of full barrier precautions during insertion of central venous catheters, skin preparation with chlorhexidine, avoidance of femoral venous catheterization when possible, and removal of unnecessary catheters (Pronovost 2008).

The quality and safety research group from the Johns Hopkins University partnered with the Michigan Health and Hospital Association Keystone Center for Safety and Quality to determine whether or not similar results could be achieved in a large number of ICUs from diverse hospitals by use of these guidelines. A collaborative cohort study of 103 Michigan ICUs reporting 375 757 catheter-days over an 18-month period between March 2004 and September 2005 demonstrated a reduction in the median rate of CRBSI per 1000 catheter-days from 2.7 at baseline to zero at 3 months after implementation of the 5 evidence-based interventions ($p <0.002$) (Pronovost et al. 2006).

A follow-up study demonstrated that the reduced rates of CRBSIs achieved in the initial 18-month study were sustained for an additional 18 months by continuing to orient staff and report CRBSIs and catheter days to the appropriate stake holders (Pronovost et al. 2010). The state-wide implementation of these five interventions to reduce CRBSIs, together with measures to reduce ventilator-associated pneumonia (recumbent positioning, daily interruption of sedatives, and prophylaxis for both peptic ulcer disease and deep venous thrombosis), were associated with a significant reduction in the mortality rate in the study group compared with the surrounding area (Lipitz-Snyderman et al. 2011). The Keystone Project studies provide evidence that CRBSIs can be significantly reduced and that the reduction can be sustained by measuring the rate of CRBSIs and providing ongoing feedback to practitioners.

PREVENTION OF CRBSIs – EVIDENCE-BASED GUIDELINES

The Centers for Disease Control (CDC) published guidelines for prevention of CRBSIs in 2011. (O'Grady et al. 2011) Recommendations were made in the areas of (1) education, training, and staffing, (2) selection of catheters and sites, and (3) hand hygiene and aseptic technique. The recommendations were categorized based on the level of supporting evidence (see Table 10.1). This chapter reviews only the recommendations based on category 1 evidence. A complete review of all recommendations is in the published guidelines (O'Grady et al. 2011).

Education, training, and staffing

Appropriate education and knowledge assessment of healthcare personnel regarding the indications, techniques of vascular catheter insertion, and infection control precautions are associated with a reduced rate of CRBSIs. Clinical privileges should be restricted to trained healthcare workers (category 1A) (Nehme 1980, Eggimann et al. 2000, Sherertz et al. 2000, Yoo et al. 2001, Coopersmith et al. 2002, 2004, Warren et al. 2003, 2004, 2006b, Higuera et al. 2005).

Selection of catheters and sites

There are a wide variety of intravascular catheters used in clinical practice (**Table 10.2**). For practical purposes, the catheters can be separated into three broad categories: Peripheral catheters, central venous catheters, and umbilical catheters (for use in neonates).

Peripheral catheters

The operator should be familiar with the selected peripheral catheter (category 1B) (Band and Maki 1980, Tully 1981, Ryder 1995). Peripheral catheters should be removed immediately if the patient develops signs of phlebitis (pain, erythema, edema, warmth. or a palpable venous cord) (category IB) (Maki et al. 1991). Metal needles ("scalp veins") should not be used for the administration of fluids and medications that can cause tissue necrosis in the event of extravasation (category 1A) (Band and Maki 1980, Tully 1981). Although not a CDC recommendation,

Table 10.2 Catheters used for venous and arterial access.

Catheter type	Entry site	Length	Comments
Peripheral venous catheters	Usually inserted in veins of forearm or hand	<3 inches (7.6 cm)	Phlebitis with prolonged use; rarely associated with bloodstream infection
Peripheral arterial catheters	Usually inserted in radial artery; can be placed in femoral, axillary, brachial, posterior tibial arteries	<3 inches (7.6 cm)	Low infection risk; rarely associated with bloodstream infection
Midline catheters	Inserted via the antecubital fossa into the proximal basilica or cephalic veins; does not enter central veins, peripheral catheters	3–8 inches (7.6–20.3 cm)	Anaphylactoid reactions have been reported with catheters made of elastomeric hydrogel; lower rates of phlebitis than short peripheral catheters
Non-tunneled central venous catheters (CVCs)	Percutaneously inserted into central veins (subclavian, internal jugular, or femoral)	>8 cm depending on patient size	Account for most CRBSIs
Pulmonary artery catheters	Inserted through a Teflon introducer in a central vein (subclavian, internal jugular, or femoral)	≥30 cm depending on patient size	Usually heparin bonded; similar rates of bloodstream infection as CVCs; subclavian site preferred to reduce infection risk
Peripherally inserted central venous catheters (PICCs)	Inserted into basilic, cephalic, or brachial veins and enter the superior vena cava	≥20 cm depending on patient size	Lower rate of infection than non-tunneled CVCs
Tunneled central venous catheters	Implanted into subclavian, internal jugular, or femoral veins	≥8 cm depending on patient size	Cuff inhibits migration of organisms into catheter tract; lower rate of infection than non-tunneled CVCs
Totally implantable	Tunneled beneath skin and have subcutaneous port accessed with a needle; implanted in subclavian or internal jugular vein	≥8 cm depending on patient size	Lowest risk for CRBSI; improved patient self-image; no need for local catheter site care; surgery required for catheter removal
Umbilical catheters	Inserted into either umbilical vein or umbilical artery	≥6 cm depending on patient size	Risk for CRBSIs similar with catheters placed in umbilical vein versus artery

CRBSIs, catheter-related bloodstream infections.

the author's own practice is to restrict infusion of medications that are thrombogenic or noxious to soft tissues (e.g., potassium chloride or calcium salts) to central venous catheters. This practice minimizes the risk of pain and phlebitis, and avoids extravasation, which can cause soft-tissue necrosis.

Care must be taken with the use of infusion pumps. Very rarely, a subfascial infusion of fluid under pressure can cause a compartment syndrome. If unrecognized and untreated, irreversible nerve injury and myonecrosis can result in addition to the risks of soft-tissue infection at the site of extravasation.

Central venous catheters

Central venous access can be achieved via a peripheral vein or the femoral, subclavian, or internal jugular veins. A peripherally inserted central catheter (PICC) placed under ultrasound guidance is the preferred site of access for long-term intravenous therapy, administration of phlebitogenic or noxious medications, or intravenous nutritional support because of the low risk of mechanical complications (e.g., pneumothorax, hemothorax, and air embolism). A femoral venous catheter should be avoided when possible because of the increased risk of CRBSIs (category Level 1A) (Goetz et al. 1998, Merrer et al. 2001, Lorente et al. 2005, Parienti et al. 2008) and deep venous thrombosis (Merrer et al. 2001).

Subclavian and internal jugular catheters may be tunneled subcutaneously or non-tunneled. Non-tunneled central venous catheters account for most CRBSIs (O'Grady et al. 2011) and should be avoided if possible.

Subclavian venous catheters are associated with a lower risk of CRBSIs and are preferable to internal jugular venous catheters for non-tunneled central venous access (category 1B) (Robinson et al.

1995, Goetz et al. 1998, Merrer et al. 2001). However, the risk of infection must be weighed against the experience and skill of the operator. Bleeding from the injured subclavian artery is difficult or impossible to tamponade. A subclavian artery injury combined with a pneumothorax can lead to massive hemothorax and exsanguination. As a general principle, the clinician should choose a catheterization technique for which she or he has the appropriate training and experience.

Ultrasound guidance for placement of central venous catheters has been shown to significantly reduce the number of cannulation attempts and the mechanical complications of central venous catheterizations (category 1B) (Randolph et al. 1996, Hind et al. 2003, Lamperti et al. 2008, Froehlich et al. 2009, Schweickert et al. 2009, Fragou et al. 2011). Reductions in cannulation attempts and mechanical complications reduce infections at the catheter site.

Occasionally central venous access must be performed in an emergency under less than ideal circumstances. If the sterility of the catheter insertion is in question, the catheter should be removed within 48 h when the patient's hemodynamic status has stabilized (category 1B) (Mermel et al. 1991, Mermel and Maki 1994, Raad et al. 1994, Capdevila et al. 1998, Abi-Said et al. 1999, National Kidney Foundation 2001). ICU patients frequently have fever associated with leukocytosis of uncertain cause, raising the question of CRBSIs. Prompt removal of the catheter, a previously recommended practice, is no longer essential (category 1A) (Lederle et al. 1992, Parenti et al. 1994, Raad et al. 1994, Berenholtz et al. 2004, Pronovost 2008). Hemodynamically stable patients can be evaluated for the cause of infection before removal of a catheter. In general, the catheter should be removed only for a definitively diagnosed infection. On occasions, a catheter can be removed after failure to identify an alternative cause of infection.

Hand hygiene and aseptic technique

Insertion of an intravascular catheter is a surgical procedure and should be treated as such. Prior hand washing with conventional soap and water or alcohol-based hand rubs (Pittet et al. 1999, Bischoff et al. 2000, Boyce et al. 2002, Coopersmith et al. 2002), with strict aseptic technique for insertion and care of the catheters, is essential (category 1B) (Mermel et al. 1991, Raad et al. 1994, Capdevila et al. 1998, Abi-Said et al. 1999). Clean, rather than sterile, gloves may be worn for insertion of peripheral venous catheters as long as the skin is not touched after sterile preparation (category 1C). Maximal sterile barrier precautions including cap, mask, sterile gown, gloves, and full body drape should be used for all insertion and guidewire exchanges of central venous catheters (category 1B) (Mermel et al. 1994, Raad et al. 1994, Sherertz et al. 2000, Carrer et al. 2005).

A solution of 70% isopropyl alcohol, tincture of iodine, or a >0.5% chlorhexidine preparation with isopropyl alcohol may be used to prepare the skin (category 1A) (Maki and Ringer 1991, Mimoz et al. 1996). There are no data comparing the efficacy of the various skin preparations. Basic surgical principles should be employed in the management of the catheter insertion site. Topical antibiotics should not be used on insertion sites, except for dialysis sites, because of the risk of fungal infections and antimicrobial resistance (category 1B) (Flowers et al. 1989, Zakrzewska-Bode 1995). There is no indication for systemic antimicrobial prophylaxis before or during intravascular catheter insertion (category 1B) (van de Wetering and van Woensel 2007).

The same principles are applied to the insertion of peripheral arterial catheters except that sterile gloves are mandated for all arterial line insertions (category 1B) (Rijnders et al. 2003, Traore et al. 2005, Koh et al. 2008). There are various recommendations for the management of the pressure monitoring system attached to the arterial catheter (O'Grady et al. 2011). The basic principles are use of disposable transducers when possible, use of a closed system, use of topical antiseptics before accessing the system, and replacement of tubing and connectors contaminated with blood.

APPROACH TO THE FEBRILE PATIENT WITH A LONG-TERM INDWELLING VASCULAR CATHETER

An ICU patient with a long-term indwelling central venous catheter who develops fever and leukocytosis usually has multiple potential sites of infection, including the central venous catheter. The clinician must determine the cause of the infection and whether the catheter should be removed. The catheter is always a consideration for infection but the risk is directly proportional to the duration of catheterization. The longer the catheter has been in place, the greater the risk of a CRBSI. Other variables to be considered include the anatomic site of catheterization, whether or not the catheter is tunneled, the condition of the skin at the insertion site, and the function of the catheter. The femoral and internal jugular venous catheters are at much greater risk for CRBSIs compared with subclavian venous catheters. Tunneled catheters are less likely to be associated with CRBSI than non-tunneled ones. Catheter insertion sites draining fluid or pus or surrounded by erythematous skin are of great concern. Percutaneous central venous catheters for hemodialysis access also have a significant risk for CRBSIs, particularly if the catheters have been in place for an extended period of time.

Making a definitive diagnosis of CRBSIs

With certain exceptions, patients without positive blood cultures do not have a CRBSI. A careful search for alternative sources of infection using microbial cultures, physical examination and appropriate imaging techniques (CT scans of the abdomen and chest), depending on the clinical problem, is essential. Neither the fever nor the white blood cell (WBC) counts are particularly helpful. Patients with leukopenia (WBCs <2000) or leukocytosis (WBCs >18 000) merit special attention. In most cases, a positive blood culture, especially with Gram-positive organisms, suggests the diagnosis. If the fever resolves after the catheter is removed, a CRBSI is highly probable. Culture of the catheter tip is usually unnecessary. Placing the catheter tip in broth media is a waste of time. The culture will be 'positive' even if only one colony grows. In the unusual case where a culture is desirable, the roll-plate method should be used. The catheter tip is rolled on a blood agar plate and the number of colonies counted. By convention, >15 colonies are considered an infection.

From an operational point of view, if the catheter is removed, the blood cultures become negative and the fever resolves, a retrospective diagnosis of CRBSI is made. In a few highly suspicious unusual cases, a quantitative culture of the catheter tip is reasonable.

Indications for catheter removal (Figure 10.1)

The catheter should be removed immediately if there are positive blood cultures and no other source of infection is identified. In general, catheters should be removed immediately if *S. aureus* or *Candida* spp are identified on blood cultures. Occasionally, a difficult-to-place essential line can be changed over a guidewire and observed while the patient is treated with antibiotics. However, in almost all cases, patients with a *S. aureus* or *Candida* spp. blood-borne infection will require catheter removal. Patients with SACRBSIs should receive an echocardiogram to exclude the infrequently associated case of endocarditis. Patients with a *Candida* spp. CRBSI should receive an ophthalmic examination to exclude candida endophthalmitis.

In selected clinical situations, including infection with *S. epidermidis*, the catheter can be temporarily preserved during antibiotic treatment. Eventually, most infections require catheter removal.

Duration of antibiotic therapy

Patients with *S. aureus* and *Candida* spp. infections require 14 days of antibiotic therapy after catheter removal. The optimal duration of treatment for CRBSIs secondary to coagulase-negative staphylococci remains unknown. Most clinicians give a minimum of 7 days of antibiotic therapy for a CRBSI in this circumstance.

CONCLUSION

Advances in clinical care have led to the proliferation of intravascular catheterizations. This has resulted in an epidemic of CRBSIs accounting for significant morbidity, mortality, and increased cost of care. Advances in bacteriology and pathophysiology have led to effective strategies that have demonstrated significant reductions in the risk of CRBSIs in both single and multi-institutional studies. Adherence to the 2011 CDC guidelines for the prevention of intravascular catheter-related infections (O'Grady et al. 2011) is essential to control the epidemic and achieve safe intravascular therapy.

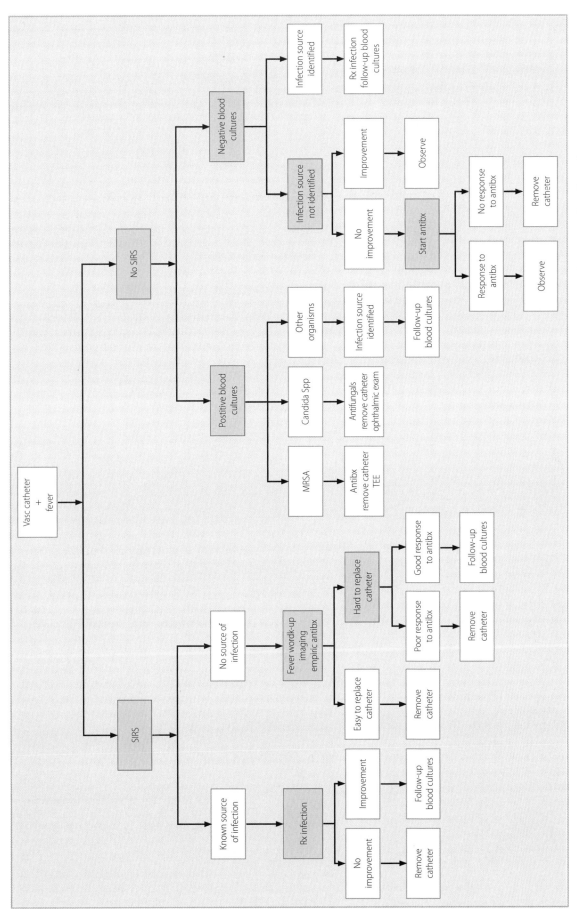

Figure 10.1 Management of patients with an indwelling vascular catheter and a fever. (Reprinted from O'Grady et al. (2011). Copyright 2011, with permission from Elsevier.)

■ REFERENCES

Abi-Said D, Raad I, Umphrey J, et al. Infusion therapy team and dressing changes of central venous catheters. *Infect Control Hosp Epidemiol* 1999;**20**:101–5.

Anaissie E, Samonis G, Kontoyiannis D, et al. Role of catheter colonization and infrequent hematogenous seeding in catheter-related infections. *Eur J Clin Microbiol Infect Dis* 1995;**14**:134–7.

Band JD, Maki DG. Steel needles used for intravenous therapy. Morbidity in patients with hematologic malignancy. *Arch Intern Med* 1980;**140**:31–4.

Berenholtz SM, Pronovost PJ, Lipsett PA, et al. Eliminating catheter-related bloodstream infections in the intensive care unit. *Crit Care Med* 2004;**32**:2014–20.

Bischoff WE, Reynolds TM, Sessler CN, et al. Handwashing compliance by health care workers: The impact of introducing an accessible, alcohol-based hand antiseptic. *Arch Intern Med* 2000;**160**:1017–21.

Blot SI, Depuydt P, Annemans L, et al. Clinical and economic outcomes in critically ill patients with nosocomial catheter-related bloodstream infections. *Clin Infect Dis* 2005;**41**:1591–8.

Boyce JM, Pittet D. Guideline for Hand Hygiene in Health-Care Settings: recommendations of the Healthcare Infection Control Practices Advisory Committee and the HICPAC/SHEA/APIC/IDSA Hand Hygiene Task Force. *Infect Control Hosp Epidemiol* 2002;**23**:S3–40.

Capdevila JA, Segarra A, Pahissa A. Catheter-related bacteremia in patients undergoing hemodialysis. *Ann Intern Med* 1998;**128**:600.

Carrer S, Bocchi A, Bortolotti M, et al. Effect of different sterile barrier precautions and central venous catheter dressing on the skin colonization around the insertion site. *Minerva Anestesiol* 2005;**71**:197–206.

Coopersmith CM, Rebmann TL, Zack JE, et al. Effect of an education program on decreasing catheter-related bloodstream infections in the surgical intensive care unit. *Crit Care Med* 2002;**30**:59–64.

Coopersmith CM, Zack JE, Ward MR, et al. The impact of bedside behavior on catheter-related bacteremia in the intensive care unit. *Arch Surg* 2004;**139**:131–6.

Cosgrove SE, Sakoulas G, Perencevich EN, et al. Comparison of mortality associated with methicillin-resistant and methicillin-susceptible *Staphylococcus aureus* bacteremia: a meta-analysis. *Clin Infect Dis* 2003;**36**:53–9.

Dimick JB, Pelz RK, Consunji R, et al. Increased resource use associated with catheter-related bloodstream infection in the surgical intensive care unit. *Arch Surg* 2001;**136**:229–34.

Dobbins BM, Kite P, Kindon A, et al. DNA fingerprinting analysis of coagulase negative staphylococci implicated in catheter related bloodstream infections. *J Clin Pathol* 2002;**55**:824–8.

Donlan RM. Role of biofilms in antimicrobial resistance. *ASAIO J* 2000;**46**:S47–52.

Douglas LJ. Candida biofilms and their role in infection. *Trends Microbiol* 2003;**11**:30–6.

Eggimann P, Harbarth S, Constantin MN, et al. Impact of a prevention strategy targeted at vascular-access care on incidence of infections acquired in intensive care. *Lancet* 2000;**355**:1864–8.

Farber BF, Kaplan MH, Clogston AG. *Staphylococcus epidermidis* extracted slime inhibits the antimicrobial action of glycopeptide antibiotics. *J Infect Dis* 1990;**161**:37–40.

Flowers RH, 3rd, Schwenzer KJ, Kopel RF, et al. Efficacy of an attachable subcutaneous cuff for the prevention of intravascular catheter-related infection. A randomized, controlled trial. *JAMA* 1989;**261**:878–83.

Fragou M, Gravvanis A, Dimitriou V, et al. Real-time ultrasound-guided subclavian vein cannulation versus the landmark method in critical care patients: A prospective randomized study. *Crit Care Med* 2011;**39**:1607–12.

Froehlich CD, Rigby MR, Rosenberg ES, et al. Ultrasound-guided central venous catheter placement decreases complications and decreases placement attempts compared with the landmark technique in patients in a pediatric intensive care unit. *Crit Care Med* 2009;**37**:1090–6.

Gaynes R, Edwards JR. Overview of nosocomial infections caused by Gram-negative bacilli. *Clin Infect Dis* 2005;**41**:848–54.

Goetz AM, Wagener MM, Miller JM, Muder RR. Risk of infection due to central venous catheters: effect of site of placement and catheter type. *Infect Control Hosp Epidemiol* 1998;**19**:842–5.

Hawser SP, Douglas LJ. Biofilm formation by Candida species on the surface of catheter materials in vitro. *Infect Immun* 1994;**62**:915–21.

Herrmann M, Suchard SJ, Boxer LA, et al. Thrombospondin binds to *Staphylococcus aureus* and promotes staphylococcal adherence to surfaces. *Infect Immun* 1991;**59**:279–88.

Higuera F, Rosenthal VD, Duarte P, et al. The effect of process control on the incidence of central venous catheter-associated bloodstream infections and mortality in intensive care units in Mexico. *Crit Care Med* 2005;**33**:2022–7.

Hind D, Calvert N, McWilliams R, et al. Ultrasonic locating devices for central venous cannulation: meta-analysis. *BMJ* 2003;**327**:361.

Kaasch AJ, Fowler VG, Jr., Rieg S, et al. Use of a simple criteria set for guiding echocardiography in nosocomial Staphylococcus aureus bacteremia. *Clin Infect Dis* 2011;**53**:1–9.

Koh DB, Gowardman JR, Rickard CM, et al. Prospective study of peripheral arterial catheter infection and comparison with concurrently sited central venous catheters. *Crit Care Med* 2008;**36**:397–402.

Lamperti M, Caldiroli D, Cortellazzi P, et al. Safety and efficacy of ultrasound assistance during internal jugular vein cannulation in neurosurgical infants. *Intensive Care Med* 2008;**34**:2100–5.

Lederle FA, Parenti CM, Berskow LC, Ellingson KJ. The idle intravenous catheter. *Ann Intern Med* 1992;**116**:737–8.

Lipitz-Snyderman A, Steinwachs D, Needham DM, et al. Impact of a statewide intensive care unit quality improvement initiative on hospital mortality and length of stay: retrospective comparative analysis. *BMJ* 2011;**342**:d219.

Lorente L, Henry C, Martin MM, et al. Central venous catheter-related infection in a prospective and observational study of 2,595 catheters. *Crit Care* 2005;**9**:R631–5.

McDevitt D, Francois P, Vaudaux P, Foster TJ. Identification of the ligand-binding domain of the surface-located fibrinogen receptor (clumping factor) of *Staphylococcus aureus*. *Mol Microbiol* 1995;**16**:895–907.

Mack D, Davies AP, Harris LG, et al. Microbial interactions in *Staphylococcus epidermidis* biofilms. *Anal Bioanal Chem* 2007;**387**:399–408.

Maki DG, Ringer M, Alvarado CJ. Prospective randomised trial of povidone-iodine, alcohol, and chlorhexidine for prevention of infection associated with central venous and arterial catheters. *Lancet* 1991;**338**:339–43.

Maki DG, Weise CE, Sarafin HW. A semiquantitative culture method for identifying intravenous-catheter-related infection. *N Engl J Med* 1977;**296**:1305–9.

Maki DG, Ringer M. Risk factors for infusion-related phlebitis with small peripheral venous catheters. A randomized controlled trial. *Ann Intern Med* 1991;**114**:845–54.

Mehall JR, Saltzman DA, Jackson RJ, Smith SD. Fibrin sheath enhances central venous catheter infection. *Crit Care Med* 2002;**30**:908–12.

Mermel LA, Maki DG. Infectious complications of Swan-Ganz pulmonary artery catheters. Pathogenesis, epidemiology, prevention, and management. *Am J Respir Crit Care Med* 1994;**149**:1020–36.

Mermel LA, McCormick RD, Springman SR, Maki DG. The pathogenesis and epidemiology of catheter-related infection with pulmonary artery Swan–Ganz catheters: a prospective study utilizing molecular subtyping. *Am J Med* 1991;**91**:197S-205S.

Mermel LA, McKay M, Dempsey J, Parenteau S. Pseudomonas surgical-site infections linked to a healthcare worker with onychomycosis. *Infect Control Hosp Epidemiol* 2003;**24**:749–52.

Merrer J, De Jonghe B, Golliot F, et al. Complications of femoral and subclavian venous catheterization in critically ill patients: a randomized controlled trial. *JAMA* 2001;**286**:700–7.

Mimoz O, Pieroni L, Lawrence C, et al. Prospective, randomized trial of two antiseptic solutions for prevention of central venous or arterial catheter colonization and infection in intensive care unit patients. *Crit Care Med* 1996;**24**:1818–23.

Murga R, Miller JM, Donlan RM. Biofilm formation by gram-negative bacteria on central venous catheter connectors: effect of conditioning films in a laboratory model. *J Clin Microbiol* 2001;**39**:2294–7.

National Kidney Foundation. KDOQI Clinical Practice Guidelines for Vascular Access, 2000. *Am J Kidney Dis* 2001;**37**(suppl 1):S137–81.

Nehme AE. Nutritional support of the hospitalized patient. The team concept. *JAMA* 1980;**243**:1906–8.

Ni Eidhin D, Perkins S, Francois P, et al. Clumping factor B (ClfB), a new surface-located fibrinogen-binding adhesin of *Staphylococcus aureus*. *Mol Microbiol* 1998;**30**:245–57.

O'Grady NP, Alexander M, Burns LA, et al. Guidelines for the prevention of intravascular catheter-related infections. *Am J Infect Control* 2011;**39**:S1–34.

Parenti CM, Lederle FA, Impola CL, Peterson LR. Reduction of unnecessary intravenous catheter use. Internal medicine house staff participate in a successful quality improvement project. *Arch Intern Med* 1994;**154**:1829–32.

Parienti JJ, Thirion M, Megarbane B, et al. Femoral vs jugular venous catheterization and risk of nosocomial events in adults requiring acute renal replacement therapy: a randomized controlled trial. *JAMA* 2008;**299**:2413–22.

Pittet D, Dharan S, Touveneau S, et al. Bacterial contamination of the hands of hospital staff during routine patient care. *Arch Intern Med* 1999;**159**:821–6.

Pronovost P. Interventions to decrease catheter-related bloodstream infections in the ICU: the Keystone Intensive Care Unit Project. *Am J Infect Control* 2008;**36**:S171 e1–5.

Pronovost P, Needham D, Berenholtz S, et al. An intervention to decrease catheter-related bloodstream infections in the ICU. *N Engl J Med* 2006;**355**:2725–32.

Pronovost PJ, Goeschel CA, Colantuoni E, et al. Sustaining reductions in catheter related bloodstream infections in Michigan intensive care units: observational study. *BMJ* 2010;**340**:c309.

Raad I, Costerton W, Sabharwal U, et al. Ultrastructural analysis of indwelling vascular catheters: a quantitative relationship between luminal colonization and duration of placement. *J Infect Dis* 1993;**168**:400–7.

Raad I, Hohn DC, Gilbreath BJ, et al. Prevention of central venous catheter-related infections by using maximal sterile barrier precautions during insertion. *Infect Control Hosp Epidemiol* 1994;**15**:231–8.

Raad I, Hanna HA, Awad A, et al. Optimal frequency of changing intravenous administration sets: is it safe to prolong use beyond 72 hours? *Infect Control Hosp Epidemiol* 2001;**22**:136–9.

Randolph AG, Cook DJ, Gonzales CA, Pribble CG. Ultrasound guidance for placement of central venous catheters: a meta-analysis of the literature. *Crit Care Med* 1996;**24**:2053–8.

Renaud B, Brun-Buisson C. Outcomes of primary and catheter-related bacteremia. A cohort and case-control study in critically ill patients. *Am J Respir Crit Care Med* 2001;**163**:1584–90.

Rijnders BJ, Van Wijngaerden E, Wilmer A, Peetermans WE. Use of full sterile barrier precautions during insertion of arterial catheters: a randomized trial. *Clin Infect Dis* 2003;**36**:743–8.

Robinson JF, Robinson WA, Cohn A, et al. 2nd. Perforation of the great vessels during central venous line placement. *Arch Intern Med* 1995;**155**:1225–8.

Rosenthal VD, Maki DG, Salomao R, et al. Device-associated nosocomial infections in 55 intensive care units of 8 developing countries. *Ann Intern Med* 2006;**145**:582–91.

Ryder MA. Peripheral access options. *Surg Oncol Clin N Am* 1995;**4**:395–427.

Safdar N, Maki DG. The pathogenesis of catheter-related bloodstream infection with noncuffed short-term central venous catheters. *Intensive Care Med* 2004;**30**:62–7.

Schweickert WD, Herlitz J, Pohlman AS, et al. A randomized, controlled trial evaluating postinsertion neck ultrasound in peripherally inserted central catheter procedures. *Crit Care Med* 2009;**37**:1217–21.

Sherertz RJ, Ely EW, Westbrook DM, et al. Education of physicians-in-training can decrease the risk for vascular catheter infection. *Ann Intern Med* 2000;**132**:641–8.

Stillman RM, Soliman F, Garcia L, Sawyer PN. Etiology of catheter-associated sepsis. Correlation with thrombogenicity. *Arch Surg* 1977;**112**:1497–9.

Traore O, Liotier J, Souweine B. Prospective study of arterial and central venous catheter colonization and of arterial- and central venous catheter-related bacteremia in intensive care units. *Crit Care Med* 2005;**33**:1276–80.

Tully JL, Friedland GH, Baldini LM, Goldmann DA. Complications of intravenous therapy with steel needles and Teflon catheters. A comparative study. *Am J Med* 1981;**70**:702–6.

van de Wetering MD, van Woensel JB. Prophylactic antibiotics for preventing early central venous catheter Gram positive infections in oncology patients. *Cochrane Database Syst Rev* 2007;(**1**):CD003295.

von Eiff C, Peters G, Heilmann C. Pathogenesis of infections due to coagulase-negative staphylococci. *Lancet Infect Dis* 2002;**2**:677–85.

Warren DK, Zack JE, Cox MJ, et al. An educational intervention to prevent catheter-associated bloodstream infections in a nonteaching, community medical center. *Crit Care Med* 2003;**31**:1959–63.

Warren DK, Zack JE, Mayfield JL, et al. The effect of an education program on the incidence of central venous catheter-associated bloodstream infection in a medical ICU. *Chest* 2004;**126**:1612–18.

Warren DK, Cosgrove SE, Diekema DJ, et al. A multicenter intervention to prevent catheter-associated bloodstream infections. *Infect Control Hosp Epidemiol* 2006a;**27**:662–9.

Warren DK, Quadir WW, Hollenbeak CS, et al. Attributable cost of catheter-associated bloodstream infections among intensive care patients in a nonteaching hospital. *Crit Care Med* 2006b;**34**:2084–9.

Wisplinghoff H, Bischoff T, Tallent SM, et al. Nosocomial bloodstream infections in US hospitals: analysis of 24,179 cases from a prospective nationwide surveillance study. *Clin Infect Dis* 2004;**39**:309–17.

Yoo S, Ha M, Choi D, Pai H. Effectiveness of surveillance of central catheter-related bloodstream infection in an ICU in Korea. *Infect Control Hosp Epidemiol* 2001;**22**:433–6.

Zakrzewska-Bode A, Muytjens HL, Liem KD, Hoogkamp-Korstanje JA. Mupirocin resistance in coagulase-negative staphylococci, after topical prophylaxis for the reduction of colonization of central venous catheters. *J Hosp Infect* 1995;**31**:189–93.

Chapter 11 | *Clostridium difficile* infection

Donald E. Fry

Clostridium difficile is an anaerobic, Gram-positive rod that was not identified until 1935 (**Figure 11.1**). It is a difficult bacterium to culture, hence the name "difficile." It was not associated with clinical disease until the late 1970s when experimental studies in guinea-pigs identified it as the pathogen of the antibiotic-associated enterocolitis syndrome. Since its identification, *Clostridium difficile* infections (CDIs) have progressively increased in frequency as a complication of hospitalized patients. In the USA, it occurs in nearly 400 000 hospitalized cases per year and exceeds 1% of all hospitalized adult patients (Agency for Healthcare Research and Quality 2011) (**Figure 11.2**). Total cases have been estimated to approach 3 million per year including ambulatory, post-discharge, and relapsing cases from prior infection. The number of deaths associated with CDIs has steadily increased as the number of cases has increased (Zilberberg et al. 2008). CDI has become an international epidemic among all cohorts of patients (Gerding 2010), but is especially problematic for patients undergoing major surgical procedures. Infections can be quite unpredictable, and occur in episodic clusters within given hospitals.

CDI has followed a clinical trajectory that can be compared with meticillin-resistant *Staphylococcus aureus* (MRSA) infection. The organism has assumed a more virulent profile in addition to being a more common cause of infections. Similar to MRSA, it is now being identified with increased frequency as a community-acquired pathogen. Preventive strategies have been inconsistently successful. Little progress has been made over the last two decades in the development of new treatments. It has rapidly become one of the most severe complications among surgical patients.

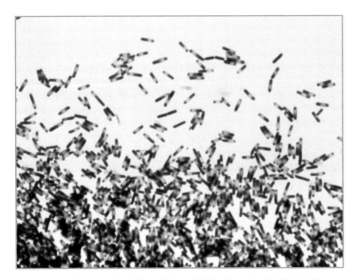

Figure 11.1 Micrograph of *Clostridium difficile*. (From the Public Health Image Library, Centers for Disease Control, courtesy of Dr Gilda Jones: http://phil.cdc.gov/phil/details.asp.)

■ PATHOGENESIS

As it is an obligate anaerobe, *C. difficile* exists as a spore when outside a host. When confronted with an unfriendly environment, the spore permits survival of the bacterium until it finds a suitable milieu to transform into the vegetative phase that leads to clinical infection.

The cell target for *C. difficile* in causing human disease is the colonocyte. The spore gains access to humans by being ingested from the external environment. The thick coat of the spore permits survival in passing through the acid environment of the stomach. The passage into the small intestine does not favor the transition to the vegetative phase because of the oxygen tension in this area. Only in the distal ileum and then in the colon are environmental anaerobic conditions within the lumen favorable for the vegetative phase of the organism. As an abundance of non-specific host defense mechanisms exist within the colon, a critical inoculum of ingested spores is necessary to yield a clinical infection.

Colonization resistance best describes the normal colonic mucosa's ability to withstand CDI because of the normal microbial constituents. The normal microflora have 10 000 anaerobes for each aerobic organism in the rectosigmoid colon, so competition for substrates to support the vegetative state for *C. difficile* is problematic. Metabolic end-products of competing microflora may be sufficiently toxic to *C. difficile* to repress the vegetative state transition. Even if the vegetative transition occurs, the competitive inhibition of the normal anaerobic population of bacteria for receptor sites on the target colonocytes may preclude binding and the resultant CDI.

In addition to colonization resistance, other non-specific host defense mechanisms protect the colon mucosa from infection mediated by *C. difficile* or other pathogenic bacteria. Surface mucins form an initial protective barrier. IgA antibody may bind to *C. difficile* surface targets to impede the binding to colonocytes. Effective gut motility can propel spores through the colon and minimize the opportunity for vegetative forms to bind to the colonocyte. Thus, in surgical patients it is easy to identify that disruption of normal feeding, anesthetics and analgesics, and non-specific ileus, which attends bowel manipulation during laparotomy, can lead to a diminished colonic transit time that favors the emergence of CDI.

Binding to the colonocyte is a critical determinant for CDIs to occur. Fimbriae and flagellae play a role in motility and binding of the vegetative form. Specific surface receptors of the bacterial cell bind to the colonocyte and have been a therapeutic focus because receptor blockade will modulate microbial virulence. The positive electrical charge of the *C. difficile* surface and the negative charge of the colonocyte surface are also considered to play a role in adhesion of the pathogen.

Once binding occurs, the *C. difficile* microorganism elaborates two unique toxins that synergistically damage the mucosa of the colon. Toxin A is an enterotoxin and toxin B a non-specific cytotoxin. The toxins bind to the plasma membrane of colonocytes, are internalized, and damage the cytoskeleton of the host cell, leading to necrosis.

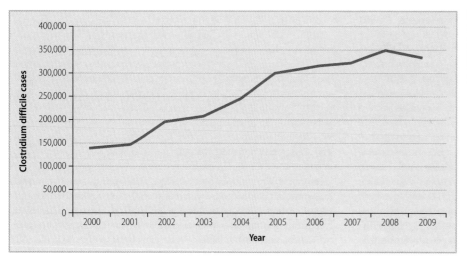

Figure 11.2 The progressive increase in *Clostridium difficile* infections among discharged patients from US hospitals over the last 10 years. (Data from the National Inpatient Sample, Healthcare Cost and Utilization Project, http://hcupnet.ahrq.gov.)

The loss of cytoskeleton leads to the observed "cell rounding" in the affected colonocyte before frank membrane disruption and necrosis. The presence of these toxins is essential for microbial virulence because *C. difficile* strains are identified that do not produce toxins and do not have virulence.

Other virulence factors facilitate CDIs once the process has been initiated by toxins A and B. Hyaluronidase and collagenase disrupt the extracellular matrix between colonocytes and in the subsequently exposed submucosal tissues. A polysaccharide capsule retards phagocytosis of the pathogen by host leukocytes. The necrosis of colonocytes and the effects of other bacteria in the heavily populated colon lead to progressive injury of the transmural population of colonic cells. With inflammatory changes of smooth muscle, poor peristalsis, increased intestinal pressure, and tissue ischemia occur as the disease progresses.

CDI has distinct pathological stages. In advanced cases it is possible to identify all four stages affecting different areas of colonic mucosa. The erythematous mucosa reflects early consequences of the toxins. At this stage, diarrhea and crampy abdominal pain begin. Patchy necrosis represents areas where toxic effects have caused cell necrosis and lysis with a robust mucosal inflammatory response. Pseudomembranes are identified at diagnostic endoscopy as inflammatory exudates form over areas of necrotic mucosa. The clinical symptoms of diarrhea and crampy abdominal pain are exacerbated. Abdominal distension reflects inflammatory effects on colonic smooth muscle. Transmural inflammation and toxic megacolon emerge as the disease progresses because of impaired and poorly coordinated colonic peristalsis. Severe abdominal pain and distension are present. The patients are systemically toxic. Diarrhea commonly ceases at this point. Transmural necrosis occurs with smooth muscle death from severe inflammation and ischemic changes of colonic distension. The microcirculation may thrombose from the intense inflammation. The adventitial layer of the colon may maintain viability, giving a deceptive external appearance to the extent of the colonic mucosal necrosis underneath. With necrosis of the overlying serosa, bacterial peritonitis and potentially even perforation of the necrotic segment may occur in very advanced cases.

Over the last decade, new hypervirulent strains (BI/NAP1/027) of *C. difficile* have emerged and are associated with unusually severe and rapidly evolving CDIs (McDonald et al. 2005). These hypervirulent strains represent mutants with loss of the regulatory gene that controls the production of toxins A and B. Mutant strains produce 15–20 times the quantity of these toxins and yields a fulminate disease

that is strongly associated with the rapid evolution of full-thickness necrosis of the colon. These variants result in such a rapidly evolving enterocolitis that the diarrhea phase of the disease may be very transient or not present at all. Surgical intervention has become much more common and mortality rates for these patients are dramatically greater than identified with conventional CDIs. In addition, these hypervirulent strains have been associated with a binary toxin known at *C. difficile* transferase (Papatheodorou et al. 2011). This binary toxin is distinct from toxins A and B, but it may be synergistic with them. Some evidence indicates that the binary toxin may enhance the adherence of *C. difficile* to the colonocyte and promote enhanced virulence by this mechanism.

RISK FACTORS

A number of patient variables and healthcare interventions are associated with the development of CDIs (Ananthadrishnan 2011). Among patient factors, increasing age is the most commonly recognized association. Despite stool detection of the toxins of *C. difficile* in 50% of neonates in intensive care settings, CDIs are very uncommon in neonates and infants. It is thought that the neonatal and infant populations have lower rates of infection because of the reduced expression of the target receptor for *C. difficile* on the immature colonocyte. The incidence of the infection increases with increasing age (**Figure 11.3**). Most CDIs occur in patients aged >60 years. Although the frequency of infection is linked to the number and duration of hospitalizations, age-adjusted profiles of hospital days by decade of life still demonstrates that CDIs increase with age as an independent variable. This association with increased age appears to be related to a progressive reduction in colonization resistance in elderly people, the increase in the use of antibiotics with each passing decade, increased hospitalization and nursing home days, and the immunosuppression of chronic diseases.

Many specific patient disease variables are being associated with an increased odds ratio for the development of CDIs (Loo et al. 2011). Patients with ulcerative colitis and regional enteritis have increased frequency and severity of CDIs. Colon cancer patients have similarly been noted to have increased rates due to either a more vulnerable colonic barrier or weight loss from the illness. Renal failure patients receiving dialysis have the immunosuppression of chronic disease, frequent antibiotics, and frequent transfusion as potential causative factors. Most patients with several chronic disease conditions have been associated with CDIs, and even pregnancy has been recognized (Rouphael et al. 2008). Vitamin

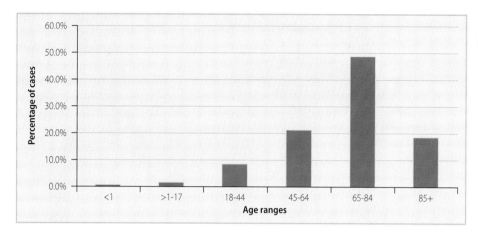

Figure 11.3 The age distribution of *Clostridium difficile* infection from a 20% national sample of patients in the USA from 2000 to 2009. (Data from the National Inpatient Sample, Healthcare Cost and Utilization Project, http://hcupnet.ahrq.gov.)

D deficiency is another recently identified variable. Probably the strongest patient characteristic is the history of prior CDIs. There is no sexual predilection for this infection.

Although selected host factors do contribute to the frequency of CDIs, it is most strongly linked to being a healthcare-associated disease. Over 90% of cases are linked to the use of systemic antibiotics. Ampicillin, amoxicillin, and clindamycin were the antibiotics associated with CDIs in the early descriptions of this infection, but the quinolone group of drugs has recently been very strongly correlated with this complication. The cephalosporin group has had a consistent association over the three decades of tracking this disease. Virtually every antibiotic has been associated with CDIs, including vancomycin and metronidazole as the drugs used to actually treat the infection. This latter paradox speaks to the complexity of the numerous variables that result in this clinical infection.

The hospital length of stay has a strong correlation with CDI infection because the hospital is the source of spores for most patients. Duration of stay in the intensive care unit (ICU) appears to have a stronger relationship than conventional ward hospitalization. The endotracheal tube of ventilator patients provides an entrance route for spore entry via the oropharynx. Enteral feeding likely provides an access route for the spore from the external environment and also neutralizes gastric acid as a primary barrier to colonization. However, enteral feeding can be viewed as a method to foster a normalization of gut colonization.

Many specific treatments are associated with CDIs. Both antifungal and antiviral chemotherapy are linked but the underlying patient disease is a likely contributor as well. Antineoplastic chemotherapy may have specific gastrointestinal toxicities that would appear to injure the colonic mucosa and increase the vulnerability for CDIs. Corticosteroids and other immunosuppressive drugs that are commonly employed in transplant recipients certainly contribute to increased rates of CDIs in this population of patients. The use of histamine antagonists and proton pump inhibitors has had the greatest association in recent years because of the loss of protective effects of gastric acidity (McCarthy 2010).

The postoperative surgical patient, particularly those undergoing major abdominal procedures, is at high risk for CDIs. Nasogastric tubes provide the avenue for spore introduction, the generous use of antibiotics disrupts the normal colonic environment, and impaired gut motility due to ileus and opiate analgesics all become synergistic effects to make CDIs a major problem. Although mechanical bowel preparation has been associated with CDIs, recent evidence has not demonstrated any correlation (Krapohl et al. 2011).

▉ DIAGNOSIS

The diagnosis of a CDI has become so common among adult hospitalized patients that virtually all patients aged >60 years and those with any duration of time in the ICU must be considered at risk. All physicians and surgeons should have a high index of suspicion for CDIs. Any of a number of different clinical signs or symptoms must trigger an evaluation.

Diarrhea has been the most frequent clinical event that heralds a CDI. A formal definition has included three unformed stools over 24 h for 2 consecutive days, or 8 unformed stools over 48 h, or 2 individual watery stools within a 24-h period. In elderly patients, in particular, the duration of the diarrhea phase of the disease may be very transient and no consolation should be taken from diarrhea that spontaneously resolves. The hypervirulent strains of *C. difficile* may not have a diarrhea phase at all. Bloody diarrhea is not a feature of CDIs and if present requires an evaluation for alternative diagnoses.

Although abdominal pain and abdominal distension are common features of patients after major surgical procedures, the new onset of crampy abdominal pain and distension is a consistent feature of patients with CDIs. This crampy abdominal pain in association with new-onset diarrhea usually differentiates the pain of CDI from that associated with diarrhea secondary to enteral feeding or other causes. Fever and leukocytosis are not consistent features of CDIs. Dehydration, electrolyte abnormalities, and hypoalbuminemia will be seen with advanced CDIs but can occur from a number of different causes in postoperative patients.

However, CDIs may be the diagnosis in only as few as 30% of diarrhea syndromes in hospitalized patients. The dramatic increase in the used of enteral feeding regimens over the last 20 years provides both an access route for the *C. difficile* spore, but provides a high-probability alternative source of diarrhea due to poor patient tolerance of feeding formulations. A host of different medications can provoke diarrhea (Ringel et al. 1995). Impaction continues to be a clinical association with diarrhea and a rectal examination is required in all of these patients.

Conventional abdominal radiographic studies are commonly used in the patient with clinical symptoms consistent with CDI. Often these are done because of concern for postoperative intestinal obstruction. Non-specific colonic distension is usually found in the CDI patient and the identification of air–fluid levels means that other diagnoses are applicable. The abdominal computed tomography (CT) scan has been useful with thickened colonic wall being a feature of transmural edema in the patient with CDI infection.

Proctosigmoidoscopy has been a traditional method for the diagnosis of CDIs. It can be a logistical problem in patients with severe diarrhea or poor cooperation. Pseudomembranes are generally considered diagnostic when present but their presence depends on the duration of illness. Finally, even with the longer, flexible proctosigmoidoscopy, the diseased segment of the colon may not be accessible with the bedside examination.

As large numbers of patients with diarrhea do not have CDIs, a specific diagnosis must be established before treatment is undertaken. Direct recovery of *C. difficile* by bacterial cultures can be performed but is a pain-staking process that is generally not performed except in research centers. Culture methods commonly employ egg yolk agar that is supplemented with cycloserine, cefoxitin, and fructose. As *C. difficile* has a consistent pattern of cefoxitin resistance, it is added to the media to suppress the growth of other anaerobic species. The plated culture medium is incubated under anaerobic conditions. Precise anaerobic culture technique is required, and recovery of *C. difficile* does not define the issue of the organism being a toxin producer. As specific sensitivities of clinical isolates have not been of value in the selection of specific antimicrobial therapy, cultures are usually not performed. Other studies such as Gram stains, fecal leukocyte detection, and occult blood detection are not of value.

The most common diagnosis method for CDIs is detection of the toxins in the diarrhea specimen using an enzyme immunoassay. Current immunoassays detect both toxin A and toxin B. As sensitivity and specificity are <95%, the study of a single diarrheal specimen may not be positive in the CDI patient. The rapidity of performance of the immunoassay is such that sequential specimens may be studied if the initial results are negative in patients in whom compelling clinical signs and symptoms are consistent with a CDI. This diagnostic method should be used only on diarrheal stools, because the accuracy of the assay is diminished in formed stool. This latter observation underscores that the immunoassay for toxins cannot be used as a screening tool in patients who are at risk for the infection but have not yet demonstrated symptoms of the disease.

The expanded use of the polymerase chain reaction (PCR) for diagnosis is available in most clinical laboratories and this method has been employed for detection of specific genes for toxins A and B. PCR has greater sensitivity and specificity than other diagnostic methods. The PCR method can be done quite rapidly. This advantage of quick diagnosis followed by prompt isolation of CDI patients has the advantage of rapid initiation of therapy and enhancement of infection control practices in the hospital (Bartlett 2010). PCR may supplant direct toxin measurement as the diagnostic method of choice.

Other diagnostic methods are uncommonly employed. The direct detection of glutamate dehydrogenase has been used as an antigen marker for the presence of *C. difficile*. This method has better sensitivity than the toxin detection method, but has lower specificity. This study is positive when patients have non-toxigenic colonization with *C. difficile*. For the latter reason, positive studies for the antigen require confirmation by the toxin assay.

The cytotoxicity assay employs the filtrate of the stool to directly determine toxic effects. The filtrate is incubated overnight with reference cell cultures to identify the typical "rounding" effects of toxins A and B. It is a direct bioassay of toxicity and may be the most accurate of studies when correctly performed. It is a technically demanding and expensive method that is not practical for routine use in the clinical setting.

PREVENTION

The prevention of CDIs requires particular attention to those clinical variables that have been clearly associated with the infection. Enhanced infection control practices are essential. If the patient is not exposed to the *C. difficile* spore, the CDI will not occur. It is essential to have enhanced hand hygiene for prevention of CDIs as well as the other pathogens (e.g., MRSA) in the hospital setting. Mechanical cleansing of the hands after patient contact is necessary. Alcohol-based hand gets and rubs do not eliminate *C. difficile* spores and give the artificial sense that infection control is being practiced when it is not. Chlorhexidine hand washes and scrubs do appear to have benefit, but it may be the mechanical scrubbing of the hands that is most important. Patients with established infection should be placed into single hospital rooms, or should be put together. Some hospitals have advocated segregating infected patients to a dedicated ward or wing of the hospital, and have dedicated nursing personnel provide the care for those patients to prevent dissemination of the spores. Patients with infection should remain isolated until diarrhea symptoms have resolved for 48 h. The use of gloves for handling and placement of indwelling oropharyngeal tubes and devices is important. Gloves and gowns are likewise necessary for all contacts with active CDI patients to avoid transmission to others.

Environmental decontamination is necessary for patient rooms, ICUs, and even the operating room after occupancy by CDI patients. Similarly, all reusable hospital equipment (e.g., endoscopes) requires the same vigilance for decontamination after each patient contact. When outbreaks occur, a greater dependence on disposable supplies is often indicated. Chlorine bleaches have the greatest effectiveness in the elimination of environmental spore contamination. Sodium hypochlorite solution at 1000 parts/million has been recommended to be effective in the reduction of CDI rates (Cohen et al. 2010).

Monitoring and surveillance of CDI cases over time within the hospital can provide useful information about targeting overall preventive strategies. Even though CDI rates are similar to those seen with MRSA, the degree of surveillance of these infections has not been given the same level of attention that MRSA infections receive. Accurate monitoring of events, establishing the hospital ward or unit responsible for the infection, and establishing control charts to quickly identify clusters of infection are very important in the evolution of an effective hospital-based preventive strategy.

More effective use of antibiotics in the surgical patient is as important as infection control practices. Despite the abundance of evidence that has demonstrated no value to extending preventive antibiotics into the postoperative time frame, the practice of multiple days of systemic antibiotics continues. Preventive antibiotics only have a role in the prevention of infection at the surgical site (see Chapter 4). Preventive systemic antibiotics do not provide patient benefit in covering open wounds or individual indwelling devices or tubes. Systemic antibiotics do not penetrate only those areas for which the clinician is using them, but they penetrate virtually all tissues of the body. Prolonged antibiotics eliminate sensitive organisms from the patient's colonization and have disruptive effects on the normal colonic microflora. Antibiotics with anaerobic activity are especially troublesome in this regard.

Therapeutic use of antibiotics has been a major influence in promoting CDIs, as have preventive drugs. When patients have established infection, the putative organism is commonly not immediately available and accordingly the initial choice of antibiotics tends to be very broad in the expectation of covering all possibilities until the culture and sensitivity data are available. This has resulted in the initiation of antibiotic combinations of three or more drugs that comprehensively cover Gram-positive, Gram-negative, and anaerobic species. Although the broad initial coverage is understandable in the setting of uncertainty about the pathogen or pathogens involved in the infection, especially in the ICU, the philosophy of de-escalation of antibiotic therapy is not uniformly obeyed and patients are continued on multiple drugs for an excessive period of time.

Furthermore, once patients are started on appropriate antibiotics there is clinical uncertainty as to when they should be discontinued. Recent studies have demonstrated benefit to earlier discontinuation of systemic antibiotics for patients with ventilator-associated pneumonia (VAP) (Pugh et al. 2011) and those with intra-abdominal infection (Solomkin et al. 2010). The duration of administration for VAP patients may be sufficient for 7–10 days instead of the traditional 14 days or more. Intra-abdominal infection patients may benefit from only 5–7 days, and patients with perforative appendicitis may require fewer days than that. The duration of antibiotic therapy for catheter-associated urinary tract infection remains poorly defined and is probably excessive (see Chapter 9). Similarly, antibiotic use for soft-tissue infections is commonly excessive when effective debridement has been achieved. Confusion continues to exist with open wounds about what constitutes infection and what is colonization that will not benefit from systemic antibiotics. In most clinical circumstances of treating established infection in the surgical patient, the tendency is to over-treat patients. The result is that the normal colonic microflora is obliterated with C. difficile and other highly resistant bacteria being the residual intraluminal colonists.

Selective gut decontamination (SGD) remains a controversial method to prevent infections including CDIs among hospitalized patients (Stoutenbeck et al. 2007). SGD is an attempt to suppress pathogenic bacteria from colonizing the gastrointestinal tract in severely ill patients. Some evidence suggests that it may be effective in reducing certain nosocomial infections where the gastrointestinal tract is thought to be a reservoir of pathogenic organisms. Others still question the utility of this method, fearing that a longer-term evolution of resistant pathogens will be the consequence. It is a concern that continued spore exposure from the external environment for patients with deliberate eradication of gut bacteria would set the stage for increased rates of CDI. Most SGD regimens attempt to preserve the anaerobic colonic microflora by using only antimicrobials against Gram-negative aerobic bacteria. SGD has not been associated with increased rates of CDI.

It is inevitable that some discussion would evolve around the use of either vancomycin or metronidazole to prevent CDIs. No current evidence has demonstrated the benefits of such a strategy. Metronidazole is absorbed from the gastrointestinal tract and may have long-term resistance implications for this antimicrobial agent. The implications of using vancomycin in such a fashion would further destabilize the precarious emergence of vancomycin-resistant Gram-positive pathogens.

TREATMENT OF CDIs

The treatment of CDIs has multiple components in addition to the use of antimicrobial chemotherapy. As these patients are commonly elderly and the volume of diarrhea can be large, extracellular fluid depletion and electrolyte imbalance can be major issues. The inflammatory response within the colonic wall can lead to dislocation of plasma proteins and extracellular water, in additional to the consequences of the diarrhea. Monitoring and managing fluid and electrolytes are important to maintain adequate perfusion of the inflamed colon.

A major component of management is to re-evaluate the antibiotics that are likely to provoke CDIs. Unnecessary postoperative preventive antibiotics and prolonged therapeutic antibiotic administration that do not have legitimate value should be discontinued. Ampicillin, amoxicillin, clindamycin, cephalosporins, and quinolone antibiotics have the strongest association with CDIs and alternative drug choices should be considered when continuation of antibiotic therapy is necessary. A minority of CDIs may resolve by simple cessation of systemic antibiotics without specific treatment addressed to C. difficile. Obviously specific antibiotic therapy will be warranted in most CDI patients but it is reasonable to expect a more difficult resolution of the infection and a higher rate of recidivism if other systemic antibiotics are being continued during the effort to treat CDIs.

A common reaction among surgeons when patients develop postoperative diarrhea is to symptomatically treat the patient with antiperistaltic agents. Diarrhea is the response of the colon to expel noxious agents, and the elimination of C. difficile toxins that are not bound to colonocytes is an appropriate response of the host. Anti-peristaltic agents lead to impaired colonic contractility, with retention of toxins, and increased intraluminal pressure. Furthermore, effective anti-peristaltic therapy can obscure the early clinical recognition of CDI, and after treatment has been started may give the false impression that therapy is effective. The risk of toxic megacolon can be expected to be enhanced from the use of diphenoxylate and atropine (Lomotil) or loperamide (Imodium).

Specific antimicrobial therapy is the most important component of treatment to eradicate the pathogen. As systemically administered antibiotics poorly penetrate the lumen of the colon, orally administered drugs that give therapeutic intraluminal concentrations are desirable for therapy. Metronidazole and vancomycin are the antimicrobial choices that have been most commonly chosen for CDI treatment (Table 11.1).

Metronidazole has been used most commonly over the last few decades, but has features that currently limit its use to mild and moderately severe CDIs. It is efficiently absorbed in the proximal gastrointestinal tract, but is eliminated in active form within the bile to yield an adequate concentration within the bowel lumen. Metronidazole has a comprehensive spectrum of activity against all intestinal anaerobic bacteria and is viewed as a disruptive intervention upon the colonic microflora. It is very inexpensive and has a long track record

Table 11.1 The current recommended antimicrobial treatment options for the initial episode of CDI.

Antimicrobial treatment	Dosage	Commentary
Metronidazole: mild-to-moderate infection	500 mg orally three times/day, 10–14 days	Food and Drug Administration (FDA) approved
Vancomycin: severe infection	125 mg orally every 6 h, 10–14 days	FDA approved
Vancomycin: severe and complicated	500 mg orally every 6 h + metronidazole 500 mg intravenously every 8 h until clinical resolution	FDA approved drugs for an unapproved dosing regimen
Fidaxomicin	200 mg orally every 12 h, 10–14 days	FDA approved

of effectiveness in the management of CDI. Metronidazole is dosed at 250–500 mg every 6 h for 10–14 days as the usual course of treatment. Higher doses used for the full 14 days of treatment are thought to reduce rates of recurrent or relapsing infection after cessation of therapy. As it is efficiently absorbed, it does have nausea, headache, alteration of taste, and peripheral neuropathy as associated adverse events. Although metronidazole should have the advantage of less induction of resistant Gram-positive overgrowth in the colon, one study identified that vancomycin-resistant enterococci (VREs) are as common with metronidazole as with vancomycin in the treatment of CDIs (Al-Nassir et al. 2008).

Based on recent studies, oral vancomycin is the recommended treatment for severe cases of CDIs (Zar et al. 2007). Vancomycin is not absorbed from the gastrointestinal tract and yields very high concentrations in the colon after oral administration. It has a focused activity against Gram-positive pathogens, and has the theoretical advantage of not influencing Gram-negative rods or Gram-negative colonic anaerobes. It will promote VREs in the colon and increase rates of VRE nosocomial infection. It does not have systemic toxicity because it is not absorbed, but it is significantly more expensive than metronidazole. The oral preparation has periodically been in short supply because it has no clinical use other than the treatment of CDIs. Vancomycin is dosed at 125 mg every 6 h for 10–14 days.

Dissatisfaction with metronidazole and vancomycin has led to the search for alternative agents that would give a better clinical response to initial treatment, but also reduce the frequency of recurrent/relapsing infection once the treatment regimen has been completed. This dissatisfaction with metronidazole and vancomycin has not been because of emerging resistance but rather because of recurrent infection. Fidaxomicin is a new oral treatment that has been approved for use by the Food and Drug Administration (FDA) in the USA, and has the promise of better results in the treatment of CDIs.

Fidaxomicin is a macrocyclic antibiotic with antimicrobial activity against *C. difficile* that exceeds that of vancomycin. This in vitro superiority is also seen against the hypervirulent strains. It has a greater post-antibiotic effect than vancomycin, and has fostered the hope that recurrence of infection will be less with this treatment. Fidaxomicin is minimally absorbed and does not appear to have any systemic toxicity. Colonic concentrations of the drug are quite high. Fidaxomicin is active against Gram-positive bacteria, which include most strains of staphylococci. It does not have activity against Gram-negative rods or anaerobes of the colon.

A multicenter randomized clinical trial of 596 patients with CDIs were treated with doses of either 200 mg fidaxomicin or 125 mg vancomycin (Louie et al. 2011). Each drug was given every 6 h and the total duration of treatment was for 10 days. Clinical resolution of CDIs at the completion of treatment was statistically the same, at 88% for fidaxomicin and 86% for vancomycin. Recurrent or relapsing infections within 36–40 days after randomization were less frequently observed with fidaxomicin in the modified intention-to-treat patients (15% vs 25%, $p = 0.005$). However, there was no difference in recurrence rate among those patients with CDI secondary to the BI/NAP1//027 strain type. These observations have been confirmed in a second large randomized trial where outcomes of initial treatment were the same, but recurrent infections were higher in the vancomycin-treated patients (Cornely et al. 2012).

A real clinical problem is the patient with severe fulminate CDI and the patient with severe ileus or toxic megacolon. Orally administered antibiotics will have little or no chance of advancing distally within the gastrointestinal tract to the level of the colon in relevant concentrations. Penetration of the colonic lumen by the intravenous route in distended colon with either metronidazole or vancomycin is suspect. A limited number of patients have been successfully treated with intravenous tigecycline at 50 mg every 12 h in the management of unresponsive cases with prior conventional therapy (Larsen et al. 2011). There is speculation that tigecycline may penetrate the colon better than alternative agents. Additional studies are needed to validate tigecycline therapy for the difficult CDI case that is refractory to conventional management.

◾ Recurrent infection

Recurrent CDI within 60 days of treatment occurs in up to 30% of cases. Recurrent infection may not even be with the same *C. difficile* strain of the original infection, which obviously implicates host issues as being of significance in this population of patients. Recurrence is generally not associated with *C. difficile* strains that were resistant to the primary antibiotic choice, because sensitivities of these bacteria to metronidazole and vancomycin have remained stable and recurrent pathogens are sensitive to the antimicrobials initially used for treatment. Recurrent infection with the hypervirulent BI/NAP1/027 strains and chronic recurrent infection among a selected subset of patients have been the major impetus for the development of more effective treatments.

It has been difficult to define patient comorbidities that are unique to the population of patients with recurrent or relapsing infection. Treatment variables associated with recurrent CDI include prior relapse of infection, inadequate dosing or duration of treatment for the initial episode, poor patient compliance with the initial treatment regimen, continued or interval reintroduction of systemic antibiotic therapy, and with certain strains of *C. difficile*. An explanation for recurrent CDIs remains very elusive for many patients.

The management of recurrent infection generally follows the guidelines of initial care with larger doses and a full 14 days of treatment. Some have advocated a longer course of treatment for recurrent cases, although success with this strategy has not been clearly documented. A host of different treatments has been employed for recurrent cases. For extraordinarily difficult cases, donor fecal enemas have been used as a desperate but not particularly popular treatment to restore normal colonic microbiota (Bakken 2009). **Table 11.2** illustrates many of the unique regimens that have been used in the management of recurrent CDIs.

An important observation has been that patients with recurrence of CDIs after apparently successful initial treatment commonly do not have an anti-toxin A antibody response compared with those patients without recurrence (Kyne et al. 2001). Indeed, the odds ratio of having recurrent disease without the appropriate IgG antibody response to toxin A was 48.0. This has led to the conclusion that the adaptive immune response may play an important role in the resolution of CDIs. It has raised the speculation that active or passive immunization of the host may facilitate the resolution of the clinical disease and reduce the incidence of recurrence. Experimental treatment with antibodies to toxins A and B have further fueled speculation of a therapeutic benefit for infected patients (Babcock et al. 2006).

A prospective randomized clinical trial with fully human monoclonal antibodies to toxins A and B has demonstrated potential benefits (Lowy et al. 2010). Antibodies were administered as a single dose at the start of treatment. Antibody treatment and placebo patients received either metronidazole or vancomycin as primary treatment

Table 11.2 A survey of alternative therapies that have been used in the treatment of recurrent and relapsing *Clostridium difficile* infection.

Antimicrobial options	Reference	Commentary
Tapered vancomycin dosing	Cohen et al. (2010)	Vancomycin continued after conventional dosing with additional 125 mg twice daily for 7 days; then 125 mg four times daily for 7 days; then 125 mg four times daily for 2–8 weeks. Do not use metronidazole
Vancomycin + rifaximin	Johnson et al. (2007)	Anecdotal data; rifaximin is a poorly absorbed rifampin derivative; it may promote resistance
Vancomycin + cholestyramine	Lagrotteria et al. (2006)	No evidence to support cholestyramine; used to bind *C. difficile* toxins. Cholestyramine binds vancomycin
Gut recolonization strategies		
Vancomycin + *Saccharomyces boulardii*	Tung et al. (2009)	Competitive inhibition of *C. difficile*; some evidence that it may be useful; risk of fungemia in host with damaged colonic mucosa?
Lactobacilli + other gut anaerobes	Venuto et al. (2010)	Probiotic strategy to restore anaerobic colonization of the colon; evidence is mixed.
Yogurt	Pochapin (2000)	Probiotic concept, inexpensive, and little evidence to support its clinical use for *C. difficile*
Brewer's yeast	Schellenberg et al. (1994)	Limited evidence; *Saccharomyces* cerevisiae has been seen as pathogen in humans
Non-toxigenic *C. difficile*	Gerding (2012)	Blocks colonocyte receptor and prevents binding of the pathogen. Currently being investigated
Enterococcus faecium SF 68	Marteau et al. (2001)	Competitive inhibition of *C. difficile* at the colonocyte receptor
Fecal bacteriotherapy	Bakken (2009)	Restores normal colonic colonization quickly; many centers are evaluating this treatment; no controlled trials
Immunomodulation		
Anti-toxin monoclonal antibodies	Lowy et al. (2010)	Binds the toxins, but does not affect *C. difficile* colonization
Intravenous immunoglobulin	Abougergi and Kwon (2011)	Passive immunization against *C. difficile* enterotoxins, but limited clinical data

of the CDI. The results demonstrated a statistically significant reduction in recurrent infection in those patients receiving the antibodies at 84 days after initiation of antimicrobial therapy. Patients with BI/NAP1/027 strain infection had a similar reduction in recurrent infections. The severity of diarrhea was interpreted to be less in the antibody-treated patients than the placebo group. The monoclonal antibody treatment did not improve the results of treatment for the primary CDI. Duration of hospitalization, time to resolution of the initial diarrhea, and severity of diarrhea were similar for the initial infection event.

The role of using monoclonal antibodies that address the toxins of *C. difficile* will require continued study and evaluation. Of interest, some treated patients still developed recurrent disease even with documented antibody titers. Whether the duration of disease and the severity of inflammation before antibody administration affected the treatment outcome is unclear. Does successful avoidance of clinically recurrent disease mean that the patient has a chronic carrier state where the toxins are neutralized but the *C. difficile* pathogen remains as a viable colonist of the colon in a non-symptomatic state? Some clinical evidence indicates this as a real possibility (Kyne et al. 2000). As this treatment is passive immunity and colonization of the host may be a consequence of treatment, longer follow-up may be necessary to identify the evolution of recurrent events.

The record of monoclonal antibody treatment in other areas has resulted in a dramatic increase in the expense of treatment. A discussion of whether this treatment will be used should be offered to all patients with CDIs if continued evaluation validates effectiveness of the antibody treatment. Offering it to all patients will be treating 70–80% of patients for no benefit. A preferable strategy may be to reserve this treatment for patients known to develop recurrent infections.

■ TREATMENT IMPLICATIONS FOR SURGEONS

The changing frequency and the changing epidemiology of CDI have implications in both preventing and managing this complication after operations, and in the previously infrequent circumstance of necessary surgical intervention. With more patients having an initial infection with *C. difficile*, it is likely that more patients will have the carrier state and will have had a prior episode of CDI. A clinical history of CDI becomes a necessary part of the evaluation of patients for major operations. Patients with a prior CDI history must understand that it is a clinical risk for any surgical procedure. Rigid restrictions in the use and selection of antibiotics become very important for the patient with a prior episode of CDIs, but also for the elderly patient who is at increased risk for this complication of care. Systemic preventive antibiotics need to be stopped in the immediate postoperative period. The changing character of CDIs means additional important issues for surgeons.

■ Community-acquired CDIs

The epidemic of CDIs among hospitalized patients has led to an increased number of patients with the asymptomatic carrier state. With 40 million hospitalizations per year in the USA and equally large numbers of hospitalizations in other countries, vast numbers of the resilient *C. difficile* spores are being transported out of the healthcare environment and into the community. It should not be surprising that the ubiquitous dissemination of spores and the equally widespread use of outpatient antibiotics for indicated and poorly indicated reasons would be a combination for community-acquired CDIs (CA-CDIs) to emerge as a clinical issue. As the ecological issue of the colonic environment that favors the emergence of CDI remains poorly defined, and knowing that CDIs can occur in the absence of antibiotic exposure, the evolution of CA-CDIs is a totally predictable event.

Numerous studies have reported large numbers of patients with CA-CDIs (Dial et al. 2005, Khanna et al. 2012). None has had infection previously as an inpatient. Small percentages have had ambulatory exposure to antibiotics. An association with proton pump inhibitors and histamine blockers would imply that a loss of gastric acidity may be a contributing variable. A different perspective indicates that 94% of CDIs have had an exposure to the healthcare environment, but that 75% of current new cases have their onset outside the hospital (Centers for Disease Control 2012).

CA-CDIs and the simultaneous evolution of the BI/NAP1/127 strain give the surgeon a new source of concern when evaluating an elderly patient arriving from home with complaints of crampy abdominal pain and distension. The differential diagnosis of this clinical scenario must add CA-CDIs to the list of intestinal obstruction, colonic impaction, non-specific ileus, and the many other sources of abdominal pain and distension seen in patients aged ≥70 years. Diarrhea may or may not be a part of the symptom complex and the hypervirulent strain makes prompt diagnosis difficult but necessary in a short time frame if a major catastrophe is to be avoided.

Fulminant CDIs

CDIs cover a vast continuum of severity. At the mild end of the disease, patients may recover by simple cessation of the antibiotics that provoked the infection and do not require any specific treatment for *C. difficile*. At the other end of the spectrum are those patients with a fulminate disease that rapidly progresses to toxic megacolon and the risk of necrosis, toxemia, and death.

Fulminate CDIs occur in about 5% of total cases but appear to be increasing in frequency. The fulminate infection occurs in two scenarios: First, in the immunosuppressed and debilitated patient or, second, in the patient with the hypervirulent BI/NAP1/127 strain of infection. The patients characteristically have a rapidly evolving disease, with a diarrhea phase that may be quite transient or non-existent in about 20% of cases. Crampy abdominal pain and distension are associated with hypotension, oliguria, hypoalbuminemia, and leukocytosis or even leukopenia. Abdominal radiographs demonstrate distension of the colon with marked thickening of the colonic wall. As the diarrhea phase of the disease is fleeting to non-existent, stool sampling for the diagnostic toxin assay may be compromised. Bedside flexible sigmoidoscopy may be necessary to identify pseudomembranes so that treatment can be initiated. Volume administration and pharmacological support of blood pressure is usually required for the fulminate CDI.

Antimicrobial therapy for the patient with fulminate disease is compromised. The loss of colonic motility yields poor delivery of the antibiotic to the lumen of the infected colon. Systemic metronidazole or vancomycin is generally chosen, but the penetration of antibiotic into the inflamed and distended colon is poor, with a similarly poor clinical response to treatment. As noted above, tigecycline may be useful in this setting. With a failure of clinical response to systemic antibiotic therapy, the clinician is confronted with the decision for the surgical option and colectomy.

Surgical management

The surgical management of CDIs has increased in frequency over the last decade because of both the increase in frequency of the infection and the hypervirulent strain. Necrosis of the mucosa extends into the submucosa and muscularis of the colon. The severe inflammatory response results in complete loss of colon motility. Increased intraluminal pressure compromises perfusion. The clinical picture of progression of disease in the face of aggressive medical therapy and the evolution of systemic inflammation and multiple organ dysfunction means that the surgical option is required. At this point in the evolution of CDI, failure to exercise surgical intervention results in a fatal outcome.

At abdominal exploration, the surgeon is confronted with a complex circumstance that requires appropriate judgment. Findings may vary from the identification of massive distended colon without evidence of transmural necrosis to long segment necrosis of the colon with or without perforation. Patchy necrosis may be encountered. Commonly necrotic mucosa is encountered at the ends of segmental resections indicating that the seromuscular coat of the colon is viable but the mucosal lining is not.

As the pattern of severe CDIs will have non-contiguous "skip" areas, segmental resection of the colon, even when one has resected to a point where retained colonic mucosa appears to be viable, is a gamble that other areas of significant necrosis remain. Best results are achieved with subtotal colectomy (Butala and Divino 2010) (**Figure 11.4**).

An innovative solution for the surgical management of the patient requiring laparotomy for advanced CDI has recently been introduced. Neal et al. (2011) have introduced the concept of performing a loop ileostomy at laparotomy for the patient with surgical indications but without transmural necrosis of the colon. The ileostomy becomes the conduit for the introduction of vancomycin irrigation directly into the colon on a continuous basis, and avoids the poor pharmacokinetics of systemic administration in the patient with toxic megacolon. Early results are favorable but additional experience with this treatment strategy is necessary.

CONCLUSION

In summary, CDIs are increasing in frequency and severity. The clinical onset of disease may be in the community or as a hospital-acquired infection. First-line oral antibiotic therapy has been effective for many cases, but surgical intervention is still necessary for selected cases. New management strategies are necessary for both prevention and management of this very important bacterial infection. CDIs have become an infection of considerable clinical significance for the practicing surgeon.

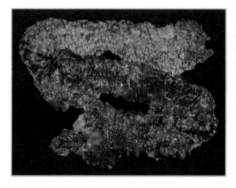

Figure 11.4 A colectomy specimen from a patient with far-advanced Clostridium difficile infection. (Figure courtesy of Dale N. Gerding, MD)

REFERENCES

Abougergi MS, Kwon JH. Intravenous immunoglobulin for the treatment of *Clostridium difficile* infection: a review. *Dig Dis Sci* 2011;**56**:19–26.

Agency for Healthcare Research and Quality. *National Inpatient Sample, Healthcare Cost and Utilization Project*. Bethesda, MA: AHRQ, 2011. http://hcupnet.ahrq.gov (accessed March 26, 2012).

Al-Nassir WN, Sethi AK, Li Y, et al. Both oral metronidazole and oral vancomycin promote persistent overgrowth of vancomycin-resistant enterococci during treatment of *Clostridium difficile*-associated disease. *Antimicrob Agents Chemother* 2008;**52**:2403–6.

Ananthadrishnan AN. *Clostridium difficile* infection: epidemiology, risk factors and management. *Natl Rev Gastroenterol Hepatol* 2011;**8**:17–26.

Babcock GJ, Broering TJ, Hernandez HJ, et al. Human monoclonal antibodies directed against toxins A and B prevent *Clostridium difficile*-induced mortality in hamsters. *Infect Immun* 2006;**74**:6339–47.

Bakken JS. Fecal bacteriotherapy for recurrent *Clostridium difficile* infection. *Anaerobe* 2009;**15**:285–9.

Bartlett JG. *Clostridium difficile*: progress and challenges. *Ann N Y Acad Sci* 2010;**1213**:62–9.

Butala P, Divino CM. Surgical aspects of fulminate *Clostridium difficile* colitis. *Am J Surg* 2010;**200**:131–5.

Centers for Disease Control. Vital signs: preventing *Clostridium difficile* infections. *Morbid Mortal Wkly Rep* 2012;**61**:1–6.

Cohen SH, Gerding DN, Johnson S, et al. Clinical practice guidelines for *Clostridium difficile* infection in adults: 2010 update by the society for healthcare epidemiology of America (SHEA) and the Infectious Diseases Society of America (IDSA). *Infect Control Hosp Epidemiol* 2010;**31**:431–55.

Cornely OA, Crook DW, Esposito R, et al. Fidaxomicin versus vancomycin for infection with clostridium difficile in Europe, Canada, and the USA: a double-blind, non-inferiority, randomised controlled trial. *Lancet Infect Dis* 2012;12:281–9.

Dial S, Delaney JA, Barkun AN, Suissa S. Use of gastric acid-suppressive agents and the risk of community-acquired *Clostridium difficile*-associated disease. *JAMA* 2005;**294**:2989–95.

Gerding DN. Global epidemiology of *Clostridium difficile* infection in 2010. *Infect Control Hosp Epidemiol* 2010;**31**(suppl 1):S32–4.

Gerding DN. *Clostridium difficile* infection prevention: biotherapeutics, immunologics, and vaccines. *Discov Med* 2012;**13**:75–83.

Johnson S, Schriever C, Galang M, Kelly CP, Gerding DN. Interruption of recurrent clostridium difficile-associated diarrhea episodes by serial therapy with vancomycin and rifaximin. *Clin Infect Dis* 2007;**44**:846–48.

Khanna S, Pardi DS, Aronson SL, et al. The epidemiology of community-acquired *Clostridium difficile* infection: a population-based study. *Am J Gastroenterol* 2012;**107**:89–95.

Krapohl GL, Phillips LR, Campbell DA Jr, et al. Bowel preparation for colectomy and risk of *Clostridium difficile* infection. *Dis Colon Rectum* 2011;**54**:810–q7.

Kyne L, Warny M, Qamar A, Kelly CP. Asymptomatic carriage of *Clostridium difficile* and serum levels of IgG antibody against toxin A. *N Engl J Med* 2000;**342**:390–7.

Kyne L, Warny M, Qamar A, Kelly CP. Association between antibody response to toxin and protection against recurrent *Clostridium difficile* diarrhea. *Lancet* 2001;**357**:189–93.

Lagrotteria D, Holmes S, Smieja M Smaill F, Lee C. Prospective, randomized inpatient study of oral metronidazole versus oral metronidazole and rifampin for treatment of primary episode of *Clostridium difficile*-associated diarrhea. *Clin Infect Dis* 2006;**43**:547–52.

Larsen KC, Belliveau PP, Spooner LM. Tigecycline for the treatment of severe *Clostridium difficile* infection. *Ann Pharmacother* 2011;**45**:1005–10.

Loo VG, Bourgault AM, Poirier L, et al. Host and pathogen factors for *Clostridium difficile* infection and colonization. *N Engl J Med* 2011;**365**:1693–703.

Louie TJ, Miller MA, Mullane KM, et al. Fidaxomicin versus vancomycin for *Clostridium difficile* infection. *N Engl J Med* 2011;**364**:422–31.

Lowy I, Molrine DC, Leav BA, et al. Treatment with monoclonal antibodies against *Clostridium difficile* toxins. *N Engl J Med* 2010;**362**:197–205.

McCarthy DM: Adverse effects of proton pump inhibitor drugs: clues and conclusions. *Curr Opin Gastroenterol* 2010;**26**:624–31.

McDonald LC, Killgore GE, Thompson A, et al. An epidemic, toxin gene-variant strain of *Clostridium difficile*. *N Engl J Med* 2005;**353**:2433–41.

Marteau PR, de Vrese M, Cellier CJ, Schrezenmeir J. Protection from gastrointestinal diseases with the use of probiotics. *Am J Clin Nutr* 2001;**73**(2 suppl):430S–6S.

Neal MD, Alverdy JC, Hall DE, Simmons RL, Zuckerbraun BS. Diverting loop ileostomy and colonic lavage: an alternative to total abdominal colectomy for the treatment of severe, complicated Clostridium difficile associated disease. *Ann Surg* 2011;**254**:423–7.

Papatheodorou P, Carette JE, Bell GW, et al. Lipolysis-stimulated lipoprotein receptor (LSR) is the host receptor for the binary toxin *Clostridium difficile* transferase (CDT). *Proc Natl Acad Sci U S A* 2011;**108**:16422–7.

Pochapin M. The effect of probiotics on *Clostridium difficile* diarrhea. *Am J Gastroenterol* 2000;**95**(1 suppl):S11–13.

Pugh R, Grant C, Cooke RP, Dempsey GP. Short-course versus prolonged-course antibiotic therapy for hospital-acquired pneumonia in critically ill adults. *Cochrane Database Syst Rev* 2011;**(10)**:CD007577.

Ringel AF, Jameson GL, Foster ES. Diarrhea in the intensive care patient. *Crit Care Clin* 1995;**11**:465–77.

Rouphael NG, O'Donnell JA, Bhatnagar J, et al. *Clostridium difficile*-associated diarrhea: an emerging threat to pregnant women. *Am J Obstet Gynecol* 2008;**198**:635.e1–6.

Schellenberg D, Bonington A, Champion CM, Lancaster R, Webb S, Main J. Treatment of *Clostridium difficile* diarrhoea with brewer's yeast. *Lancet* 1994;**343**:171–2.

Solomkin JS, Mazuski JE, Bradley JS, et al. Diagnosis and management of complicated intra-abdominal infection in adults and children: guidelines by the Surgical Infection Society and the Infectious Diseases Society of America. *Surg Infect* 2010;**11**:79–109.

Stoutenbeek CP, van Saene HK, Little RA, Whitehead A. The effect of selective decontamination of the digestive tract on mortality in multiple trauma patients: a multicenter randomized controlled trial. *Intensive Care Med* 2007;**33**:261–70.

Tung JM, Dolovich LR, Lee CH: Prevention of *Clostridium difficile* infection with *Saccharomyces boulardii*: a systematic review. *Can J Gastroenterol* 2009;**23**:817–21.

Venuto C, Butler M, Ashley ED, Brown J. Alternative therapies for *Clostridium difficile* infections. *Pharmacotherapy* 2010;1266–78.

Zar FA, Bakkanagari SR, Moorthi KM, Davis MB. A comparison of vancomycin and metronidazole for the treatment of *Clostridium difficile*-associated diarrhea, stratified by disease severity. *Clin Infect Dis* 2007;**45**:302–7.

Zilberberg MD, Shorr AF, Kollef MH: Increase in adult *Clostridium difficile*-related hospitalizations and case-fatality rate, United States, 2000–2005. *Emerg Infect Dis* 2008;**14**:929–31.

Chapter 12 Burn wound infections

David N. Herndon, Noe A. Rodriguez, Katrina Blackburn Mitchell, James J. Gallagher

Infection is a common and problematic outcome of burn injury. Burn injury predisposes individuals to infection in three main ways. The most obvious is through the loss of skin, which serves as the primary barrier to infection. Second, larger burns can induce immunosuppression and weaken cellular and humoral defenses. Finally, damaged tissue can provide a fertile substrate for pathogen growth. This chapter discusses definitions of infection, potential pathogens, and treatment options for successful management of the burn patient.

■ PATHOBIOLOGY OF THE BURN WOUND

Thermal injury kills both the bacteria and tissue cells on the skin surface. Accordingly, initial cultures are usually sterile. However, subsequent cultures will be positive because of the survival of bacteria present in the hair follicles and sebaceous glands. Indeed, the number of bacteria (10^3/g) may be equal to pre-injury levels (Teplitz et al. 1964, Robson and Krizek 1973a, Pruitt et al. 1998). Given that bacterial doubling time is only about 20 min, a single bacterial cell can generate 10 billion cells within a 24-h period (Robson 1979). Viable resident bacteria and secondary contamination from the environment become the early potential pathogens of the burn wound. In the absence of burn treatment, bacterial proliferation may lead to vessel thrombosis and necrosis of any remaining dermal elements. This may transform partial-thickness burns to full-thickness burn injuries. Continued proliferation will result in a greater risk of viable tissue invasion and septicemia (Burke et al. 1977, Artz and Moncrief 1979). Invasive infections are histologically characterized by the presence of bacteria and hemorrhage in unburned tissue, small-vessel thrombosis with ischemic necrosis of unburned tissue, and dense bacterial growth in the subeschar space. Advancement of the infection is usually associated with the progression of colonization from early Gram-positive to later Gram-negative bacteria. In fact, almost two-thirds of burn wounds that are still open at 21 days will contain extended-spectrum β-lactamase-producing *Pseudomonas* spp. Fortunately, effective topical wound management usually blocks this natural progression of bacteria multiplication and tissue invasion. However, even contemporary burn care practice may still ineffectively control virulent pathogens that have arisen early after injury, leading to invasive burn wound infections and necrotizing soft-tissue infection.

Severe burn injury triggers a profound response to injury. This includes a hypermetabolic response, which can mimic multiple aspects of the systemic inflammatory response syndrome (SIRS) and make detection of the infection more difficult. Challenges such as this have prompted international forums to create definitions of infection so that the diagnosis and management of patients can be standardized. In 2007, a consensus conference was formed within the American Burn Association (ABA) to define sepsis and infections in burn injury (Greenhalgh et al. 2007). This consensus conference relied on methodology use by other societies (Bone et al. 1992, Levy et al. 2003) to develop general definitions of SIRS and sepsis (**Box 12.1**).

Box 12.1 American Burn Association sepsis criteria (from Greenhalgh et al. 2007).

1. Temperature: >39°C or <36.5°C
2. Progressive tachycardia:
   - Adults: >110 beats/min
   - Children: >2 standard deviations (SD) above age-specific norms
3. Progressive tachypnea:
   - Adults: >25 breaths/min if not ventilated, or minute ventilation >1 l/min on the ventilator
   - Children: >2 SD above age-specific norms
4. Thrombocytopenia (3 days post initial resuscitation)
   - Adults: <100 000/μl
   - Children: >2 SD below age-specific norms
5. Hyperglycemia (applies only to non-diabetic patients)
   - Untreated plasma glucose >200 mg/dl, or
   - Insulin resistance (>7 U insulin/h IV drip or >25% increase in insulin requirements over 24 h
6. Inability to continue enteral feedings >24 h because of:
   - Abdominal distension, or
   - Residual twice the feeding rate for adults or >150/h in children, or
   - Uncontrolled diarrhea

This conference also developed useful definitions to differentiate infectious and non-infectious clinical issues in the burn wound (**Table 12.1**).

■ RECOGNITION AND DIAGNOSIS OF INFECTION IN THE BURN WOUND

■ Use of burn wound cultures

Colonization or infection of major burn wounds usually occurs within 3–5 days of admission. Infection often arises from the patient's own bacterial flora. Burn wounds should be inspected daily by the burn surgeon, and any area of the wound that has changed in appearance should undergo biopsy with pathological assessment. Histological evidence of burn wound infection correlates with quantitative cultures showing high bacterial counts in approximately 80% of cases (Pruitt et al. 1998, Mayhall 2003). Bacterial counts exceeding 10^3 organisms/g tissue require a change in topical therapy, whereas those exceeding 10^5 organisms/g tissue require localized burn wound infection to be considered and a histological examination to be performed. Histological evidence of invasion requires wound excision and systemic antibiotics. The burn wound must be closely assessed for these manifestations

Table 12.1 Definitions for differentiating between non-infectious and infectious complications of the burn wound (from Greenhalgh et al. 2007).

Syndrome	Clinical and pathological criteria
Wound erythema	Redness surrounding the burn injury that is not a first-degree burn; redness appears 2–3 days after burn and dissipates by 5 or 6 days after burn; not infectious
Wound colonization	Isolation of low levels of bacteria ($<10^5$ bacteria/g tissue) from the wound surface; no invasive infection
Wound impetigo	Small multifocal superficial abscesses that can cause extensive loss of epithelium from previously healed split-thickness skin grafts and that manifest as graft "melting or ghosting" or scalp folliculitis; *Staphylococcus aureus* associated
Wound infection	Isolation of high levels of bacteria ($>10^5$ bacteria/g tissue) in the excised burns, donor site, or wound eschar; no invasive infection
Invasive infection	Pathogens present in the burn wound at a sufficient concentration (frequently $>10^5$ pathogens/g tissue), depth, and surface area to cause suppurative separation of the eschar or graft loss, invasion of unburned tissue, or sepsis syndrome
Cellulitis	High levels of bacteria (>105 bacteria/g tissue) present in the wound and/or wound eschar, with surrounding tissue revealing erythema, induration, warmth, and/or tenderness
Necrotizing infection, fasciitis	Aggressive, invasive infection with underlying (beneath the skin) tissue necrosis

of bacterial sepsis and fungal invasion. Changes in the color, odor, or exudate will frequently precede bacterial sepsis. A rapidly emerging and spreading dark discoloration signals fungal invasion.

The routine use of wound cultures varies considerably. Robson and Krizek (1973b) demonstrated that burn wound colony counts $>10^5$/g tissue led to only a 19% graft survival rate. On the other hand, colony counts $<10^5$/g tissue had a 94% chance of graft survival. This led to widespread use of burn wound biopsies and cultures. Steer et al. (1996) demonstrated that a wide variation exists in the bacterial densities within a wound at any given time. This finding challenged the value of clinical management based on routine burn wound culturing. Barret and Herndon (2003) investigated the effect of burn wound excision on bacterial colonization and invasion. They discovered that preoperative colony counts $>10^5$ were reduced to counts $<10^4$ when wounds were treated aggressively through surgery. This type of treatment led to excellent skin graft take. This difference may be attributable to changes in the surgical paradigm and technique. Barret and Herndon (2003) identified a subgroup with preoperative colony counts exceeding 10^6 organisms/g tissue. Although this group had post-excision, pre-grafting cultures that averaged 10^4 organisms/g tissue, they suffered a 75% infection rate and graft loss. Although burn wound colony counts have significant value in guiding patient care, they may also be unreliable and inaccurate due to sample site variation. The reasons and uses for burn wound cultures are described in **Box 12.2**.

Several major benchmarks must be achieved to ensure reliable clinical microbiology (Heggers and Robson 1991). Effective microbiological diagnosis depends on appropriate specimen selection, specimen collection, and transport of specimens to the laboratory. Appropriate specimen management affects patient care in several significant ways:

- It is key for accurate laboratory diagnosis.
- It influences therapeutic decisions.
- It affects hospital infection control, the length of the patient's stay, and overall hospital costs.
- It plays a major role in laboratory costs and efficiency.

Before analysis, the specimen collection site must be selected. This site must represent a location of active disease. The area of the wound with the worst clinical appearance is an optimal location from which to culture pathogens. In addition, an appropriate device must be used for sample collection.

With burn wounds, obtaining a culture that is not contaminated with the normal surface flora of the injured skin is particularly important. In addition, the size or amount of the specimen plays an essential role in the appropriate identification of the etiological agent. The use

---

Box 12.2 Burn wound cultures in burn care.

- Early cultures should be negative or have low counts, with sensitive Gram-positive organisms. Therefore, positive cultures or high counts suggest early **contamination** of the burn
- If invasive burn wound infection is suspected, then wound culture and histological analysis can aid in confirmation of the clinical diagnosis
- Routine culturing and identification of colonization may aid in **empirical** antimicrobial coverage if the patient subsequently becomes ill
- Increasing colony counts may indicate a need to change topical antimicrobial agents
- Not all organisms are created equal. Wound colonization with particularly virulent or resistant organisms may be a predictor of coming invasive burn wound infection
- Operative wound colony counts $>10^6$ suggest a high risk of infectious complication and graft failure
- Burn wound culture results may aid in the evaluation of nosocomial spread of organisms and guide **infection control** practice

of prophylactic antimicrobials (both topical and systemic) should also be noted so that appropriate inhibitors and sufficient dilutions can be prepared or reagents added to void any effects of drug interactions. The specimen should be collected and placed in a sterile container containing appropriate transport media. All specimens must be promptly transported to the laboratory. Direct communication with the microbiologist can often be very helpful.

■ Definitions for the burn patient

Small burns (<10%) are common and typically clean when examined for early treatment. Fever alone does not indicate infection, because burn injury increases the body temperature set point. Fever can accompany burns of any size. Moreover, the frequency or severity of fever is not proportional to the burn size or depth. Evaluating burns for possible infection requires an awareness of *burn wound erythema* (**Figure 12.1**). This redness usually appears 2–3 days after injury and dissipates by 5–6 days. Burn wound erythema is not a first-degree burn and is not infectious. It results in local inflammatory cytokines and mediators. Burn wound erythema is normally non-tender to palpation, as opposed to infectious cellulitis.

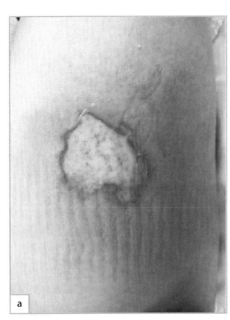

Figure 12.1 Burn wound erythema on post-burn day 2 (a) and its spontaneous resolution on day 12 (b).

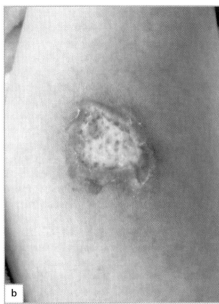

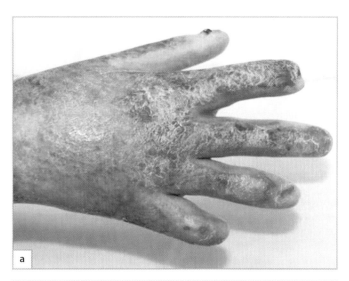

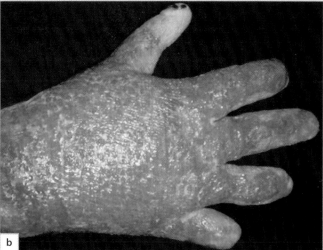

Figure 12.2 (a) Successful skin grafting pictured 2 months post burn. (b) At 3 months, a new open wound has formed from burn wound impetigo.

Burn wound impetigo

Burn wound impetigo (**Figure 12.2**) refers to small multifocal superficial abscesses. These may present as folliculitis on the scalp. These abscesses can extensively damage previously healed split-thickness skin grafts and donor sites (Pruitt et al. 1998). This phenomenon has been termed "graft melting" or "ghosting." *Staphylococcus aureus,* particularly meticillin-resistant *S. aureus* (MRSA), is commonly seen in these conditions. Successful treatment requires frequent cleansing with disinfectants, unroofing of any abscesses, and twice-daily application of a topical antimicrobial such as silver nitrate, Dakin solution, or mupirocin.

Burn wound colonization

Burn wound colonization (**Figure 12.3**) is defined as the presence of low concentrations of bacteria on the wound surface, the absence of

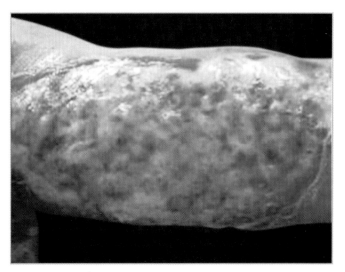

Figure 12.3 The appearance of burn wound colonization.

any invasive infection, and <10^5 bacteria/g tissue (Greenhalgh et al. 2007). Burn wound colonization is treated through continued burn care with cleaning, topical antimicrobials, and surgery. If serial colony counts increase, the topical agent may need to be changed.

Burn wound infection

This is characterized by >10^5 bacteria/g tissue. The presence of cellulitis forms the basis for this diagnosis. In early burns, painless and surrounding blanching erythema is seen. It is an not infection, and antibiotics are not needed. Cellulitis is characterized by pain, advancing erythema, warmth, and tenderness. In addition, pathological colors and odors often signal the presence of an infection. Infected burn wounds are usually treated with thorough cleansing, topical antimicrobials, and systemic antibiotics. Antibiotic therapy is guided by culture and sensitivity results. Gram-positive organisms (e.g., *S. aureus*) are suspected early and then Gram negatives later in the patient's management. Neglected wounds may have fluctuant pus beneath the eschar and progress to a full-thickness injury. Similar to any abscess, these areas should be opened and drained. Evaluation of burn wounds in elderly and diabetic individuals requires special care, as the inflammatory response can be blunted and wound severely underestimated.

Invasive burn wound infection

This is defined as "the presence of pathogens in a burn wound at sufficient concentrations in conjunction with depth, surface area involved and age of patient to cause suppurative separation of eschar or graft loss, invasion of adjacent unburned tissue, or cause the systemic response of sepsis syndrome" (Greenhalgh et al. 2007). Burn wounds with invasive infections have many different colors and distinct odors. However, because time and some topical agents also produce color changes, the most reliable sign of invasive burn wound infection is conversion of an area of partial-thickness burn to full-thickness necrosis or the necrosis of previously viable tissue in an excised wound bed. As indicated by the definition above, a burn wound infection does not need to be accompanied by sepsis to be considered invasive. Nevertheless, many invasive burn wound infections are life threatening and require immediate surgical treatment. Invasive infections can progress very rapidly and affect normal skin, causing erythema and pain followed by hemorrhagic bulla and possibly necrotic satellite lesions.

Invasive infection of burn wounds, particularly large burns, can be prevented through removal of dead tissue. Once an invasive infection has been established, it must be aggressively treated. To this end, surgeons must eliminate all dead tissue, including dead muscle, to control the infection and ensure that wound sites will support grafting. Such aggressive surgical intervention can include conversion of a tangential excision to the fascial level or even amputation of a limb. For treatment of the wound surface, dead tissue is completely removed, and the wound is treated with topical antimicrobial soaks such as silver nitrate, sulfamylon, and Dakin solution. If fungus is a concern, these soaks can be used in combination topical nystatin. More frequent soaking dressing changes (four times a day) may also be necessary. Effective antibiotics are administered based on culture and sensitivity information.

Toxic shock syndrome

Toxic shock syndrome (TSS) in the burn wound is a form of severe soft-tissue infection from TSS toxin (TSST)-1-producing *S. aureus*. TSS commonly occurs in young children (mean age 2 years) with small burns (<10%) and has an incidence of 2.6%. The prodromal period lasts 1–2 days and is associated with pyrexia, diarrhea, vomiting, malaise,

and often a rash, although the burn appears clean. If the infection is left untreated, shock ensues, usually around 2–4 days after the burn injury. During this time, the mortality rate can reach 50%. Knowledge of TSS and aggressive treatment are the best defenses against preventing this condition (Tompkins and Rossi 2004). TSST infections are commonly caused by MRSA, so administration of empirical anti-MRSA antimicrobials is advised in all cases of suspected TSS (White et al. 2005, Napolitano 2009).

BACTERIA AND THEIR TREATMENT
Gram-positive organisms

Staphylococcus aureus is the most important cause of bacterial burn wound infections (Murray 2003). Septicemia, cellulitis, impetigo, scalded skin syndrome, surgical site infections, and many other conditions are associated with *S. aureus*. Staphylococci, including *S. aureus*, produce a large variety of toxic metabolites including proteases, collagenases, and hyaluronidase. These factors digest the extracellular matrix, which is essential for wound healing. Pathogenic strains of staphylococci also produce pyrogenic exotoxins, leukocidins, and TSST-1. TSST-1, along with the other staphylococcal by-products, causes TSS in susceptible patients (Edwards-Jones and Greenwood 2003). Patients with TSS experience a sudden onset of fever, vomiting, diarrhea, and shock. They also have a diffuse macular erythematous rash. Hyperemia of various mucous membranes and desquamation on the hands and feet then occur. However, the role of TSS has not been completely elucidated in the burn patient. We have observed that, although burn patients may be infected with TSST-producing *S. aureus*, they do not always develop TSS.

All staphylococci produce penicillinases. These enzymes hydrolyze the penicillin β-lactam ring. Accordingly, these types of infections are treated with penicillinase-resistant penicillins. Parenteral antibiotics in this category include nafcillin, meticillin, and oxacillin. Cephalosporins are also used. MRSA infections are resistant to all β-lactam drugs and are commonly treated with vancomycin. Vancomycin acts on bacteria at a different site from the penicillins. Vancomycin is eliminated at a greater rate in hypermetabolic burn patients, who exhibit an increased glomerular filtration rate. Furthermore, a wide variability in vancomycin elimination exists among burn patients. Thus, dosages must be adjusted for each patient to optimize time-dependent serum concentrations. The peak and trough levels are determined using the minimum inhibitory concentration (MIC) for a particular bacterial organism. A trough level of 10–15 µg/ml is normally used for vancomycin monitoring, with care being taken to ensure that this serum level is maintained between dosing intervals. Maintaining appropriate trough levels is important for effective treatment of the infected patient, but also to avoid the emergence of resistant bacterial strains. For burn-associated MRSA pneumonia, a vancomycin trough concentration of 15–20 µg/ml should be the target (Rybak 2006). Treatment of microorganisms in burn wound infections may also require higher vancomycin trough serum concentrations due to "vancomycin MIC creep."

Streptococci are virulent pathogens in the burn patient and are associated with invasive cellulitis of the burn wound and skin graft losses. *Streptococcus pyogenes* (group A streptococci) and *S. agalactiae* (group B streptococci) are the major species of burn infection interest. These bacteria can be treated with penicillins (i.e., phenoxymethylpenicillin) or the first-generation cephalosporins (cefazolin).

Enterococci are resistant to the cephalosporin class of antibiotics, and have become important causes of burn wound infection for that reason. Enterococci as a group are significant pathogens during the hospitalization of the burn patient (Law et al. 1994). Vancomycin is effective against most enterococcal bacteria. However, a combination of agents such as ampicillin and aminoglycosides may be used. Vancomycin-resistant enterococci (VREs) have emerged in burn units, causing major concern. VREs are best treated with linezolid or daptomycin (see Chapter 2). Specific sensitivities are needed to validate therapy for VREs.

■ Gram-negative organisms

A distinctive group of Gram-negative rods contributes to burn wound infections. These include *Pseudomonas* spp., *Acinetobacter* spp., and the *Enterobacteriaceae*. The *Pseudomonas* spp. are the most frequently encountered burn wound pathogens. Wound infections due to *P. aeruginosa* are particularly troublesome. *Pseudomonas* spp. can produce disease ranging from superficial skin infections to fulminate sepsis. Invasive *Pseudomonas* spp. produce ecthyma gangrenosum (**Figure 12.4**), which appears as a purple–blue–blackish area in previously healthy tissue. These organisms survive in aqueous environments and prefer moist environments. For this reason, they have become problematic in the hospital environment. Indeed, *P. aeruginosa* is the leading cause of nosocomial respiratory tract infection.

Acinetobacter sp. is another significant Gram-negative pathogen commonly associated with burn infection. These microorganisms are normal colonists of human skin and the respiratory, gastrointestinal, and genitourinary tracts. These pathogens are problematic for burn patients, not only for burn wound infection, but also for pulmonary, intravenous catheter, and urinary tract infections. These organisms have a low intrinsic virulence and occur in the most immunosuppressed of the burn population. They also tend to acquire a high degree of resistance, most likely associated with previous antimicrobial therapy (Albrecht et al. 2006).

Enterobacteriaceae such as *Escherichia coli*, *Klebsiella* spp., *Enterobacter* spp., *Serratia marcescens*, and *Proteus* spp. are additional Gram-negative organisms infecting burns and other sites in the burn patient. These organisms often cause nosocomial pneumonia in patients with inhalational injury. They are also responsible for urinary tract infections associated with indwelling urinary catheters (Patel and Williams-Bouyer 2009).

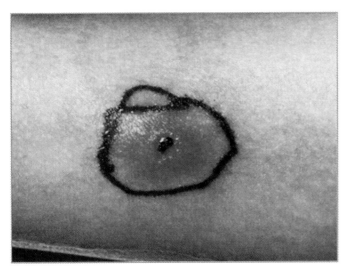

Figure 12.4 Ecthyma gangrenosum.

Gram-negative infections are typically treated based on culture and sensitivity data, but empirical choices while awaiting culture information may be selected from the antibiogram specific for the unit or hospital. Antibiotic synergism may result in multiple drugs for treatment of these organisms. Historically, the antibiotics of choice for treating Gram-negative infections were the aminoglycosides, particularly gentamicin. Quinolones, carbapenems, aztreonam, and others become choices when the sensitivity data is available (see Chapter 2).

Serious systemic infections caused by multidrug-resistant Gram-negative bacteria are treated with polymyxins. From 2000 to 2004, the pediatric burn hospital, Shriners Hospitals for Children in Galveston, TX, reviewed the use of colistimethate sodium in 109 patients (72 boys and 37 girls, median and mean age of 9 years) with a total body surface area (TBSA) burn ranging from 21% to 99% (median 60% and mean 62%). The overall survival rate was 80% in these patients, who had incompletely treated and life-threatening Gram-negative infections. Polymyxin B binds, via its free amino acid groups, to negatively charged phospholipids. Binding is greatest in the kidney and brain, followed by the liver, muscle, and lung. Repeated administration of this drug causes it to accumulate in tissues, with concentrations reaching four to five times peak serum concentrations and persisting for at least 5–7 days. The extensive tissue binding of this drug makes removal by dialysis difficult. For these reasons, nephrotoxicity and central nervous system toxicity should be monitored during systemic use of this drug. The adverse effects of colistimethate sodium occur in proportion to the length of its use and include *Clostridium difficile*-associated colitis, renal dysfunction, and neuropathies (unpublished data).

Sensitive organisms are commonly treated using aminoglycoside antimicrobials. These agents may be more effective and less toxic at single daily doses than multiple daily doses. Randomized, controlled studies have revealed that, in adults, efficacy (e.g., bacteriological and/or clinical cure), nephrotoxicity, and ototoxicity are similar or improved after a single daily dosing of aminoglycosides compared with multiple daily dosing. Decreasing the frequency of dosing may counter aminoglycoside-induced adaptive resistance (i.e., reversible refractoriness to the antimicrobial effects of subsequent aminoglycoside doses because of decreased uptake of the drug after the initial dose). It may also help prevent selection of aminoglycoside-resistant subpopulations of Gram-negative bacteria by providing a recovery period in which serum aminoglycoside concentrations are negligible. Despite these findings, once-daily dosing of aminoglycosides may not be advisable in burn patients with serious infections and impaired host defenses (e.g., patients with *P. aeruginosa* infections and neutropenia) or in patients exhibiting rapid clearance or unpredictable aminoglycoside pharmacokinetics (e.g., extensive burns, cystic fibrosis, massive ascites). If aminoglycosides are used in burn patients with any dosing strategy, pharmacokinetic dosing is essential.

Extended-spectrum penicillins are less toxic alternatives in burn patients with Gram-negative bacterial infections. The most frequent adverse reactions of extended-spectrum penicillin are hypersensitivity reactions, gastrointestinal effects, and local reactions. Gram-negative infections may be treated with fourth-generation cephalosporins such as cefepime, extended-spectrum β-lactamase inhibitor penicillins (piperacillin/tazobactam and ticarcillin/clavulanate), and the carbapenems (imipenem/cilastatin, meropenem, ertapenem). These antibiotics are most effective when the serum concentrations between dosing intervals are maintained at once or twice the MIC. Thus, more frequent dosing or longer infusions may be necessary to maintain this MIC.

Anaerobes

Of the anaerobes, *Bacteroides* and *Fusobacterium* spp. are the most commonly seen and may play a role in burn wound infections. These anaerobes are normally present in the body. In burned patients, anaerobic infections are usually associated with avascular muscle seen in electrical injuries, frostbite, or cutaneous flame burns with concomitant crush-type injuries. The incidence of anaerobic infections has been considerably decreased by early excision and grafting. In cases of suspected anaerobic infection, appropriate collection methods to maintain anaerobic conditions for transport to the laboratory are necessary. Metronidazole has continued to be the drug of choice for the treatment of anaerobic soft tissue infections.

Fungi: Yeasts and molds

Fungal infections were not common in burned patients until the advent of topical antimicrobial agents. The incidence of mycotic invasion has doubled since the implementation of topical antimicrobial agents. Fungal infections most commonly affect the burn wound, with an increasing number of local or disseminated fungal infections being seen in the urinary tract, respiratory tract, vagina, and gastrointestinal tract (Sheridan 2005). Special media are required for fungal isolation, and special biochemical tests are necessary for identification of the several possibilities for fungal infection. Of fungi, Candida spp. most commonly colonizes burn wounds. Positive blood cultures or positive cultures from three organs (wound, urine, bronchial washings, retina) are usually required for the diagnosis of candidal sepsis. The addition of nystatin to topical silver sulfadiazine has considerably decreased candida sepsis (Desai et al. 1992). Early diagnosis may be aided by antibody detection. (Desai et al. 1987). Unfortunately, less than 40% of infected patients received a timely diagnosis (Kobayashi et al. 1990).

Other fungi such as *Aspergillus, Penicillium, Rhizopus, Mucor, Rhizomucor, Fusarium*, and *Curvularia* spp. may also be present and cause burn wound infection. In severely immunosuppressed patients, these lesser-known fungi may have a greater invasive potential than yeasts (Horvath et al. 2007).

Early diagnosis of fungal infection can be difficult, because symptoms frequently mimic bacterial infections. Routine culture techniques may require from 7 days to 14 days to identify fungal contaminants, delaying the initiation of treatment. Correlation between histopathological and culture identification has been shown to be inconsistent. Therefore, histopathology alone can be inadequate for determining the best antifungal agent (Schofield et al. 2007). Arterial blood cultures and retinal examination for characteristic candidal lesions can be useful. Unlike candidal infections, true fungal infections occur early in the hospital course of patients with specific predisposing characteristics. Most frequently, burned patients infected with fungi are exposed to spores from either rolling on the ground or jumping into contaminated surface water at the time of injury. Other environmental sources have been cited for nosocomial fungal infection, including bandaging supplies, heating and air-conditioning ducts, and floor drains (Becker et al. 1991). Once colonized, fungi invade subcutaneous tissue with non-branching hyphae, stimulating an inflammatory response. This phenomenon is diagnostic of fungal wound infection. Vascular invasion is common and often accompanied by thrombosis and avascular necrosis, clinically observed as rapidly advancing dark discolorations of the wound margins with well-demarcated lesions. Systemic dissemination of the infection occurs with invasion of the vasculature. Yeast isolation from the wound may not represent infection and should be validated by clinical observations. Clinically observed lesions from molds confirm the diagnosis. Infection with mold is often invasive and requires very aggressive treatment, with topical medication, surgery, and intravenous (IV) medication. It is common to work with a pathologist to ensure that margins are free of hyphae at the conclusion of a debridement. Amphotericin B has been the standard choice for IV treatment of invasive mold infection. Currently, there are five classes of systemic antifungal medications: the polyenes, azoles, nucleoside analogs, echinocandins, and allylamines. These new drugs offer improved side-effect profiles over amphotericin B.

Although amphotericin B dexolate (AmBd) has been the standard choice for IV treatment of life-threatening invasive mold, this drug is associated with significant toxicity, including infusion-related events and dose-limiting renal dysfunction. Three new lipid formulations of amphotericin B (AmB lipid complex [ABLC], AmB colloidal dispersion, and liposomal AmB [AmB-L]) offer several advantages over AmBd. These advantages include increased daily doses of the parent drug (up to 1- to 15-fold), high tissue concentrations in reticuloendothelial organs, decreased infusion-related events (especially ABLC and AmB-L), and a marked decrease in nephrotoxicity. These lipid drugs are more expensive than AmBd, but cost is best assessed pharmacoeconomically (cost of drug acquisition as well as cost of hospital stay, monitoring, complications, etc.).

For most patients with systemic candidiasis, cryptococcosis, and the endemic mycoses (e.g., blastomycosis, histoplasmosis, and coccidioidomycosis), AmBd or azole drugs (voriconazole, fluconazole, itraconazole, or posaconazole) should be used as initial therapy. Initial treatment with a lipid drug for these patients cannot be justified, unless the patients require AmB therapy and have pre-existing renal dysfunction. Invasive aspergillosis is treated with voriconazole due to its efficacy and lower toxicity profile. AmBd may still be used as an alternative treatment agent. Posaconzole is an effective treatment for aspergillosis. The azoles (fluconazole, itraconazole, voriconazole, and posaconazole) demonstrate similar activity against most *Candida* spp. But each of the azoles has less activity against *C. glabrata* and *C. krusei*. The echinocandins (caspofungin, anidulafungin, micafungin) have very good efficacy against most *Candida* spp., but may have less activity against *C. parapsilosis*. Flucytosine has limited clinical indications and may be used with AmBD in selected life-threatening candida syndromes.

Viral infection of the burn wound

The diagnosis and treatment of viral infections in burned patients have received increasing attention. Subclinical viral infection is extremely common, as seen by prospective and retrospective assays of sera. Linnemann and MacMillan (1981) conducted a large retrospective study of stored sera from burned children. They found that 22% of patients exhibited a fourfold increase in antibodies to cytomegalovirus (CMV). They also found that 8% had increased herpes simplex titers and 5% had increased varicella-zoster titers. Follow-up revealed that CMV infection developed in 33%, herpetic infection in 25%, and adenovirus infection in 17%.

CMV infection rarely alters the clinical course of the patient. This type of infection frequently accompanies bacterial and fungal infections. Primary CMV infection or reactivation of CMV occurs at an overall frequency of 33%. CMV inclusions have been detected in multiple organs, although they have not been reported to be found in the burn wound itself (Deepe et al. 1982). Prospective analyses conducted by Linnemann and MacMillan (1981) revealed that CMV infection is directly correlated with more severe burns, more skin grafts, and subsequently higher numbers of blood transfusions. Patients with burns covering <50% of the TBSA rarely manifest clinical signs of CMV infection. Infection with CMV occurs about 1 month after burn injury and appears as an unexplained fever and lymphocytosis, which is associated with a concomitant rise in specific antibodies.

CMV infection frequently occurs in immunocompromised patients and produces an array of adverse conditions. These conditions range from febrile illness to systemic infections with organ involvement (e.g., lungs, brain, liver, colon, and pancreas) (Ljungman et al. 2002). Up to 23% of severely burned patients who are seronegative seroconvert, whereas more than half of seropositive patients undergo CMV reactivation based on a fourfold or greater rise in antibody titer (Kealey et al. 1987, Bale et al. 1990). Systemic CMV infection in severely burned patients has been described in only two reports (Nash and Foley 1970, Hamprecht et al. 2005). This suggests that severely burned patients rarely contract systemic infections. However, severely burned patients frequently have increased CMV antibodies, which suggests that these infections are subtle and have been overlooked. CMV-associated pathological changes have been detected in endothelial and periendothelial cells present in generalized, non-healing burn wounds (Swanson and Feldman 1987). In one reported case of CMV infection, a cadaver allograft from a CMV-positive donor was transplanted onto a severely burned adult. Immunohistochemical staining of the allograft revealed the presence of inclusion bodies consistent with CMV infection as well as CMV antigens; however, there was no clear relationship between CMV infection and the necrosis, inflammation, and increased vascularity present in the infected skin (Bale et al. 1992). In experimental animals, severe burn injury increases the risk of CMV infection, and CMV infection is associated with a greater susceptibility to sepsis (Hamilton and Overall 1978, Bale et al. 1982).

Cadaver skin may transmit CMV infection, as do blood transfusions. Often, burn patients who contract CMV infection have received multiple blood transfusions. Tennenhaus et al. (2006) conducted surveys in US and German burn centers to investigate awareness, perceptions, diagnosis, and treatment of CMV in burn patients. They found that the incidence of CMV infection was 1:870 in US burn centers and 1:280 in German burn centers. An analysis of testing methods revealed that 19% of US and 70% of German burn centers used serology, 25% of US and 52% of German centers used body fluid viral isolation, and 6% of US and 43% of German centers relied on leukocyte CMV DNA analysis. Half the US centers distinguished infection from clinical disease, whereas only two-thirds of the German centers did. Moreover, 19% of the US and 43% of the German centers surveyed would treat the established infection.

Herpes simplex virus is another problematic viral pathogen encountered in burn patients (Haik et al. 2011). In healing partial-thickness burns or split-thickness donor sites, herpes simplex infections usually appear as vesicles (**Figure 12.5**). However, in immunocompromised burn patients, they are barely noticeable and appear as red macules. After the appearance of these macules, the infection rapidly progresses, spreading over entire donor sites and previously healed areas. This can lead to a near-total loss of epidermal coverage. In addition, this infection can sometimes affect other epithelial surfaces such as the oral or intestinal mucosa, potentially causing erosion and perforation. Patients usually experience an unexplained fever unresponsive to routine antibiotic coverage before the appearance of herpes simplex lesions. Burn patients with herpetic infections have been found to experience greater mortality, extensive visceral involvement, and necrotizing tracheobronchitis. Herpes infection of partial-thickness burns and donor sites may eventually produce full-thickness injuries that require skin grafting for closure. Herpes infections may also lead to multisystem organ failure by producing

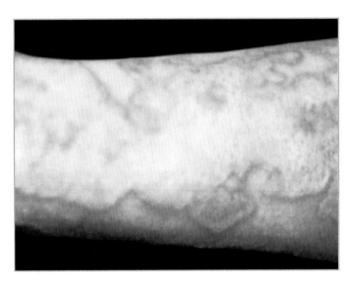

Figure 12.5 Herpetic burn wound infection.

necrotizing hepatic and adrenal lesions. Patients with a disseminated herpes infection have a morality rate that is twice as high as that in patients with a similar age and burn size. Previously infected herpetic wounds can be adequately covered by split-thickness grafts, although secondary graft loss often occurs and reoperation with patch grafting is needed.

Chickenpox (varicella-zoster) can be life-threatening to immunocompromised hosts, such as burn patients. These infections are rapidly spread through inhalation of the virus. Indeed, small chickenpox epidemics have occurred in pediatric burn units. This type of infection manifests itself as fluid-filled lesions. In some cases, they may present as hemorrhagic, oozing pockmarks, which are prone to secondary infection and scarring. Vesicles can be present in uninjured epithelium, mucus membranes, and healed or healing partial-thickness burns. These vesicles are much more destructive to injured skin than uninjured skin, because newly healed or healing skin is particularly fragile. Damage can be inflicted on neovascularized skin grafts with resultant graft loss.

■ Tetanus

Routine prophylaxis for tetanus (*Clostridium tetani*) is part of the admission protocol for the burn center. Patients receive 0.5 ml tetanus toxoid if it has not been received in the previous 3 years. If the patient's last booster was more than 10 years ago, 250 U tetanus antitoxin is also administered.

■ TOPICAL ANTIMICROBIAL COMPOUNDS AND AGENTS

The proper use of prophylactic topical agents has been achieved in burn wound management. Maintaining low concentrations of bacterial colonization diminishes the frequency and duration of septic episodes. Topical antimicrobial agents have significantly reduced burn mortality. However, no single agent is completely effective against all organisms, and each possesses its own advantages and disadvantages. Although most topical agents retard wound healing, the application of some antimicrobial agents may increase metabolic rate. Their effectiveness is measured by their ability to inhibit bacterial growth in vitro and reduce wound colony counts in vivo. Studies have demonstrated that some agents used in the past are ineffective in inhibiting bacterial growth in vitro (Kucan and Smoot 1993). If quantitative cultures demonstrate bacterial concentrations >10^2 organisms/g, then a change in the topical agent is strongly recommended.

■ Sodium hypochlorite (NaOCl)

The most effective topical antibacterial for cleansing a wound is NaOCl. This agent has superior topical antimicrobial effects and lower tissue toxicity than such products as povidone–iodine, acetic acid, and hydrogen peroxide. Although povidone–iodine is bactericidal at concentrations of 1% and 0.5%, it is toxic to fibroblasts. Acetic acid is toxic to fibroblasts, but not bactericidal, when used at a concentration of 0.25%. Hydrogen peroxide is toxic to fibroblasts at 3% and 0.3% concentrations, but is bactericidal at only the 3% concentration. Heggers et al. (1991) have reported the efficacy of NaOCl at a concentration of 0.025%. A 0.025% NaOCl solution is a tenth of the concentration of "half-strength Dakin," the formulation that is used by many hospitals as a topical antimicrobial agent. It is an excellent cleansing agent that is bactericidal, non-toxic to fibroblasts, and does not inhibit wound healing. However, the 0.025% NaOCl solution is only effective over a 24-hour time frame after the buffer (0.3 mol/l NaH_2HPO_4) is added to the NaOCl (Holder et al. 1979).

Soaks in buffered 0.025% NaOCl solution are beneficial in reducing the bacterial numbers in a wound. The 0.025% NaOCl solution is a broad-spectrum antiseptic and is bactericidal against *P. aeruginosa* and *S. aureus*, as well as other Gram-negative and Gram-positive organisms (Nash et al. 1971, Strock et al. 1990). It is effective against meticillin-resistant staphylococci and enterococci. A 0.025% NaOCl solution may be used separately or together with other antibacterial agents to control colonization or infection. This solution also enhances wound healing compared with mafenide acetate (Strock et al. 1990).

■ Silver nitrate (AgNO₃)

$AgNO_3$ is now used as a 0.5% solution that is non-toxic, does not injure regenerating epithelium in the wound, and is bacteriostatic against *S. aureus*, *Escherichia coli*, and *P. aeruginosa*. $AgNO_3$ is most effective when the wound is debrided of all dead tissue and carefully cleansed of emollients and debris. Multilayered coarse-mesh dressings should be placed over the wound and saturated with the $AgNO_3$ solution. Similar to silver sulfadiazine, $AgNO_3$ has limited eschar penetration (Moncrief 1968, Fuller et al. 1971, Heggers et al. 1991). As it is hypotonic it can result in hyponatremia and hypochloremia. Serum electrolytes must be monitored very carefully. A 0.5% $AgNO_3$ solution is light sensitive and turns black on contact with tissues and other chloride-containing compounds when it is allowed to dry. Hyperpyrexia may also occur if $AgNO_3$ becomes dry and is covered with an impervious dressing. Some institutions have combined $AgNO_3$ with miconazole powder. The resulting 0.5% $AgNO_3$ and 2% miconazole aqueous solution is effective in preventing fungal overgrowth in burn wounds. *Klebsiella* spp., *Providencia* spp., and other *Enterobacteriaceae* have lesser susceptibility to 0.5% $AgNO_3$ solution. A 0.5% $AgNO_3$ solution with *Enterobacter cloacae* and other nitrate-positive organisms may cause methemoglobinemia by converting nitrate to nitrite in the body.

■ Silver sulfadiazine

Silver sulfadiazine (Silvadene, Thermazine, Flamazine, and SSD) is available as a 1% water-soluble cream. The silver ion binds with DNA of the microbe, releasing the sulfonamide. This agent is most effective against *P. aeruginosa* and the *Enterobacteriaceae*. It is also equally effective as any antifungal drug against *C. albicans*. However, some strains of *Klebsiella* spp. have been less effectively controlled. Recently, *P. aeruginosa* resistance to silver sulfadiazine has been reported. Silver sulfadiazine is equally effective when applied using either the closed or the open method. Antimicrobial effectiveness has been observed to last for up to 24 h, and it still is considered by most to be the first line prophylaxis against Gram-negative organisms. More frequent changes are required if a creamy exudate forms on the wound. Some of the benefits of this topical agent are its ease of use and that it is pain free. Tissue penetration is limited to the surface epidermal layer (Heggers et al. 1991). Nevertheless, it is not associated with acid–base disturbances or pulmonary fluid overload. Silver sulfadiazine can be used in combination with other antibacterials and enzymatic escharotomy compounds. It can be combined with nystatin to enhance antifungal activity. Silver sulfadiazine has been shown to retard wound healing. An adverse reaction to this drug may be a reversible granulocyte reduction.

■ Mafenide acetate (Sulfamylon)

Mafenide acetate is available as an 8.5% water-soluble cream or a 5% aqueous solution. This agent has more bacteriological data supporting efficacy than other topical agents. Mafenide acetate has been shown to be effective against a broad range of microorganisms, especially all strains of *P. aeruginosa*. After wound debridement, 8.5% mafenide acetate cream is applied to the wound like "butter" (Lindberg butter) (Lindberg et al. 1968). The treated burn surface is left exposed for maximal antimicrobial potency. The cream is applied a minimum of twice a day and reapplied between applications if rubbed off the wound. Advantages of the cream are its ability to control *P. aeruginosa* wound infections, ease of application, and the absence of the need for dressings. It effectively penetrates burn eschar and prevents colonization of the burn.

The 5% solution is used to saturate an eight-ply gauze dressing and is applied to the burn wound area. The dressing should be kept saturated with the 5% mafenide acetate solution to produce maximal antimicrobial effects. The dressings may be changed every 8 h. Shortcomings of mafenide acetate include overgrowth with *C. albicans*, it being a carbonic anhydrase inhibitor that causes a metabolic acidosis, and pain from application on partial-thickness wounds. However, it is quite effective in burn wounds with poor perfusion such as on the ear. The 5% aqueous solution of mafenide acetate can be used in a wet dressing covered by a splint. The 5% mafenide acetate solution in major burn patients reduces fatalities by 33% (Pruitt and Foley 1973, Desai et al. 1987). Mafenide acetate can be used together with other antimicrobials. It does retard wound healing.

■ Povidone–iodine (Betadine)

A 10% ointment of povidone–iodine has been in use for over half a century after the active agent demonstrated a broad spectrum of antimicrobial activities in liquid form. Povidone–iodine has a broad spectrum of antibacterial and antifungal activities. Povidone–iodine ointment can be used effectively in both the closed and the open techniques. Quantitative bacteriological data show that it is most efficacious when applied every 6 h. Adverse effects associated with topical povidone–iodine include pain with application; absorption causing iodine toxicity, renal failure, and acidosis; and cytotoxicity to fibroblasts. It remains a highly effective when used on intact skin.

Gentamicin sulfate (Garamycin)

Gentamicin sulfate is available as a 0.1% water-soluble cream. It has a broad spectrum of antimicrobial activity. Its popular use in wounds is based on its antimicrobicidal efficacy against *P. aeruginosa*. Gentamicin resistance rapidly develops when used as a topical antimicrobial agent. A new gentamicin-eluting bioresorbable core/shell fiber-structured burn wound dressing shows promise in topical treatment of burns. In initial trials, these drug-eluting fiber structures have shown a significant decrease in bacterial viability and no survival of bacteria after 2 days of treatment.

Bacitracin/polymyxin (Polysporin)

Topical bacitracin/polymyxin is used to "butter" bolsters that are used to prevent mechanical shearing of newly grafted tissue. This topical ointment barrier has not been shown to control infection. It is commonly used as topical coverage for small face burns and for skin graft coverage because it is easily applied. It is not documented to reduce infections. Prolonged use is associated with hypersensitivity.

Nitrofurantoin (Furacin)

Topical nitrofurantoin has been used extensively but has had questionable therapeutic value. Recent research has shown effectiveness in treating MRSA. Nitrofurantoin has also been shown to be 75% effective against Gram-negative bacterial isolates other than *P. aeruginosa*, whereas bacitracin/polymyxin is only 21% effective (Greenhalgh et al. 2007).

Mupirocin (Bactroban)

Mupirocin was introduced as a topical antibiotic by Fuller et al. (1971). In vitro studies have established that mupirocin has broad inhibitory activity against Gram-positive microbes, specifically *S. aureus* and *S. epidermidis*. Mupirocin has been shown to be efficient in treating infection or colonization due to *S. aureus* in various clinical settings. Rode et al. (1989) have shown that mupirocin is efficacious in the treatment of established wound infections resulting from *S. aureus* that is resistant to systemic meticillin, topical mafenide acetate, and povidone–iodine. In addition, recent in vitro and in vivo endeavors have shown mupirocin to be equally efficacious in meticillin-resistant burn wound infections.

Acticoat A.B.

Acticoat A.B. Dressing consists of two sheets of high-density polyethylene mesh coated with ionic silver and a rayon/polyester core. Acticoat A.B. Dressing provides broad-spectrum bactericidal coverage against VREs, MRSA, *P. aeruginosa*, *Candida* spp., and many other pathogens. This dressing can remain intact on the wound for several days if exudation is minimal. Acticoat must remain moist to be active. Rewetting with water is recommended.

Nystatin (Mycostatin, Nilstat)

Nystatin is an antifungal antibiotic produced by *Streptomyces noursei*. Nystatin has fungistatic or fungicidal activity against a variety of pathogenic and non-pathogenic strains of yeasts and fungi. In vitro, nystatin concentrations of 3 µg/ml inhibit *C. albicans* and *C. guilliertnondi*. Concentrations of 6.25 µg/ml are required to inhibit *C. krusei* and *Geotrichum lactis*. In general, there is little difference between inhibitory and fungicidal concentrations for a particular organism. Nystatin is not active against bacteria, protozoa, or viruses.

Nystatin is not absorbed systemically and is used orally for the treatment of intestinal candidiasis. In our burn population, nystatin 'swish and swallow' is used prophylactically to prevent the oral or perineal overgrowth of yeast and fungi in patients receiving two or three systemic antibiotics. In patients with coexisting intestinal candidiasis and vulvovaginal candidiasis, nystatin may be administered orally, together with the intravaginal application of an antifungal agent. Most evidence suggests that combined therapy does not substantially reduce the risk of recurrence of vulvovaginal candidiasis compared with intravaginal therapy alone. However, limited evidence suggests that the reduction of intestinal candidal colonization in combination with intravaginal antifungal therapy may provide some improvement in mycological response and reduction in the recurrence rate of vulvovaginal candidiasis. For the treatment of cutaneous or mucocutaneous candidal infections, 100 000 U/g nystatin may be applied topically as a cream, lotion, or ointment to affected areas two to four times daily. The cream or lotion formulations are preferred to the ointment for use in moist, intertriginous areas. The use of occlusive dressings and ointment formulations should be avoided in the treatment of candidiasis because they favor the growth of yeast and the release of its irritating endotoxin. Concomitant therapy should include proper hygiene and skin care. In addition, the affected areas should be kept dry and exposed to air whenever possible.

The topical treatment of burn wounds with nystatin powder at a concentration of 6 000 000 U/g has been shown to eradicate invasive fungal infections. This topical treatment is effective for superficial and deep burn fungal wound infections. The powder is easily applied, does not produce pain or discomfort, and does not impair wound healing. Nystatin powder may be combined with 1% silver sulfadiazine cream or 5% mafenide acetate aqueous solution to enhance fungal activity.

INFECTION CONTROL BEST PRACTICE

The microorganisms initially populating the burn wound consist of a mixture of endogenous, airborne, and environmental sources of pathogens. The most elaborate methods of isolation have failed to eliminate infection, although they have significantly reduced the incidence of cross-contamination. The most effective means of decreasing exposure of burned patients to exogenous bacteria is strict observation of appropriate hand washing among the healthcare providers. Universal contact isolation is often a routine practice in burn centers. Facemasks, waterproof gowns, and gloves should be worn whenever direct contact with body fluids and wound exudates is possible so that both the patient and the healthcare provider are protected from inadvertent contamination. All dressing materials should be maintained as patient specific. IV pumps and poles, blood pressure devices, monitoring equipment, bedside tables, and beds should be cleaned with antibacterial solutions at least daily. Decontamination of the patient room after discharge should be undertaken with detergents. At Shriners Hospitals for Children, Galveston, TX, Hepa air filters with 99.99% efficiency on 0.3 µm-sized particles are used and changed regularly. Most units now house major burn patients within individual, self-contained positive-pressure isolation rooms. However, these units contain common bathing or showering facilities. These areas should be consciously cleaned between patients with an effective bactericidal agent. Disposable liners for cleaning surfaces are encouraged, and sterilizable instruments should be used for debridements.

■ REFERENCES

Albrecht MC, Griffith ME, Murray CK, et al. Impact of *Acinetobacter* infection on the mortality of burn patients. *J Am Coll Surg* 2006;**203**:546–50.

Artz CP, Moncrief JA. *The Treatment of Burns*, 2nd edn. Philadelphia: Saunders, 1969.

Bale JF Jr, Gay PE, Madsen JA. Monitoring of serum amylase levels during valproic acid therapy. *Ann Neurol* 1982;**11**:217–18.

Bale JF Jr, Kealey GP, Massanari RM, Strauss RG. The epidemiology of cytomegalovirus infection among patients with burns. *Infect Control Hosp Epidemiol* 1990;**11**:17–22.

Bale JF Jr, Kealey GP, Ebelhack CL, Platz CE, Goeken JA. Cytomegalovirus infection in a cyclosporine-treated burn patient: case report. *J Trauma* 1992;**32**:26367.

Barret JP, Herndon DN. Effects of burn wound excision on bacterial colonization and invasion. *Plast Reconstr Surg* 2003;**111**:744–50; discussion 751–42.

Becker WK, Cioffi WG Jr, McManus AT, et al. Fungal burn wound infection. A 10-year experience. *Arch Surg* 1991;**126**:44–8.

Bone RC, Balk RA, Cerra FB, et al. Definitions for sepsis and organ failure and guidelines for the use of innovative therapies in sepsis. The ACCP/SCCM Consensus Conference Committee. American College of Chest Physicians/ Society of Critical Care Medicine. *Chest* 1992;**101**:1644–55.

Burke JF, Quinby WC, Bondoc CC, Sheehy EM, Moreno HC. The contribution of a bacterially isolated environment to the prevention of infection in seriously burned patients. *Ann Surg* 1977;**186**:377–87.

Deepe GS Jr, MacMillan BG, Linnemann CC Jr. Unexplained fever in burn patients due to cytomegalovirus infection. *JAMA* 1982;**248**:2299–301.

Desai MH, Herndon DN, Abston S. *Candida* infection in massively burned patients. *J Trauma* 1987;**27**:1186–8.

Desai MH, Rutan RL, Heggers JP, Herndon DN. *Candida* infection with and without nystatin prophylaxis. A 11-year experience with patients with burn injury. *Arch Surg* 1992;**127**:159–62.

Edwards-Jones V, Greenwood JE. What's new in burn microbiology? James Laing Memorial Prize Essay 2000. *Burns* 2003;**29**:15–24.

Fuller AT, Mellows G, Woolford M, Banks GT, Barrow KD, Chain EB. Pseudomonic acid: an antibiotic produced by *Pseudomonas fluorescens*. *Nature* 1971;**234**:416–17.

Greenhalgh DG, Saffle JR, Holmes JHT, et al. American Burn Association consensus conference to define sepsis and infection in burns. *J Burn Care Res* 2007;**28**:776–90.

Haik J, Weissman O, Stavrou D, et al. Is prophylactic acyclovir treatment warranted for prevention of herpes simplex virus infections in facial burns? A review of the literature. *J Burn Care Res* 2011;**32**:358–62.

Hamilton JR, Overall JC Jr. Synergistic infection with murine cytomegalovirus and Pseudomonas aeruginosa in mice. *J Infect Dis* 1978;**137**:775–82.

Hamprecht K, Pfau M, Schaller HE, Jahn G, Middeldorp JM, Rennekampff HO. Human cytomegalovirus infection of a severe-burn patient: evidence for productive self-limited viral replication in blood and lung. *J Clin Microbiol* 2005;**43**:2534–6.

Heggers JP, Robson MC. *Quantitative Bacteriology : Its role in the armamentarium of the surgeon*. Boca Raton, FL: CRC Press, 1991.

Heggers JP, Sazy JA, Stenberg BD, et al. Bactericidal and wound-healing properties of sodium hypochlorite solutions: the 1991 Lindberg Award. *J Burn Care Rehabil* 1991;**12**:420–4.

Holder IA, Schwab M, Jackson L. Eighteen months of routine topical antimicrobial susceptibility testing of isolates from burn patients: results and conclusions. *J Antimicrob Chemother* 1979;**5**:455–63.

Horvath EE, Murray CK, Vaughan GM, et al. Fungal wound infection (not colonization) is independently associated with mortality in burn patients. *Ann Surg* 2007;**245**:978–5.

Kealey GP, Bale JF, Strauss RG, Massanari RM. Cytomegalovirus infection in burn patients. *J Burn Care Rehabil* 1987;**8**:543–5.

Kobayashi K, Mukae N, Matsunaga Y, Hotchi M. Diagnostic value of serum antibody to *Candida* in an extensively burned patient. *Burns* 1990;**16**:414–17.

Kucan JO, Smoot EC. Five percent mafenide acetate solution in the treatment of thermal injuries. *J Burn Care Rehabil* 1993;**14**(2 Pt 1):158–63.

Law EJ, Blecher K, Still JM. Enterococcal infections as a cause of mortality and morbidity in patients with burns. *J Burn Care Rehabil* 1994;**15**:236–9.

Levy MM, Fink MP, Marshall JC, et al. 2001 SCCM/ESICM/ACCP/ATS/SIS International Sepsis Definitions Conference. *Crit Care Med* 2003;**31**:1250–6.

Lindberg RB, Moncrief JA, Mason AD Jr. Control of experimental and clinical burn wounds sepsis by topical application of sulfamylon compounds. *Ann N Y Acad Sci* 1968;**150**:950–60.

Linnemann CC Jr, MacMillan BG. Viral infections in pediatric burn patients. *Am J Dis Child* 1981;**135**:750–3.

Ljungman P, Griffiths P, Paya C. Definitions of cytomegalovirus infection and disease in transplant recipients. *Clin Infect Dis* 2002;**34**:1094–7.

Mayhall CG. The epidemiology of burn wound infections: then and now. *Clin Infect Dis* 2003;**37**:543–50.

Moncrief JA. The status of topical antibacterial therapy in the treatment of burns. *Surgery* 1968;**63**:862–7.

Murray PRBEJ. *Manual of Clinical Microbiology*. 8th edn. Washington, DC: ASM Press, 2003.

Napolitano LM. Severe soft tissue infections. *Infect Dis Clin North Am* 2009;**23**:571–91.

Nash G, Foley FD. Herpetic infection of the middle and lower respiratory tract. *Am J Clin Pathol* 1970;**54**:857–63.

Nash G, Foley FD, Goodwin MN Jr, Bruck HM, Greenwald KA, Pruitt BA Jr. Fungal burn wound infection. *JAMA* 1971;**215**:1664–6.

Patel JA, Williams-Bouyer NM. Infections in burn patients. In: Feigin RD, Cherry JD, Demmler-Harrison GJ, Kaplan SL (eds), *Feigin & Cherry's Textbook of Pediatric Infectious Diseases*, Vol 1, 6th edn. Philadelphia, PA: Saunders/ Elsevier, 2009: Chapter 87, pp. 1139–53.

Pruitt BA Jr, Foley FD. The use of biopsies in burn patient care. *Surgery* 1973;**73**:887–97.

Pruitt BA Jr, McManus AT, Kim SH, Goodwin CW. Burn wound infections: current status. *World J Surg* 1998;**22**:135–45.

Robson MC. Bacterial control in the burn wound. *Clin Plast Surg* 1979;**6**:515–22.

Robson MC, Krizek TJ, Heggers JP. Biology of surgical infection. *Curr Probl Surg* 1973a:1–62.

Robson MC, Krizek TJ. Predicting skin graft survival. *J Trauma* 1973b;**13**:213–17.

Rode H, Hanslo D, de Wet PM, Millar AJ, Cywes S. Efficacy of mupirocin in methicillin-resistant *Staphylococcus aureus* burn wound infection. *Antimicrob Agents Chemother* 1989;**33**:1358–61.

Rybak MJ. The pharmacokinetic and pharmacodynamic properties of vancomycin. *Clin Infect Dis* 2006;**42**(suppl 1):S35–9.

Schofield CM, Murray CK, Horvath EE, et al. Correlation of culture with histopathology in fungal burn wound colonization and infection. *Burns* 2007;**33**:341–6.

Sheridan RL. Sepsis in pediatric burn patients. *Pediatr Crit Care Med* 2005;**6**(3 suppl):S112–19.

Steer JA, Papini RP, Wilson AP, McGrouther DA, Parkhouse N. Quantitative microbiology in the management of burn patients. I. Correlation between quantitative and qualitative burn wound biopsy culture and surface alginate swab culture. *Burns* 1996;**22**:173–6.

Strock LL, Lee MM, Rutan RL, et al. Topical Bactroban (mupirocin): efficacy in treating burn wounds infected with methicillin-resistant staphylococci. *J Burn Care Rehabil* 1990;**11**:454–9.

Swanson S, Feldman PS. Cytomegalovirus infection initially diagnosed by skin biopsy. *Am J Clin Pathol* 1987;**87**:113–16.

Tenenhaus M, Rennekampff HO, Pfau M, Hamprecht K. Cytomegalovirus and burns: current perceptions, awareness, diagnosis, and management strategies in the United States and Germany. *J Burn Care Res* 2006;**27**:281–8.

Teplitz C, Davis D, Mason AD Jr, Moncrief JA. Pseudomonas burn wound sepsis. I Pathogenesis of experimental pseudomonas burn wound sepsis. *J Surg Res* 1964;**4**:200–16.

Tompkins D, Rossi LA. Care of out patient burns. *Burns* 2004;**30**:A7–9.

White MC, Thornton K, Young AE. Early diagnosis and treatment of toxic shock syndrome in paediatric burns. *Burns* 2005;**31**:193–7.

Chapter 13   Fungal infections of surgical significance

Joseph S. Solomkin, Jianan Ren, Donald E. Fry

The contemporary population of surgical patients represents vulnerable hosts for the increased frequency of fungal infections. Aggressive surgical care in cancer patients and the expansion of transplantation interventions means that more immunosuppressed patients are in the surgical intensive care unit (ICU). Continued progress in supportive care, including the development of antibiotics with increasingly broad spectra of activity, has increased fungal colonization and resultant rates of infections among injured and other complex postoperative patients. The understanding and treatment of these fungal infections are not fully understood, but progress has been made and newer prevention and treatment strategies are evolving. This chapter provides an overview of those fungal infections that are most likely to be encountered by surgeons in the care of patients. It can be certain that additional species of fungal pathogens will be added to those discussed in the upcoming decades.

■ CANDIDA INFECTIONS

Candidemia and other candida infection syndromes are diseases of medical and surgical progress. Surgical patients are at considerable additional risk because perforations of the gastrointestinal (GI) tract at any level, but especially of the colon, result in release of colonizing Candida organisms into a previously sterile body site in approximately 20% of cases. Further, there is considerable evidence that GI dysfunction, including ileus and changes in the intestinal microflora, increases the density of candida and the probability of mucosal invasion. All of the other major risk factors, including the presence of central venous catheters, exposure to broad-spectrum antibiotics, and use of parenteral nutrition, are also present.

Despite the application of prophylaxis and early therapy strategies, these infections are not declining, but rather appear to have reached a stable plateau (Vincent et al. 1998, Kett et al. 2011). An important issue is whether these infections are epiphenomena, appearing in patients who are fated to die, or whether there is the effect of an attributable mortality that can be reduced by various therapeutic strategies.

Candida albicans, C. glabrata, and other species are pathogens and not commensals requiring failure of host defenses alone to cause infection. We provide recommendations for the identification of patients at risk to warrant prophylaxis, and then discuss treatment strategies in established infection.

■ Epidemiology of candida infections

Candida spp. remain the fourth leading cause of nosocomial bloodstream infection, preceded only by coagulase-negative staphylococci, Staphylococcus aureus, and enterococci (Zilberberg et al. 2008). Furthermore, in infections occurring after previous intra-abdominal surgery, Candida spp. are cultured from approximately 20% of these patients. In multicenter observational studies, overt candida infection is encountered in about 0.8–1% of patients in ICUs (Kett et al. 2011).

Candida spp. are the most common fungal pathogens causing serious hospital-acquired infections, especially in patients admitted to ICUs (Hidron et al. 2008) (**Figure 13.1**). A recent study using the National Hospital Discharge Survey estimated the incidence rate of invasive candidiasis to have increased from 23 per 100 000 US population in 1996 to 29 per 100 000 in 2003 (Pfaller and Diekema 2007). Candidemia represents about a third of these infections. In addition, more resistant non-albicans Candida spp. are increasingly identified as etiological agents in candidemia. The best incidence data come from a European study from multiple ICUs examining the point prevalence of specific infections (Vincent et al. 2009).

Matched cohort and case–control studies in various hospitalized patient populations, including those in the ICU, report attributable mortality rates for candidemia in the range 20–30% (Morgan et al. 2005, Zaoutis et al. 2005, Falagas et al. 2006). The attributable morbidity and mortality of other forms of candida infections have a similar range of increased mortality and an increased length of stay of 5–7 days (Prowle et al. 2011). On surgical services, candida peritonitis represents approximately 80% of the candida infection syndromes seen, and has a 30% excess attributable mortality rate (Leroy et al. 2009).

■ Microbiology of candida infection

Although there are more than 100 described species of Candida only four are commonly associated with infection: C. albicans, C. tropicalis, C. parapsilosis, and C. glabrata (Falagas et al. 2006). Of these, C. albicans has long been the most common (>60% of infections); the other three major species are seen at rates varying from 5% to 20%. C. tropicalis is a virulent organism and mucosal colonization by this organism frequently leads to invasive infection.

An evolution of the epidemiology of candidiasis has been recently described with a reduction in the incidence of C. albicans in favor of the non-albicans species, in particular C. glabrata and to a lesser extent C. krusei (Vincent et al. 1995). This appears to have occurred because of wide usage of fluconazole, and is important because several strains of C. glabrata have reduced susceptibility to fluconazole. C. krusei is highly resistant to all triazoles. In a study of 2618 blood isolates, 10% (232/2441) of the patients had recently (≤30 days) been treated with antifungal drugs. Pre-exposure to either fluconazole or an echinocandin resulted in a decreased prevalence of C. albicans in favor of less drug-susceptible species (Lortholary et al. 2011).

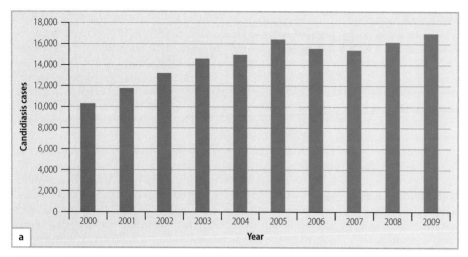

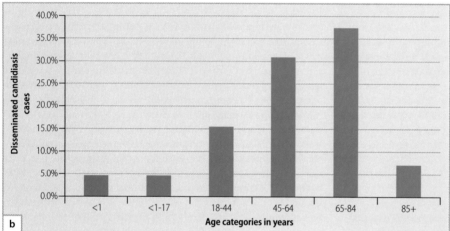

Figure 13.1 (a) The annual hospital discharges of patients with disseminated candida infection in the USA. (b) Age of patients with disseminated candida infection who were discharged from hospitals in the USA from 2000 to 2009. (Agency for Healthcare Research and Quality, HCUPnet database, accessed March 8, 2012: http://hcupnet.ahrq.gov.)

▪ Pathogenicity and virulence factors for Candida spp.

Four virulence factors have been demonstrated for *Candida* spp. (Brown et al. 1999, de Repentigny et al. 2000, Haynes 2001, Naglik et al. 2003):

- Adherence to epithelial and endothelial cells
- Secretion of proteases that degrade connective tissue proteins and facilitate invasion
- Production of cell-surface mannans that serve to attach the yeast to host tissues and suppress host response
- Resistance to oxidative killing by neutrophils.

The transition from yeast (**Figure 13.2**) to filamentous growth is a critical step in the subsequent expression of several virulence mechanisms for *C. albicans*. The yeast-to-hyphal transition of *C. albicans* can be triggered by a wide variety of factors, suggesting that hyphal growth is a response to nutrient deprivation, especially low nitrogen, and that filamentous growth enables the fungus to forage for nutrients more effectively (Hostetter 1998, Mitchell 1998, Brown et al. 1999, Naglik et al. 2003). Of considerable importance to the pathogenicity of candida infections is the ability of these organisms to produce and participate in biofilms (Albuquerque and Casadevall 2012, Nobile et al. 2012).

Although *C. glabrata* is an important human pathogen, its pathogenicity mechanisms are different, and center on altering events after phagocytosis by macrophages and neutrophils. Immune evasion strategies seem to play key roles during infection, because

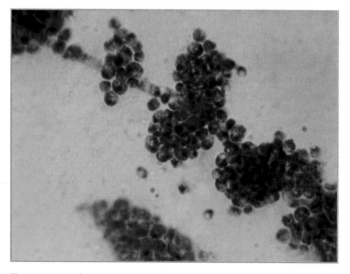

Figure 13.2 A photomicrograph of *Candida albicans*. (From the Public Health Image Library, Centers for Disease Control, courtesy of Dr Gordon Roberstad: http://phil.cdc.gov/phil/details.asp.)

reduced inflammatory responses are observed in animal models. Furthermore, *C. glabrata* multiplies intracellularly after engulfment by macrophages. Similar mechanisms explain *C. parapsilosis* virulence (Horvath et al. 2012).

Clinical aspects of candida infection

The GI tract is an important portal of entry for microorganisms, including yeasts, into the bloodstream. The passage of endogenous fungi across the mucosal barrier is referred to as fungal translocation (by analogy with bacterial translocation). There is considerable clinical evidence for transmigration of yeast in non-neutropenic humans, and appears to occur in profoundly immunocompromised patients who have received bone marrow transplantation (Blijlevens 2005, Niscola 2010). Although yeast cells have no intrinsic motility, they are able to translocate across the intestinal mucosa within a few hours of ingestion if present in high enough concentrations.

Candida spp. are commensals in the gut lumen and on mucocutaneous surfaces in the immunocompetent host with normal GI colonization. In critically ill patients, colonization with *Candida* spp. precedes and leads to infection. If multiple body sites are colonized, there will be an increased risk of severe infection in high-risk patients, and the chance of invasion can be predicted by the extent of pre-existing colonization.

Pittet et al. (2005) performed a 6-month prospective cohort study among patients admitted to surgical and neonatal ICUs. Routine microbiological surveillance cultures at different body sites were performed. A candida colonization index was determined daily as the ratio of the number of distinct body sites colonized with identical strains over the total number of body sites tested; a mean ratio of 5.3 was obtained. All isolates ($n = 322$) sequentially recovered were genotyped which allowed strain delineation among *Candida* spp. Twenty-nine patients met the criteria for inclusion; all were at high risk for candida infection; 11 patients (38%) developed severe infections (8 candidemia); the remaining 18 patients were heavily colonized, but never required intravenous antifungal therapy. Candida colonization always preceded infection with genotypically identical strains of *Candida* spp.. The proposed colonization indexes reached threshold values at 6 days before candida infection and demonstrated high positive predictive values (66–100%). The intensity of candida colonization helps to predict subsequent infections with identical strains in critically ill patients.

Prior antibiotic therapy is commonly viewed as an independent risk factor for candida infection, but this may not be uniformly correct. In a case–control study, antibiotic administration was shown to be only marginally associated with candidemia, and substantially less important than prior candida colonization (Borzotta and Beardsley 1999). There are multiple other factors that result in changes in the GI flora. These include intestinal ileus, antacid therapy, and contamination with hospital flora. The point of emphasis is that appropriate anti-infective therapy for a bacterial infection should not be stopped because *Candida* spp. are identified at one or more sites. In intra-abdominal infections, mixed flora infections with *Candida* spp. and bacteria are commonly observed.

Candida prophylaxis

A meta-analysis of studies employing ketoconazole or fluconazole prophylaxis has been performed (Cruciani et al. 2005). These authors found 9 studies (seven double blind) with a total of 1226 patients that compared ketoconazole or fluconazole to no prophylaxis. Prophylaxis with azole antifungals was associated with reduced rates of candidemia, mortality attributable to candida infection, and overall mortality. From the fluconazole studies, it was apparent that prior colonization was the major determinant of successful imidazole prophylaxis (Pelz et al. 2001).

Prophylaxis is a consideration in transplant recipients. The incidence and mechanism of microbial entry vary in different groups of transplant recipients, depending on the following:

- The organ transplanted
- The donor source
- The type of surgical procedure performed
- The recipient's age and general condition at the time of the procedure.

Other influential factors are the conditioning regimen, the type and duration of immunosuppressive therapy, and the presence or absence of organ rejection and graft-versus-host disease. In heart transplant recipients, for example, aspergillus infection is a major problem, whereas, in other organ transplant recipients, most fungal infections are attributable to *Candida* spp. (Warnock 1995, Pappas et al. 2006). The infection is usually located at the surgical site: an intra-abdominal abscess in liver or pancreas transplantation, the mediastinum or the lungs in heart or heart–lung transplantation, and the urinary tract in kidney transplantation.

Several studies have documented the efficacy of amphotericin B, liposomal amphotericin B, and fluconazole in preventing candida infections. The incidence of candida infection in patients not receiving prophylaxis varies between 10 and 20%, and prophylaxis is cost-effective, particularly if provided with imidazoles (Avery 2011, San-Juan et al. 2011).

There is an increasing appreciation of the role of *Candida* spp. in infections after acute pancreatitis (Warnock 1995, Pappas et al. 2006). A large series of patients undergoing surgery for infected pancreatic necrosis found *Candida* sp. present in approximately 10% of the patients at their initial surgery for infection (Gotzinger et al. 2000). These patients had received prophylaxis with amoxicillin/clavulanate, a factor that might explain intestinal overgrowth and translocation of *Candida* spp. This is a particular issue because of the interest in the use of broad-spectrum antibiotics, especially imipenem/cilastatin, as prophylaxis for patients with necrotizing pancreatitis. There is consistent and substantial data *against* this practice, and there are no data on fungal prophylaxis in patients not receiving antimicrobial prophylaxis (de Vries et al. 2007). We believe that the appropriate prophylaxis strategy is to provide low-dose oral fluconazole.

Management of specific infections
Candidemia

Many if not most candidemias seen in the ICU are catheter-related bloodstream infections (CRBSIs). This is defined as candidemia in one or separate venopunctures, occurring in a patient with an intravascular catheter and no other obvious site for infection after careful clinical and laboratory evaluation. Several procedures have been developed to aid in the diagnosis of catheter-associated candidemia. If the catheter is removed, a quantitative culture of the tip should recover at least 15 colony-forming units (CFU) of the same *Candida* spp. as found in blood culture by the roll-plate technique, or at least 100 CFU of the same *Candida* sp. as found in blood culture by the sonication technique. The issue, compared with Gram-positive bacterial CRBSIs, is the source of the fungi. In most cases, they are not identified at the insertion site, and likely result from hematogenous infection after GI overgrowth. There is compelling evidence that catheter removal is a central component of therapy.

Echinocandins are now considered the treatment of choice for candidemia, with fluconazole added if *C. albicans* is suspected. This recommendation is based on recent IDSA (Infectious Diseases Society of America) guidelines (Pappas et al. 2009). Aside from evidence that fluconazole is synergistic with echinocandins, a major concern for monotherapy with fluconazole for empirical therapy has to do with the possibility that a resistant strain may be present, and the observation that the echinocandins are fungicidal, which may be more efficacious in patients with shock or other severe physiological responses to infection. Patients who have previously received fluconazole for either prophylaxis or therapy should be treated with an echinocandin.

Choice of antifungal

All patients with candidemia should receive antifungal therapy. We recommend initial therapy with intravenous echinocandin or fluconazole for 3 days, particularly if the infecting organism is likely to be *C. albicans*. If the patient responds rapidly to this regimen, the dosage may be decreased and administered orally. For patients with hematogenous candidiasis that are known to be colonized with *C. krusei* or *C. lusitaniae*, amphotericin B (0.5–0.7 mg/kg per day) should be the treatment of choice.

Duration of therapy

Duration of therapy depends on the extent and seriousness of the infection. Therapy can be limited to 7–10 days for patients with catheter-related and low-grade fungemia, without evidence of organ involvement or hemodynamic instability. Those patients with high-grade fungemia, evidence of organ involvement, or hemodynamic instability need to receive antifungal therapy for 10–14 days after resolution of all signs and symptoms of infection.

Candidemia in non-neutropenic patients

Fluconazole (loading dose of 800 mg [12 mg/kg], then 400 mg [6 mg/kg] daily) plus an echinocandin (caspofungin: loading dose of 70 mg, then 50 mg daily; micafungin: 100 mg daily; anidulafungin: loading dose of 200 mg, then 100 mg daily) is recommended as initial therapy for most adult patients. Transition from an echinocandin to fluconazole is recommended for patients who have isolates with likely susceptibility to fluconazole (e.g., *C. albicans*) and who are clinically stable. For infection due to *C. glabrata*, an echinocandin is preferred. For infection due to *C. parapsilosis*, treatment with fluconazole is recommended. The recommended duration of therapy for candidemia without obvious metastatic complications is 2 weeks after documented clearance of *Candida* spp. from the bloodstream and resolution of symptoms attributable to candidemia. Intravenous catheter removal is strongly recommended for non-neutropenic patients with candidemia.

Suppurative thrombophlebitis

A rare but serious consequence of hematogenous candidemia is suppurative thrombophlebitis, which results from infection of a vessel traumatized by prolonged catheterization. Endothelial disruption exposes the basement membrane and leads to thrombus formation and propagation. Suppurative thrombophlebitis is particularly serious because intravascular infection results in a persistent high-density fungemia. Management of this disease consists of high-dose antifungal therapy, removal of the central venous catheter, and excision of the infected vein, when possible. Typically, blood cultures remain positive for several days; sometimes, they remain positive for as long as 3–4 weeks despite appropriate antifungal therapy, if the infected vein is not excised.

Peritonitis and Intra-abdominal abscess

Systemic therapy is required to eradicate *Candida* spp. found within intra-abdominal abscesses, peritoneal fluid, or fistula drainage. *Candida* spp. are not uncommonly cultured from intra-abdominal infectious foci but should be considered a serious threat only in specific patient groups. Four risk factors for intra-abdominal candida infection have been identified including failed treatment for intra-abdominal infection, anastomotic leakage after elective or urgent surgery, surgery for acute pancreatitis, and splenectomy.

Systemic antifungal therapy should be provided for these patients found to have *Candida* spp. at the site of recurrent intra-abdominal infection or previous surgery, and those with either fistulae or drain tracts. Antibacterial therapy should be provided if bacteria are identified by either Gram stain or culture. Most of these patients will have polymicrobial infection. Occasionally, *Candida* spp. may be associated with acalculous cholecystitis or cholangitis. This is increasingly found in patients with percutaneously placed drainage catheters for malignancy. Such patients must be given systemic therapy for clinical evidence of infection, including candidemia, and the drainage catheter must be changed.

Urinary tract infection

The recovery of *Candida* spp. from the urinary tract most commonly results from contamination from the perirectal or genital area. Colonization of the bladder is usually seen with prolonged catheterization, diabetes mellitus, or other diseases associated with incomplete bladder emptying. In addition, *Candida* spp. usually colonize ileal conduits. Persistent candidemia in the surgical ICU may, however, be an early marker of disseminated infection in critically ill high-risk patients. Replacing or removing the bladder catheter is preferable. If candida colonization persists, particularly if the patient has a risk factor for cystitis (e.g., diabetes mellitus or a disease that leads to incomplete bladder emptying) or hematogenous dissemination (e.g., immunosuppression or manipulation of the genitourinary system), antifungal therapy should be considered. Amphotericin B bladder irrigation provides only temporary clearance of fungemia and systemic treatment is usually needed.

■ COMMUNITY-ACQUIRED FUNGAL PATHOGENS

■ Blastomycosis
Pathogenesis

Infections with *Blastomyces dermatitidis*, also known as North American blastomycosis, are principally pulmonary (Smith and Kauffman 2010). The fungus is found in the soil primarily in the USA, but is seen in the other continents. The spores are airborne and lodgment is in the lung (**Figure 13.3**). Infection occurs 4–6 weeks or longer after exposure. Person-to-person transmission is not thought to occur. The vigorous inflammatory response results in lesions that are mistaken for primary lung cancer. The skin is the most common site for extrapulmonary involvement.

Diagnosis

Acute pulmonary infection presents with productive cough, fever, and pleuritic chest pain. Chronic infections have multiple weeks of cough and chest discomfort. Chest radiographs will show infiltrates in acute infection, and chronic infection shows fibronodular infiltrates that portray carcinoma. Cavitation and miliary appearances can be seen. Organisms can be seen from expectorated or bronchoscopic secretions by KOH preparation. Cultures require many weeks for growth. Biopsy of suspected skin lesions and lung biopsy will identify the organism. Urine antigen studies have been useful, but cannot replace fungal identification.

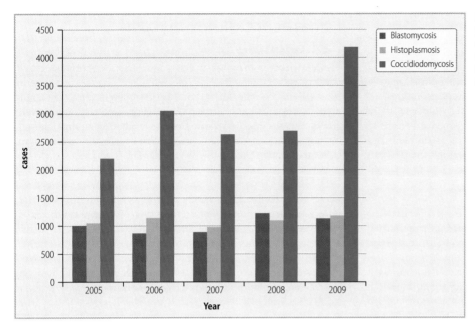

Figure 13.3 This annual frequency of inpatient pulmonary blastomycosis, histoplasmosis, and coccidioidomycosis from 2005 to 2009. (Agency for Healthcare Research and Quality, HCUPnet database, accessed March 8, 2012: http://hcupnet. ahrq.gov.)

Treatment

Mild acute blastomycosis requires no antifungal therapy. Oral itraconazole and ketoconazole are used for outpatient therapy of chronic pulmonary infection (Chapman et al. 2008). Severe and disseminated cases of acute and chronic cases are treated with intravenous amphotericin B. Large lung lesions may be resected in expectation of carcinoma. If the diagnosis is established before thoracotomy, chemotherapy alone is the treatment. In severe cases requiring hospitalization and intravenous treatment, mortality rates are approximately 25% in immunocompetent patients and 40% in HIV infection.

■ Coccidioidomycosis

This highly infectious dimorphic fungal infection is secondary to *Cocccidioides immitis and C. posadasii* which are endemic to the south-western USA (Anstead and Graybill 2006) (see Figure 13.3). It is caused by inhalation of soil-based fungal spores. There is a vigorous inflammatory response with pulmonary lodgment that is similar to acute bacterial infection. Subacute infection is characterized by granuloma formation and even caseation. Scaring and fibrosis replace granuloma in the chronic phase, and may result in chronic obstructive lung disease and cavitation. An inadequate host response (e.g., corticosteroid therapy, HIV) may result in dissemination. The systemic disease may give cutaneous lesions, musculoskeletal manifestations with osteolytic bone lesion, and meningitis.

Diagnosis

The acute pulmonary infection follows a broad continuum of disease with half the infections being minimally symptomatic. Most severe acute cases will have fever, malaise, and pleuritic chest pain. In less than 10% of cases, symptoms can be severe with myalgias, fatigue, headache, and weight loss. Respiratory failure can occur in extreme pulmonary infections. Severe or persistent symptoms beyond 4–6 weeks may herald miliary disease. Skin and bone lesions will occur with dissemination, and meningitis can also be a complication of systemic disease. Endophthalmitis may occur as evidence of dissemination. Chest radiographs show alveolar infiltrates initially which

progress to nodular lesions in the granulomatous phase. Complete resolution is the rule for acute pulmonary lesions with only a small number (<5%) developing calcified or cavitated lesions.

The diagnosis is made by culture of the fungus or by direct histopathological identification. Surgical biopsy of solitary lesions may be necessary for diagnosis. Skin lesions may have the appearance of basal cell carcinoma and diagnosis is established with excisional biopsy. Disseminated disease can be confirmed with cytological or tissue cultures of liver and bone marrow biopsies. Blood cultures may be positive in immunosuppressed patients. Detection of antibodies by immunodiffusion complement fixation or ELISA methods is used by reference laboratories.

Treatment

In immunocompetent patients, no specific therapy for acute pulmonary infection is necessary unless symptoms persist for 4–6 weeks (Limper et al. 2011). Fluconazole or itraconazole is used for persistent cases or for pulmonary infection in immunosuppressed patients or those with risk factors (chronic lung disease) for severe infection. Diffuse pulmonary disease or disseminated infections are initially treated with an amphotericin B lipid preparation and followed with a full year of oral therapy with fluconazole or itraconazole. Surgical resection of pulmonary cavities may be necessary for hemoptysis or secondary infection of the cavity itself. Occasionally, empyema may develop and require drainage. Bronchopleural fistulae from ruptured pleural blebs may require surgical repair.

■ Cryptococcal infections
Pathogenesis

Cryptococcus neoformans and *C. gattii* are the pathogens most identified with human disease (Li and Mody 2010). This encapsulated fungus is inhaled and may cause a mild pulmonary infection, but is disseminated from the lung. Meningitis is the clinical infection of interest. *C. neoformans* infection is associated with lymphomas, leukemias, transplantation, HIV infection, and patients on high-dose corticosteroid therapy. *C. gattii* infections occur in immunocompetent patients.

Diagnosis

Headache, fever, and meningeal signs are customary and similar to aseptic meningitis. Symptoms are commonly chronic and persistent. Skin lesions may rarely be seen. India ink preparation of cerebrospinal fluid is usually the best diagnostic method. Special stains are required for identification in tissue biopsies. Cultures of infected body fluids will usually be positive, but centrifugation of cerebrospinal fluid may be necessary to optimize recovery from the sediment. Negative cultures are common, and repeated cultures are often necessary. Biopsies of bone or skin lesions will yield an unexpected *C. neoformans.*

Treatment

Mild pulmonary infections in selected patients are treated with fluconazole or itraconazole (Limper et al. 2011). Cryptococcal meningitis and disseminated infections are treated with combination therapy of amphotericin B and flucytosine, followed by maintenance oral fluconazole. Asymptomatic disease is identified on sputum cultures or an excised pulmonary nodule and do not require antimicrobial therapy.

◼ Histoplasmosis
Pathogenesis

Histoplasmosis is caused by *H. capsulatum* (Kauffman 2009). It is an airborne pathogen and causes acute pulmonary infections (see Figure 13.3). The reservoir for the pathogens appears to be wild birds. The pulmonary infection is usually mild or completely asymptomatic. It has the potential to cause disseminated disease in susceptible hosts. The spores are ingested by and proliferate within macrophage cells. *H. capsulatum* forms granulomas in tissue and yields calcified lesions in the lung and mediastinal lymph nodes. Most acute cases completely resolve. Upper lobe cavitations occur and resemble tuberculosis. These cavities may become secondarily infected and are associated with lung carcinoma. Histoplasma endophthalmitis is a recognized complication of disseminated disease. The disseminated and chronic forms of the disease are associated with chronic steroid therapy, HIV, and immunosuppressed hosts.

Diagnosis

Acute pulmonary symptoms are fever, chills, and cough. Infiltrates are seen on chest radiographs. Acute fulminant disease in children may lead to severe infection with respiratory distress. Chronic disseminated infection may have intermittent fever, weight loss, and hepatosplenomegaly.

Excised tissue will demonstrate the microorganisms on hematoxylin and eosin sections. The organisms can usually be cultured from sputum specimens and bone marrow aspirates. Similar to many fungi, 4 weeks may be required for cultures. Blood cultures are positive in over 50% of disseminated infections. Antibody and antigen detection methods are used to supplement cultures and histopathological detection of the fungus.

Treatment

Acute pulmonary histoplasmosis is a self-limited disease (Wheat et al. 2007). Mild-to-moderate cases of pulmonary infection and chronic cavitating disease are treated with itraconazole. Only severe cases require treatment with amphotericin B, which is followed with itraconazole for 12 months. Surgical management is not generally part of the management of histoplasmosis. Solitary lung lesions and cavitating lesions may require surgical resection to rule out the presence of lung cancer.

◼ Paracoccidioidomycosis
Pathogenesis

Also known as South American blastomycosis, *Paracoccidioides brasiliensis* causes acute pulmonary infection after inhalation of airborne spores (Ramos-e-Silva and Saraiva 2008). Pulmonary paracoccidioidomycosis is usually asymptomatic but can cause an acute suppurative or granulomatous infection. Cavitation can occur. Dissemination results in mucocutaneous lesions and head–neck adenopathy. It is endemic to South America and most cases are in men.

Diagnosis

Acute infection has non-specific symptoms of fever and cough. Fibronodular lesions and cavitation can be seen on chest radiograph. Oropharyngeal, cutaneous lesions and cervical adenopathy herald disseminated disease. The organism can be seen in sputum and typically requires long incubation times for cultures. Histological identification can be made from oropharyngeal or cutaneous biopsies. Complement fixation, immunodiffusion, and other antibody detection studies are available.

Treatment

The majority of diagnosed cases have disseminated disease (Limper et al. 2011). Systemic amphotericin B is required for severe cases, followed by 6–12 months of oral therapy with ketoconazole, itraconazole, or sulfadiazine. Surgical treatment plays a role in the biopsy only of lesions or nodes for diagnosis.

◼ Sporotrichosis
Pathogenesis

The pathogen of sporotrichosis, *Sporothrix schenckii,* is found in soil and on plants. It causes infection after contamination of cutaneous wounds and abrasions. Nodular granulomas form at the site of injury, and the infection spreads as lymphangitis. Satellite granulomas may develop along the path of lymphangitis. Deeper wounds can cause tendon and bone joint infections. Dissemination is uncommon, but is associated with central nervous system (CNS), pulmonary, cutaneous, or bone infections.

Diagnosis

Persistent papular lesions with discharge and ulceration on the upper extremity are the common scenario. Culture of the serosanguineous discharge may identify the fungus. Punch or excisional biopsy of cutaneous lesions with culture and identification of granulomas on histology is usually diagnostic.

Treatment

Itraconazole is the treatment for cutaneous sporotrichosis (Limper et al. 2011). A saturated solution of potassium iodide (SSKI) has been commonly employed for the cutaneous infection, but there is no good clinical evidence to support this treatment (Xue et al. 2009). Difficult cutaneous infection and extracutaneous sporotrichosis are treated with intravenous amphotericin B, followed by several months of itraconazole.

◼ NON-CANDIDA HEALTHCARE-ASSOCIATED INFECTIONS

◼ Aspergillus fumigatus

Among the *Aspergillus* spp., *Aspergillus fumigatus* is of greatest concern as a human pathogen. It is a ubiquitous fungus that is an opportunistic pathogen in hospitalized patients with immunosuppression, neutropenia, and severe debilitation.

It is an airborne pathogen that is typically associated with cavitating infections of the lung, and other associated infections of the upper airway, including the sinuses and the external/middle ear. The lung is the most common site for this unusual infection (**Figure 13.4**) and forms a matted collection of vegetations commonly referred to as an "aspergilloma." This fungus has a very low virulence profile, generally does not demonstrate invasion of adjacent tissues, and does not elicit a significant inflammatory response from the host. These infections will result on occasion with endocarditis, solid organ lesions (liver, spleen, brain), and rarely a metastatic endophthalmitis similar to *Candida albicans* can be seen.

The diagnosis of aspergillus infection is suspected in immunosuppressed patients with hemoptysis and a cavitated lesion of the lung. Hemoptysis can be massive and life threatening. A necrotizing pneumonitis is seen in patients with chronic obstructive pulmonary disease. Sinus infections can be very subtle and may have few symptoms. Proptosis from adjacent extension of infection into the orbital area from the sinuses can be seen. This can appear similar to mucormycosis. Infections of the external or middle ear require a high index of suspicion.

The diagnosis is made by culture identification of *Aspergillus* spp. from a site with an accompanying clinical picture of infection. *Aspergillus* spp. are not difficult to culture and positive lung cultures may reflect colonization rather than true infection. Sinus aspirates and cultures from ear specimens are reliable. In selected cases, tissue biopsy may be required to definitively establish the diagnosis. In pulmonary infections, this may mean transtracheal or lung biopsy. The infection is rarely established from blood cultures.

Voriconazole is currently the recommended first-line treatment for aspergillus infection (Walsh et al. 2008). Lung resection may be necessary in cases of severe hemophysis. Drainage and debridement may be necessary in sinus infections.

■ Mucormycosis

Formerly called the phycomycoses and then the zygomycetes, this collective group of hundreds of different fungi are is collectively called the mucormycoses. This group of opportunistic pathogens includes *Mucor, Rhizopus, Cunninghamella, Apaphyhsomyhces,* and *Absidia* spp., and many others.

Pathogenesis

Infections of the nasal sinuses and rarely the lung occur by inhalation of these ubiquitously-found fungi in immunocompromised or diabetic individuals (Sun and Singh 2011). Rarely, burn wounds or open traumatic wounds may become secondarily infected after long periods of hospitalization and sustained illness.

The nasal infections can result in severe nasofacial necrosis and extension into the orbit, eye, and even the brain (**Figure 13.5**). Necrotizing pulmonary infections result from invasion of the pulmonary vasculature, with lung infarction and even massive hemoptysis being the consequence. Patients with diabetes are most susceptible because of the affinity of these microorganisms for a high concentration of glucose.

Dissemination can occur from the lung or nasosinus routes, and may yield cutaneous or visceral lesions. Even GI and CNS infections can be seen. The invasion of these fungi into arterioles yields the necrotizing feature, which combined with the immunosuppressed or susceptible host leads to a usually fatal outcome for disseminated disease.

Diagnosis

The diagnosis is usually made by identification of the species on tissue biopsy. Black discharge suggests the diagnosis and organisms may be seen on KOH preparations. Tissue biopsies with histological demonstration of invasion of the organism are the most reliable. Cultures must be interpreted carefully and are notoriously negative. When only a few colonies are identified on culture, this may reflect airborne contamination and not infection.

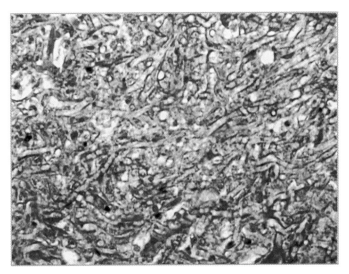

Figure 13.4 A hematoxylin and eosin stain of avian lung tissue infected with *Aspergillus* spp. (From the Public Health Image Library, Centers for Disease Control, courtesy of CDC/Dr William Kaplan: http://phil.cdc.gov/phil/details.asp.)

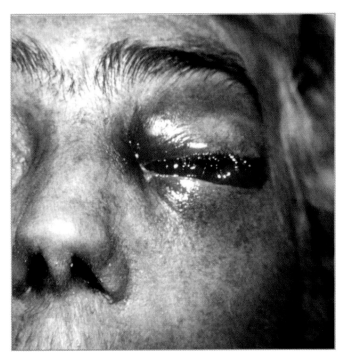

Figure 13.5 A case of periorbital mucormycosis. (From the Public Health Image Library, Centers for Disease Control, courtesy of Dr Thomas Sellers, Emory University: http://phil.cdc.gov/phil/details.asp.)

Treatment

The treatment of mucormycosis is surgical debridement of dead tissue, medical control of underlying medical conditions, and antifungal chemotherapy. There has been considerable study into the development of effective antifungal treatments for this difficult infection (Spellberg et al. 2009). Lipid formulations of amphotericin B are the standard systemic treatment. These fungi are usually resistant to the azoles and echinocandins. Results are poor with most patients dying from severe local or disseminated infection. Effective surgical debridement of necrotic tissue is essential for patient survival.

■ Pneumocystis pneumonia

Pneumocystis jiroveci, formerly known as *P. carinii*, is primarily a pulmonary pathogen of immunosuppressed hosts that became a source of considerable interest from infections in AIDS patients in the early 1980s. Considered formerly to be a paracytic pathogen, it is now classified as a fungal organism (**Figure 13.6**). It does not have the typical ergosterol within the plasma membrane as other fungi do, and thus has resistance to those antifungal therapies directed at ergosterol synthesis.

It is acquired by airborne transmission and may reside as a colonist within the lung for prolonged periods of time (Carmona and Limper 2011). The clinical pneumonitis emerges with immunosuppression of the host. Many of the pathophysiological features of this pathogen are poorly understood because in vitro culture has been elusive and inhibited effective study. Although initially considered only a pulmonary pathogen, *P. jiroveci* has been identified in lymph nodes, liver, spleen, bone marrow, and other tissues. Similar to other fungi, it can be found in the retina.

The diagnosis is suspected in vulnerable patients with a nonproductive cough, fever, shortness of breath, and diffuse bilateral infiltrates in the perihilar region on chest radiograph. Histopathological identification is required for diagnosis. Cultures cannot be done in the clinical microbiology laboratory. Induced sputum may identify the pathogen, but bronchoalveolar lavage has yielded the diagnosis in up to 90% of cases. Transbronchial biopsy or even open lung biopsy has been required in selected cases. Antigen or antibody detection methods have not been successful.

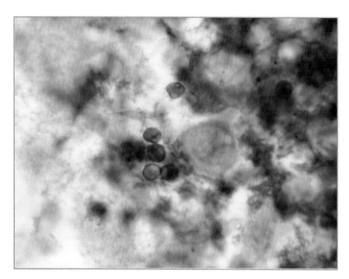

Figure 13.6 A photomicrograph of *Pneumocystis* jiroveci in lung with toluidine blue stain. (From the Public Health Image Library, Centers for Disease Control, courtesy of Dr Peter Drotman: http://phil.cdc.gov/phil/details.asp.)

Treatment of pneumocystis pneumonia is managing the underlying predisposing illness (e.g., HIV antiretroviral treatment) and specific therapy to target *P. jiroveci*. Trimethoprim–sulfamethoxazole given orally or intravenously for 14 days in non-HIV patients, and 21 days for HIV patients, is the current therapy. Primaquine, an anti-malarial agent, is used with clindamycin as a second choice. Pentamidine has been used but can be given only intravenously for established infection. Pentamidine aerosol is used for prevention of recurrent infection. Complications of pneumocystis pneumonia include recurrent infections and pneumothorax. Mortality rates for this infection depend on the constellation of risk factors in the patient. Improvement has been seen in HIV patients with this infection, but remains at 30–50% for non-HIV-associated infections (Sepkowitz 2002).

■ ANTIFUNGAL AGENTS

The number of antifungal agents continues to expand. The dosage schedule for the current systemic agents is identified in **Table 13.1**. The dosing identified is primarily of adult patients. The frequency and amount of drug administered may exceed that noted in the table based on the degree of illness identified by the clinician.

■ Amphotericin B deoxycholate

Amphotericin B is an antifungal produced by *Streptomyces nodosus*. Despite the many problems that are associated with administration and toxicity of the drug, it continues to be a commonly employed systemic antifungal agent.

Amphotericin B binds to the ergosterol component within the membrane. Cholesterol in human membranes is also bound, but the affinity of the drug is much greater for fungal ergosterol. Binding of amphotericin B to the fungal plasma membrane results in cylindrical channels which permit loss of cytoplasmic enzymes (Vertut-Croquin et al. 1983). Amphotericin B is also thought to cause oxidative damage to the fungal cell, and may actually stimulate B-lymphocyte function in the host. Changes in the binding characteristics of ergosterol may be a mechanism of resistance.

Amphotericin B is administered only by the intravenous route, and has no appreciable absorption from the GI tract when given orally. The antibiotic is highly protein bound (>90%). It penetrates the CNS poorly. It has an initial biological elimination half-life of 24 h, but, after therapy is completed, has a terminal half-life of 15 days. Drug is identified in the urine for over 6 weeks after cessation of treatment. The prolongation of drug elimination after treatment is related to cell membrane binding of the drug to host cells.

Administration of amphotericin B poses some special problems (Carlson and Condon 1994). The compound is unstable if exposed to heat, prolonged sunlight, or an acid pH <4.2, and will precipitate in electrolyte solutions. Acute reactions to amphotericin B are common and require the administration of a 1-mg test dose. Fever and chills, dyspnea, and even hypotension can be encountered, with the acute reaction identified with a peak response by 4 h after administration due to the release of proinflammatory cytokines (Laniado-Laborin and Cabrales-Vargas 2009).

Amphotericin B has toxicity that is linked to total dose and duration of therapy. Renal toxicity secondary to renal vasoconstriction results in renal tubular damage. Saline loading by the administration of 500 ml of 0.9% saline before and 500 ml after amphotericin B administration may reduce nephrotoxicity. Additional renal toxicity includes anemia, renal tubular acidosis, and renal losses of potassium. Potassium supplementation is commonly required.

Table 13.1 Antifungal drugs and dosing schedules used in adult patients (unless otherwise indicated) without renal failure.

Drug	Dosage	Comments
Amphotericin B deoxycholate	0.5–1.0 mg/kg per day	This preparation has been used for 50 years in the treatment of severe fungal infections
Liposomal amphotericin	3–6 mg/kg per day	Amphotericin in incorporated into a true liposome for drug delivery
Amphotericin lipid complex	5 mg/kg per day	The active amphotericin B is complexed with two separate phospholipids in this preparation
Amphotericin colloidal suspension	3–4 mg/kg per day	Amphotericin is complexed with cholesteryl sulfate. Colloidal complex is broken down by macrophages to release active drug
5-Fluorocytosine	100–150 mg/kg per day in four divided doses	Oral antifungal that is ordinarily used in combination with amphotericin B
Fluconazole	200 mg on day 1, followed by 100 mg daily for *Candida* sp.; 400 mg on day 1, and 200 mg daily for cryptococcal infection	Commonly used antifungal that is both an intravenous and an oral preparation
Itraconazole	200–400 mg daily	The azole antifungal with a role in the treatment of aspergillus, blastomycosis, and histoplasmosis infection
Voriconazole	6 mg/kg every 12 h for 24 h; then 4 mg/kg every 12 h	Used for aspergillus and candidal infections
Posaconazole	100–400 mg 2–3 times per day	Higher doses are used for invasive oropharyngeal infections that are refractory to other azole antifungal agents.
Ketoconazole	100–200 mg daily in adults; 3.3–6.6 mg/kg daily in children	Only available as an oral preparation and used for oral pharyngeal candida infections with sensitive organisms
Caspofungin	50 mg daily after a loading dose of 70 mg on day 1	Used for invasive candida infections
Anidulafungin	100–200 mg loading dose for day 1, followed by 50–100 mg daily	Used for invasive candida infections
Micafungin	50–150 mg daily	Used for invasive candida infections

Amphotericin B forms stable complexes with lipids, which permit the development of new formulations that reduce the toxic profile of this treatment. Three lipid formulations of amphotericin B are approved for use: Amphotericin B lipid complex (Abelcet), amphotericin B colloidal dispersion (Amphotec), and liposomal amphotericin B (AmBisome). Functionally, these lipid formulations are sustained-release methods to maintain drug concentration without excessive and toxic peak concentrations. Clinical experience has demonstrated reductions in both nephrotoxicity and other adverse effects. The daily dosing of these lipid preparations is much greater than the deoxycholate preparation (see Table 13.1).

5-Fluorocytosine

As the first orally administered antifungal agent, 5-fluorocytosine has been primarily used in the treatment for *Candida* spp. (not *C. krusei*) and *Cryptococcus neoformans*. It is ordinarily used in combination with amphotericin B.

The mechanism of action for 5-fluorocytosine requires that the drug be deaminated to 5-fluorouracil within the target fungal microorganism. The 5-fluorouracil is incorporated into the RNA of the fungus and inhibits protein synthesis. The 5-fluorouracil may be phosphorylated through a series of reactions which results in the inhibition of thymidine synthetase, and the resultant inhibition of DNA synthesis. Mechanisms of resistance include loss of permeability or failure of mutants to deaminate the parent compound to 5-fluorouracil.

Leukopenia and thrombocytopenia are complications directly attributable to 5-fluorocytosine and may be amplified by the simultaneous use of amphotericin B. The drug does not cause renal failure. Nausea, vomiting, and diarrhea may be seen as consequences of deamination of the parent drug to 5-fluorouracil. Hepatic toxicity has also been identified. Hypersensitivity can also be seen.

Azole antifungal drugs

The azole compounds inhibit cytochrome P450 with resultant reduction in ergosterol and defective membrane synthesis by the targeted fungal pathogen. They may have a direct action on the cytoplasmic membrane as well. The inhibition of cytochrome 450 results in a large number of drug interactions in using these drugs (**Box 13.1**)

Box 13.1 Drugs of surgical interest that have significant interactions with the azole antifungals.

This listing in not complete, but identifies drugs of surgical significance.
Decreased azole serum concentration
H$_2$ receptor antagonists
Proton pump inhibitors
Sulcrafate
Increased azole metabolism
Rifampin
Phenyltoin
Phenobarbital
Increased concentration: coadministered drug
Oral hypoglycemics
Warfarin
Ciclosporin
Tacrolimus
Phenyltoin
Benzodiazepines
Statin drugs
Rifampin
Selected cancer chemotherapy drugs
Digoxin

(Brüggeman et al. 2009, Gubbins and Heldenbrand 2010). The mechanisms for the emergence of resistance include pathogen development of efflux pumps to reduce intracellular drug concentrations, point mutations of the gene encoding the target enzyme of drug action, and the development of bypass pathways that eliminate drug effects (Pfaller 2012). The need to maintain drug concentrations above the minimum inhibitory concentration (MIC) range and the unpredictable pharmacology of the azoles have led to some recommending therapeutic monitoring to achieve optimum outcomes (Kontoyiannis 2012).

Fluconazole has a broad range of antifungal activity. This compound can be given orally or by intravenous administration. It has over a full decade of use in the treatment of candida infections, and is approved for use in cryptococcal infections. It has also been used for coccidioidomycosis. Fluconazole is employed for the prevention of candida infections in bone marrow transplantation, and for patients undergoing chemoradiation. Resistant organisms are identified with sustained use. Drug-associated adverse events are very low. Elevation of hepatic enzymes and alopecia are seen and are reversible with cessation of the drug. Hypersensitivity and anaphylaxis are uncommon.

Itraconazole is an oral preparation that is used in the long-term management of patients with aspergillosis, blastomycosis, and histoplasmosis. It is not available as a parenteral preparation. GI complaints are the most common adverse events. Similar to other azoles, hypersensitivity can be seen but is uncommon.

Voriconazole is an intravenous and oral antifungal preparation. It is used in invasive aspergillosis, candida infections in non-neutropenic patients, and candidal esophagitis. Selection of this drug is always confirmed by specific sensitivity validation. Adverse outcomes leading to discontinuation of treatment have been elevated hepatic enzymes, rash, and visual disturbances.

Posaconazole is an oral suspension that is used for the treatment of oropharyngeal candida infection, and for prophylaxis in immunocompromised patients who are considered at risk for invasive candida or aspergillus infection. Hypersensitivity, arrhythmias and prolonged Q–T interval, and hepatic toxicity are the major adverse events.

Ketoconazole is an oral preparation that has poorer tissue penetration and a less desirable adverse event profile than the other azole antifungals. It is used for oral candida infections, and can be used for less severe infections of blastomycosis and coccidioidomycosis. It is used as a topical cream for cutaneous fungal infections.

■ Echinocandins

The echinocandins are large lipopeptide molecules that are inhibitors of β-1,3-glucan synthesis, an action that results in disruption of the fungal cell wall and osmotic stress, lysis, and death of the microorganism (Denning 2003). Available echinocandins include caspofungin, anidulafungin and micafungin. They are intravenous drugs. The echinocandins are fungicidal against most Candida spp. and fungistatic against Aspergillus spp. No drug target is present in mammalian cells.

Results of studies of echinocandins in candidemia and invasive candidiasis suggest equivalent efficacy to amphotericin B, with substantially fewer toxic effects. The IDSA guidelines for the treatment of candidiasis specifically suggest the use of echinocandins preferentially among patients with moderate-to-severe disease (Pappas et al. 2009). Absence of antagonism in combination with other antifungal drugs suggests that combination antifungal therapy could become a general feature of the echinocandins, particularly for invasive aspergillosis. Echinocandins exert concentration-dependent killing in many different in vitro and animal models of disseminated fungal infection. Fewer than 50 cases of echinocandin-resistant infections with species such as *C. albicans*, *C. glabrata*, *C. tropicalis*, and *C. krusei* have been described in limited series or case reports (Lortholary et al. 2011). All species were found in patients pre-exposed to echinocandins.

The echinocandins have few adverse events. They are associated with histamine release on administration. They do not have the hepatotoxicity or drug interaction problems that are seen with the azole antifungals.

■ REFERENCES

Albuquerque P, Casadevall A. Quorum sensing in fungi – a review. **50**:337–45.

Anstead GM, Graybill JR. Coccidioidomycosis. *Infect Dis Clin N Am* 2006;**20**:621–43.

Avery RK. Antifungal prophylaxis in lung transplantation. *Semin Respir Crit Care Med* 2011;**32**:717–26.

Blijlevens NM. Implications of treatment-induced mucosal barrier injury. *Curr Opin Oncol* 2005;**17**:605–10.

Borzotta AP, Beardsley K. Candida infections in critically ill trauma patients: a retrospective case-control study. *Arch Surg* 1999;**134**:657–64; discussion 64–5.

Brown DH Jr, Giusani AD, Chen X, Kumamoto CA. Filamentous growth of *Candida albicans* in response to physical environmental cues and its regulation by the unique CZF1 gene. *Mol Microbiol* 1999;**34**:651–62.

Brüggemann RJ, Alffenaar JW, Blijlevens NM, et al. Clinical relevance of the pharmacokinetic interactions of azole antifungal drugs with other coadministered agents. *Clin Infect Dis* 2009;48:1441–58.

Carlson MA, Condon RE. Nephrotoxicity of amphotericin B. *J Am Coll Surg* 1994;**179**:361–81.

Carmona EM, Limper AH. Update on the diagnosis and treatment of pneumocystitis pneumonia. *Ther Adv Respir Dis* 2011;**5**:41–59.

Chapman SW, Dismukes WE, Proia LA, et al. Clinical practice guidelines for the management of blastomycosis: 2008 update by the Infectious Diseases Society of America. *Clin Infect Dis* 2008;**46**:1801–12.

Cruciani M, de Lalla F, Mengoli C. Prophylaxis of Candida infections in adult trauma and surgical intensive care patients: a systematic review and meta-analysis. *Intensive Care Med* 2005;**31**:1479–87.

Denning DW. Echinocandin antifungal drugs. *Lancet* 2003;**362**:1142–51.

de Repentigny L, Aumont F, Bernard K, Belhumeur P. Characterization of binding of *Candida albicans* to small intestinal mucin and its role in adherence to mucosal epithelial cells. *Infect Immun* 2000;**68**:3172–9.

de Vries AC, Besselink MG, Buskens E, et al. Randomized controlled trials of antibiotic prophylaxis in severe acute pancreatitis: relationship between methodological quality and outcome. *Pancreatology* 2007;**7**:531–8.

Falagas ME, Apostolou KE, Pappas VD. Attributable mortality of candidemia: a systematic review of matched cohort and case-control studies. *Eur J Clin Microbiol Infect Dis* 2006;**25**:419–33.

Gotzinger P, Wamser P, Barlan M, Sautner T, Jakesz R, Fugger R. Candida infection of local necrosis in severe acute pancreatitis is associated with increased mortality. *Shock* 2000;**14**:320–3.

Gubbins PO, Heldenbrand S. Clinically relevant drug interactions of current antifungal agents. *Mycoses* 2010;**53**:95–113.

Haynes K. Virulence in *Candida* species. *Trends Microbiol* 2001;**9**:591–6.

Hidron AI, Edwards JR, Patel J, et al. NHSN annual update: antimicrobial-resistant pathogens associated with healthcare-associated infections: annual summary of data reported to the National Healthcare Safety Network at the Centers for Disease Control and Prevention, 2006–2007. *Infect Control Hosp Epidemiol* 2008;**29**:996–1011.

Horvath P, Nosanchuk JD, Hamari Z, Vagvolgyi C, Gacser A. The identification of gene duplication and the role of secreted aspartyl proteinase 1 in *Candida parapsilosis* virulence. *J Infect Dis* 2012.;**205**:923–33.

"]

Hostetter MK. Linkage of adhesion, morphogenesis, and virulence in *Candida albicans*. *J Lab Clin Med* 1998;**132**:258–63.

Kauffman CA: Histoplasmosis. *Clin Chest Med* 2009;**30**:217–25.

Kett DH, Azoulay E, Echeverria PM, Vincent JL. Candida bloodstream infections in intensive care units: analysis of the extended prevalence of infection in intensive care unit study. *Crit Care Med* 2011;**39**:665–70.

Kontoyiannis DP. Invasive mycoses: strategies for effective management. *Am J Med* 2012;**125**:S25–38.

Laniado-Laborin R, Cabrales-Vargas MN. Amphotericin B: side effects and toxicity. *Rev Iberoam Micol* 2009;**26**:223–7.

Leroy O, Gangneux JP, Montravers P, et al. Epidemiology, management, and risk factors for death of invasive Candida infections in critical care: a multicenter, prospective, observational study in France (2005–2006). *Crit Care Med* 2009;**37**:1612–8.

Li SS, Mody CH. Cryptococcus. *Proc Am Thorac Soc* 2010;**7**:186–96.

Limper AH, Knox KS, Sarosi GA, et al. An official American Thoracic Society Statement: Treatment of fungal infections in adult pulmonary and critical care patients. *Am J Respir Crit Care Med* 2011;**183**: 96–128.

Lortholary O, Desnos-Ollivier M, Sitbon K, Fontanet A, Bretagne S, Dromer F. Recent exposure to caspofungin or fluconazole influences the epidemiology of candidemia: a prospective multicenter study involving 2,441 patients. *Antimicrob Agents Chemother* 2011;**55**:532–8.

Mitchell AP. Dimorphism and virulence in *Candida albicans*. *Curr Opin Microbiol* 1998;**1**:687–92.

Morgan J, Meltzer MI, Plikaytis BD, et al. Excess mortality, hospital stay, and cost due to candidemia: a case-control study using data from population-based candidemia surveillance. *Infect Control Hosp Epidemiol* 2005;**26**:540–7.

Naglik JR, Challacombe SJ, Hube B. *Candida albicans* secreted aspartyl proteinases in virulence and pathogenesis. *Microbiol Mol Biol Rev* 2003;**67**:400–28, table.

Niscola P. Mucositis in malignant hematology. *Expert Rev Hematol* 2010;**3**:57–65.

Nobile CJ, Fox EP, Nett JE, et al. A Recently evolved transcriptional network controls biofilm development in *Candida albicans*. *Cell* 2012;**148**:126–38.

Pappas PG, Andes D, Schuster M, et al. Invasive fungal infections in low-risk liver transplant recipients: a multi-center prospective observational study. *Am J Transplant* 2006;**6**:386–91.

Pappas PG, Kauffman CA, Andes D, et al. Clinical practice guidelines for the management of candidiasis: 2009 update by the Infectious Diseases Society of America. *Clin Infect Dis* 2009;**48**:503–35.

Pelz RK, Hendrix CW, Swoboda SM, et al. Double-blind placebo-controlled trial of fluconazole to prevent candidal infections in critically ill surgical patients. *Ann Surg* 2001;**233**:542–8.

Pfaller MA. Antifungal drug resistance: mechanisms, epidemiology, and consequences for treatment. *Am J Med* 2012;**125**:S3–13.

Pfaller MA, Diekema DJ. Epidemiology of invasive candidiasis: a persistent public health problem. *Clin Microbiol Rev* 2007;**20**:133–63.

Prowle JR, Echeverri JE, Ligabo EV, et al. Acquired bloodstream infection in the intensive care unit: incidence and attributable mortality. *Crit Care* 2011;**15**:R100.

Pittet D, Monod M, Suter PM, Frenk E, Auckenthaler R. Candida colonization and subsequent infections in critically ill surgical patients. *Ann Surg* 1994;**220**:751–8.

Pittet D, Allegranzi B, Sax H, et al. Consideration for a WHO European strategy on health-care-associated infection, surveillance, and control. *Lancet Infect Dis* 2005;**5**:242–50.

Ramos-e-Silva M and Saraiva LDE. Paracoccioidomycosis. *Dermatol Clin* 2008;**26**:257–69.

San-Juan R, Aguado JM, Lumbreras C, et al. Universal prophylaxis with fluconazole for the prevention of early invasive fungal infection in low-risk liver transplant recipients. *Transplantation* 2011;**92**:346–50.

Sepkowitz KA. Opportunistic infections in patients with and patients without acquired Immunodeficiency Syndrome. *Clin Infect Dis* 2002;**34**:1098–107.

Smith JA, Kauffman CA: Blastomycosis. *Proc Am Thorac Soc* 2010;**7**:173–80.

Spellberg B, Walsh TJ, Kontoyiannis DP, Edwards J Jr, Ibrahim AS. Recent advances in the management of mucormycosis: from bench to bedside. *Clin Infect Dis* 2009;**48**:1743–51.

Sun H-Y, Singh N. Mucormycosis: Its changing face and management strategies. *Lancet Infect Dis* 2011;**11**:301–11.

Vertut-Croquin A, Bolard J, Chabbert M, Gary-Bobo C. Differences in the interaction of the polyene antibiotic amphotericin B with cholesterol- or ergosterol-containing phospholipid vesicles. A circular dichroism and permeability study. *Biochemistry* 1983;**22**:2939–44.

Vincent JL, Bihari DJ, Suter PM, et al. The prevalence of nosocomial infection in intensive care units in Europe. Results of the European Prevalence of Infection in Intensive Care (EPIC) Study. EPIC International Advisory Committee. *JAMA* 1995;**274**:639–44.

Vincent JL, Anaissie E, Bruining H, et al. Epidemiology, diagnosis and treatment of systemic Candida infection in surgical patients under intensive care. *Intensive Care Med* 1998;**24**:206–16.

Vincent JL, Rello J, Marshall J, et al. International study of the prevalence and outcomes of infection in intensive care units. *JAMA* 2009;**302**:2323–9.

Walsh TJ, Anaissie EJ, Denning DW, et al. Treatment of aspergillosis: guidelines of the Infectious Diseases Society of America. *Clin Infect Dis* 2008;**46**:327–60.

Warnock DW. Fungal complications of transplantation: diagnosis, treatment and prevention. *J Antimicrob Chemother* 1995;**36**(suppl B):73–90.

Wheat LJ, Freifeld AG, Kleiman MB, et al. Clinical practice guidelines for the management of patients with histoplasmosis: 2007 update by the Infectious Diseases Society of America. *Clin Infect Dis* 2007;**45**:807–25.

Xue S, Gu R, Wu T, Zhang M, Wang X. Oral potassium iodide for the treatment of sporotrichosis. *Cochrane Database Syst Rev* 2009;**7**:CD006136.

Zaoutis TE, Argon J, Chu J, Berlin JA, Walsh TJ, Feudtner C. The epidemiology and attributable outcomes of candidemia in adults and children hospitalized in the United States: a propensity analysis. *Clin Infect Dis* 2005;**41**:1232–9.

Zilberberg MD, Shorr AF, Kollef MH. Secular trends in candidemia-related hospitalization in the United States, 2000–2005. *Infect Control Hosp Epidemiol* 2008;**29**:978–80.

Chapter 14 Viral infections of surgical significance

Donald E. Fry

The number of viruses that participate in human disease is steadily increasing. The problem of viral infection has proven to be more elusive than bacterial disease because these microbes have not been readily identifiable with conventional microscopy or by culturing techniques. Different viral infections share many common clinical characteristics that make differentiation of disease expression very difficult. Antiviral chemotherapy and other treatments of viral diseases have generally lagged behind those of bacterial infections.

Surgeons need an expanded understanding of those viral illnesses that impact surgical care. Viruses are causes of neoplasia, opportunistic infections in immunosuppressed surgical patients, and important potential sources of occupational infections for the surgeon.

HUMAN IMMUNODEFICIENCY VIRUS

It has been 30 years since the first HIV/AIDS cases were identified in young males with pneumocystis pneumonia. During the following years, HIV infection has been a major international issue with considerable efforts to understand, prevent, and treat this disease. Despite this effort, there are 33.3 million people living with HIV infection in the world, 2.6 million new cases were identified in 2009, and 1.8 million people died from HIV during that same year (World Health Organization 2009). During the last 4 years, an average of 50 000 new cases of HIV infection per year were transmitted in the USA despite attention focused on preventive measures (Prejean et al. 2011).

HIV is a retrovirus. Its primary cellular target is the CD4 lymphocyte. Penetration of the target cell results in the synthesis of a complementary DNA to the native viral RNA by the enzyme reverse transcriptase. The complementary DNA becomes the genetic template for the production of viral proteins. An important clinical feature of the infection is its latency. There is commonly an acute viral syndrome associated with viremia of the acute infection, but the infection may exist for a decade or more before immunosuppression and life-threatening illness emerge. During this latent period, the virus is replicating and exhausting the host's reservoir of CD4 cells. During the evolution of the disease CD8, B cells, monocytes/macrophages, dendritic cells, and natural killer cells are all affected.

An important feature of HIV is hypermutation. This dynamic process of constantly changing the viral genome results in specific antigenic changes. The constantly changing viral antigens have been a major reason for failure in vaccine development.

HIV is identified throughout the world in two types. HIV-1 is most common and appears to be the most virulent and has the greatest efficiency in transmission. HIV-2 is much less common and is identified primarily in West Africa. HIV-2 is less likely to progress to clinical AIDS (Centers for Disease Control and Prevention [CDC] 2011).

Transmission of HIV infection is secondary to exposure from blood or blood products of infected individuals. Transfusion was a significant cause before effective screening methods were instituted. Intravenous drug abuse and sexual exposure remain common modes of transmission. Vertical transmission from infected mothers to neonates remains a potential route of transmission, although effective prevention has been achieved with the third trimester recognition and treatment of HIV-positive mothers. There is no evidence for transmission by saliva or casual interpersonal contact.

The natural history of HIV infection leads to clinical AIDS. The reduction of the CD4 lymphocyte count and other immune consequences result in opportunistic infections and neoplasia that constitute the case definition of AIDS (CDC 1992). These conditions are identified in Table 14.1. The morbidity and deaths from AIDS are generated by the immunosuppression rather than direct consequences of the clinical infection.

The diagnosis of HIV infection is made by screening individuals with high-risk exposures. The diagnosis is made by detection of specific antibodies or antigens. The enzyme-linked immunosorbent assay (ELISA) test for HIV-specific antibodies is highly (99%) accurate. A positive ELISA leads to a western blot evaluation of host antibodies to specific HIV antigens. The number of indeterminate diagnostic studies requiring direct viral detection has become less frequent.

Laboratory monitoring of the patient becomes an important feature during management. CD4 cell counts have been most commonly used with $<200/\mu l$ being the threshold to indicate potential emergence of AIDS. Direct measurement of HIV RNA in blood is used to monitor therapy. Monitoring warrants quantitative assessment of viral RNA every 3–4 months. Resistance monitoring of viral strains is commonly done either by evaluating genomic sequences of clinical isolates or by demonstrating inhibition of viral growth by specific agents in vitro.

The prevention of HIV infection has been the focus of a large effort by national and international health agencies. Rates of new HIV infection have declined in developed countries but continue to occur at unacceptable rates. In developing countries, safe sex programs have had a small impact and an increasing number of new cases continue to be identified. An effective vaccine has been aggressively pursued but not achieved.

The treatment of HIV infection has rapidly progressed over the last 20 years. Highly effective antiretroviral therapy has evolved with dramatic prolongation of quality life for many HIV patients (Department of Health and Human Services 2011). Current therapy is for life, although specific combinations of drugs may be changed over time. Regimens are selected based on the comorbid conditions of the patient (e.g., coexistent hepatitis virus B [HBV] or C [HCV] infection), pregnancy, drug resistance, and other variables. Table 14.2 highlights the six categories of antiretroviral drugs that are currently available. Treatment philosophy usually leads to three or more drugs being

Table 14.1 Details the surveillance conditions associated with the diagnosis of AIDS and common diagnostic methods.

Conditions of AIDS surveillance case definition	Diagnostic methods
Candidiasis of bronchi, trachea, lungs, esophagus	Typical endoscopic appearance; microscopic fungal mycelia filaments; positive cultures
Invasive cervical carcinoma	Biopsy
Coccidioidomycosis	Culture or antigen detection
Cryptococcosis	Culture or antigen detection
Cryptosporidiosis	Histology or cytology
Cytomegalovirus disease (not liver, spleen, or nodes)	Culture or antigen detection
Encephalopathy, HIV associated	Clinical association in HIV-positive patient
Herpes simplex: chronic ulcer (>1 month), bronchitis, pneumonitis, esophagitis	Culture or antigen detection
Histoplasmosis: disseminated or extrapulmonary	Culture or antigen detection
Isosoporiasis, intestinal (>1 month)	Histology or cytology
Kaposi sarcoma	Histology or cytology
Lymphoma: Burkitt, immunoblastic, or brain primary	Biopsy
Mycobacterium avium complex, M. kansasii, or other atypical species (disseminated or extrapulmonary)	Cytology, cultures, typical clinical presentation
Mycobacterium tuberculosis, any site	Cytology, cultures, typical clinical presentation
Pneumocystis jiroveci pneumonia	Clinical picture without bacteria; biopsy
Pneumonia, recurrent	Cultures; clinical recurrent pneumonia
Progressive multifocal leukoencephalopathy	Histology or cytology
Salmonella septicemia, recurrent	Cultures
Toxoplasmosis of brain	Imaging of brain; positive antibody detection
Wasting syndrome due to HIV	Clinical association of >10% loss of body mass in HIV-positive patient

used for naïve cases, with agents chosen from groups with a different mechanism of action. The extensive number of treatment options, differences in drug-associated complications, different number of associated chronic illnesses (e.g., HBV or HCV), and differences in responsiveness mean that physicians with extensive experience in the management of HIV infection are required.

In the 1980s and 1990s, there was considerable concern about occupational risks of HIV infection for surgeons and healthcare workers. Uncertainty about the efficiency of transmission of HIV infection resulted in implementation of universal precautions and reductions in blood exposure during operations. These precautions continue to be recommended and are discussed with hepatitis below (Fry 2007). In the USA, 57 documented cases of HIV transmission have occurred among healthcare workers and another 139 cases are considered as probable transmissions based upon epidemiologic evidence (CDC 2002). No cases have occurred in the sterile environment of the operating room. The current risk of HIV transmission from a percutaneous injury is identified at 0.3% (CDC 2003).

HEPATITIS

Hepatitis continues to be an international viral pathogen in millions of patients annually. Each hepatitis virus has a unique natural history and different consequences. For surgeons, hepatitis B and C are associated with cirrhosis of the liver, hepatocellular carcinoma, and portal hypertension. The risks of hepatitis as an occupational infection continue at present. Reported hepatitis viruses of interest are identified in **Table 14.3**. Each is discussed.

Hepatitis A

Hepatitis A virus (HAV) continues to be the most clinically identified cause of hepatitis worldwide. HAV is an RNA virus that is transmitted via the fecal–oral route from contaminated water or food products. The ingested virus adheres to the upper aerodigestive tract mucosa, accesses the circulation, and binds specifically to the hepatocyte. The viral RNA replicates within the hepatocyte cytoplasm, which then leads to lysis of the host cell and liberation of new virions to continue the cycle. The bile becomes a rich source of viruses which enter the intestinal tract, and the viral particles are passed from the gut to contaminate other food and water sources.

HAV causes a severe and incapacitating infection. Fever, malaise, nausea, vomiting, and marked jaundice are the usual clinical findings. Mild leukocytosis is usually present with dramatic increases in the serum concentrations of aspartate aminotransferase (AST) and alanine aminotransferase (ALT). The clinical hepatitis syndrome may last 2–3 weeks, but several months may be required for full recovery. Although the acute hepatitis syndrome is severe, deaths from acute HAV infection are quite uncommon but can be seen in pregnant women, elderly people, and immunocompromised individuals. HAV infection does not have a chronic phase of infection. Resolution of the acute infection results in complete eradication of the virus. There is no post-hepatitis cirrhosis. HAV infection is not a risk for occupational infection.

The diagnosis is customarily made by clinical criteria. Acute and convalescent sera for HAV antibody confirm the diagnosis. The virus can be isolated form blood and stool. Reverse transcriptase polymerase

Table 14.2 The six groups of currently available antiretroviral agents that are available for the treatment of HIV infection (Department of Health and Human Services 2011).

Nucleoside/nucleotide reverse transcriptase inhibitors		
Generic name	**Brand name**	**Dosage (adults)**
Abacavir	Ziagen	300 mg twice daily, or 600 mg four times daily
Didanosine	Videx EC	400 mg four times daily
Emtricitabine	Emtriva	200 mg four times daily
Lamivudine	Epivir	150 mg twice daily, or 300 mg four times daily
Stavudine	Zerit	40 mg twice daily
Tanofovir disoproxil fumarate	Viread	300 mg four times daily
Zidovudine	Retrovir	300 mg twice daily, or 200 mg three times daily
Non-nucleoside reverse transcriptase inhibitors		
Delaviridine	Rescriptor	400 mg three times daily
Efavirenz	Sustiva	600 mg at bedtime
Etravirine	Intelence	200 mg twice daily
Nevirapine	Viramune	400 mg four times daily
Rilpivirine	Edurant	25 mg four times daily
Protease inhibitors		
Atazanavir	Reyataz	400 mg QD
Darunavir	Prezista	600–800 mg four times or twice daily not alone
Fosamprenavir	Lexiva	1400 mg twice daily
Indinavir	Crixivan	800 mg three times daily
Lopinavir/Ritonavir	Kaletra	400 mg/100 mg twice daily, or 800 mg/200 mg four times daily
Nelfinavir	Viracept	1250 mg twice daily or 750 mg three times daily
Ritonavir	Norvir	100-400 mg four times daily with other protease inhibitors
Saquinavir	Invirase	1000 mg twice daily not alone
Tipranavir	Aptivus	500 mg twice daily not alone
Fusion inhibitors		
Enfuvirtide	Fuzeon	90 mg (1 ml) subcutaneously twice daily
CCR5 antagonists		
Maraviroc	Selzentry	150–600 mg twice daily based on companion drugs
Integrase inhibitor		
Raltegravir	Isentress	400 mg twice daily

The drugs are given as combinations of multiple agents. Dosages are adjusted depending on companion treatments and patient tolerance. Drug interactions with other therapy and the toxicities of the agents are complex.

Table 14.3 Those viruses proven or suspected to cause hepatitis in humans.

Hepatitis type	Nucleic acid	Route of transmission	Clinical commentary
A	RNA	Fecal–oral	Severe acute hepatitis, but infrequently fatal: not associated with chronic hepatitis disease; an effective vaccine is available
B	DNA	Blood borne	5% of infections become lifetime chronic disease: associated with end-stage liver disease and hepatocellular carcinoma; a safe and effective vaccine is available
C	RNA	Blood borne	60–80% of infections become lifetime chronic infection; a variable natural history of chronic infection; no vaccine
D	RNA	Blood borne	Requires acute or chronic hepatitis B infection to infect humans; exacerbates severity of chronic hepatitis B; no vaccine
E	RNA	Fecal–oral	Many common features similar to hepatitis B; not associated with chronic hepatitis disease; no vaccine
G	RNA	Blood borne	Associated with hepatitis B and C patients but unproven to actually cause infection of the hepatocyte
TT	DNA	Blood borne	Transfusion-associated infection but of unproven clinical relevance for hepatitis
SEN	DNA	Blood borne	Transfusion-associated virus: unproven as a hepatitis virus

chain reaction (rtPCR) will identify the viral RNA. No specific treatment other than supportive care is required for the acute infection. HAV infection can be prevented by use of the HAV vaccine which is highly effective for international travelers going to endemic areas.

Hepatitis B

Hepatitis B virus (HBV) infection has traditionally been of greatest concern to surgeons. Chronic HBV infection has been a recognized cause of end-stage liver disease and its related manifestations. HBV infection has been recognized for over 60 years as an occupational risk to healthcare workers after blood exposure from infected patients (Kuh and Ward 1950, Trumbell and Greiner 1951).

HBV is a DNA virus. It is transmitted by percutaneous or mucous membrane exposure to contaminated blood or other body fluids. HBV is transmitted by sexual contact and intravenous drug abuse. Blood and blood product transfusion has been eliminated as a source of transmission with effective screening methods. Internationally millions of new cases occur annually. It is currently estimated that 350 million people have chronic HBV infection worldwide (Dienstag 2008).

Following entry of the virus into the circulation, it binds to hepatocytes. The viral DNA replicates new particles from the infected cell. Only 25% of acute infections are characterized with icterus, elevated hepatic enzymes (e.g., AST, ALT), and the clinical hepatitis syndrome, whereas all others are subclinical. Unfortunately, 5% of all HBV infections are associated with chronic infection. In chronic HBV infection the patient is positive for the virus for life and remains a reservoir for infection to others. The chronic HBV patient will progress to post-necrotic cirrhosis, portal hypertension, and even hepatocellular carcinoma. The natural history of chronic infection commonly requires over 20 years from acute infection to chronic manifestations of the disease.

The diagnosis is established by the detection of antibodies or HBV antigen in the patient. The acute infection will develop both the surface and core antibody to HBV. Identification of the core antibody is indicative of current or prior HBV infection, because surface antibody alone may reflect prior HBV immunization. Identification of the HBV antigen confirms that active disease is present. Persistence of the antigen reflects chronic hepatitis.

Prevention of HBV infection is an international objective with the safe and effective HBV vaccine. A three-dose regimen is used via intramuscular administration, with the second and third dose given 1 and 6 months after the initial dose. An antibody response should be documented to identify the 5–10% of non-responders, who should undergo a second course of immunization. For non-responders following revaccination, prevention of exposure remains the only recourse. Successful immunization is currently believed to confer lifetime immunity.

Dramatically improved treatment of patients with chronic HBV infection has occurred over the last 10–15 years. Seven different drugs are currently employed in the management of these patients (**Table 14.4**). Interferon-α may be used as a conventional formulation or pegylated with polyethylene glycol. All other therapies are nucleoside analogs. Interferon-α therapy is used for 48 weeks whereas the nucleosides are used over many years. Each has different toxicity and different rates of effectiveness. All require dosing modifications for renal failure. The goal of therapy is to reduce the viral load and prevent progression of the disease. Current trends in treatment have been to use drugs that have lowest resistance trends and lower toxicity profiles, and yield the best results in the elimination of HBV DNA. Therapeutic choices are modified when patients have concurrent HIV infection. The current treatments are not considered curative and patients must be monitored for viral breakthrough (Bhattacharya and Thio 2010, Kwon and Lok 2011).

Surgeons and other healthcare workers (HCWs) have contracted occupational HBV infection from percutaneous exposure to blood. There is a 30% risk for acute HBV infection after percutaneous injury by needlestick from a chronically infected patient. The generalized use of the HBV vaccine is reducing the risk in the USA, but occupational HBV infection remains an international risk for surgeons and HCWs. All should be immunized.

When exposure to a known HBV-infected patient occurs, a post-exposure prophylaxis protocol should be implemented. First, a current HBV serology should be obtained. If a positive HBV surface antibody is obtained, then the prior immunization is still effective. If the serology is positive for HBV core antibody, then remote HBV infection

Table 14.4 Drugs currently used or being evaluated for the treatment of patients with chronic hepatitis B infection.

Drug	Mode of action	Dose	Comments
Interferon-α-2a	Enhanced immune response	180 µg s.c. weekly for 48 weeks	>25% rate of fever, headache, etc. Contraindicated in decompensated cirrhosis Eliminates HBV DNA in 30–60% of treated patients
Lamivudine	Cytidine analog	100 mg daily	Rapid development of resistance Associated with hepatic steatosis, lactic acidosis 40–70% loss of HBV DNA
Emtricitabine	Cytidine analog	200 mg daily	High resistance rates Similar features to lamivudine Not FDA approved in the USA
Telbivudine	Thymidine analog	600 mg daily	Similar effects and adverse events as lamivudine Longer elimination half-life 60–85% loss of HBV DNA
Adefovir	Adenosine monophosphate analog	10 mg daily	Very nephrotoxic 20–50% loss of HBV DNA
Tenofovir	Adenosine monophosphate analog	300 mg daily	Nephrotoxicity 75–90 % loss of HBV DNA
Entecavir	Guanosine analog	1 mg daily	Headaches, diarrhea, arthralgia, lactic acidosis 70–90% loss of HBV DNA

FDA, Food and Drug Administration; HBV, hepatitis B virus; s.c., subcutaneous administration.

has occurred and no additional preventive measures are necessary. However, a positive core antibody requires documentation of current antigen status because chronic HBV infection may exist. If the exposed individual is antibody-negative and has not previously been immunized, then a dose of the HBV immune globulin should be given and the initial does of the HBV vaccine given as the first step in full immunization. If the individual has had prior immunization but is weakly positive for surface antibody, then a dose of the immune globulin and a single booster dose of the vaccine should be administered. No recommendations are currently available about routine booster doses of the vaccine, but this may be prudent for surgeons in high-risk specialties to consider. Surgeons with chronic HBV infection and are "e" antigen positive are an infectious risk to patients and should follow the recommendations of the American College of Surgeons (**Box 14.1**).

Hepatitis C

Before 1989, only HAV and HBV were identified hepatitis viruses. A third virus was suspected, and these infections were collectively referred to as non-A, non-B hepatitis. The identification of HCV and the development of the HCV antibody test allowed effective diagnosis and represented the virus of the non-A, non-B hepatitis. Screening of blood donations has documented HCV to be more common than HBV infection.

Box 14.1 The recommendations of the American College of Surgeons in the Statement on the Surgeon and Hepatitis (www.facs.org/fellows_info/statements/st-22.html).

- **Relevant to all blood-borne pathogens:** Surgeons should use the highest standards of infection control, including the use of barriers and practices to avoid blood exposure. This should be practiced in all sites where surgical care is rendered. Maximum effort should be extended to avoid blood exposure for all members of the surgical team
- **Relevant to hepatitis infected patients:** Surgeons have the ethical obligation to provide care to all patients, including those infected with hepatitis
- **Relevant to hepatitis B:** Surgeons should know their antibody status. Surgeons with natural antibodies without prior immunization should be evaluated for chronic HBV infection and if positive should be evaluated for the "e" antigen of HBV. Those surgeons who are "e" antigen positive or have high viral counts for HBV should have an expert panel convened to make recommendations about the continuation of clinical practice. Surgeons with chronic HBV infection should seek expert medical care to receive current treatment for their illness
- **Relevant to hepatitis B:** All surgeons should be immunized against HBV if they have not previously had HBV infection. Surgeons must know that they have seroconverted at the completion of the immunization process. A failed initial immunization effort requires a second immunization attempt. A failed second immunization means particular adherence to practices to avoid blood exposure
- **Relevant to hepatitis C:** Surgeons should know their antibody status for HCV. Avoiding blood exposure is the only preventive strategy in the absence of a vaccine against HCV infection. Surgeons with chronic HCV infection should adhere to strict infection control practice and use of barrier precautions. They should seek expert medical counsel for treatment of their infection

---

Even though it is an RNA virus, HCV shares many characteristics of HBV infection. It is transmitted by blood exposure and intravenous drug abuse, and it is associated with multiple sexual partners. Associations with blood transfusion have largely disappeared with effective screening of the blood supply. There remain about 15–30% of HCV infections that do not have identified clinical associations (Rosen 2011). It is not transmitted by the oral route. Similar to HBV, HCV infection is identified with an acute hepatitis syndrome in about 20–30% cases. Unfortunately, HCV infection results in chronic infection in >60% of acute infections. At present over 3 million chronic HCV infections exist in the USA.

HCV gains access to the blood, binds to specific receptors on the hepatocyte, is internalized into the cell, and replicated viral particles are the result. There are at least six genotypes of HCV, of which genotype-1 is most common in the USA and western Europe. HCV infection has a worldwide distribution with the greatest prevalence in sub-Saharan Africa (Cowan et al. 2011).

The natural history of chronic HCV infection is quite variable. Selected chronic infections will spontaneously resolve whereas others result in a persistently positive state of chronic infection with little clinical progression. About 20–30% of chronic cases develops cirrhosis over 30 or more years, and are expected to create an enormous future disease burden worldwide. Once cirrhosis develops, a 1–3% per year risk of hepatocellular carcinoma is observed.

The diagnosis of chronic HCV infection is recognized by the identification of persistent HCV antibody. Chronic infection is validated and the specific genotype is defined by rtPCR. The degree of liver fibrosis is best established with liver biopsy, but several liver biomarkers (e.g., AST, ALT) are used to estimate ongoing injury to the liver.

The treatment for chronic HCV infection is pegylated interferon-α and ribavirin for 48 weeks. Ribavirin is an orally administered nucleoside anti-metabolite. It is dosed as 800–1200 mg/day in divided doses. Interferon-α treatment has the expected proinflammatory effects of fever, arthralgias, malaise, and other related symptoms. Ribavirin is associated with hemolytic anemia and an increased rate of myocardial infarction. Ribavirin is considered to be teratogenic and effective contraception is recommended for patients of reproductive age. Genotype-1 patients have a 40% sustained response rate with no detectable viral RNA at 24 weeks after completion of treatment. Response rates are 70–80% for patients with genotype-2 or -3 infection.

The introduction of new protease inhibitors have demonstrated improved outcomes compared with interferon-α and ribavirin. Telaprevir (Zeuzem et al. 2011) and boceprevir (Bacon et al. 2011) have demonstrated overall response rates of 80% and 60% for genotype-1 infection. Although these newer treatments are exciting, they have introduced a dramatic increase in the cost of therapy. As not all chronic HCV infection progresses to cirrhosis and hepatocellular carcinoma, better selection criteria are necessary to define who should be treated and who may not be harmed by observation.

No HCV vaccine is currently approved in the prevention of occupational infection. Only uniform precautions to avoid percutaneous or mucous membrane exposure will prevent HCV infection. Percutaneous needlestick injuries are associated with about a 2% risk of seroconversion. As large numbers of patients are unaware of their infection status, uniform application of precautions will provide protection from HCV and other unappreciated blood-borne pathogens.

Universal precautions should include personal protective equipment and the avoidance of high-risk operating room behaviors associated with percutaneous injury. Eye protection should always be worn to avoid splash exposures. Double gloving should be employed in all thoracic and abdominal operations. This is best done by having the inside glove half a size larger than the external glove to avoid constriction of the hands and digits. Double gloving will not interfere with tactile discrimination or manual dexterity (Fry et al. 2010). Other than the hands, the forearms are the area of highest blood "strike through" and warrant the use of sleeve reinforcements for trauma, obstetrical cesarean sections, and cardiac surgery. A reinforced anterior panel of the gown or a water-impervious apron under the surgical gown will prevent strike through in high-risk procedures, and knee-length foot covers are justified in trauma cases.

Technical modifications in operating room behavior will reduce rates of intraoperative blood contamination of the surgical team. Wire suture material should be used only in very specific circumstances (e.g., sternal closure) and must be used with caution to avoid injury. Double gloving will avoid shear injury of the digits from tying large monofilament suture material (e.g., 0 or no. 1 polypropylene) under tension. Palpation of the needle tip in blind suturing techniques should be avoided. Swaged needles should be removed before tying suture material. Blunt needle technology appears to potentially reduce injuries. A "way" station can be established with a Mayo stand between the instrument nurse/technician and the surgeon to prevent direct passing of loaded needle holders. Increased use of the electrocautery for opening body cavities has been recommended but may increase infection at the surgical site.

Despite all the barrier enhancement and technical modifications, attitudes about avoiding injury in the operating room remain the most important area for prevention. Many percutaneous injuries in the operating room are the result of carelessness. An increased sense of awareness of sharp instruments and needles is essential. Percutaneous injury is preventable but only when sensitivity to the use of "sharps" has been increased.

Blood exposure and percutaneous injury continue to occur in the operating room and require a prompt response. Even though the surgeon may believe that the skin of the hands or forearm is intact, blood contact from breaks in the gloves or penetration of the surgical gown should be promptly managed. For blood contact or percutaneous injury of the hands or forearm, rescrubbing is desirable, but often not practical because of the circumstances in the operation. Irrigation of the local area with povidone–iodine or isopropyl alcohol is recommended because of their known viricidal activity. With percutaneous injuries, an acute HCV antibody should be done to establish that the exposed individual has not previously had HCV infection. Seroconversion should be documented by periodic reassessments of the HCV antibody. If seroconversion occurs and the individual is positive for HCV RNA, then the treatment protocol of active HCV infection identified above is recommended. Post-exposure treatment with the HCV antiviral therapy before documentation of actual infection is not recommended. The administration of HCV immune globulin does not provide post-exposure prevention.

Are surgeons with HCV infection a threat for transmission of infection to their patients? Although this has been rarely documented, the biggest threat to patients is from contaminated needles or multi-use vials of pharmaceuticals that have been contaminated by violations of infection control practices. The general consensus at this time is that surgeons who are HCV positive may continue to practice as long as they adhere to standards of infection control (see Box 14.1).

Hepatitis D

Hepatitis D virus (HDV), or hepatitis D, is an incomplete RNA virus that is solely a pathogen with coexistent HBV infection. HDV is transmitted by the same behaviors as HBV and may be transmitted simultaneously with HBV infection (Hughes et al. 2011). It may occur following chronic HBV infection. There are multiple different genotypes of HDV. The presence of HDV infection results in more rapid and severe progression to liver failure than expected from chronic HBV infection alone. The diagnosis of chronic HDV infection requires identification of the specific antigen or the viral RNA of the virus. The treatment of HDV infection has been difficult because it requires the treatment of two chronic viruses at the same time. Treatment with interferon-α for 48 weeks has resulted in observed virus-free states followed by relapse. The viral response of HDV appears to be linked to the effective reduction in HBV. The treatment of end-stage liver disease with combined HDV and HBV infection has been liver transplantation, with evidence of effectiveness when the antigenemia of the HBV is suppressed with HBV immunoglobulin. HDV has not been identified as an occupational risk for surgeons and the risk is eliminated by effective HBV immunization.

Hepatitis E

Hepatitis E virus (HEV) is an RNA virus that is transmitted by the fecal–oral route. Epidemic outbreaks of this infection are identified in Asia and Africa, but clinical infection is a sporadic event in developed countries and associated with international travel. Clinical epidemics demonstrate the typical hepatitis syndrome. Acute infection usually resolves without a chronic viral persistence except in very immunosuppressed individuals. Acute infection is rarely fatal except in pregnancy and in very young children. Infection is suspected in patients with an acute hepatitis syndrome who are negative for the conventional hepatitis antibodies. There are four genotypes of HEV but only a single serotype. Commercial assays for anti-HEV antibody are available and detection of the viral RNA occurs at the onset of the viral syndrome. A vaccine for HEV is currently not available. Treatment of clinical infection is supportive care only. HEV rarely is transmitted by transfusion and is not considered an occupational risk.

Other hepatitis viruses

The search for additional hepatitis viruses continues. A putative orally transmitted hepatitis virus was labeled hepatitis F but has not been validated. As no virus has been identified in up to 20% of patients with transfusion-associated hepatitis, the search for additional blood-borne hepatitis viruses has continued.

Hepatitis G (HGV) was reported in 1996 (Linnen et al. 1996). This virus was associated with chronic hepatitis and was commonly identified with HBV, HCV, and HIV infections. HGV is blood borne, and has been identified in about 2% of studied individuals. At the same time, an entire group of GB viruses (GBV) were being identified as human and primate pathogens. The "GB" came from the initials of the surgeon with non-A, non-B, non-C hepatitis which was the index case from which the virus was recovered. Of the four GB viruses, only GBV-C appears to cause infection in humans. GBV-C and the aforementioned HGV, although potentially having some unique genomic features, are the same class of virus (Stapleton et al. 2011). Despite early association with chronic hepatitis, neither GBV-C nor HGV has been proven to infect hepatic cells and may actually infect and replicate within lymphocytes.

Additional viruses have been associated with transfusion-associated hepatitis and have been found as potentially additional viral pathogens with HBV and HCV infection. Both the Torqueteno (TT) virus (Hino and Miyata 2007) and the SEN virus (Sagir et al. 2004) are single-stranded DNA viruses that are transmitted by transfusion but have not been documented to cause hepatitis. Both are found in patients without clinical disease and may simply be commensal viruses.

HUMAN PAPILLOMAVIRUS

Human papillomavirus (HPV) causes a chronic infection of the human epithelium and mucosa. It is a double-stranded DNA virus with over 100 different strains of differing virulence. These ubiquitous viruses are not inactivated with prolonged exposure to the environment. Infection occurs in association with traumatic events (e.g., cuts, abrasions) that permit viral access to the basal cell layer. The complete viral particle is found only in the fully mature keratinocyte where they are released with superficial sloughing of these cells. The different serotypes of HPV result in different disease phenotypes. Specific strains are associated with incorporation of the viral DNA into the host genome and result in malignant transformation.

Infection with HPV is not associated with the acute symptoms of inflammation but rather becomes clinically expressed as neoplasia. For most patients who acquire HPV, the infection is latent or subclinical, and becomes a clinical illness only from symptoms attendant on local growth of a lesion. HPV infections have varying degrees of clinical consequences for the patient and are classified according to the anatomic site where infection occurs. The three major groupings of HPV infection are anogenital, upper aerodigestive tract, and nongenital cutaneous sites.

Anogenital HPV
Cervical carcinoma

Cervical carcinoma is the HPV-associated disease of greatest concern. Virtually 100% of cervical carcinoma cases are secondary to HPV infection. Infection of the female genital tract is secondary to sexual transmission of the virus. The HPV virus infects the squamous epithelium of the cervical canal. Population studies have identified that 35% of women have HPV virus with differing prevalence by age (**Figure 14.1**) (Dunne et al. 2007). Infection with HPV occurs and then spontaneously resolves within 2 years among most women. About 10% of women have long-term persistence of the sexually acquired infection and are at risk for the development of cervical carcinoma. Infection may exist with more than one viral strain of HPV. Resolution of infection from one strain does not affect infection from a second strain. Reactivation of HPV infection from immunosuppression (e.g., HIV infection) or aging, but without interval sexual exposure, indicates that these infections are not eradicated but rather become latent within the host.

HPV infections occur in up to 80% of women studied over a lifetime. Persistence of the virus or transformation into invasive cervical carcinoma requires the presence of other cofactors. Factors associated with the malignant transformation are early menarche, early age sexual intercourse, multiple child births, multiple sexual partners, other sexually transmitted infections, and tobacco use.

HPV does not cause acute symptoms from the sexually transmitted infection itself. The traditional method of evaluating patients has been with the Papanicolaou smear from a cervical scraping, which identifies the consequences of HPV infection rather than early identification of the virus. DNA detection and typing of the virus are done in research settings and have been useful in the identification of specific strains (types 16, 18) associated with cervical cancer. Serological tests may be positive for antibodies to specific HPV strains, but may reflect the history of infection rather than the infection that is currently active. Positive smears for abnormal cytology necessitate cervical biopsy.

The histological change of cervical intraepithelial neoplasia (CIN) is the precursor lesion for invasive cancer (Kahn 2009). CIN (formerly known as cervical dysplasia) is graded on the depth of cellular abnormality on the cervical biopsy. CIN-1 involves the lower third of the cervical epithelial cells, CIN-2 involves the lower two-thirds, and CIN-3 involves the full thickness of the cervical epithelium. CIN-1 will spontaneously resolve in >90% of cases, whereas CIN-2/-3 is associated with the development of invasive cervical cancer in most cases. CIN-2/3 cases typically undergo conization or a loop electrical excision procedure (LEEP). If invasive cancer is identified, then oncological management of the uterus is pursued. Globally, nearly 500 000 women have the diagnosis of cervical carcinoma with deaths identified in half of them.

Enhanced understanding of the role of HPV in cervical carcinoma has led to the development of an effective vaccine (Harper et al. 2004, Villa et al. 2005). The recombinant vaccine has antibodies for types 6, 11, 16, and 18 (Gardasil or Silgard) or for types 16 and 18 alone (Cervarix). Both vaccines are administered in three doses over 6 months. The immunization is recommended for females aged 9–26, and ideally before first sexual exposure. Infection that is already established with types 16 and 18 does not benefit from immunization against these HPV types. Clinical trials have demonstrated a reduction in CIN frequency, but a reduction in invasive cervical carcinoma has not been documented. As 30% of CIN is caused by HPV types not covered by the vaccine, and the duration of protection has not been documented, cervical cancer screening is still recommended.

Vulvovaginal carcinoma

Vulvar and vaginal cancers are less common than cervical cancer, but share many clinical risk factors. In the USA, vulvovaginal squamous

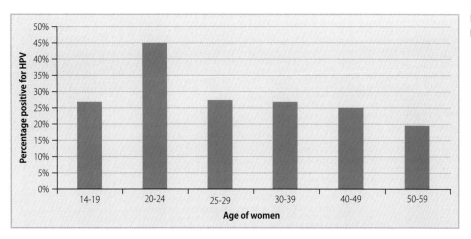

Figure 14.1 Prevalence by age of human papillomavirus in women.

carcinoma occurs in only 1–2 /100 000 women. About 40% of vulvar cancers and 65% of vaginal cancers are secondary to HPV infection. HPV type 16 is most commonly associated with vulvovaginal carcinoma (Smith et al. 2009).

Similar to cervical carcinoma, there are premalignant dysplastic lesions of vulvar intraepithelial neoplasia (VIN) and vaginal intraepithelial neoplasia (VAIN). They have similar grading systems of 1–3 with similar histological criteria to cervical carcinoma. VIN-2/-3 lesions have an 80% association with HPV and VAIN-2/-3 have over a 90% association. A differentiated VIN variant is seen in older patients with vulvar carcinoma that is not associated with HPV and is histologically distinct. VIN and vulvar cancer appear to be increasing with increased prevalence of HPV as the putative agent.

Vulvovaginal cancer and premalignant lesions present with dyspareunia and pelvic discomfort. Many are asymptomatic and identified with screening examinations. Biopsy confirms the diagnosis. Surgical excision of invasive cancer and premalignant VIN-2/-3 or VAIN-2/-3 lesions has been the treatment. Vulvar cancer has a better prognosis than vaginal carcinoma, likely because of earlier recognition.

Imiquimod (Aldara) as a 5% cream is an alternative treatment for VIN-2/-3 lesions and has benefit when compared with a placebo (van Seters 2008). Additional clinical trials are needed with comparisons to surgical intervention. As HPV types 16 and 18 are the most common strains associated with vulvovaginal squamous carcinoma, it is hoped that the quadrivalent vaccine may impact the frequency of the dysplastic and malignant lesions.

Male genital carcinoma

Penile squamous carcinoma is uncommon in the USA and western Europe where the incidence is about 1 case per 100 000 adult males per year. About 50% of these carcinomas are associated with HPV DNA. The HPV types identified in penile carcinoma are the same as those in female cervical carcinoma. Risk factors for penile carcinoma are early age sexual activity, multiple sexual partners, anogenital warts, and tobacco use (Giuliano et al. 2010). Circumcision is considered protective against penile cancer. The carcinoma begins as erosions or sores on the distal penile skin. These cancers are diagnosed by biopsy. Treatment is surgical excision. The association of HPV with penile squamous carcinoma is of interest because current evidence suggests that these subclinical viral infections in men are as frequent as they are in women (Smith et al. 2011). HPV immunization of males for the prevention of penile carcinoma has not been validated because of the very low incidence, but it is recommended for the prevention of genital warts discussed subsequently.

Anal carcinoma

Squamous cell carcinoma of the anal canal has increased in frequency in recent years. There are about 6000 cases per year in the USA. A total of 90% are attributable to HPV disease, and types 16 and 18 are identified in these HPV cancers (Parkin and Bray 2006). Risk factors include anal receptive intercourse, HIV disease, numbers of sexual partners, anogenital warts, and tobacco use. The diagnosis is by tissue biopsy. Therapy is primarily chemoradiation. As a result of the high frequency of type 16 and 18 HPV, prevention may accrue from the use of the HPV vaccine.

Genital warts

Benign anogenital warts (condylomata accuminata) are the most common genital lesions attributable to HPV infection. These lesions can be only a few millimeters in size or very large. The lesions occur at sites of epithelial injury and are usually from an infected sexual partner. Lesions occur around the labia in women, on the penis and scrotum of men, and in the perianal areas of both sexes. HPV types 6 and 11 are the associated pathogens. Anogenital warts have the same risk factors as other HPV infections, but are especially troublesome for HIV and immunosuppressed patients. The diagnosis is made by the identification of the typical skin lesion. Biopsy may be necessary to eliminate the possibility of squamous carcinoma.

The treatment of anogenital warts has many options. Lesions that are 1 cm in diameter are best treated with medical options (**Table 14.5**). Somewhat larger lesions can be treated with liquid nitrogen or electrocautery. Lesions with very board bases and considerable size (>3 cm) commonly result in the patient being taken to the operating room for removal by excision or electrocauterization. All treatment options are employed to manage the symptomatic lesions and are not curative of the underlying HPV infection. Patients should be counseled that the condylomata may recur.

Table 14.5 None of medical therapies is proven safe for pregnant women.

Treatment	Commentary
Imiquimod 5% cream	Self-administered three times a week for up to 16 weeks. Treated area should be washed 6–10 h after application. Treatment is immune enhancer and will have local inflammatory reactions
Podofilox 0.5% solution or gel	Self-administered application twice a day for 3 days with 4 days off. Repeated for four cycles if necessary. Mild pain and discomfort. Only for wart burden <10 cm²
Podophyllin resin 10–25% in tincture of benzoin	Applied weekly by healthcare provider. Applied to only 10 cm² per treatment episode. Air drying is necessary at application to avoid contact with normal skin from clothing. Area of treatment should be washed 1–4 h after application
Sinecatechin 15% ointment	Self-administered green tea extract. Applied three times daily for up to 16 weeks. Local burning and pain. Not recommended for immunosuppressed (e.g., HIV) patients
Trichoroacetic or bichloroacetic acid 80–90%	Chemical coagulation of proteins. Applied by healthcare provider once a week. Must dry to avoid injury to adjacent tissues. Pain and irritation
Cryotherapy	Liquid nitrogen application by healthcare provider. Care must be taken to avoided injury to adjacent tissues. Effective therapy will have pain. Repeat applications are commonly necessary
Surgical removal	Surgical removal by excision or electrocautery is reserved for large burden of warts. Topical therapy may be required for small residual lesions

From Centers for Disease Control and Prevention. Sexually transmitted diseases: treatment guidelines 2010, genital warts: www.cdc.gov/std/treatment/2010/genital-warts.htm.

The quadrivalent HPV vaccine does have efficacy for type 6 and 11 viruses and is approved for use in females and males for the prevention of anogenital warts (Liddon et al. 2010). Prospective randomized administration of the vaccine in males aged 16–26 years resulted in significantly fewer HPV type 6, 11, 16, and 18 infections, and fewer anogenital warts (Giuliano et al. 2011). As condylomata are associated with other types of HPV, all anogenital lesions will not be prevented. Prevention of HPV type 16 and 18 infections in males has the epidemiological advantage of potentially reducing the transmission of these strains to others.

Aerodigestive tract HPV infection

Of considerable interest to surgeons is the evolving role of HPV infection in the genesis of head and neck squamous cancers. Traditional associations have linked squamous carcinoma of the mouth, tongue, pharynx, and larynx to tobacco and alcohol use. Recently, patients with head and neck cancers have been identified with reduced or no tobacco use, and the results of treatment have been better than historical cases. These epidemiological observations led to the identification of HPV as the etiological agent, and that the type 16 strain associated with squamous cancers in the anogenital region was the most common HPV identified. Most current squamous head and neck cancers are HPV-linked cancers and HPV head and neck cancer is projected to exceed cervical carcinoma in frequency by 2020 (Chaturvedi et al. 2011).

Clinical associations with HPV head and neck cancer include multiple sexual partners, oral sexual contact, but less of a tobacco history than has been traditionally noted for these squamous carcinomas. HIV patients are at increased risk for these cancers (Stelow et al. 2010). The cancers present as primary masses of the head and neck with the usual associated symptoms. The HPV-associated lesion will present with neck metastases that have a cystic character. HPV lesions are less likely to be multifocal. The clinical management of these carcinomas remains surgical removal with traditional adjunctive measures. HPV type 16 has been associated with esophageal cancer, although this link to squamous cancer of the esophagus appears to be identified more in Asia than in the USA or Europe (Eslick 2010). Although rates of HPV have inconsistently been identified in lung cancers, type 16 virus may play a role in squamous carcinoma of the lung (Rezazadeh et al. 2009).

Respiratory papillomatosis is a recurring and difficult disease that occurs in both children (age <5) and adult populations between ages 20 and 30 (Chadra and James 2010). It consists of papilloma developing in the larynx, trachea, and bronchi. It is seldom associated with invasive cancer (<5%). In children the infection is the consequence of airway contamination with HPV at birth. It is poorly understood in adults and may relate to sexual practices. It is associated with HPV types 6 and 11, but has been seen with other types. Clinical symptoms consist of hoarseness, stridor, and upper airway obstruction. Laryngobronchoscopy establishes the diagnosis of usually numerous papillomas. The treatment has been endoscopic removal of the lesions. Systemic antiviral therapies have been used (interferon-α, indole 3-carbinol, cidofovir) and intralesional treatment with cidofovir is currently being explored. Photodynamic therapy is also being evaluated.

Non-genital cutaneous HPV infection

Cutaneous warts occur in many locations but most predictably on the digits and palms of the hands, and on the volar surface of the feet (plantar wart). These are also the consequences of HPV infection, but usually reflect different types of viruses from those identified with anogenital lesions. The hand warts are associated with HPV types 1, 3, 26, and 27, and plantar warts with types 2, 3, 4, 27, and 28.

The diagnosis of the cutaneous wart is ordinarily made by observing the typical dry, raised, rough, and crusty lesion of the hands or plantar surface of the foot. Warts with an atypical or moist appearance may require biopsy. In most cases, the diagnosis is obvious.

Treatment is necessary when the location (e.g., bottom of the foot) causes discomfort or functional impairment. Multiple different preparations of podophyllin resin are available. Podophyllin resin gives a burning sensation at the site of application. Imiquimod as a 5% cream application is effective, well tolerated locally, but very expensive. Topical salicylic acid, which is at a very high concentration in the compound used, has also been used effectively. Many other treatments have been advocated but are usually reserved for refractory cases (Lipke 2006).

Epidermodysplasia verruciformis (EV) is a rare genetic disorder associated with cutaneous malignancy secondary to HPV infections. These patients have flat, wart-like lesions with a predilection for developing HPV infection. HPV types 5, 8, and 14 have been associated with the transition of these lesions to invasive squamous carcinoma. Surgical management of documented squamous cancer is the treatment, but many topical agents are used in an attempt to control the constantly erupting EV skin lesions (Gewirtzman et al. 2008).

Bowen disease is an *in situ* squamous carcinoma of the skin. It is an irregular, flat erythematous plaque. It is associated with HPV types 16, 18, 31, 33, and 51, but is also linked to solar exposure, carcinogens, and immunosuppression in HIV infection. It can occur over any skin area. It is most often seen in women, but is seen in penile skin involvement (erythroplasia of Queyrat). It is not seen in patients aged <30 years. Excision is the traditional treatment, but newer treatments include photodynamic therapy, cryotherapy, and local chemotherapy (Cox et al. 2007). Imiquimod treatment is being evaluated.

HUMAN HERPESVIRUSES

Human herpesviruses (HHVs) are double-stranded DNA viruses that are common human pathogens. Over 90% of adults have been infected with one or more of the eight classes of HHV (Fry 2001). They are ubiquitous and commonly transmitted by saliva, airborne droplets, or direct lesion contact. They are associated with clinical infection in transplant recipients and immunosuppressed patients (e.g., HIV infection). The HHVs have a role in oncogenesis. An important feature of HHV infection is that the host harbors the virus for life after the acute infection and clinical events are the consequence of remote infection.

HHV-1 (herpes simplex)

Herpes simplex infection is best known for the perioral "cold sore" and for acute viral conjunctivitis. The infection typically occurs in the oropharynx, eyes, and face, and severe cases may extend into the central nervous system (CNS). The infection is easily transmitted by contact with an infected person even though that person may not have current symptoms. Virus from the initial infection is chronically harbored in the sensory ganglion cells (commonly the trigeminal ganglion) and is not eradicated. The acute infection has a broad array of severity, only to be repeatedly reactivated in selected patients.

The acute infections clinically present with stomatitis and pharyngitis of 3 days' to 3 weeks' duration. Vesicular perioral lesions proceed to a crusted lesion that may persist for several weeks. Occasionally a herpetic whitlow may be seen after a puncture wound, and have been reported with healthcare occupational needlesticks. Herpes gladiatorum represents mucocutaneous herpetic lesions identified after cutaneous skin trauma, with wrestlers being an index group for this infection. Herpes simplex keratitis may lead to corneal damage and a chorioretinitis may evolve in immunosuppressed or HIV patients. Similarly, immunosuppressed patients may develop viral encephalitis, esophagitis, and pneumonia with herpes simplex.

The diagnosis of herpes simplex infections is made by identification of the characteristic vesicular lesions of the skin. In adult patients the clinical diagnosis is usually confirmed by historical information of prior perioral lesions. When a specific viral diagnosis is required in serious cases, scrapings of the lesions for DNA detection, antigen detection, or cell culture is used. PCR detection methods are most common. When visceral or CNS infections are suspected, then acute and convalescent sera for antibody detection are employed.

Antiviral treatment of herpes simplex infection is used. Dosing and drug selection vary with the severity of the disease. Mucocutaneous infection is managed with aciclovir (400 mg by mouth four times daily), famciclovir (500 mg by mouth three times daily), or valaciclovir (500 mg by mouth twice daily) for a total of 7–10 days. Other sites of infection and recurrent infection have various other doses and durations, and are discussed elsewhere (Cernik et al. 2008).

HHV-2 (genital herpes)

Genital herpes occurs from HHV-2 which is distinctly different from HHV-1, even though the two viruses share a 50% genetic homology and have common clinical features (Gupta et al. 2007). Transmission occurs from sexual contact. The virus is harbored in sensory nerves similar to other herpesvirus types. The infected partner may or may not have evidence of clinical disease because shedding of the virus may be a chronic process. Primary infection may have symptoms of an acute viral infection but also be associated with sacral pain. Acute infections may be subclinical, with clinical disease not being expressed until much later. Reactivation occurs with stressor events and may recur for no explainable reason. High rates of reactivation are seen in immunocompromised patients. Over 25% of adults are seropositive for HHV-2. Vertical transmission to neonates with the birthing process is a particular problem with infected mothers.

The preliminary diagnosis of genital herpes is usually made by recognition of the typical vesicular rash of the perineum. The infection needs to be documented because of the common appearance of these genital lesions with other infections. A swab specimen is submitted for viral culture, antigen detection, or PCR to detect viral DNA. Aciclovir, famciclovir, and valaciclovir are the antiviral agents chosen. The dosing and duration of treatment are dependent on whether the current episode is the first episode, a recurrent episode, or a sustained episode requiring suppressive therapy, and whether the patient is immunosuppressed (Gupta et al. 2007). Vaccines to prevent this infection are under investigation but have not been validated as beneficial.

HHV-3 (varicella-zoster)

HHV-3 causes the infections of varicella (chickenpox) and herpes zoster (shingles). Varicella is the acute infection and herpes zoster is the recurrent infection decades later (Heininger and Seward 2006, Dworkin et al. 2007). The acute infection is acquired from airborne virus that adheres to the mucosa of the upper respiratory tract, proliferates and spreads to regional lymph nodes. The systemic infection results in the erythematous vesicular rash known as chickenpox. The infection occurs approximately 2 weeks after exposure and the patients are contagious for 7–10 days until the crusted lesions have separated. The pruritic vesicular rash is occasionally the source of secondary streptococcal or staphylococcal infections. The infection can infrequently extend to pneumonia, encephalitis, myocarditis, and other unusual manifestations. In most cases it is a self-limited disease that requires only supportive care. As with all herpesviruses, the virus remains dormant in the dorsal root ganglia after acute clinical infection.

Herpes zoster generally occurs in the sixth decade of life or later. It is associated with any acute illness, immunocompromised patients, HIV, or corticosteroid therapy. It can be a spontaneous clinical event without other associated clinical disease. It characteristically occurs unilaterally in a thoracic or lumbar dermatome. Pain in the dermatomal distribution is followed by a maculopapular rash 1–2 days later, which is then succeeded by the vesicular rash. Occasionally zoster will occur in a cranial nerve distribution and is very painful. Ocular zoster is a rare but severe reactivation. The duration of pain with herpes zoster is variable and may extend well beyond resolution of the rash. Post-herpetic neuralgia can be a longstanding source of chronic pain.

The diagnosis of varicella-zoster is made by the distinct clinical presentation. Viral cultures, PCR detection of DNA, and other antigen detection techniques can be used but are infrequently necessary. An effective vaccine has dramatically reduced the frequency of acute chickenpox in western societies and is expected to reduce the frequency of herpes zoster.

Clinical chickenpox in children is managed with supportive care. Adolescents and adults are commonly treated for 5–7 days with aciclovir, famciclovir, or valaciclovir to reduce the duration of the rash. For herpes zoster, the use of valaciclovir is more effective at relieving pain and resolving the rash. Immunization of children with the varicella-zoster vaccine is recommended with one dose at about 1 year of age, and a second at age 4–6. Immunization of individuals age >60 years is recommended to prevent the frequency and the severity of zoster.

HHV-4 (EBV)

Epstein–Barr virus (EBV) is most frequently associated with mononucleosis (Oludare et al. 2011). It is also associated with Burkitt lymphoma, nasopharyngeal carcinoma, some gastric lymphomas, and other lymphoproliferative diseases. EBV is transmitted by human saliva as the common source of infection. Blood transfusion and organ transplantation are other causes. Targeted host cells include lymphocytes and endothelial cells, with the site of original transmission occurring in tonsillar tissues. The proliferation of EBV leads to clinical infection at 5–7 weeks later in most cases. Others have a mild or subclinical infection. The patient carries the virus for life within B cells.

The acute mononucleosis syndrome is characterized by malaise, fever, fatigue, sore throat, cervical lymphadenopathy, and splenomegaly. Hepatic enzyme abnormalities are usually present. Symptoms last for more than 2 weeks. Recovery from fatigue takes a longer course. Protracted chronic EBV infection lasting for more than 6 months is also seen after acute infections. Complications of acute EBV infection may include pancreatitis, parotitis, pericarditis, pneumonia, and rarely splenic rupture.

The diagnosis of acute EBV mononucleosis is made by the heterophile antibody test. Elevations of AST, ALT, and bilirubin reflect the hepatitis syndrome that accompanies mononucleosis. In situ hybridization and PCR can be used to detect RNA transcripts and DNA of EBV. These viral detection methods are used in transplant recipients and HIV patients with immunosuppression. Aciclovir, ganciclovir, and valaciclovir are used for the treatment of established infection.

Oncogenesis from EBV remains an incompletely understood phenomenon (Grunhe et al. 2009). B-cell lymphoma may be an event after acute infection such as Burkitt lymphoma in children, or it may occur many years later with immunosuppression such as seen in transplantation or HIV patients. Immunosuppression may lead to an often fatal post-transplant lymphoproliferative disorder that is characterized by B-cell and plasma cell hyperplasia, and then the development of lymphoma. The successful treatment of this lymphoproliferative disorder is to reverse the immunosuppression regimen.

Treatment of EBV-associated lymphoma is a combination of chemotherapy regimens. The monoclonal antibody to CD20 (rituximab) of the B cell may be added to the chemotherapeutic regimen (Aldoss et al. 2008). After tissue diagnosis and staging, localized nasopharyngeal cancer is treated with radiation, whereas locally advanced disease and cervical metastatic adenopathy are managed with additional chemotherapy. Other monoclonal antibodies are being explored.

As 90% of patients have latent EBV, prevention of reactivation of the disease is of significance in transplantation recipients. Use of the aciclovir derivatives covers both EBV and cytomegalovirus infection. Development of an EBV vaccine to prevent reactivation in transplant recipients and other patient populations with severe immunosuppression is being pursued.

HHV-5 (cytomegalovirus)

Cytomegalovirus (CMV) is an infection of relevance in the care of transplantation and increasingly among critically ill patients with immunosuppression (Cook and Trgovcich 2011). CMV is present in over 50% of patients from prior clinical infection which results in latency within the salivary glands and other tissues. CMV infection is transmitted in the birthing process and in breast milk. It is transmitted in saliva, by sexual contact, blood products, and transplanted organs. The acute infection may be analogous to mononucleosis, but for many patients the acute infection is subclinical. Severe acute or reactivation disease may result in clinical hepatitis, retinitis, encephalitis, pneumonitis, and myocarditis. Reactivation disease is associated with gastrointestinal hemorrhage or perforation in transplant recipients and HIV patients.

The clinical diagnosis is difficult because of the absence of characteristic findings. Fever, leukopenia, and hepatosplenomegaly may be present. Reactivation disease in transplantation recipients may have clinical features of the systemic inflammatory response syndrome from any other cause, and requires an index of suspicion. Viral isolation, antigen detection, and PCR identification of DNA are the usual methods employed. Serological assays have been problematic because increases in antibodies may not occur for up to 4 weeks after the onset of symptoms and antibody titers may remain high from a prior reactivation.

Prevention of new infection or reactivation of pre-existent CMV has been an area of interest in transplant recipients. Knowledge of the patient's status with respect to prior CMV infection is important. Blood products and transplanted organs from CMV-positive donors into naïve recipients require preventive antiviral therapy for 3–6 months after transplantation. Ganciclovir, valaciclovir, and valganciclovir are used to prevent transmission or reactivation events (De Keyzer et al. 2011). Ganciclovir and valganciclovir are used for the treatment of clinical CMV infection.

HHV-6

HHV-6 clinically infects 95% of people within 2 years of birth (Abdel Massih and Razonable 2009). Similar to other herpesviruses, it then becomes latent and is present for life. Reactivation disease is identified in transplant recipients and HIV-infected patients. There are two variants: HHV-6A and HHV-6B. HHV-6 replicates within the salivary gland and saliva is the likely source of transmission. The T lymphocyte is the primary target cell and repository of latent virus.

Primary HHV-6 infection in infants is better known as roseola. It is a febrile viral illness that is self-limited in most cases. Its primary source of concern in adults is reactivation disease, in particular among transplant recipients (Kumar 2010). Reactivation disease is characterized by fever and rash, a hepatitis syndrome, especially if HCV is present, myelosuppression, pneumonitis, neurological illness, and an increased rate of graft rejection. Ganciclovir, foscarnet, and cidofovir have been proposed as antiviral treatments.

HHV-7

HHV-7 is understood the least of any herpesviruses. The primary infection is during childhood and is similar to that of HHV-6. The lymphocyte is the target cell population but its presence in saliva is established and plays a role in transmission. It remains latent after acute infection within lymphocytes. Definition of the frequency of reactivation disease remains unclear. Transplantation recipients are considered a population of patients at risk for this reactivation infection (Shiley and Blumberg 2010). Ganciclovir and foscarnet are the accepted antiviral treatments.

HHV-8

HHV-8 is the virus of Kaposi sarcoma (KS). Transmission is from saliva, but has been documented to be transmitted via blood transfusion and organ transplantation. Serological studies indicate that as many as 25% of patients may be positive for this virus. It is latent after acute infection in endothelial cells. HHV-8 is also associated with Castleman disease as an uncommon lymphoproliferative disease. Immunosuppression, commonly from HIV disease, is the clinical cofactor that results in KS, although KS can be seen in transplant recipients and cancer chemotherapy patients. The association between KS and HHV-8 is so strong that viral identification is unnecessary.

The treatment of HHV-8 and KS is to control the commonly underlying HIV disease. Highly active antiretroviral therapy will cause regression of the skin lesions but may not affect complete resolution. KS is not cured and recurs over time. Interferon-α, rapamicin, interleukin-12, thalidomide, lenalidomide, cytotoxic agents, and others have been explored for KS (Uldrick and Whitby 2011).

POLYOMA VIRUSES

The polyoma viruses are double-stranded DNA viruses that are associated with experimental neoplasia. The five different polyoma viruses that are associated with human disease are identified in Table 14.6. The BK and JC viruses are most recognized with human infection (Jiang et al. 2009, Raghavender and Brennan 2010). These two viruses share 75% homology in their respective genomes. The BK polyoma virus is recognized as a significant pathogen in immunosuppressed transplant recipients. The JC virus is associated with progressive multifocal leukoencephalopathy (PML). The other three polyoma viruses (**Table 14.6**) have been cultured from the human respiratory tract (KI and WU viruses) or from Merkel cell carcinoma. The role of these latter three viruses in causing infection or neoplasia has not been defined. This discussion focuses on the BK and JC viruses.

Table 14.6 Details for five types of known polyoma viruses and their potential role in human infection.

Polyoma virus type	Cellular target	Clinical commentary
BK virus	Renal and urinary tract epithelium	BK polyoma virus nephropathy is associated with over-immunosuppression in renal transplant recipients, and loss of 50% of kidney grafts when clinical infection occurs
JC virus	Lymphocytes, oligodendrocytes, renal epithelium	JC polyoma viruses are associated with progressive multifocal leukoencephalopathy seen in immunosuppressed HIV patients and transplant recipients
KI virus	Respiratory epithelium	Recovered from the respiratory tract, but of uncertain pathological significance
WU virus	Respiratory epithelium	Recovered from the respiratory tract, but of uncertain pathological significance
Merkel cell virus	Skin	Associated with Merkel cell cancer, but has an uncertain role in the causation of the tumor

Current evidence indicates that polyoma virus infection occurs in childhood, and remains as a chronic but inactive virus in the host. Routes of transmission remain unclear and may be the result of fecal–oral, airborne, transplacental, or other physical contract with individuals shedding the virus. Seroprevalence of either JC or BK virus is identified in up to 80% of adults, and nearly 20% of individuals will shed the virus in their urine. The JC virus is more prevalent than the BK virus. During latency after childhood infection, the JC virus resides within the lymphoid, neural, and renal tissues. The BK virus resides within the epithelial cells of the collecting system of the urinary tract.

Primary infection occurs when the polyoma virus binds to membrane receptor sites at the target cell population. Primary infection is thought to be asymptomatic or a mild respiratory infection. The virus is internalized by endocytosis. Cytoplasmic trafficking results in the virus residing within the nucleus. It remains in this latent state until immunosuppression leads to reactivation. New virions are produced at this point with resultant lysis of the host cell and release of new particles.

BK polyoma infection

Reactivation infection with BK polyoma virus appears as a nephropathy, hemorrhagic cystitis, pneumonia, retinitis, hepatic dysfunction, or meningoencephalitis. BK nephropathy occurs with profound immunosuppression in transplant recipients, or in those with advanced HIV infection. Although an association in transplant recipients has been made with specific immunosuppression agents, it is the degree of immunosuppression and not the agent that is identified with BK polyoma nephropathy.

BK nephropathy occurs in the transplanted kidney, and is highly unusual in the native kidney of patients who have received non-renal solid organ transplants. The specificity of the transplanted kidney for this reactivated infection suggests that the virus may actually be within the renal epithelium of the donor kidney and not the recipient. The disease starts as an interstitial nephritis, is detected about 1 year after transplantation, and results in loss of kidney grafts in 50% of cases depending on the severity of the infection.

The diagnosis of BK nephropathy is by biopsy of the transplanted kidney, because rejection of the kidney from other causes is clinically similar. Typical histological changes are observed in the biopsy and specific immunohistochemistry antibodies confirm the diagnosis. As a result of lack of homogeneity in tissue changes, two biopsy specimens are performed. Urine screening demonstrates the presence of the BK virus at 3–6 months after kidney transplantation. The JC virus is identified within 5 days but not associated with clinical disease (Saundh et al. 2010).

As clinical reactivation of disease is recognized only with interstitial nephritis or failure of the kidney graft, methods for screening the patients to detect early viral activation is important in kidney transplant recipients during the first 2 years (Hirsch et al. 2005). Detection of "decoy" cells in the urine of the kidney transplant recipient has an almost 100% sensitivity but only a 20% specificity for detecting active infection. The decoy cells represent sloughed renal tubular epithelial cells which have viral inclusions. DNA PCR in blood or urine and mRNA PCR in urine have higher specificities in the diagnosis.

The treatment of BK polyoma nephropathy is to reduce the patient's level of immunosuppression. The obvious risk is to reduce immunosuppression without triggering graft rejection. Reduction or elimination of mycophenolate has been one strategy that is employed but no standard for reduction in immunosuppression has been established. Early reductions in immunosuppression based on evidence from screening the patient yields better results than waiting until nephropathy occurs. Current evidence does not support the use of cidofovir or leflunomide to treat BK nephropathy (Johnston et al. 2010).

JC polyoma infection

PML is a demyelinating disease of the white matter of the brain. Similar to BK nephropathy, it is seen in patients with severe immunosuppression and is most commonly seen in advanced HIV infection. It is also seen in transplant recipients and in patients receiving monoclonal antibody treatment for autoimmune diseases (Tan and Koralnik 2010). B lymphocytes carry the virus to the CNS with the resultant damage to glial cells. Clinical symptoms include mental status changes, ataxia, paresis, and other focal neurological deficits. Asymmetrical brain lesions are identified by imaging. Toxoplasmosis and lymphoma are differential diagnoses. Identification of viral DNA by PCR of the spinal fluid may be negative in 20% of PML cases, and will require brain biopsy to establish the diagnosis. The treatment of PML in HIV infection is enhanced antiretroviral therapy to achieve better control of the infection. In transplant recipients and other patients on immunosuppressive therapy, reduction or cessation of immunosuppression may be necessary. Antiviral chemotherapy against the JC virus has not been successful. The prognosis for the PML patient is poor, with survival being only a few months, although longer survivals are achieved in HIV patients with successful antiretroviral treatment. Newer clinical syndromes associated with JC virus include granule cell neuropathy of the cerebellum, JC virus encephalopathy, and JC viral meningitis.

Rabies

Once a common disease among homeothermic animals and humans, rabies is an uncommon disease in the USA and western Europe because of effective immunization of animal populations at risk (e.g., dogs) and effective post-exposure prophylaxis in humans. Rabies is caused by the single-stranded RNA lyssavirus. However, over 50 000 deaths occur worldwide per year, with dogs the most likely source of the human infection. Bats, skunks, and raccoons account for rabies transmission to humans in the USA, where the annual incidence of human infection is only about 1/100 million people (CDC 2009).

Human transmission typically follows a soft-tissue bite from an infected animal. Human-to-human transmission can occur from bites from infected patients. A total of 16 cases of fatal rabies have occurred after corneal, solid organ, and vascular tissue transplantation from infected donors (Manning et al. 2008). Virus from the soft-tissue exposure enters into peripheral nerves, and then migrates into the CNS where the encephalitis and viral syndrome of the infection evolve. Exposure to clinical disease commonly requires 2 weeks to 2 months, but longer intervals for infection are seen. Proliferation of the virus within the CNS leads to the clinical syndrome of confusion, agitation, and hallucinations, and other evidence of cerebral dysfunction. Increased salivation and lacrimation are associated with high concentrations of the virus. Muscle paralysis leads to ineffective swallowing and the association of hydrophobia with this infection.

Prevention of infection begins with local wound management. Non-viable tissue is debrided and local irrigation with isopropyl alcohol or povidone–iodine is used. Irrigation with viricidal solutions is not scientifically validated as preventing infections but is intuitive and may also avoid other animal bite-associated infections. Post-exposure prophylaxis (PEP) is effective and is employed after exposure events where rabies is suspected (Manning et al. 2008). The original vaccine by Pasteur and Roux was attenuated virus derived from rabbit tissue. Vaccines in recent years have been derived from human diploid and purified chick embryo cell cultures after viral deactivation. PEP is initiated within 10 days of exposure. Human rabies immunoglobulin (20 units/kg) from hyperimmune human donors is infiltrated as much as possible around the soft injury, with the remainder given intramuscularly at a site remote from the exposure site. The administration of the immunoglobulin is not recommended more than 7 days after exposure. The first dose of the vaccine is given at the time of exposure with four additional doses given on days 3, 7, 14, and 28 after exposure. Current vaccines have replaced the well-chronicled and painful abdominal injections of early generations of rabies vaccines.

The diagnosis of rabies is established from viral cultures or PCR of infected brain tissues or body fluids. Skin, cerebrospinal fluid, saliva, and urine may yield the identification of the virus. The index animal may be a source to confirm that rabies is present. Light microscopic methods have been employed to establish the diagnosis in areas without access to high-tech methods.

Clinical rabies has traditionally been viewed as uniformly fatal. Antiviral chemotherapy has not been considered of any benefit although it has been used. Survivors of rabies have been identified in the last decade with the so-called "Milwaukee" protocol where patients have been treated with a pharmacologically induced coma and drug therapy of ketamine, midazolam, ribavirin, and amantadine (Willoughby 2007). Prolonged ventilator supportive care is necessary. Survival with this protocol has been about 8%. Survivors do not appear to have significant neurological sequelae. Survival remains unlikely, and PEP remains the needed strategy to prevent this infection.

REFERENCES

Abdel Massih RC, Razonable RR. Human herpesvirus 6 infections after liver transplantation. *World J Gastroenterol* 2009;**15**:2561–9.

Aldoss IT, Weisenburger DD, Fu K, et al. Adult Burkitt lymphoma: advances in diagnosis and treatment. *Oncology* 2008;**22**:1508–17.

Bacon BR, Gordon SC, Lawitz E, et al. Boceprivir for previously treated chronic HCV genotype-1 infection. *N Engl J Med* 2011;**364**:1207–17.

Bhattacharya D, Thio CL. Review of hepatitis B therapeutics. *Clin Infect Dis* 2010;**51**:1201–8.

Centers for Disease Control and Prevention. 1993 revised classification system for HIV infection and expanded surveillance case definition for AIDS among adolescents and adults. *MMWR Weekly Rep* 1992;**41**(RR-17):1–18.

Centers for Disease Control and Prevention. Surveillance of healthcare personnel with HIV/AIDS, as of December 2002. Available at: www.cdc.gov/ncid0d/dhqp/bp_hiv_hp_with.html. (accessed August 15, 2012)

Centers for Disease Control. Exposure to blood-what health-care workers need to know, 2003. Available at: www.cdc.gov/ncidod/dhqp/pdf/bbp/Exp_to_Blood.pdf.

Centers for Disease Control and Prevention. Rabies in the U.S., 2009. Available at: www.cdc.gov/rabies/location/usa/index.html (accessed September 30, 2011).

Centers for Disease Control and Prevention. HIV-2 infection surveillance-United States, 1987–2009. *MMWR Weekly Rep* 2011;**60**:985–8.

Cernik C, Gallina K, Brodell RT. The treatment of herpes simplex infections: an evidence-based review. *Arch Intern Med* 2008;**168**:1137–44.

Chadha NK, James A. Adjuvant antiviral therapy for recurrent respiratory papillomatosis. *Cochrane Database Syst Rev* 2010;(**4**):CD005053.

Chaturvedi AK, Engels EA, Pfeiffer RM, et al. Human papillomavirus and rising oropharyngeal cancer incidence in the United States. *J Clin Oncol* 2011;**29**:4294–301.

Cook CH, Trgovcich J. Cytomegalovirus reactivation in critically ill immunocompetent hosts: a decade of progress and remaining challenges. *Antiviral Res* 2011;**90**:151–9.

Cowan ML, Thomas HC, Foster GR. Therapy for chronic viral hepatitis: current indications, optimal therapies and delivery of care. *Clin Med* 2011;**11**:184–9.

Cox NH, Eedy DJ, Morton CA. Guidelines for management of Bowen's disease: 2006 update. *Br J Dermatol* 2007;**156**:11–21.

De Keyzer K, Van Laecke S, Peeters P, Vanholder R. Human cytomegalovirus and kidney transplantation: a clinician's update. *Am J Kidney Dis* 2011;**58**:118–26.

Department of Health and Human Services. Guidelines for the use of antiretroviral agents in HIV-1-infected adults and adolescents, 2011. Available at: http://aidsinfo.nih.gov/contentfiles/AdultandadolescentGL.pdf. (accessed August 15, 2012)

Dienstag JL. Hepatitis B viral infection. *N Engl J Med* 2008;**359**:1486–1500.

Dunne EF, Unger ER, Sternberg M, et al. Prevalence of HPV infection among females in the United States. *JAMA* 2007;**297**:813–19.

Dworkin RH, Johnson RW, Breuer J, et al. Recommendations for the management of herpes zoster. *Clin Infect Dis* 2007;**44**(suppl 1):S1–26.

Eslick GD. Infectious causes of esophageal cancer. *Infect Dis Clin N Am* 2010;**24**:845–52.

Fry DE. Herpesviruses: Emerging nosocomial pathogens? *Surg Infect* 2001;**2**:121–30.

Fry DE. Occupational risks of blood exposure in the operating room. *Am Surg* 2007;**73**:637–46.

Fry DE, Harris WE, Kohnke EN, Twomey CL. The influence of double-gloving on manual dexterity and tactile sensation of surgeons. *J Am Coll Surg* 2010;**210**:325–30.

Gewirtzman A, Bartlett B, Tyring S. Epidermodysplasia verruciformis and human papilloma virus. *Curr Opin Infect Dis* 2008;**21**:141–6.

Giuliano AR, Anic G, Nyitray AG. Epidemiology and pathology of HPV disease in males. *Gynecol Oncol* 2010;**117**:S15–19.

Giuliano AR, Palefsky JM, Goldstone S, et al. Efficacy of quadrivalent HPV vaccine against HPV Infection and disease in males. *N Engl J Med* 2011;**364**:401–11.

Gruhne B, Kamranvar SA, Masucci MG, Sompallae R. EBV and genomic instability – a new look at the role of the virus in the pathogenesis of Burkitt's lymphoma. *Semin Cancer Biol* 2009;**19**:394–400.

Gupta R, Warren T, Wald A. Genital herpes. *Lancet* 2007;**370**:2127–37.

Harper DM, Franco EL, Wheeler C, et al. Efficacy of a bivalent L1 virus-like particle vaccine in prevention of infection with human papillomavirus types 16 and 18 in young women: a randomised controlled trial. *Lancet* 2004;**364**:1757–65.

Heininger U, Seward JF. Varicella. *Lancet* 2006;**368**:1365–76.

Hino S, Miyata H. Torque teno virus (TTV): current status. *Rev Med Virol* 2007;**17**:45–57.

Hirsch HH, Brennan DC, Drachenberg CB, et al. Polyomavirus-associated nephropathy in renal transplantation: interdisciplinary analyses and recommendations. *Transplantation* 2005;**79**:1277–86.

Hughes SA, Wedemeyer H, Harrison PM. Hepatitis delta virus. *Lancet* 2011;**378**:73–85.

Jiang M, Abend JR, Johnson SF, Imperiale MJ. The role of polyomaviruses in human disease. *Virology* 2009;**384**:266–73.

Johnston O, Jaswal D, Gill JS, et al. Treatment of polyomavirus infection in kidney transplant recipients: a systematic review. *Transplantation* 2010;**89**:1057–70.

Kahn JA. HPV vaccination for the prevention of cervical intraepithelial neoplasia. *N Engl J Med* 2009;**361**L271–8.

Kuh C, Ward WE. Occupational viral hepatitis: an apparent hazard for medical personnel. *JAMA* 1950;**143**:631–35.

Kumar D. Emerging viruses in transplantation. *Curr Opin Infect Dis* 2010;**23**:374–8.

Kwon H, Lok AS. Hepatitis B therapy. *Nat Rev Gastroenterol Hepatol* 2011;**8**:275–84.

Liddon N, Hood J, Wynn BA, Markowitz LE. Acceptability of human papillomavirus vaccine in males: a review of the literature. *J Adolesc Health* 2010;**46**:113–23.

Linnen J, Wages J, Zhang-Keck Z-Y, et al. Molecular cloning and disease association of hepatitis G virus: a transfusion-transmissible agent. *Science* 1996;**271**:505–8.

Lipke MM. An armamentarium of wart treatments. *Clin Med Res* 2006;**4**:273–93.

Manning SE, Rupprecht CE, Fishbein D, et al. Human rabies prevention – United States, 2008: recommendations of the Advisory Committee on Immunization Practices. *MMWR* 2008;**57**(RR-3):1–28.

Odumade OA, Hogquist KA, Balfour HH Jr. Progress and problems in understanding and managing primary Epstein-Barr virus infections. *Clin Microbiol Rev* 2011;**24**:193–209.

Parkin DM, Bray F. The burden of HPV-related cancers. *Vaccine* 2006;**24**(suppl 3):S3/11–25.

Prejean J, Song R, Hernandez A, et al. Estimated HIV incidence in the United States, 2006–2009. *PLoS One* 2011;**6**:e17502.

Raghavender B, Brennan DC. Human polyoma viruses and disease with emphasis on clinical BK and JC. *J Clin Virol* 2010;**47**:306–12.

Rezazadeh A, Laber DA, Ghim S-J, Jensen BA, Kloecker G. The role of human papillomavirus in lung cancer: a review of the evidence. *Am J Med Sci* 2009;**338**:64–67.

Rosen HR. Chronic hepatitis C infection. *N Engl J Med* 2011;**364**:2429–38.

Sagir A, Kirschberg O, Heintges T, Erhardt A, Häusinger D. SEN virus infection. *Rev Med Virol* 2004;**14**:141–8.

Saundh BK, Tibble S, Baker R, et al. Different patterns of BK and JC polyomavirus reactivation following renal transplantation. *J Clin Pathol* 2010;**63**:714–8.

Shiley K, Blumberg E. Herpes viruses in transplant recipients: HSV, VZV, human herpes viruses, and EBV. *Infect Dis Clin North Am* 2010;**24**:373–93.

Smith JS, Backes DM, Hoots BE, Kurman RJ, Pimenta JM. Human papillomavirus type-distribution in vulvar and vaginal cancers and their associated precursors. *Obstet Gynecol* 2009;**113**:917–24.

Smith JS, Gilbert PA, Melendy A, Rana RK, Pimenta JM. Age-specific prevalence of human papillomavirus infection in males: a global review. *J Adolesc Health* 2011;**48**:540–52.

Stapleton JT, Foung S, Muerhoff AS, Bukh J, Simmonds P. The GB viruses: a review and proposed classification of GBV-A, GBV-C (HGV), and GBV-D in class Pegivirus within the family Flaviviridae. *J Gen Virol* 2011;**92**:233–46.

Stelow EB, Jo VY, Stoler MH, Mills SE. Human papillomavirus-associated squamous cell carcinoma of the upper aerodigestive tract. *Am J Surg Pathol* 2010;**34**:e15–24.

Tan CS, Koralnik IJ. Progressive multifocal leukoencephalopathy and other disorders caused by JC virus: clinical features and pathogenesis. *Lancet Neurol* 2010;**9**:425–37.

Trumbell ML, Greiner DJ. Homologous serum jaundice: an occupational hazard to medical personnel. *JAMA* 1951;**145**:965–67.

Uldrick TS, Whitby D. Update on KSHV epidemiology, Kaposi sarcoma pathogenesis, and treatment of Kaposi sarcoma. *Cancer Lett* 2011;**305**:150–62.

van Seters M, van Beurden M, ten Kate FJW, et al. Treatment of vulvar intraepithelial neoplasia with topical imiquimod. *N Engl J Med* 2008;**358**:1465–73.

Villa LL, Costa RL, Petta CA, et al. Prophylactic quadrivalent human papillomavirus (types 6, 11, 16, and 18) L1 virus-like particle vaccine in young women: a randomised double-blind placebo-controlled multicentre phase II efficacy trial. *Lancet Oncol* 2005;**6**:271–8.

Willoughby RE Jr: A cure for a rabies? *Sci Am* 2007;**296**:88–95.

World Health Organization. *Global summary of the AIDS epidemic*, 2009. Available at: www.who.int/hiv/data/2009_global_summary_png. (accessed August 15, 2012)

Zeuzem S, Andreone P, Pol S, et al. Teleprevir for retreatment of HCV infection. *N Engl J Med* 2011;**364**:2417–28.

Chapter 15 Cardiothoracic surgical infections

Jorge A. Wernly, Charles A. Dietl, Jess D. Schwartz

◼ THORACIC EMPYEMA

◼ Definition

An empyema is a collection of pus within the pleural cavity. Empyemas follow bacterial contamination of the pleural space. The most common source of pleural infection is a pneumonic process. Approximately 40% of all patients with pneumonia develop a parapneumonic pleural effusion (PPE) but only a small percentage result in a "complicated" empyema (Koegelenberg et al. 2008). Empyemas may also result from lung abscesses, postoperative contamination, trauma, or extension of an abscess from below the diaphragm.

Thoracic empyemas have three phases of development: The acute or exudative stage, the transitional or fibrinopurulent stage, and the chronic or organizing stage. The acute stage is characterized by accumulation of pleural fluid secondary to a contiguous pulmonary infection. If not treated appropriately it may evolve into the fibrinopurulent stage, characterized by bacterial invasion, increased white blood cells, and fibrin deposition. The organizing stage occurs when fibroblasts and capillaries grow into a thick, firm fibrin layer known as pleural peel.

◼ Clinical presentation and diagnosis

Patients usually present with fever, malaise, pleuritic chest pain, and dyspnea. The diagnosis of empyema must be suspected in patients who describe these symptoms after bronchopneumonia, or a recent surgical procedure involving the lungs, esophagus, or mediastinum, recent chest trauma, or an intra-abdominal operation.

On examination patients usually appear ill and debilitated. Some are tachypneic and hypoxic, and present with respiratory distress or generalized sepsis. Breath sounds are typically decreased on the side of the empyema. The chest radiograph is characterized by a large pleural effusion, which raises the index of suspicion of empyema. Lateral decubitus films are useful to determine if the pleural effusion is free flowing or loculated.

The diagnosis of empyema should be established by thoracocentesis and sampling the pleural fluid, which is usually cloudy and foul smelling. Gram stain with culture and sensitivity testing is the most important initial laboratory test for the diagnosis. However, the presence of a thin serous fluid or a negative Gram stain does not exclude infection of the pleural space. The pleural fluid should also be analyzed for neutrophil count, pH, glucose level, and lactate dehydrogenase (LDH). If the pleural fluid contains neutrophils ($>15\,000/mm^3$), and has a low pH (<7.20), low glucose level (<60 mg/dl), or high LDH (>1000 IU/l), there is strong evidence of pleural infection (Koegelenberg et al. 2008). Pleural fluid pH is the preferred study because it has the highest diagnostic accuracy, and requires only a blood gas analyzer. Alternative diagnostic tests for detecting nonpurulent PPE

include tumor necrosis factor-a, myeloperoxidase, matrix metalloprotease-2, neutrophil elastase, interleukin-8, lipopolysaccharide-binding protein, and other biomarkers (Porcel 2010). Bacteriological and chemical analysis of the pleural fluid is necessary to categorize parapneumonic effusions and to identify which require drainage for optimal outcomes (Colice et al. 2000).

Ultrasonography is the preferred method for guiding thoracocentesis because of loculation of the effusion, and better definition of the diaphragm than with a chest radiograph. Furthermore, ultrasonography is extremely helpful for accurate placement of a pigtail catheter drainage or tube thoracostomy. The routine use of ultrasound-guided aspiration and drainage should be encouraged, because of patient safety and better sampling of the pleural effusion. It also provides additional diagnostic and prognostic information, and more effective pleural drainage (Lee et al. 2010).

Computed tomography (CT) may be helpful to differentiate empyemas from lung abscesses, and to evaluate effectiveness of a drainage procedure. A contrast-enhanced CT scan may demonstrate multiloculated effusions, as well as a thick pleural peel or an entrapped lung. Fluid collections in the fissures or those located in the paramediastinal or paravertebral regions may be detected only by CT scan (Heffner et al. 2010). CT also allows more accurate identification of life-threatening complications after pulmonary resection, such as empyema and bronchopleural fistulas that require prompt management. Magnetic resonance imaging (MRI) and positron emission tomography (PET) have limited use in pleural space infections (Heffner et al. 2010).

◼ Pathogenesis and bacteriology

Fluid in the pleural space predisposes to secondary bacterial contamination. Empyema may occur when bacteria in high concentrations access the sterile pleural space. The most common source of pleural infection is a pneumonic process. Bacterial contamination of pleural effusions or hemothorax may also follow blunt or penetrating chest trauma. Not infrequently, empyemas follow postoperative pleural effusions. This complication is usually secondary to bronchopleural fistulas after lung resection, and anastomotic leaks after esophagectomy. Traumatic, iatrogenic, or spontaneous perforations of the thoracic esophagus may result in empyema and fulminant sepsis which are lethal if not managed promptly.

Bacteriological assessment of pleural fluid is inconsistent. Falguera et al. (2011) observed successful cultures in only 60% of patients with an uncomplicated PPE and 72% of complicated PPE. *Streptococcus pneumoniae* was the most frequently pathogen identified in 36% of uncomplicated PPEs and 48% of complicated PPEs. Other Gram-positive cocci, (*Staphylococcus aureus* and *Streptococcus viridians*), Gram-negative bacilli (*Haemophilus influenzae, Pseudomonas aeruginosa* and *Klebsiella* spp.), and anaerobes (*Bacteroides* and *Fusobacterium* spp.) were also identified in complicated PPEs.

Polymicrobial infections were more common in complicated PPEs (Falguera et al. 2011).

The rate of parapneumonic empyemas requiring hospitalization in the USA from 1996 through 2008 has increased 1.8-fold in adults (Grijalva et al. 2011). The main reason for this increase was due to a 3.3-fold increase in the rate of staphylococcal empyema. The mean length of hospitalizations was longer for staphylococcal empyema than for other pathogens. The increase in staphylococcal empyema may also be responsible for the increased rate of fatal parapneumonic empyema hospitalizations observed.

Isolation of *Candida* spp. in patients with empyema is extremely rare, and may be an important clue for suspecting gastrointestinal tract perforation (Ishiguro et al. 2010).

Prevention

Patients with a small-to-moderate free-flowing pleural effusion, negative cultures, and a normal pleural fluid (with pH >7.2) are at lowest risk of poor outcome, and do not require drainage of the pleural effusion. It will resolve after effective antibiotic therapy of the underlying pneumonia (Table 15.1). Conversely, patients with frank pus on aspirate, loculated or large free-flowing pleural effusion, those with positive cultures or Gram stains, or an abnormal pleural fluid (with pH <7.2) are at high risk of poor outcome, and will require effective drainage of the pleural effusion, in addition to antibiotics and supportive measures (**Table 15.1**) (Colice et al. 2000).

Postoperative pleural space infections are the second most common cause of empyema. The appropriate preoperative administration of prophylactic antibiotics is effective in prevention and cannot be overemphasized. However, bacterial contamination of pleural fluid after thoracotomy is usually related to bronchopleural fistulas or esophageal anastomotic leaks. Technical prevention of these serious postoperative complications is essential. The use of a pedicled intercostal muscle flap to buttress the bronchial stump and the esophagogastric anastomosis may reduce the risk of bronchopleural fistulas after pulmonary resection and the risk of intrathoracic anastomotic leaks after esophagectomy (Cerfolio et al. 2005). Prevention also includes drainage of retained blood or clots in post-traumatic hemothorax with a thoracostomy tube or thoracoscopy.

Supportive measures

Patients with empyema are usually catabolic and immunodeficient. Hypoalbuminemia is associated with poor outcome. For this reason, adequate nutritional support should be provided as soon as the diagnosis of empyema is established. Enteral feeding is often desirable. Other supportive measures include respiratory care and management of associated comorbidities (e.g., diabetes). Patients who present with hypoxia and respiratory distress require intubation and ventilator support, and those who appear toxic will need adequate fluid resuscitation and hemodynamic support including sepsis management protocols.

Antibiotic treatment

The recommended guidelines of the American College of Chest Physicians for the treatment of parapneumonic effusions are evidenced-based methods. The initial step is to recognize risk for poor outcome, and to identify which patients should undergo a drainage procedure (see Table 15.1) (Colice et al. 2000). Regardless of the categorizing risk, empirical antibiotic therapy should be dictated by the underlying pneumonic process, and modified based on culture results. (Koegelenberg et al. 2008).

Whenever possible, empirical antibiotics should be based on the Gram stain and adjusted for culture/sensitivity results. Gram-positive bacteria are usually susceptible to a combination of b-lactam/b-lactamase inhibitors such as intravenous amoxicillin with clavulanic acid, whereas carbapenem provides excellent coverage for both Gram-negative and Gram-positive bacteria.

A combination of intravenous cefuroxime and metronidazole is usually recommended for the 30% of cases of community-acquired culture-negative pleural infections. Hospital-acquired but culture-negative infections require broader-spectrum antibiotic coverage with intravenous piperacillin and tazobactam (Davies et al. 2003). Additional empirical anaerobic antibiotic coverage with metronidazole is generally advisable because anaerobic organisms are difficult to culture (Chapman and Davies 2004). Aminoglycosides are not recommended because of poor pleural penetration. Treatment with vancomycin or linezolid is indicated for meticillin-resistant Staphylococcus aureus (MRSA) infections. For patients who are allergic to penicillin and cephalosporins, a combination of ciprofloxacin and clindamycin is usually effective. Little evidence supports the duration of antibiotic treatment. Most clinicians would agree that 3 weeks of intravenous antibiotics is appropriate, provided that there is adequate drainage of the pleural fluid (Davies et al. 2003). Similar recommendations are made for postoperative and post-traumatic infections.

Drainage procedures

Thoracocentesis should be used only for diagnosis. Effective drainage should be accomplished with a tube thoracostomy (24 or 28 French [Fr]) or pigtail catheters (10–14 Fr) inserted under ultrasonic or CT guidance (Koegelenberg et al. 2008). The infected pleural space should be promptly and effectively drained after diagnosis of a complicated PPE or empyema (risk category 3 or 4; see Table 15.1). Correct positioning of the chest tube or catheter is assured with imaging rather than blind insertion without radiological guidance, irrespective of the drain size (Koegelenberg et al. 2008).

There is no consensus on the optimal size of the chest drainage tube. A large multicenter prospective study on chest tube size found

Table 15.1 Risk categorization for poor outcome in patients with parapneumonic pleural effusions.

Risk category	Radiographic appearance of pleural effusion	Bacteriology	Chemical analysis	Risk of poor outcome	Drainage procedure
1	Minimal free-flowing effusion	Unknown	pH unknown	Very low	Not indicated
2	Small-to-moderate free-flowing effusion	Negative Gram stain *and* culture	pH >7.2	Low	Not indicated
3	Large free-flowing or loculated effusion	Positive Gram stain *or* culture	pH <7.2	Moderate	Yes
4	Large free-flowing or loculated effusion	Frank pus	pH <7.0	High	Yes

no difference in outcomes between small catheters (<14-Fr gauge) and large bore (>20-Fr gauge) chest tubes (Rahman et al. 2010). In addition to providing adequate drainage, the small catheters (12 or 14 Fr) are more comfortable and easier to insert (Chapman and Davies 2004). To ensure patency, most clinicians recommend regular flushing with 30 ml of saline every 6 h, in addition to connection to suction (-20 cmH$_2$O).

According to evidence-based guidelines of the American College of Chest Physicians the use of drainage procedures alone for complicated PPE is associated with higher mortality when compared to treatment plans that include fibrinolytic or surgical approaches (Colice et al. 2000). Patients with PPE who have persistent sepsis or ineffective chest tube drainage should be considered for intrapleural fibrinolytic therapy or surgical treatment.

Intrapleural fibrinolytic therapy

Fibrinolytic agents in the pleural cavity can lyse the fibrinous septations within the infection, improve drainage, and are not associated with systemic fibrinolysis or bleeding complications (Koegelenberg et al. 2008). In a randomized double-blind study, intrapleural streptokinase (250 000 IU in 100 ml 0.9% saline) and urokinase (100 000 IU in 100 ml 0.9% saline) introduced through the chest tube over 6 days are equally effective, and both agents reduced the need for surgical treatment (Bouros et al. 1997). In another study, surgical intervention was significantly reduced to 13% for the streptokinase group compared with 45% for control participants (Diacon et al. 2004).

However, a controversial article from the First Multicenter Intrapleural Sepsis Trial (MIST-1) showed that intrapleural streptokinase did not improve mortality, the rate of surgery, or the length of hospital stay (Maskell et al. 2005). A possible explanation for the negative results is that chest tubes were usually inserted without guidance, and fibrinolytic therapy was initiated 8–28 days (median 14 days) after onset of symptoms. However, a more recent randomized study showed that intrapleural fibrinolytics decrease the rate of surgical interventions and the hospital stay, if used early in the fibrinopurulent stage (Misthos et al. 2005).

Improved results have recently been observed in the MIST-2 trial (Rahman et al. 2011) using combined intrapleural tissue plasminogen activator (tPA) and deoxyribonuclease (DNAase). The DNAase reduces viscosity in purulent exudates (Maskell et al. 2005). It is necessary to liquefy the deoxyribose nucleoproteins in the solid sediment of pus (Koegelenberg et al. 2008). The MIST-2 trial showed that the combination of tPA and DNAase significantly reduced surgical referral and hospital stay, whereas surgical referral was not significantly reduced in patients treated with either tPA or DNAase alone (Rahman et al. 2011).

In the MIST-1 trial (Maskell et al. 2005) 16% of patients died and 16% needed surgery at 3 months in the streptokinase group. However, the MIST-2 trial (Rahman et al. 2011) showed that the mortality rate at 3 months was 8%, and surgical referral was only 4% in patients treated with intrapleural tPA and DNAase.

Surgical treatment

Based on expert recommendations, the American College of Chest Physicians recommends fibrinolytics, video-assisted thoracoscopic surgery (VATS), or open surgery for managing patients with category 3 or 4 PPE (Colice et al. 2000). In a recent retrospective study, the procedure success rates were significantly lower for chest tube drainage (38%) and pigtail catheter drainage (40%), when compared with (81%) VATS or open thoracotomy (89%). Success was defined as resolution

of empyema with lung re-expansion, no sepsis, and no additional procedures (Wozniak et al. 2009).

The only randomized controlled trial comparing VATS with intrapleural streptokinase showed that VATS was more effective than fibrinolytics (Wait et al. 1997). Also, a historically controlled series showed VATS with the same success as open thoracotomy (Mackinlay et al. 1996). However, the total patients in these studies were too few to support any conclusion.

Although no significant difference in mortality was observed between surgical (10%) versus nonsurgical (16%) management of empyema in a retrospective review (Anstadt et al. 2003), deaths from several randomized controlled trials was significantly lower with open thoracotomy (1.9%), VATS (4.8%), or fibrinolytic therapy (4.3%) when compared with drainage procedures alone (8.8%) (Colice et al. 2000). Based on expert opinion, patients should be referred to surgical treatment (VATS or open thoracotomy) for ineffective chest tube drainage or persistent sepsis (Davies et al. 2003).

Thoracoscopic debridement may be considered for incompletely drained or loculated PPE, if performed during the fibrinopurulent stage (Koegelenberg et al. 2008). The objectives of VATS are to evacuate purulent collections, disrupt loculations, and remove fibrinous deposits to permit lung re-expansion. However, when empyema is in the organizing phase, VATS debridement is ineffective to remove the visceral peel encasing the lung (Lardinois et al. 2005).

Open thoracotomy may be indicated at several stages of complicated PPE or empyema (Koegelenberg et al. 2008). During the acute or exudative phase, the main indication for open surgical drainage is persistent sepsis from residual pleural fluid collections, despite drainage and antibiotics (Davies et al. 2003). Open thoracotomy should be used liberally for decortication during the chronic or organizing stage (>2 weeks) and for Gram-negative organisms (Lardinois et al. 2005). Decortication is a major surgical procedure that consists of resecting all the fibrous layers causing entrapment to effect lung re-expansion (Koegelenberg et al. 2008). Most patients who undergo decortication can be discharged in 1 or 2 weeks without chest tubes. The reported mortality rate of open decortication ranges from 2% to 10% (Colice et al. 2000, Anstadt et al. 2003).

However, in elderly debilitated and immunocompromised patients, open decortication is associated with significant morbidity and mortality. An open thoracic window is a safer alternative to provide adequate drainage in poor-risk patients. This procedure should be delayed until the lung surface is adhered to the parietal pleura to avoid pneumothorax. The open thoracic window, or modified Eloesser flap, is usually performed under general anesthesia and consists of resecting portions of two or three ribs, and creating an inverted U-shaped flap of skin and subcutaneous tissue to marsupialize the most dependent portion of the empyema cavity (Thourani et al. 2003). The procedure is safe, effective, and definitive for poor-risk patients with chronic empyema. The 30-day mortality rate in this high-risk group of patients was 5%, with no long-term morbidity from the procedure. Other surgical indications for the modified Eloesser flap include post-resectional, post-traumatic, and tuberculosis-related empyemas (Thourani et al. 2003).

In patients with post-pneumonectomy empyema, the infected pleural space can be initially sterilized with daily antibiotic irrigation of the thoracic cavity as described by Clagett and Geraci (1963), followed by skeletal muscle transposition to obliterate the residual pleural space. When a bronchopleural fistula is present, a modified Clagett technique consisting of pedicled skeletal muscle to cover the stump at open drainage is associated with an 80% survival rate (Deschamps et al. 2001).

STERNAL WOUND INFECTIONS

Definition

Sternal wound infection is an uncommon but potentially devastating complication of cardiac surgery. Sternal wound infections are classified as superficial or deep. Deep sternal wound infections (DSWIs) may involve the sternum, retrosternal space, or both. A precise distinction between the two types of infection is crucial, because the therapeutic approach is different. Superficial infections have good prognosis, whereas DSWIs are associated with significant morbidity and mortality, prolonged hospitalization, and increased costs. Several publications in the 1980s included sterile wound dehiscence, and the terms "sternitis" and "mediastinitis" were used synonymously to define sternal wound infections. To standardize the definition of DSWIs, the Oakley classification of mediastinitis includes five subtypes: Type I within 2 weeks, type II 2–6 weeks after surgery, type III is the presence of risk factors, type IV is failed prior treatment, and type V is presentation more than 6 weeks after the operation (El Oakley and Wright 1996).

Incidence

The current incidence of DSWIs in large series of patients ranges from 0.59% to 2.6% (**Table 15.2**). Most of these are retrospective analyses of cardiac operations using midline sternotomy incisions. According to the STS database, the rate of mediastinitis was 0.6% among 331 429 coronary artery bypass graft (CABG) cases. However, it primarily captures acute events, and many later infections may not be recorded (Fowler et al. 2005b). Although some suggest that the rate of DSWIs may be increasing because of increasing patient risk, recent data suggest that DSWIs are actually decreasing due to better management of patient risk (Matros et al. 2010).

The Dutch multicenter surveillance study (Manniën et al. 2011) found that sternal surgical site infections (SSIs) were more frequently associated with diabetes, obesity, preoperative length of stay, and reoperations. Multivariate analysis demonstrated the following risk factors as independent predictors of DSWIs: Diabetes (odds ratio [OR] = 1.7), obesity (OR = 2.2), chronic lung disease (OR = 2.3), preoperative length of stay >3 days (OR = 1.9), respiratory failure (OR = 3.2), combined valve/CABG procedures (OR = 1.9), and re-exploration for bleeding (OR = 6.3) (Filsoufi et al. 2009). The same authors observed that the mortality rate was 14.2% in patients who had DSWIs compared with 3.6% in the control group. The 5-year survival rate was also decreased in patients who developed DSWIs (55.8% ± 5.6% vs 82.0% ± 0.6%) (Filsoufi et al. 2009). Thus, risk assessment and proper prevention are important.

Pathogenesis and bacteriology

Infections occur in cardiac surgical procedures because of multiple incisions and ports, prolonged anesthesia time, and impaired immune responsiveness among many patients (El Oakley and Wright 1996). An additional risk to increase infections includes reduction of sternal blood supply from harvesting of the internal mammary artery (IMA), especially if bilateral IMAs are utilized. Excessive use of electrocautery, foreign bodies (including wax), hematoma, and sternal instability have been implicated. Blood transfusion increases infections due to transfusion-induced immunosuppression.

Most DSWIs are caused by Gram-positive bacteria, particularly *S. aureus* and *S. epidermidis*. Polymicrobial infections are not uncommon, and Gram-negative bacteria may account for up to 35% of DSWIs. Gårdlund et al. (2002) identified three different types of DSWIs according to the microbiology and pathogenesis:

1. DSWIs associated with obesity or chronic obstructive lung disease secondary to coagulase-negative staphylococci and with sternal dehiscence
2. DSWIs caused by perioperative contamination of the mediastinal space by *S. aureus* in patients usually with stable sternums
3. DSWIs caused by spread from concomitant infections, often secondary to Gram-negative rods (*Klebsiella* and *Enterobacter* spp.).

Outbreaks of mediastinitis from Gram-negative organisms such as *Pseudomona* or *Serratia* spp. are usually secondary to nosocomial spread (Gårdlund et al. 2002).

Candida spp. infections are very infrequent, and have been associated with prolonged mechanical ventilation, and in those with a reoperation before the diagnosis of a DSWI (Modrau et al. 2009). DSWIs secondary to candida infection are associated with a very high mortality. The in-hospital all-cause mortality rate was 35% in patients with candida DSWIs compared with 15% in bacterial infections, and the 1-year all-cause mortality rate was 41% with candida DSWIs compared with 23% in patients with bacterial infection.

Prevention

The Surgical Care Improvement Project (SCIP) was created in 2006 with the goal of reducing surgical complications by 25% by the year 2010 (Bratzler et al. 2006). SCIP is a national campaign and partnership of leading public and private healthcare organizations. Several SCIP measures were introduced to reduce the incidence of SSI. Six of the nine performance measures are related to SSI prevention (Bratzler et al. 2006) and five have relevance to cardiac surgery (**Table 15.3**).

Table 15.2 Incidence of DSWIs in recent series.

First author	Year	Patients	Patients with DSWIs (%)
Gårdlund	2002	9557	126 (1.32)
Gummert	2002	9303	134 (1.44)
Lu	2003	4228	109 (2.60)
Crabtree	2004	4004	73 (1.80)
Friedman	2007	4987	62 (1.33)
Filsoufi	2009	5798	106 (1.80)
Ariyaratnam	2010	7602	44 (0.59)
DSWIs, deep sternal wound infections.			

Table 15.3 SCIP-Infection module and outcome measures.

SCIP-Inf module	Core measures
SCIP-Inf-1	Prophylactic antibiotic received within 1 h before surgical incision
SCIP-Inf-2	Prophylactic antibiotic selection for surgical patient
SCIP-Inf-3	Prophylactic antibiotic discontinued within 24 h of surgery end time (48 h after cardiac surgery end time)
SCIP-Inf-4	Cardiac surgery patients with controlled 6am postoperative blood glucose level (<200 mg/dl)
SCIP-Inf-5	Postoperative surgical site infection diagnosed during index hospitalization
SCIP-Inf-6	Surgery patients with appropriate hair removal
Inf, infection; SCIP, Surgical Care Improvement Project.	

Appropriate administration of prophylactic antibiotics is covered in the first three SCIP measures (see Chapter 4) (Fry 2008).

In addition to appropriate administration of prophylactic antibiotics, SCIP-4 and SCIP-6 have special significance for cardiac surgery. SCIP-4 requires perioperative glycemic control of cardiac cases because of the increased risk of DSWIs in patients with diabetes and poorly controlled hyperglycemia. Furnary and associates (2003) demonstrated that appropriate glycemic control (<200 mg/dl) with continuous insulin infusion reduces DSWIs and mortality in patients with diabetes who undergo cardiac surgical procedures. Glycemic control before and during the operation, and over the entire postoperative course, should be universally applied to all cardiac surgical patients to reduce the risk of SSIs. The increased use of perioperative intravenous insulin may explain the reduction of DSWIs in recent studies (Matros et al. 2010).

Another core measure, SCIP-6, refers to appropriate hair removal with electric clippers immediately before the skin incision. Advanced hair removal should not be done and straight razors should not be used at all because microbial growth in skin abrasions may lead to wound colonization.

An association between SCIP performance and clinical outcomes has not been demonstrated on individual SCIP measures. However, adherence to all-or-none SCIP-Inf measures was associated with decreased likelihood of developing an SSI (Stulberg et al. 2010).

In a recent retrospective study, Trussell et al. (2008) observed that timely perioperative antibiotic administration, tight blood glucose control, and hair removal with clippers significantly decreased SSI rates in CABG patients.

As the patient's skin is a major source of pathogens that may cause SSIs, effective skin decolonization can be accomplished with a 4% chlorhexidine shower the evening and morning before surgery, followed by a chlorhexidine–alcohol scrub instead of a povidone–iodine scrub or paint for skin preparation in the operating room (Darouiche et al. 2010).

A well-controlled, multicenter, randomized study by Bode et al. (2010) demonstrated the efficacy of preoperative screening of nasal carriers of *S. aureus* followed by decontamination with intranasal mupirocin twice a day over 5 days, in addition to daily baths with chlorhexidine soap. According to the Society of Thoracic Surgeons' practice guidelines, routine mupirocin administration is recommended for all patients undergoing cardiac surgical procedures in the absence of a documented negative testing for staphylococcal colonization. In fact, most cardiac surgical programs have instituted a routine protocol for intranasal mupirocin beginning at least the day before surgery (sooner, if elective) and continuing for 2–5 days after surgery (Engelman et al. 2007).

In addition to the SCIP measures, the avoidance of blood transfusions, the judicious use of electrocautery, and selective use of bilateral IMA are practices that should decrease DSWIs. Sternal ischemia may be minimized by skeletonization of one or both IMAs during harvesting, which has been associated with a reduction in DSWI rates. The application of topical vancomycin to the cut sternal edges may also reduce postoperative DSWI, although evidence is currently not available.

Clinical presentation and diagnosis

Sternal wound infections may present acutely with generalized sepsis during the first or second week after the operation (type I). The diagnosis of mediastinitis may be difficult to establish during the early stages. After cardiac surgery, patients who present with septicemia and positive blood cultures frequently have mediastinitis, and evidence of SSIs may not become evident until the second postoperative week. In a prospective infection control surveillance study at Duke University, mediastinitis occurred in 76.7% of patients with blood cultures positive for *S. aureus*, but only in 11.9% patients with blood cultures positive for other pathogens, suggesting that *S. aureus* bacteremia after CABG strongly predicts the presence of mediastinitis, whereas other bacteremias did not alter the clinical suspicion of mediastinitis (Fowler et al. 2005).

Mortality rates can be >50% in patients who present with generalized sepsis. The risk of death is significantly higher for patients with persistently positive bacteremia, non-CABG cardiac surgery, and receiving prolonged mechanical ventilation. Mortality is usually higher with sepsis due to Gram-negative bacteria and *S. aureus* (Olsen et al. 2008).

Thus, a timely diagnosis is essential. Unfortunately, imaging studies such as CT and radioisotope scans are usually non-diagnostic during the early stages. Mediastinal fluid collections or free gas bubbles are not specific during the early postoperative period, because these findings may be present in patients without mediastinitis. However, these observations could be indicative of mediastinitis when present >21 days after surgery (Yamashiro et al. 2008). Clinical correlation with imaging may dictate the need to explore the wound to obtain multiple cultures and tissue sampling to confirm the diagnosis. Multiple tissue samplings before administration of antibiotics are necessary to ensure a microbiologically correct diagnosis that identifies the primary pathogen (Tammelin et al. 2002).

A more common scenario for presentation of DSWIs is between the second and sixth postoperative weeks (types II, II, or IV), usually with purulent drainage and sternal instability. These physical findings are usually diagnostic. However, in some patients fever and leukocytosis may be the only clinical manifestations during several days before the diagnosis can be established. Other non-specific symptoms may be increasing wound pain, with localized redness and tenderness. A CT scan combined with granulocyte antibody scintigraphy may be of help to distinguish between deep and superficial sternal infections (Bitkover et al. 1996).

Sternal wound infections may also present more than 6 weeks postoperatively as chronic or recurrent osteomyelitis (type V). Imaging studies are important to confirm or exclude the diagnosis of chronic osteomyelitis. MRI and CT lack specificity in chronic osteomyelitis (Prandini et al. 2006) and, although leukocyte scintigraphy has acceptable accuracy to diagnose chronic osteomyelitis in the peripheral skeleton, fluorodeoxyglucose (FDG) PET has the highest diagnostic accuracy for detecting chronic osteomyelitis in the axial skeleton (Termaat et al. 2005) (**Figure 15.1**). In addition, PET is a valuable tool that allows accurate assessment of residual activity after medical or surgical treatment (Prandini et al. 2006).

Treatment

Type I mediastinitis can usually be treated with thorough debridement and a closed mediastinal irrigation–suction system. A safe and effective initial step for rapid control of sepsis consists of reopening the entire incision, removal of all sternal wires, and debridement of necrotic tissue. However, in mediastinitis types II and III, wound debridement and closed mediastinal irrigation have been associated with high failure rates and up to 35% mortality rates, whereas open wound packing followed by pedicle flap closure has a significantly lower mortality. More recently the vacuum-assisted closure (VAC) device has been applied to open sternal wounds to facilitate granulation tissue formation after aggressive sternal debridement or total

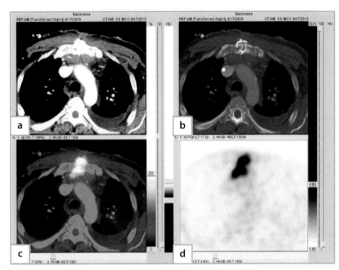

Figure 15.1 **CT/PET scan performed 6 weeks after coronary artery bypass graft demonstrates infection** (using intravenous 15.1 mCi fluorodexoyglucose [FDG]; computed tomography (CT)/positron emission tomography (PET) fusion images were obtained 1 h after FDG administration). (a,b) The CT scan fails to reveal involvement of the sternum. (c,d) PET scan shows FDG-avid soft tissue phlegmon and sternal involvement, with phlegmon extending into the mediastinum.

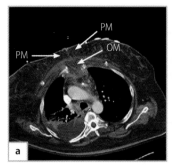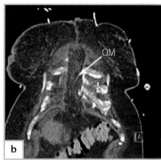

Figure 15.2 **Computed tomography (CT) scan of the chest shows satisfactory reconstruction.** The study was performed 7 days after chest wall reconstruction using a pedicled omental flap (OM) and bilateral pectoralis major muscle flaps (PM). Scanning was performed after administration of 100 ml Isovue-300 intravenous contrast. Images were reconstructed at 3-mm increments. (a) Axial view; (b) coronal view.

sternectomy (Scholl et al. 2004). Some have identified improved stabilization of open sternal wounds and decreased need for paralysis and mechanical ventilation with the VAC.

Definitive treatment requires flap reconstruction with viable tissue after debridement or sternectomy, whether the wound is initially packed open, or temporarily covered with a VAC device. Staged sternectomy and delayed flap reconstruction are also indicated after other treatment methods have failed (type IV), or in chronic sternal infections (type V). The choice of flap closure depends on the experience of the surgical team, and plastic surgeons familiar with these procedures. Bilateral pedicled pectoralis major muscle flaps have been used successfully to cover the entire wound (Scholl et al. 2004). However, coverage of the lower third of the open sternal wound may not be feasible using pectoralis muscles only.

Other reconstructive options include the use of a pedicled rectus abdominis muscle flap as an adjunct to a unilateral pectoralis major muscle flap (Roh et al. 2008), or a combination of omental flap and pectoralis major flaps (Kobayashi et al. 2011) (**Figure 15.2**). Omental flaps have the advantage that they are technically easy to harvest and the procedure can be performed by cardiac surgeons (Van Wingerden et al. 2011). Furthermore, omental transposition flaps are significantly less likely than muscle flaps to require a reoperation in patients with diabetes. In our experience, the use of a pedicled omental flap and partial mobilization of bilateral pectoralis muscles to cover the omentum have been very effective to treat DSWIs.

INFECTIONS OF THE MEDIASTINUM

Mediastinal infections are some of the most vexing and challenging problems that a physician can face. Effective treatment requires an understanding of the anatomy and pathophysiology, and a thorough knowledge of the literature. Infections of the mediastinum can be divided into acute and chronic categories. Acute mediastinitis is often the result of iatrogenic injury or spontaneous perforation of the aerodigestive tract. Chronic infections tend to be self-limiting but may progress into the clinical entity of chronic fibrosing mediastinitis as a result of fungal or tubercular infections.

The low incidence of these infections and their clinical heterogeneity precludes the scrutiny of large, stratified, double-blind, placebo-controlled, clinical trials to help the clinician with treatment options. To obtain sufficient material to allow statistical testing, "contemporary" reviews span decades of evolving clinical experiences (Freeman et al. 2000, Richardson 2005). The literature about the management of patients with mediastinitis in the past was therefore often anecdotal, confusing, and controversial. Finally, the clinical picture of these infections is changing. Once the exclusive domain of the thoracic surgeon, mediastinal infections are now often treated by minimally invasive means. Advanced endoscopy, invasive radiology, and particularly video-assisted thoracic procedures are altering currently held paradigms.

Anatomic considerations of the mediastinum

The mediastinum is defined as the space between the two lateral pleural sacs, posterior to the sternum and anterior to the vertebral column, inferior to the thoracic inlet and superior to the diaphragm. Important anatomic considerations include the fact that the fascial planes in the neck are continuous with those in the mediastinum and allow extension of infection from the neck to the chest. Deep cervical fascial layers separate the neck into three compartments: Retrovisceral, pretracheal, and perivascular. Each of these fascial planes allows direct extension downward into the mediastinum. Gravity, respiration, and negative intrathoracic pressure are all believed to facilitate intrathoracic spread of the infectious process. The posterior mediastinum is also continuous with the retroperitoneum inferiorly. Mediastinal infections can spread to the retroperitoneum via this route, whereas spread from the mediastinum to the neck is unusual. Spread of infection from the retroperitoneum or subphrenic areas to the mediastinum has been described for many years and remains an important though infrequent cause of acute mediastinitis. Finally, the lack of an esophageal serosa allows bacteria and alimentary contents direct access to the mediastinum when a perforation occurs.

Descending necrotizing mediastinitis

Descending necrotizing mediastinitis (DNM) is a form of acute mediastinitis spreading from the cervical region to the mediastinal connective tissue via the cervical facial planes. Pearse (1938) described 110 patients with suppurative mediastinitis from descending cervical infection and recorded 21 instances secondary to oropharyngeal infection. This report had an overall mortality rate of 55% with 86% occurring in nonsurgical patients and 35% in surgical patient. Although uncommon, this condition remains a life-threatening form of acute mediastinitis. Until the introduction of modern antimicrobial therapy, CT, and aggressive surgical intervention, this form of mediastinitis has continued to produce reported mortality rates between 25% and 40% (Freeman et al. 2000).

Etiology and incidence

Acute mediastinitis may results from oral, odontogenic, and peritonsillar infections that cause oropharyngeal abscesses (Ludwig angina) with severe cervical infection spreading along to the fascial planes into the mediastinum (Estrera et al. 1983). Inadvertent iatrogenic esophageal intubations, instrumentation, and penetrating trauma may cause cervical infections which may also extend to the mediastinum. Furthermore, any surgical procedure on the neck, including lymph node biopsy, thyroidectomy, tracheostomy, and mediastinoscopy, can rarely cause subsequent mediastinitis.

The bacteriological features of DNM have been well documented as polymicrobial with both aerobic and anaerobic bacteria reflecting the flora of the oral cavity (Brook et al. 1996). A synergistic effect occurs as the aerobes cause a change to the local blood supply to the deep tissues of the neck thereby allowing anaerobes to grow without oxygen. In this sense, these infections are similar to other aggressive necrotizing infections such as necrotizing fasciitis and Fournier gangrene, in which aggressive surgical debridement and drainage is life saving (Freeman et al. 2000). Antibiotics alone will not suffice. Furthermore, conditions that predispose certain patient populations to this serious infection have been characterized and include: Diabetes (13.3%), alcoholism (17.7%), neoplasm (4.4%), and radiation necrosis (3.3%).

Diagnosis

In 1983, Estrera et al. (1983) formalized the description of an acute purulent mediastinal infection arising as the result of a severe oropharyngeal infection as "descending necrotizing mediastinitis." Inclusion criteria for such a diagnosis include the following:

1. Clinical manifestation of severe oropharyngeal infection
2. Demonstration of characteristic radiological features of mediastinitis
3. Documentation of necrotizing mediastinitis at surgery or postmortem examination or both
4. Establishment of relationship between oropharyngeal infection and development of necrotizing mediastinal process

Diagnosis of DNM mandates that the relationship between mediastinitis and oropharyngeal infection be clearly established. A high index of suspicion in any patient with a deep cervical infection is warranted and should prompt rapid evaluation with the appropriate diagnostic studies. Clinical features that may help the clinician include substernal chest pain, stridor, brawny or pitting edema overlying the neck and chest, and crepitus. With progression of the disease, pleural and pericardial effusion occur which may lead to diminished breath sounds and oxygen saturations, and even pericardial tamponade. CT is the most useful test to rapidly establish a diagnosis of a deep cervical infection from one of the previously mentioned causes. Radiographic findings are likely to demonstrate soft-tissue edema with distortion of normal fascial planes. As mentioned above, pleural and pericardial fluid collections are also often present. Clinical findings have been categorized by (1) widening of the retrocervical space with or without an air–fluid level, (2) anterior displacement of the tracheal air column, (3) mediastinal emphysema, and (4) loss of the normal lordosis in the cervical spine (**Figure 15.3**). These same authors also recommended addition of thoracotomy to cervicotomy whenever the inflammatory process descended to the level of the carina anteriorly or the T4 vertebra posteriorly. Repeat neck, chest, and abdominal CT scans are recommended for any patient with clinical deterioration, even if an adequate surgical intervention was undertaken to identify disease progression.

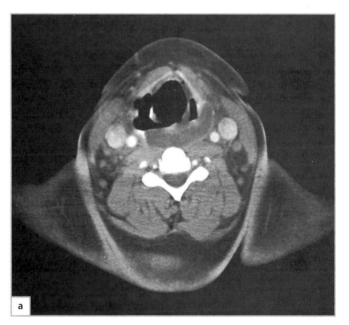

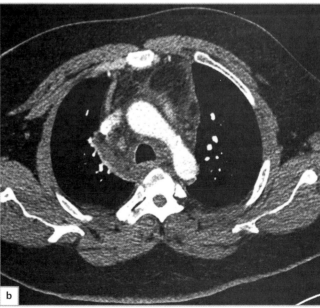

Figure 15.3 Computed tomography (CT) scan of the neck and chest with intravenous contrast demonstrates descending necrotizing mediastinitis from cervical pharyngeal infection. (a) Representative neck images showing large retropharyngeal collection. (b) Chest image showing extensive air infiltration of all mediastinal compartments.

Treatment

The treatment of DNM includes broad-spectrum antimicrobial therapy with the intention to cover both aerobes and anaerobes of oropharyngeal origin. In addition, particular care must be placed on ensuring and maintaining an adequate airway because there may be respiratory embarrassment with the ongoing swelling within the cervical region. These measures alone will not, however, suffice, and appropriate and aggressive surgical debridement and drainage are essential to reduce mortality. There is consensus that an aggressive cervical approach by either a unilateral or bilateral sternocleidomastoid muscle incision or a collar incision is appropriate. Important surgical pearls of such an approach are to open all three compartments of the neck, i.e., pretracheal, prevertebral, and perivascular. Whether to add a transthoracic approach is a bit more controversial. Estrera et al. (1983) have championed the concept that, if the preoperative radiological findings demonstrate infection at or below the level of the carina anteriorly or the T4 vertebrate posteriorly, then a transthoracic approach is mandated.

Since the 1990s, however, most authors, including Temes et al. (1998) from our institution, have reported superior outcomes with a combined transcervical and transthoracic approach. Corsten et al. (1997) solidified this view with a comprehensive literature review over the era beginning with the availability of CT scans. This consisted of 36 previous reports including a total cohort of 69 patients. When subjected to meta-analysis, this study found that 47% of patients died when surgery was limited to transcervical drainage alone, whereas the mortality rate was only 19% when a thoracic incision was added ($p <0.05$). Freeman et al. (2000) published their results on 10 patients with zero mortality. They attribute their results to an aggressive multidisciplinary effort involving head and neck, thoracic, and oral-maxillofacial surgeons. The mean number of surgical procedures was 6 ± 2 procedures per patient, reflecting aggressive attitudes toward reoperation. The preferred thoracic approach to use, whether posterolateral thoracotomy, sternotomy, clamshell, or VATS appears to be of less importance, so long as all the compartments of the mediastinum are widely debrided and drained. But, clearly, a standard posterolateral thoracotomy provides very good exposure to the pleural cavity, and the pericardium prevertebral and paraesophageal planes without the risk of sternal osteomyelitis. This aggressive approach has lead to a decrease in the overall mortality rate to 19% (Corsten et al. 1997).

◼ Esophageal perforation

Esophageal perforation is a rare but potentially catastrophic event with mortality rates in the past as high at 80% (Kuppusamy et al. 2011). The successful management requires prompt recognition and sound clinical judgment, because the consequences of delayed or incorrect decisions can be devastating.

Care of these patients therefore requires a thorough understanding of both esophageal pathophysiology and anatomy. The esophagus is a unique structure that lies within the cervical, mediastinal and abdominal compartments of the body. Unlike other viscera of the digestive tract it has no mesentery and lacks a serosal layer, which allows perforation to develop into an extensive infection. This results from the leakage of ingested material and gastrointestinal secretions leading to an intense combined chemical and infectious mediastinitis. Injuries to this organ that go unrecognized or are not treated expeditiously can lead to extremely high mortality rates. Historically, surgical therapy was considered the standard of care with improved outcomes linked to surgical interventions within the first 24 h after injury (Brinster et al. 2004). Nonsurgical management was first reported by Cameron et al. (1979) and this has expanded endoscopic and minimally invasive therapies over the last three decades. With greater experience, improved technologies and critical care recent series report mortality rates ranging from 2% to 20% (Kuppusamy et al. 2011).

Etiology and incidence

In the USA and Europe most esophageal injuries (60%) are iatrogenic (Brinster et al. 2004). Most have acute presentations, but subacute and chronic courses have been reported. Different inclusion criteria prevent concrete statements regarding incidence, but two conclusions appear to be justified: (1) Esophageal disruptions are rare and (2) they are most often caused by medical intervention usually as part of an endoscopic procedure as therapy for a stricture or achalasia. Although the rate of injury from esophagoscopy alone is very low (0.03%), perforations after dilation for peptic stricture occur in 1% of patients, and 5% after balloon dilation of achalasia (Silvis et al. 1976). Barotrauma or Boerhaave syndrome account for 15–30% of cases with trauma, foreign body ingestion, and surgical injury making up the remaining benign causes of perforations. Non-iatrogenic rupture of a normal esophagus usually follows forceful vomiting (Boerhaave syndrome), but is also associated with defecation, lifting, seizure, pregnancy, and childbirth. Any instrument placed in the pharynx, especially in emergency situations, can perforate the esophagus. Thus, nasogastric, Sengstaken–Blakemore, and endotracheal tubes in high-risk populations (elderly, bedridden, swallowing impaired patients) can be responsible. Even ingestion of certain pills (antibiotics, anti-inflammatory agents, potassium, and quinidine) can lead to esophageal perforation.

Anastomotic leaks account for most of the esophageal problems associated with surgical procedures (Richardson 2005). Inadvertent injuries during thyroidectomy, pneumonectomy, vagotomy, and antireflux procedures have been reported. External trauma can involve the esophagus, but in salvageable patients it is usually limited to the cervical region. Traumatic injury to the thoracic esophagus most often involves serious associated injuries that preclude survival. An abnormal esophagus is at increased risk of perforation. Malignant perforation is ominous and usually rapidly fatal, although under certain conditions it can be palliated. Perforations after lye ingestion or during fulminant esophageal infections are also well documented. With caustic injuries it is important to distinguish between acid and alkali ingestion: Alkali typically injures the esophagus and spares the stomach; acid does the opposite. Although mediastinitis can occur after acid ingestion and esophagogastrectomy may be required, gastric rather than esophageal injury is the hallmark of acid ingestion. An impressive variety of foreign bodies accounts for a large percentage of esophageal perforations. Innocuous items such as carbonated beverages or tortilla chips have caused perforations in patients with occult esophageal disease. Brinster et al. (2004) reported in 559 patients that 59% were caused by esophageal instrumentation, 15% were spontaneous perforations, foreign body ingestion in 12%, trauma in 9%, surgical injury in 2%, tumor in 1%, and others were 2%. This compared similarly with the prior comprehensive review of 511 perforations of Jones and Ginberg (1992). They found 43% were secondary to instrumentation, 19% by trauma, 16% spontaneous, 7% by foreign bodies, 8% from surgical injury, and 7% from other causes. In this review, endoscopy alone accounted for 35% of perforations by instrumentation, pneumatic dilation caused 25%, and bougienage caused 20%. Faulty endotracheal intubation, Sengstaken–Blakemore tubes, nasogastric tubes, sclerotherapy, and endoesophageal prostheses caused 20% of iatrogenic perforations.

It is important to maintain the distinction between esophageal perforation and mediastinitis, because it is the potential source of considerable confusion. An esophageal perforation may or may not develop into mediastinitis. Small mucosal rents can usually heal spontaneously. Although large tears that communicate with the pleura often require surgical intervention, leaks associated with slow erosion such as foreign bodies are more likely to be contained by local inflammatory reaction without invasive mediastinitis. A subset of lesser perforations, if discovered early, can be prevented from progressing to mediastinitis by non-invasive or endoluminal stenting. Furthermore, the mere presence of mediastinal air (pneumomediastinum) does not necessarily equate with mediastinitis. This entity is typically the result of some form of barotrauma and, although an expeditious diagnostic workup with an esophagram is indicated in any patient with pneumomediastinum to rule out a perforation, very often these studies are negative (Caceres et al. 2008). Again, the preceding history, inciting events, and clinical presentation can help aid diagnostic and treatment decision-making.

Finally, bacteriology is non-specific. Cultures are usually polymicrobial reflecting normal oral flora and can include Gram-negative, Gram-positive, aerobic, anaerobic organisms, and even yeasts. The most common are streptococci, *Pseudomonas* spp., and *Candida* spp. (Brook et al. 1996).

Diagnosis

Clinical presentation depends on the cause and site of injury along with the length of time from perforation. The diagnosis of esophageal perforation should obviously be considered in any patient presenting with suspicious symptoms after endoscopy or instrumentation. Chest pain, dyspnea, odynophagia, and dysphagia are often present. Associated fevers and signs of sepsis or shock are particularly ominous. The differential diagnosis includes myocardial infarction, pulmonary embolism, pneumonia, spontaneous pneumothorax, aortic dissection, pancreatitis, peptic ulcer, and esophagitis. Pain is the most frequent symptom. It varies with the location of injury and may be found in the neck, chest, back, or abdomen. It can be constant or pleuritic. A history of dysphagia, vomiting, or dyspnea may be present and physical findings are usually non-specific. Cervical crepitus is common with cervical injuries (Pate et al. 1989). Surprisingly, leukocytosis and fever are not uniform findings. Pleural effusion with a strongly acid pH, bile, or gross food particles establishes the diagnosis.

During the initial evaluation it is critical to determine the physiological stability of the patient. This is done together with treatment of any pain, and resuscitation of any hypotension or sepsis before choosing the necessary diagnostic workup. Once resuscitation has commenced and stability has been assured, diagnostic radiology with an esophagram (**Figure 15.4**) and/or a CT scan (**Figure 15.5**) is extremely valuable. Chest radiographs appear abnormal in >90% of patients although they must be carefully interpreted (Han et al. 1985). Common findings include pneumothorax, pleural effusion, mediastinal emphysema, air–fluid levels, and foreign bodies. Mediastinal widening may be present. Pneumothorax is usually on the left, but right or even bilateral accumulations are reported. Although these non-specific findings are common, they represent advanced manifestations. Definitive diagnosis can be made with a contrast esophagram in 90% of patients. In the past controversy existed as to whether to use a water-soluble contrast such as Gastrografin or barium should be employed (White and Morris 1992). However, barium contrast is 22% more accurate than water-soluble contrast (Buecker et al. 1997). Although there are concerns that barium contamination increases mediastinal or pleural inflammation, these have been found to be inaccurate. Barium should not, however, be used as the first-line contrast simply because large-volume extravasation can impair subsequent

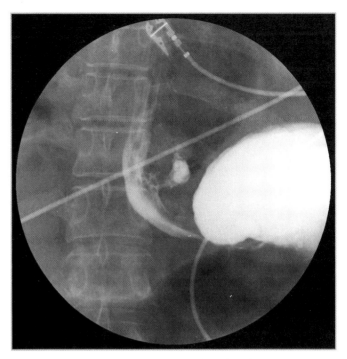

Figure 15.4 Barium swallow showing esophageal perforation. Image revealed large collection of barium outside the lumen of the distal esophagus.

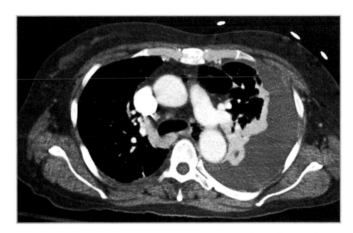

Figure 15.5 Computed tomography (CT) scan of the chest showing large left pleural effusion. There is mediastinal air next to the esophagus and a large effusion with compression of the lung.

swallows and CT scans. Most authors recommend an initial study with water-soluble contrast followed by a barium study only for patients who had negative findings (Brinster et al. 2004, Strauss et al. 2010).

A CT scan immediately after a contrast swallow may be valuable if the esophagram is equivocal in patients whose clinical presentation is consistent with perforation. Furthermore, they are often necessary in patients with intubation and septic shock in whom a contrast esophagram cannot be performed. In addition to demonstrating the perforation, the CT scan may also demonstrate the site of perforation and assist in decisions about the surgical approach.

In the past, the diagnostic utility of esophagoscopy was controversial. Certain authors found that it adds little to the esophagograms (Bladergroen et al. 1986). However, with the increasing use of non-operative endoluminal treatments, esophagoscopy has become extremely important as a means of both diagnosis and therapy.

Certainly, patients with a trapped foreign body that has perforated benefit from endoscopic removal. Intraluminal assessment of the extent of injury defines whether minimally invasive management is appropriate. Panendoscopy is also part of the standard workup for evaluation of patients with penetrating neck trauma. Several series of such patients have found that the sensitivity and specificity are >90% (Arantes et al. 2009). These results are much better than barium contrast swallow studies, which have a 10% false-negative result (Wu et al. 2007). Lastly, if pleural fluid seen can be drained by thoracocentesis, finding undigested food, a pH <6, or salivary amylase confirms the diagnosis of perforation in the proper clinical setting (Attar et al. 1990).

The diagnosis can be difficult and is often delayed beyond 24 h in up to half of all patients (Pate et al. 1989, Jones and Ginsberg 1992, White et al. 1992). The most common reasons for delay are failure to recognize symptoms (55%), misinterpretation of chest radiographs (25%), and atypical or mild symptoms (9.5%) (Jones and Ginsberg 1992). False-negative water-soluble and barium swallows do occur, and a negative test does not definitively mean that there is not a leak. However, it does support an initial nonsurgical approach unless there are severe signs and symptoms. Exploration is justified despite negative radiological and endoscopic findings if the clinical suspicion remains high (Bladergroen et al. 1986).

Treatment

Immediate, aggressive supportive therapy should be instituted in all patients with esophageal perforation. This includes ensuring an adequate airway, intravenous hydration, empirical broad-spectrum intravenous antibiotics, gastric decompression, pharyngeal aspiration, and chest physiotherapy (Jones and Ginsberg 1992). It is unfortunate that this high level of active intervention is commonly called "conservative management" in the literature. Goals of therapy for esophageal perforations of any type include the classic principles of:

- prevention of further contamination
- elimination of infection
- restoration of gastrointestinal integrity if possible
- provision of nutritional support, ideally enteral.

This of course can include wide debridement of infected and necrotic tissue, removal of distal obstruction, broad-spectrum antimicrobial therapy, and either closure or diversion of the perforation (Pate et al. 1989). Although certain general principles may exist, treatment of an individual patient must be directed by specific analysis of the cause, anatomic location, diagnostic delay, underlying pathology, and physiological condition (White et al. 1992).

Nonsurgical management

Nonsurgical management of esophageal perforation is appropriate in select patients with well-contained perforations and minimal mediastinal and pleural contamination. Expectant nonsurgical therapy limited to aggressive supportive measures alone should be reserved for patients with small, contained, minimally symptomatic esophageal perforations that drain back into the esophagus (Cameron et al. 1979). These patients do not have mediastinitis; rather they have contained processes that may or may not progress to fulminant infection. As such, therapy is intended to prevent, rather than treat, mediastinitis. Criteria for nonsurgical management have been suggested (Altorjay et al. 1997) including:

1. Early diagnosis or leak contained if diagnosis delayed
2. Leak contained within neck or mediastinum, or between mediastinum and visceral lung pleura
3. Drainage into esophageal lumen as evidenced by contrast imaging
4. Injury not in neoplastic tissue, not in abdomen, not proximal to obstruction
5. Symptoms and signs of septicemia absent
6. Contrast imaging and experienced thoracic surgeon available.

The last decade has seen a rapidly increasing interest and use of minimally invasive and endoscopic management of esophageal perforation. These newer treatment strategies include stent placement, tube thoracostomy, feeding gastrostomy, and/or jejunostomy. The outcomes without traditional surgical repair have been encouraging. Historically, endoluminal stenting began as a treatment for malignant esophageal strictures decades ago. Newer covered metal and plastic stents have been used to treat a variety of benign conditions including esophageal perforations.

Recent data would suggest that the development of esophageal stent technology has been a significant advance in minimally invasive management of esophageal perforation. Vogel et al. (2005) reported no deaths among 32 patients (4 with cervical, 28 with thoracic perforation) treated without surgical repair. Utilizing an "aggressive conservative" approach with repetitive radiographic studies and image-guided drainage, as well as surgical intervention when indicated, they documented esophageal healing in 96% of patients and an impressive overall survival rate of 96% ($n = 47$). Even in the group with spontaneous perforation, they achieved a remarkable 93% survival rate. Notably, 30% of the patients required surgical intervention for drainage or esophageal repair. In contrast, van Heel et al. (2010) reported the largest series of stenting benign perforations, including 10 patients with Boerhaave syndrome, in which healing of the perforation occurred in 23 of 33 patients. There was an overall perforation-related mortality rate of 21%, mostly due to sepsis. This experience confirms that minimally invasive therapy is not appropriate in all patients. Sepesi et al. (2010) reviewed the use of esophageal stents and found the mortality rate ranged from 0% to 16%. Most patients had iatrogenic injuries that were recognized early, and, although open surgical therapy was not the primary treatment, stenting was often done together with an attempted primary repair and/or debridement/decortication and drainage. Freeman et al. (2009) reported treatment via placement of silicone-coated stents in 17 patients with iatrogenic esophageal perforation after endoscopy or surgery. Patients with malignancy were excluded from the study; 94% of leaks were successfully sealed on barium esophagogram. Complications included respiratory failure, myocardial infarction, and deep venous thrombosis in three patients; there were no deaths. After a mean of 52 days, all stents were successfully retrieved. This "hybrid approach" warrants a randomized controlled trial.

Surgical management

Although small, contained, minimally symptomatic perforations can be treated nonsurgically, frank mediastinal suppuration, major leak, or perforation through an ulcer or tumor requires urgent, complete drainage in addition to aggressive supportive care. When one considers the therapeutic options, the condition of the esophagus is of paramount importance. This is obviously influenced by any underlying pathology in addition to the local inflammatory reaction. Local inflammation can increase rapidly over time, precluding direct repair in as short a period as 12–36 h. Finally, careful judgment is required for the elderly or seriously compromised patient. Contemporary therapeutic options include primary or reinforced primary repair, wide debridement with irrigation and drainage, exclusion and diversion, T-tube drainage, and esophagectomy with or without immediate reconstruction.

Patients with cervical perforations down to the level of the carina can usually be treated with wide surgical drainage and irrigation of the retrovisceral and pretracheal spaces because these perforations will heal without repair (Bladergroen et al. 1986). Although the large majority of cervical perforations do not spread to the mediastinum, the surgeon should be aware of "descending necrotizing mediastinitis," discussed above. With mediastinitis, a cervical approach alone may prove to be inadequate and may require additional transthoracic drainage. A cervical CT scan, performed before initial exploration, is recommended to identify patients with superior mediastinal extensions of cervical infections.

The preferred approach is primary repair. Collis et al. (1944) were early champions of primary repair for esophageal perforations. They demonstrated the need for wide debridement of necrotic tissue, myotomy to expose the full extent of the mucosal injury, complete closure of the mucosal injury, and adequate drainage of the contaminated area. Mucosal repair is critical and additional myotomy may be required for adequate exposure. In most cases, primary closure, usually with buttressing of the suture line, is recommended. Reinforcement of the repair has been found to be essential for success and primary reinforced repair within 24–26 h of rupture is usually successful (Grillo et al. 1975, Gouge et al. 1989). The choice of the pedicle tissue flap can include pleura, intercostal muscle, pericardial fat, or gastric fundus. Alternatively muscle pedicles from the diaphragm, latissimus dorsi, or sternocleidomastoid can be very effective in reinforcing the repair, depending on the location of the perforation. Our preference is a vascularized pedicle of intercostal muscle if available. Wright et al. (1995) validated buttressing primary repair of thoracic esophageal perforations with the pedicled intercostal muscle flap. They achieved primary healing in 89% of the 28 patients, 13 of whom were treated more than 24 h after perforation. In the seven patients with postoperative leaks, only one required reoperation.

Intrinsic esophageal pathology can be found in at least half the patients and merits thoughtful consideration. Moghissi and Pender (1988) identified a 100% mortality rate if repair of proximal perforations was undertaken without addressing distal obstruction. Perforations associated with achalasia are found in 5% of patients and can be directly repaired when combined with a myotomy (Urbani and Mathisen 2000). Perforations associated with simple "anatomic lesions" such as diverticula, webs, and rings occur in 10% of patients and can be treated with excision and reanastomosis if found early. When perforations occur in the presence of severe gastroesophageal reflux, an antireflux procedure should be performed to enhance the repair. A Belsey Mark IV is recommended for thoracic perforations, whereas a Nissen fundoplication is the procedure of choice for an intra-abdominal perforation (Brinster et al. 2004).

Perforations more than 24–36 h old and those associated with previous surgery or significant esophageal pathology may not be amenable to direct repair. If the patient is an acceptable surgical risk, and if the esophagus has extensive irreversible changes (cancer, previous surgery, or caustic injury), total thoracic esophagectomy, cervical esophagostomy, closure of gastric cardia, gastrostomy, and feeding jejunostomy with delayed reconstruction are indicated These can be accomplished by a either a left or a right thoracotomy or transhiatal approach. Tunneling a long segment of viable proximal esophagus onto the anterior chest wall, rather than a short cervical esophagectomy, can simplify postoperative care and facilitate future reconstruction (White et al. 1992).

Esophagectomy with immediate reconstruction has, however, been very successful in treating this same population (Orringer and Stirling 1990). Although this increases the complexity of the initial procedure, it can be accomplished safely, reduces postoperative morbidity, and eliminates a second major reconstructive procedure. This is impor-

tant when one considers that secondary reconstructions have been associated with a mortality rate as high as 10% (Skinner et al. 1980).

Debridement, irrigation, and drainage are appropriate when local inflammatory reaction or the physical condition of the patient contradicts more definitive options (Skinner et al. 1980, Pate et al. 1989). In patients with acute perforations and pleural contamination, intercostal drainage can be an important temporizing measure. Drainage includes multiple pleural catheters, distal (naso)gastric drainage, and proximal pharyngoesophageal aspiration. Drainage may or may not require thoracotomy and may be facilitated by CT-guided placement of percutaneous catheters. Decortication is generally indicated in patients with extensive collapsed lung and intrapleural contamination. If adequate (extensive) communication exists between the pleural space and the esophagus, the proximal esophageal catheter can be used for topical and continuous antibiotic irrigation (Santos and Frater 1986). Treating the esophagus through the rent with a 10- to 12-mm Montgomery tracheal T-tube together with pleural, nasogastric, and gastric drainage has been reported to be successful (Linden et al. 2007). This approach is reasonable if the diagnosis has been delayed and primary repair is not feasible.

Finally, an intermediate approach of esophageal diversion has been suggested. In this procedure, the perforated but "nonfunctional" esophagus is left *in situ*. This is accomplished by complete occlusion of the esophagogastric junction and creation of a cervical esophagostomy. Theoretically, the retained nonfunctional remnant is not a source of continued contamination. Gastrointestinal continuity is re-established after several weeks of healing. Suggested advantages include esophageal preservation and reduced surgical insult. Although some authors have been satisfied with this technique in selected circumstances (Urschel et al. 1974, Pate et al. 1989), others have abandoned it (Orringer et al. 1990, Richardson 2005). Reconstructions following this controversial procedure may be quite challenging. Thoracoscopic approaches for the management of esophageal perforations have been limited (Brinster et al. 2004).

Finally, although delay in the repair of an acute perforation may create increased soilage and subsequently greater fibrosis, it is this degree of fibrosis/necrosis that matters most and not the exact number of hours that have passed (Wang et al. 1996). Surgical judgment is paramount when deciding whether to undertake primary repair versus drainage alone, diversion and exclusion, or resection.

Results of treatment

Esophageal perforation remains a lethal condition. The mortality rate varies widely, with a mean of 18% from one meta-analysis from 1990 and 2003 (Brinster et al. 2004). However, standards for expected survival are difficult because homogeneous series do not exist. Mortality statistics for esophageal perforations decrease with the inclusion of cervical lesions and minor instrumentation tears or with the exclusion of malignant disruptions. There is, however, uniform agreement that (1) delay from time of perforation to repair multiplies mortality fivefold to ninefold for any procedure and (2) when primary repair is attempted the suture line should be buttressed with a vascularized pedicle flap (Bladergroen et al. 1986, Attar et al. 1990, Richardson 2005).

Gouge et al. (1989) reviewed 10 series of primary suture of thoracic perforations: Fistulas developed in 39% of 158 patients, with a 25% mortality rate. This included patients repaired before and 24 h after perforation. In those operated on 24 hours after perforation, the esophageal repair leaked in 50% of cases. In contrast, in 99 patients who had a buttress repair, the leakage rate was 13% and the mortality rate 6%. They also reported mortality rates as 36% for T-tube drainage, 35% for exclusion–diversion, and 26% for resection.

Abbas et al. (2009) published the largest single institution experience of 119 esophageal perforations over an 11-year period; 44 patients presented with Boerhaave syndrome. Most of these patients (34/44 or 77%) were treated with surgical primary repair. Although not statistically significant, they demonstrated better outcomes for those treated nonsurgically (4% vs 15%, $p = 0.19$). In addition, length of stay (24 days vs 13 days, $p = 0.032$) and overall complications (62% vs 6%, $p = 0.018$) favored nonsurgical therapy. In addition they identified a higher mortality rate (18% vs 3%, $p = 0.18$) with T-tube drainage.

Kuppusamy et al. (2011) reported on 81 patients presenting from 1989 to 2009; 48 patients (59%) were treated surgically, 33 patients (41%) nonsurgically, and 10 patients received a hybrid approach; 57 patients were treated <24 h and 24 patients >24 h from presentation. Overall length of stay was less in the early treatment group (11 days vs 20 days, $p = 0.003$), but overall mortality was the same. Similarly, mortality was not significantly different in those treated surgically versus nonsurgically.

Ultimately, optimal results will come from the timely application of the technique most appropriate for the specific situation, rather than adopting a standard approach. Increasing experience with thoracoscopy may dramatically change management of these patients.

■ Chronic fibrosing mediastinitis

Chronic fibrosing mediastinitis represents a benign proliferation of dense fibrotic tissue deposition within the visceral mediastinal compartment from chronic infection. The most common cause of chronic infections of the mediastinum is pulmonary granulomatous disease, although incompletely treated acute infections may also be a cause. Fungi such as *Histoplasma capsulatum* and *Coccidioides immitis* have replaced tuberculosis as the major causative organism. Clinically these chronic infections encase and entrap mediastinal structures such as the superior vena cava, trachea, and esophagus. Chronic deposition leads to restriction or local erosion of these structures. Diagnosis is suggested by calcified mediastinal lymph nodes or a wide mediastinum. The extent of involvement is defined by CT or MRI. Etiology of the causative organism is established by skin tests, serum antibodies, and culture. Treatment is appropriate systemic antifungal agents and corticosteroid. As reported by Mathisen and Grillo (1992), this approach is supported by case reports and small series, with no prospective, randomized controlled trials. Surgical procedures are usually reserved for diagnostic purposes, but can be directed toward reopening occluded or stenotic airways, pulmonary arteries, or the vena cava.

■ INFECTIVE ENDOCARDITIS

Infective endocarditis (IE) is usually caused by bacteria but fungal, rickettsial, chlamydial, and even viral infection can occur. Although any endothelial surface can be affected, valves are most common. Endocarditis has traditionally been classified as *acute* or *subacute* based on the pathogenic organism and clinical presentation. The term "acute bacterial endocarditis" refers to virulent infection that rapidly destroys the valve and often seeds to other areas of the body. It most commonly is caused by *S. aureus*. Subacute bacterial endocarditis is a more indolent process that evolves over weeks to months and is caused by more indolent pathogens such as *S. epidermidis* or *Streptococcus viridans*. This distinction is not, however, clear and the general term "infective endocarditis" is more commonly used. More importantly, IE is subcategorized into native valve endocarditis (NVE) and prosthetic

valve endocarditis (PVE). Factors that determine the clinical presentation are the infecting organism, the presence of pre-existing cardiac abnormalities, and the source of infection (**Box 15.1**).

The incidence of IE is between 1.8 and 6.2 per 100 000 persons per

---

Box 15.1 Common definitions of infective endocarditis (IE).

IE according to localization of infection and presence or absence of intracardiac material

- Left-sided native valve IE
- Left-sided prosthetic valve IE (PVE)
  - Early PVE: <1 year after valve surgery
  - Late PVE: >1 year after valve surgery
- Right-sided IE (RSIE)
- Device-related IE (permanent pacemaker or cardioverter–defibrillator)

IE according to the mode of acquisition

- Healthcare-associated IE (HCA)
  - Nosocomial: IE developing in a patient hospitalized >48 h before the onset of signs/symptoms consistent with IE
  - Non-nosocomial: Signs and/or symptoms of IE starting <48 h after admission in a patient with healthcare contact defined as:
    1. home-based nursing or intravenous therapy, hemodialysis, or intravenous chemotherapy <30 days before the onset of IE
    2. hospitalized in an acute care facility <90 days before the onset of IE
    3. resident in a nursing home or long-term care facility
- Community-acquired IE: Signs and/or symptoms of IE starting <48 h after admission in a patient not fulfilling the criteria for healthcare-associated infection
- Intravenous drug abuse-associated IE: IE in an active injection drug user without alternative source of infection

Active IE

- IE with persistent fever and positive blood culture or
- Active inflammatory morphology found at surgery or
- Patient still under antibiotic therapy or
- Histopathological evidence of active IE

Recurrence

Relapse: Repeat episode of IE caused by the same microorganism <6 months after the initial episode:

- Reinfection: Infection with a different microorganism or
- Repeat episode of IE caused by the same microorganism >6 months after the initial episode

---

year and increases significantly over age 50 (Acar and Michael 2010). The incidence of PVE is between 0.3 and 1.2% during the first year, with a subsequent annual risk of late IE of 0.5%. Epidemiology of IE has geographic variations driven by factors such as access to dental and medical care, the prevalence of intravenous drug abuse (IVDA), and HIV (Habib et al. 2009).

The overall impact of endocarditis is quite significant. Approximately 20 000 patients are hospitalized each year (8000 new patients) at an estimated cost of $100 million in direct medical expenses alone (Baddour et al. 2005). Before antibiotic therapy, IE was a uniformly fatal disease. Even with current treatment, there is a 30–38% risk of death within 1 year of diagnosis. Prevention of IE is of paramount importance (Acar and Michael 2010).

Pathogenesis

IE begins with sterile vegetations composed of extracellular matrix, platelets, and fibrin. This subclinical condition is called *non-bacterial thrombotic endocarditis* (NBTE). Endothelium damage can be caused by high-velocity turbulent blood flow secondary to valvular or structural abnormalities, electrodes, or catheters, or local inflammatory or degenerative changes. The vegetation can be seeded by microorganisms. Infected vegetations contain a large inoculum of bacteria often enclosed in a layer of polysaccharides that hampers antibiotic penetration. Experimentally it is nearly impossible to produce IE without pre-existing vegetations. However, it is unknown whether the presence of vegetations is essential to the development of IE in humans. The degree of valvular destruction depends on the bacteria, duration of the infection, and anatomic site. Lesions include ulcerations, tears, perforation, rupture, and abscess formation.

Current clinical reports indicate that left-sided IE constitutes 85% of cases (isolated aortic lesions in 55–60%, isolated mitral lesions in 25–30%, and mitral and aortic lesions in 15% of cases). Right-sided IE (RSIE) accounts for only 10–15% of all cases, and is commonly the tricuspid valve (80%) (Acar and Michael 2010).

As virtually all IE cases are seeded by venous bacteremia, what explains the predilection for left-sided endocarditis? Is it just the increased mechanical stress associated with the higher pressure of the left heart? Several pathogenic differences have been identified in laboratory animals:

- After catheter-induced endothelial trauma and inoculation with bacteria, the left-sided valves are more susceptible to bacterial contamination than those on the right side.
- The density of bacteria per gram of tissue is much higher in left-sided valves.
- Antibiotic inhibition and killing of *bacteria* were significantly decreased at an oxygen pressure (PO_2) of 80 mmHg (10.6 kPa) than at a PO_2 of 40 mmHg (5.3 kPa), conditions simulating the PO_2 tension of the left and right sides, respectively.
- More exopolysaccharide in the bacterial capsule is produced at a higher PO_2, perhaps explaining the reduced antibiotic efficacy.

Although RSIE may occur in association with congenital heart disease (CHD) and the implantation of medical devices, it is overwhelmingly a disease associated with IVDA which accounts for most cases (Moss and Munt 2003). Damage from particulate material, and the direct toxic effect of the illicit drug or diluents on the right-sided valves, make them more susceptible (Habib et al. 2009). Valvular damage by a previous IE is a recognized risk factor in many of the RSIE cases.

Host susceptibility

Spontaneous cases of IE have underlying cardiac disease (often undiagnosed), although this is frequently not the case with IVDA and healthcare-associated (HCA) infections. Structural abnormalities predisposing to IE include congenital and valvular heart disease. Degenerative valve disease is becoming more important as the incidence of rheumatic disease continues to decline. A previous cardiac operation such as a valve replacement or other intracardiac implants, or prior NVE, is a significant risk factor.

IVDA is an important risk factor. The probability of IE in this population is several times higher than with any other predisposing factors (1.5–5% per year). Other important non-cardiac risk factors include indwelling intravascular catheters, chronic hemodialysis, and advanced HIV disease. In many urban centers, IE in IVDA is now the dominant form of the disease (Fowler et al. 2005a). Recent reports

indicate that 50–75% of IE IVDA patients were HIV positive (Moss and Munt 2003). Patients with chronic inflammatory bowel disease, alcoholism, poor dental hygiene, and diabetes mellitus are also at increased risk (Wilson et al. 2007).

Age is another important host factor. Not only valve disease is more prevalent in elderly people but also more patients with prosthetic valves or prior CHD repair are surviving into old age. In addition, older patients make up a disproportionate share of hospital admissions; they have more invasive monitoring catheters and more invasive procedures that predispose to HCA endocarditis (Acar and Michael 2010).

Transient bacteremia is relatively common after dental procedures but also occurs after gastrointestinal, urological, or gynecological diagnostic or surgical procedures. More importantly, spontaneous bacteremia frequently occurs with tooth brushing, flossing, and chewing, particularly in patients with poor oral health and in many other situations. This explains why less than a quarter of all patients with IE (excluding IVDA) have an identifiable origin of bacteremia.

Bacteriology

The infecting organism is usually a single species, most commonly a Gram-positive coccus. The typical IE pathogens adhere to damaged endothelium, trigger local procoagulant activity, and nurture the infected vegetations in which they survive. They are consistently resistant to platelet microbicidal proteins. The continuing evolution of antimicrobial resistance, the increased rates of HCA *S. aureus* bacteremia, and the large number of patients with cardiac or intravascular access devices have changed the epidemiology of IE. In many areas of the world, staphylococci have surpassed streptococci as a cause of NVE (Baddour et al. 2005, Fowler et al. 2005a). Coagulase-negative staphylococci, the most common cause of PVE, are now a recognized occasional cause of NVE. *Streptococcus viridans*, a normal component of oropharyngeal flora, continues to account for more than half of all streptococcal IE. Enterococci are frequently implicated in HCA endocarditis in elderly people (Mylonakis and Calderwood 2001).

Endocarditis in IVDA results mainly from skin contaminants, because approximately 60% of cases are caused by *S. aureus*. Streptococci, enterococci, and Gram-negative organisms make up the rest of the usual isolated agents. *Pseudomonas spp.*, a rare cause of endocarditis, are almost always associated with IVDA, as are cases with fungi. Polymicrobial IE is infrequent.

HCA endocarditis

In the last decade endocarditis caused by HCA infections accounts for 15–25% of all cases. HCA infection is defined as *nosocomial* or *non-nosocomial* depending on well-established criteria (see Box 15.1). Risk factors include intravascular/intracardiac devices, hemodialysis, genitourinary or gastrointestinal procedures, and surgical wound infections. Predominant pathogens are *S. aureus* (frequently meticillin resistant) and enterococci (often multidrug resistant). Overall mortality is high (Baddour et al. 2005, Fowler et al. 2005a).

PVE

PVE is a devastating complication that accounts for 5–15% of all cases of IE. It has been divided into *early infections* (within 60 days of operation*) and late infections* (>12 months after surgery). Early infections are commonly due to *S. epidermidis* and *S. aureus,* with an increasing number being meticillin resistant. A variety of Gram-negative aerobic organisms, fungi, and streptococci cause the remainder (David et al.

2007). In *late* PVE the bacteriology is characteristic of community-acquired NVE and is usually due to *Strep. viridans* or *Staph. epidermidis*. Cases presenting between 2 and 12 months, still frequently called *early PVE* by many authors, are a mixture of less virulent HCA infections and community-acquired episodes.

The risk of PVE clearly shows an early peak at about 6 weeks after operation and then declines sharply over the next 6 months. After the first year, the risk of PVE remains low (0.2–0.5% per year) throughout the remainder of the lifespan of the valve. No specific mechanical or bioprosthetic valve has been associated with any increased infectious risk. Allograft aortic valves are unique in that they are not associated with early risk of IE, and have a low risk of infection throughout the valve's lifespan. The most important risk factors for PVE are valve operations for NVE and prosthetic valve reoperations.

Diagnosis

The clinical manifestations of IE are varied, from acute and fulminant to chronic and indolent. Symptoms develop within 2 weeks of infection. Most patients present with a febrile illness. Nonspecific symptoms such as shaking chills, night sweats, fatigue, and anorexia are common. Weight loss, diffuse arthralgias, and myalgias are not infrequent in patients with subacute IE. Occasionally patients will follow a prolonged course with few specific signs or symptoms, making recognition difficult. Heart murmurs are almost always present except with acute infections, mural infections, or RSIE. A number of microembolic manifestations have been described, ranging from stroke to splinter hemorrhages of the nail beds to splenomegaly. Clinically apparent emboli occur in 15–35% of patients but autopsy studies detect emboli more frequently. CHF is the most serious presentation of IE and usually indicates valve destruction (Acar and Michael 2010).

Emboli are more likely with large mobile vegetations and especially when the mitral valve is affected. Embolic complications tend to be recurrent if vegetations persist on echocardiography. Up to 65% of embolic events involve the central nervous system, most involving the middle cerebral artery, and have a high mortality rate (Sila 2010).

Patients with RSIE present with multiple pulmonary emboli, followed by infarcts, lung abscesses, and pleural effusions. Hemoptysis can be fatal. Peripheral emboli and immunological vascular phenomena are unusual in right-sided disease. Their presence suggests left-sided involvement or paradoxical embolism.

In acute endocarditis, leukocytosis is common; in subacute IE, anemia and a normal white blood cell count are the rule. Hematuria, proteinuria, and renal dysfunction may result from emboli, immunologically mediated nephritis, or antibiotic toxicity.

Blood cultures

The mainstay in establishing the diagnosis of IE is the demonstration of bacteremia or fungemia by blood cultures. Blood cultures are positive in 90–95% of patients not already receiving antibiotics. In general three sets of cultures should be obtained from different sites 60 min apart, irrespective of body temperature, to prove that the bacteremia is continuous. Antimicrobial therapy should not be delayed more than a few hours. Several microorganisms such as the *HACEK group* (**Box 15.2**), *Brucella* spp., and anaerobes may require special culture techniques. Fungal organisms can be extremely difficult to grow in culture media and in fact some may never be isolated from the blood (Baddour et al. 2005).

Negative blood cultures have been reported in 5–10% of patients with IE often delaying diagnosis and treatment. Failure to isolate the organism is usually prior antibiotic therapy (Acar and Michael 2010). Importantly, the suppression of bacteremia persists for many days after

---

Box 15.2 Modified Duke criteria for the diagnosis of infective endocarditis (IE) (adapted from Li et al. 2000).

Major criteria

Blood cultures positive for IE:

- Typical microorganisms consistent with IE from two separate blood cultures:
  - Viridans streptococci, *Streptococcus bovis*, HACEK[a] group, *Staphylococcus aureus*; or community-acquired enterococci, in the absence of a primary focus, or
- Persistently positive blood cultures with microorganisms consistent with IE from:
  - at least two positive blood cultures of blood samples drawn >12 h apart; or
  - all of three or a majority of four or more separate cultures of blood (with first and last sample drawn at least 1 h apart), or
  - Single positive blood culture for *Coxiella burnetii* or phase I IgG antibody titer >1:800

Echocardiographic evidence of endocardial involvement

- Echocardiography findings typical of IE:
  - Vegetation – abscess – new partial dehiscence of prosthetic valve
- New valvular regurgitation

Minor criteria

- Predisposing heart condition or injection drug use
- Fever: temperature >38°C
- Vascular phenomena: Major arterial emboli, septic pulmonary infarcts, mycotic aneurysm, intracranial hemorrhages, conjunctival hemorrhages, Janeway lesions
- Immunological phenomena: Glomerulonephritis, Olser nodes, Roth spots, rheumatoid factor
- Microbiological evidence: Positive blood culture but does not meet a major criterion or serological evidence of active infection with organism consistent with IE

Diagnosis of IE is DEFINITE in the presence of

- 2 major criteria, or
- 1 major and 3 minor criteria, or
- 5 minor criteria

Diagnosis of IE is POSSIBLE in the presence of

- 1 major and 1 minor criteria, or
- 3 minor criteria

Diagnosis of IE is REJECTED if:

Firm alternate diagnosis for manifestations of endocarditis, or resolution of manifestations of endocarditis with antibiotic therapy for ≤4 days or less, or no pathological evidence of IE at surgery or autopsy after antibiotic therapy for ≤4 days, or does not meet criteria as above

[a]HACEK group: *Haemophilus* spp.: *Hemophilus parainfluenzae*, *H. aphrophilus*, and *H. paraphrophilus*, *Actinobacillus actinomycetemcomitans*, *Cardiobacterium hominis*, *Eikenella corrodens*, and *Kingella kingae*

---

antibiotic discontinuation. A frequent cause of culture-negative (CN) IE is infections caused by nutritionally variant streptococci, fastidious organisms of the HACEK group, and *Brucella* and *Candida* spp. that do not grow in commonly used media. Importantly, the blood cultures of IE caused by intracellular bacteria such as *Bartonella*, *Coxiella*, *Chlamydia*, and *Aspergillus* spp. are constantly negative and considered true CNIE. In patients suspected of having IE, cultures in special media to recover fastidious organisms, long incubation times, cell cultures, and serological tests for *Coxiella*, *Bartonella* spp. should be performed if there is no growth after 7 days.

Echocardiography

The most important diagnostic study is echocardiography which should be done as soon as possible to establish diagnosis and identify patients at risk of complications. By demonstrating vegetations as small as 5 mm in diameter, the echocardiogram can indicate which valve is involved and the degree of valve dysfunction. Myocardial and valve ring abscesses also can be identified. Serial examinations provide prognostic and management information.

The increased accuracy of transesophageal echocardiography (TEE) over transthoracic echocardiography (TTE) is accepted (Li et al. 2000). TEE has the relative disadvantage of being a somewhat invasive, uncomfortable and time-consuming procedure. However, it is the diagnostic method of choice in patients with suspected IE and negative or inconclusive TTE.

Coronary angiography.

Cardiac catheterization not routinely is performed in IE patients but also is of value in patients with risk factors or history of coronary disease. Alternatively, high-resolution CT cardiac angiography may be used in patients with large aortic vegetations.

Diagnosis criteria of IE

Diagnostic criteria for integration of clinical, echocardiographic, and laboratory information have evolved and modified (Li et al. 2000). These "Duke criteria" have been validated by many studies. Cases are defined as **definite IE** if they fulfill two major criteria, one major plus three minor criteria, or five minor criteria; cases are defined as **possible IE** if they fulfill one major and one minor criterion or three minor criteria, or they are **rejected** if they do not meet above criteria. The definitions of these criteria are summarized in Box 15.2. The Duke criteria are meant to be a clinical guide for diagnosing IE and should not replace medical judgment.

◼ Medical management

The principal treatment for IE is antimicrobial therapy, which should be initiated on an empirical basis as soon as the presumptive diagnosis has been made and blood cultures have been drawn. Isolation of the organism and determination of antibiotic susceptibility are extremely important in choosing the proper agent and for monitoring therapy. Once the results of the cultures are available treatment can be modified appropriately.

Cure of IE requires sterilization of the vegetations; any surviving bacteria will rapidly repopulate the vegetations. This generally requires parenteral therapy in order to ensure high serum concentrations and tissue penetration. The exact choices of drug, dosage, and duration of treatment are based on the antimicrobial susceptibility of the organism responsible.

Most Streptococcus viridans and S. bovis organisms are susceptible to penicillin. Medical treatment with penicillin or ceftriaxone for 4 weeks can be expected to cure 98% of the patients. Treatment for enterococci is more difficult. Most strains are resistant to penicillin alone. Susceptibility to penicillin derivatives, vancomycin, and gentamicin should be determined in order to select therapy. Standard recommendations consist of penicillin or ampicillin plus gentamicin for 4–6 weeks. Relapses can occur in 8–20% of cases. Newer agents such as linezolid are indicated in multidrug-resistant enterococci.

NVE caused by meticillin-sensitive S. aureus (MSSA) usually responds to 4–6 weeks of a nafcillin and gentamicin. For patients with MRSA infections, vancomycin is used and may be combined with gentamicin. S. epidermidis is meticillin resistant and rifampicin is often added to vancomycin. It is important that vancomycin is not an effective agent for MSSA. Patients with Gram-positive bacteremia should receive both nafcillin and vancomycin in addition to gentamicin, until proper identification of the organism has been obtained. No standard therapies exist for MRSA or S. epidermidis resistant to vancomycin

Most HACEK organisms are ampicillin resistant but are susceptible to a third-generation cephalosporin given for 4–6 weeks. Other Gram-negative bacilli such Enterobacteriaceae and Pseudomonas spp. cannot be treated with antibiotics alone. Valve replacement after 7–10 days of therapy in combination with prolonged combination therapy has been recommended for these difficult infections.

Guidelines for unusual organisms include bartonella IE treated with a b-lactam and aminoglycoside. Brucella endocarditis requires prolonged therapy with doxycycline and rifampin for at least 8 weeks. Q fever sometimes responds to a combination of doxycycline and hydrochloroquine for prolonged periods of time until the antibody titers decrease. Fungal infections usually require surgery in addition to amphotericin B.

Culture-negative IE patients should be treated empirically based on epidemiological features and the course of infection. Usually a combination of penicillin (or vancomycin or ceftriaxone) with an aminoglycoside is recommended. Therapy should be adjusted if results of serology and special cultures techniques reveal another cause. Alternatively, if fever persists after empirical therapy, surgery should be considered for debridement and obtaining microbiological and pathological specimens.

There is significant debate about the duration of therapy. Advocates for shorter treatments cite compliance and cost issues, whereas proponents of longer regimens focus on efficacy and emphasize the consequences of relapse. The duration of therapy varies with the organism but usually is a minimum of 2 weeks and often 6 weeks (Baddour et al. 2005).

◼ Outcome considerations

Although 70% of patients with NVE can be cured with appropriate antibiotics, as many as 60% of "cured" patients eventually require repair or replacement of a damaged cardiac valve. For PVE, the prognosis is much worse. Early PVE is a much more virulent disease and carries a 75–80% overall mortality rate with medical treatment alone (David et al. 2007). Late PVE has a better prognosis but still carries a 20–50% mortality rate. Late PVE is often due to S. epidermidis or streptococci, which occasionally can be cured by antibiotics alone if there is no periprosthetic infection.

The response to medical treatment of IE in IVDA depends on the organism and location. A right-sided infection with Gram-positive organisms can be cured in 90% of patients, whereas left-sided lesions are significantly worse. Gram-negative infections are significantly worse, with only a 20% cure rate. Relapse usually occurs within 2 months of treatment (Mylonakis and Calderwood 2001).

Overall mortality depends on the pathogen and the presence of complications or coexisting conditions. Representative mortality rates are 4–16% for *Streptococcus viridans* and *S. bovis*; 15–25% for enterococci, 25–40% for staphylococci, and >50% for *Enterobacteriaceae*, *Pseudomonas* spp., and fungi.

Surgical management

The accepted indications for surgical intervention in IE are congestive heart failure (CHF), myocardial or valve ring abscess, uncontrolled infection, prosthetic valve dysfunction or dehiscence, and infections caused by fungal or Gram-negative organisms (**Box 15.3**). Other relative indications for surgery include all cases of PVE, emboli (or recurrent emboli), large vegetations (particularly when vegetations remain after an embolic episode or increase in size despite therapy), and infections caused by *S. aureus* (Di Salvo et al. 2001).

Box 15.3 Accepted Indications for surgical treatment of Infective endocarditis.

Native valve endocarditis
- Heart failure due to valve dysfunction
- Evidence of perivalvular extension of infection[a]
- Aortic, mitral regurgitation, or both, with hemodynamic evidence of elevated left ventricular end-diastolic or left atrial pressure, or moderate or severe pulmonary hypertension
- Persistent infection after 7–10 days or adequate antibiotic therapy, infection due to fungal or other resistant organisms with a poor response to antibiotic treatment
- Recurrent embolism and persistent vegetation despite appropriate antibiotic therapy

Prosthetic valve endocarditis
- Heart failure due to prosthetic dysfunction
- Evidence of periprosthetic extension of infection[a]
- Prosthetic valve with evidence of increasing obstruction or worsening regurgitation
- Prosthetic valve with dehiscence evident by cinefluoroscopy or echocardiography
- Persistent infection after 7–10 days or adequate antibiotic therapy, infection due to fungal or other resistant organisms with a poor response to antibiotic treatment
- Recurrent emboli despite appropriate antibiotic treatment
- Prosthetic valve with relapsing infection

[a]Evidence of perivalvular extension: Heart blocks; annular or aortic abscess; destructive penetrating lesions; sinus of Valsalva to right atrium, right ventricle, or left atrium fistula; mitral leaflet perforation with aortic valve endocarditis

---

The presence of shock or severe CHF is an ominous development, with a reported mortality rate of almost 90% with medical therapy alone. It can result from a variety of causes such as sepsis, valve dysfunction, intracardiac shunts, and myocardial dysfunction. Echocardiography can give a rapid assessment of cardiac hemodynamics, providing valuable preoperative information. TEE is especially well suited for this because of its better accuracy for IE manifestations, and it can also be used intraoperatively to assess the adequacy of repair.

The general consensus is that IE with CHF is best treated by surgery. Cautious delay should be considered in patients who have not yet received any antimicrobial treatment, to allow for better control with antibiotics for at least 72 h. However, in many emergency cases, it is not always possible.

Abscesses of the annulus or myocardium occur most often in patients with PVE (40–75%) compared with NVE (26–30%). The aortic position is the most common site in either PVE or NVE, accounting for the majority of all abscesses. The extent of annular or myocardial destruction is variable but extension of aortic annular abscess to involve the mitral valve is not uncommon. The conduction system is another nearby structure sometimes involved and new-onset heart block in the patient with PVE should raise the suspicion for IE with abscess. There is increased mortality in patients with annular or myocardial abscess (Baddour et al. 2005). Early and repeated TEE in patients not responding to medical therapy permits earlier diagnosis of annular or myocardial abscess and should result in lower mortality rates through earlier surgical intervention (David et al. 2007)

Although infrequent, persistent sepsis despite appropriate treatment is the second most common indication for surgical treatment. The blood cultures of patients who respond to medical therapy typically become sterile within 2 weeks. Patients who have persistent bacteremia should be considered for surgical intervention despite lack of other indications. Patients with CNIE and a continuing septic state associated with clinical and echocardiographic findings of IE should undergo surgery for both diagnostic and therapeutic reasons.

Fungal and Gram-negative organisms are unusual causes of IE (**Figure 15.6**). These patients are seldom cured with medical therapy alone. Although a few less aggressive Gram-negative bacilli may respond to combination therapy based on susceptibility and synergy testing, fungal and most Gram-negative organisms are virtually an absolute indication for valve replacement.

Other surgical indications of large vegetations, emboli, or recurrent emboli, *S. aureus* infection, and non-streptoccocal PVE are more controversial. The data on these conditions are not as clear but there is certainly a significant body of data to justify an aggressive approach.

The correlation between size of vegetation and risk of embolization is controversial, with some studies showing no correlation and others showing an increased risk with larger vegetations. Several have reported a vegetation diameter >10 mm to be an independent predictor of a new embolic event, especially at the mitral valve (Mugge et al. 1989, Di Salvo et al. 2001, Thuny et al. 2007, 2011). The risk is even higher with very large (>15 mm) and mobile vegetations.

PVE is usually considered a surgical disease. However, conservative management can be offered in patients with streptococcal infection, small or absent vegetations, and no periprosthetic abscesses.

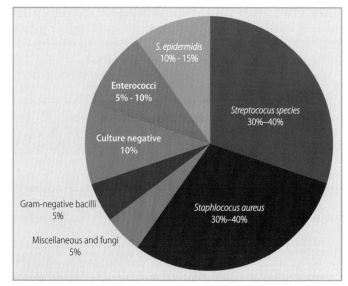

Figure 15.6 Relative prevalence of different microorganism causing infective endocarditis (IE). The pie chart depicts the relative prevalence of different microorganisms causing IE-based on reports from last decade.

Bioprostheses in the mitral position are more likely to respond to medical therapy than aortic or mechanical p. The presence of periannular extension, fistulas, new onset of heart block, S. *aureus*, Gramnegative, or fungal infection mandates early surgical intervention.

Aortic root abscesses and combined mitral and aortic ring abscesses are a challenging problem. Surgical mortality ranges from 22% to 33% (David et al. 2007). Many surgeons advocate aortic root replacement using homograft valves after radical debridement (David et al. 2007). Homografts are ideal for the reconstruction of the aortic root, the intervalvular curtain, and the anterior leaflet of the mitral valve. Alternatively, aggressive debridement and reconstruction followed by valve replacement with conventional prosthetic valves have been successfully used.

Special situations

Patients with septic cerebral emboli from IE present a difficult clinical problem. Brain imaging helps direct the timing of surgery. Patients with ischemic infarcts without hemorrhage, midline shift, or clinical coma can be safely operated on within a week. The presence of a hemorrhagic infarct indicates a very high risk of perioperative neurological complications. The operation should be delayed at least for three weeks following repeat brain imaging (Sila 2010). CT angiography and MRI can reliably recognize the presence of intracranial mycotic aneurysms.

RSIE in IVDA generally responds well to medical therapy alone, especially with Gram-positive infections. However, patients with Gram-negative or fungal infections are rarely cured with antibiotics alone (Moss and Munt 2003). There are at least three surgical options to consider in tricuspid valve IE: Valvectomy, repair, and valve replacement. Simple excision of the valve and debridement of periannular abscesses without replacement are a fast and somewhat simpler operation that avoids placing any prosthetic material in an infected field. Prosthetic valve implantation can be electively performed later. Replacement of the tricuspid valve with a mechanical prosthesis is problematic due to issues of compliance with anticoagulation and the high rate of valve thrombosis. Accordingly, the authors prefer the use of a bioprosthesis. The third option in this group of patients is vegetectomy and tricuspid valve repair, which should always be preferred when technically feasible.

As mentioned previously, IE in IVDA patients who are also HIV positive is becoming a more frequent problem. Reasonable indications for operation in these patients include urgent conditions such as a ruptured valve, shock, or cardiac failure.

Surgical outcome

Outcome depends on the indication for surgery, the valve(s) infected, the type of replacement valve, and the infecting organism. Early versus late infection is important in PVE. The surgical mortality rate for all types of IE ranges between 4.8 and 8.7% for NVE and 4 and 20% for PVE (early 25% and late 15%) (David et al. 2007). CHF remains a grim prognostic finding, with a recent series reporting a 41% surgical mortality rate in these patients. Other indicators of poor prognosis include persistent fever, extra-annular extension, non-streptococcal infection,

renal failure, and early PVE. The risk of PVE after valve replacement performed for NVE is between 3 and 7%.

The overall problem of IVDA-induced IE is significant. Sadly, many IVDA patients continue using drugs and recurrence of IE is common (Habib et al. 2009). Return to drug use is one of the most important factors in long-term survival which is only 10% over 5–10 years.

Prognostic information for those IVDA patients who are also HIV positive is limited. Although some reported no significant difference in outcome of IE in HIV-positive and HIV-negative drug users, others noted markedly increased early postoperative mortality in HIV-positive patients with active infection at the time of operation, particularly those with a CDC 4 count <200 cells/mm^3). Most of these patients died of persistent or early recurrent IE, which may be a sign of immunodeficiency despite the clinical absence of AIDS (Moss and Munt 2003).

Long-term outcome of IE

There are two types of recurrences: Relapse and reinfection (see Box 15.1). Relapse refers to a repeat episode caused by the same organism. Reinfection is used to describe infection with a different organism. Molecular techniques help identify a true relapse when the new organism is of the same species. Relapses are most often due to insufficient duration of the original treatment, suboptimal choice of antibiotics, or a persistent focus of infection. Reinfections are more frequent in IVDA, PVE, and patients undergoing chronic dialysis. With the exception of homographs in their first year, it is generally agreed that the type of valve implanted has no effect on the risk of recurrence.

A small number of studies have addressed the overall long-term prognosis of IE patients after hospital discharge. The reported survival rate after NVE is approximately 90%, 80%, 65%, and 50% at 1, 5, 10, and 15 years, respectively, whereas for PVE it is 78%, 70%, 50%, and 25% for the same intervals (David et al. 2007, Martinez-Selles et al. 2008). Factors associated with better long-term prognosis are age <55 years, lack of heart failure, NVE, and early surgical treatment (Habib et al. 2009).

Prophylaxis

Although prevention would appear to be the best way to deal with the problem of IE, several factors contribute to the failure of this approach. Overall, less than half of IE patients have a previously recognized cardiac risk and, excluding IVDA patients, less than a quarter have an identifiable cause of bacteremia (Nishimura et al. 2008). It is estimated that less than 10% of IE cases are avoidable and only a fraction of them are caused by dental procedures. Updated guidelines have recently published by several professional societies from the USA and Europe (Wilson et al. 2007, Stokes et al. 2008, Habib et al. 2009). Interestingly, although based on the same body of evidence, each guideline significantly differs in its recommendations. In common there is a general trend against empirical use of antibiotics, limiting prophylaxis to patients "with the highest risk of IE undergoing the highest risk procedures." Current American Heart Association (AHA) guidelines are summarized in **Box 15.4**. The reader is referred to the excellent review article on the rationale for revised guidelines (Gopalakrishnan et al. 2009).

Box 15.4 Summary of American Heart Association infective endocarditis prophylaxis recommendations.

High-risk cardiac conditions in which prophylaxis is reasonable
- Prosthetic cardiac valve or prosthetic material used for cardiac valve repair
- Previous infective endocarditis
- Congenital heart disease (CHD):
    - unrepaired cyanotic CHD, including shunts and conduits
    - completely repaired congenital heart defect with prosthetic material or device, during the first 6 months after the procedure
    - repaired CHD with residual defects at or adjacent to site of prosthetic patch or device inhibiting endothelialization
- Post-cardiac transplant valvulopathy

High-risk procedures for which prophylaxis is reasonable, only in patients with above listed high-risk cardiac conditions
- All dental procedures that involve manipulation of gingival tissue or the periapical region of teeth or perforation of oral mucosa
- Invasive procedure of the respiratory tract that involves incision or biopsy of respiratory mucosa
- Procedures involving infected skin, skin structures, or musculoskeletal tissue

Antibiotic prophylaxis solely to prevent infective endocarditis is not recommended for gastrointestinal or genitourinary tract procedures

REFERENCES

Abbas G, Schuchert MJ, Pettiford BL, et al. Contemporaneous management of esophageal perforation *Surgery* 2009;**146**:749–56.

Acar J, Michel PL. Infective endocarditis. In: Crawford MH, DiMarco JP, Paulus WJ (eds). *Cardiology*, 3rd edn. Philadelphia, PA: Mosby Elsevier, 2010: 1321–43

Altorjay A, Kiss J, Voros A, Bohak A. Nonoperative management of esophageal perforations. Is it justified? *Ann Surg* 1997;**225**:415–21.

Anstadt MP, Guill CK, Ferguson ER, et al. Surgical versus nonsurgical treatment of empyema thoracis: an outcomes analysis. *Am J Med Sci* 2003;**326**:9–14.

Arantes V, Campolina C, Valerio SH, et al. Flexible esophagoscopy as a diagnostic tool for traumatic esophageal injuries. *J Trauma* 2009;**66**:1677–82.

Ariyaratnam P, Bland M, Loubani M. Risk factors and mortality associated with deep sternal wound infections following coronary bypass surgery with or without concomitant procedures in a UK population: a basis for a new risk model? Interact Cardiovasc Thorac Surg 2010;**11**:543–6.

Attar S, Hankins JR, Suter CM, et al. Esophageal perforation: A therapeutic challenge. *Ann Thorac Surg* 1990;**50**:45–9.

Baddour LM, Wilson WR, Bayer AS, et al. Infective endocarditis. Diagnosis, antimicrobial therapy, and management of complications: a statement for healthcare professionals from the Committee on Rheumatic Fever, Endocarditis, and Kawasaki Disease, Council on Cardiovascular Disease in the Young, and the Councils on Clinical Cardiology, Stroke, and Cardiovascular Surgery and Anesthesia, American Heart Association – Executive Summary: endorsed by the Infectious Diseases Society of America. *Circulation* 2005;**111**:e394–434.

Bitkover CY, Gårdlund B, Larsson SA, et al. Diagnosing sternal wound infections with 99mTc-labeled monoclonal granulocyte antibody scintigraphy. *Ann Thorac Surg* 1996;**62**:1412–16.

Bladergroen MR, Lowe JE, Postlehwait RW. Diagnosis and recommended management of esophageal perforation and rupture. *Ann Thorac Surg* 1986;**42**:235–9.

Bode LGM, Kluytmans JAJW, Wertheim HFL, et al. Preventing surgical-site infections in nasal carriers of *Staphylococcus aureus. N Engl J Med* 2010;**362**:9–17.

Bouros D, Schiza S, Patsourakis G, et al. Intrapleural streptokinase versus urokinase in the treatment of complicated parapneumonic effusions: a prospective, double-blind study. *Am J Respir Crit Care Med* 1997;**155**:291–5.

Bratzler DW. The Surgical Infection Prevention and Surgical Care Improvement Projects: promises and pitfalls. *Am Surg* 2006;**72**:1010–16.

Brinster CJ, Singhal S, Lee L, et al. Evolving options in the management of esophageal perforation. *Ann Thorac Surg* 2004;**77**:1475–83.

Brook I, Frazier EH. Microbiology of mediastinitis. *Arch Intern Med* 1996;**156**:333.

Buecker A, Wein BB, Neuerburg JM, et al. Esophageal perforation: comparison of use of aqueous and barium-containing contrast media. *Radiology* 1997;**202**:683–686.

Caceres M, Ali SZ, Braud R, et al. Spontaneous pneumomediastinum: A comparative study and review of the literature. *Ann Thorac Surg* 2008;**86**:962–6.

Cameron JL, Kieffer RF, Hendrix TR, et al. Selective non-operative management of contained intrathoracic esophageal disruptions. *Ann Thorac Surg* 1979;**27**:404–8.

Cerfolio RJ, Bryant AS, Yamamuro M. Intercostal muscle flap to buttress the bronchus at risk and the thoracic esophageal-gastric anastomosis. *Ann Thorac Surg* 2005;**80**:1017–20.

Chapman SJ, Davies RJO. Recent advances in parapneumonic effusion and empyema. *Curr Opin Pulm Med* 2004;**10**:299–304.

Clagett OT, Geraci JE. A procedure for the management of postpneumonectomy empyema. *J Thorac Cardiovasc Surg* 1963;**45**:141–5.

Colice GL, Curtis A, Deslauriers J, et al. Medical and surgical treatment of parapneumonic effusions. *Chest* 2000;**118**:1158–71.

Collis JL, Humphreys DR, Bond WH. Spontaneous rupture of the esophagus. *Lancet* 1944;**ii**:179.

Corsten MJ, Shamji FM, Odell PF, et al. Optimal treatment of descending necrotizing mediastinitis. *Thorax* 1997;**52**:702–8.

Darouiche RO, Wall MJ, Itani KMF, et al. Chlorhexidine-alcohol versus povidone-iodine for surgical-site antisepsis. *N Engl J Med* 2010;**362**:18–26.

David TE, Gavra G, Feindel CM, Regesta T, Armstrong S, Maganti MD. Surgical treatment of active infective endocarditis: A continued challenge. *J Thorac Cardiovasc Surg* 2007;**133**:144–9.

Davies CWH, Gleeson FV, Davies RJO. BTS guidelines for the management of pleural infection. *Thorax* 2003;**58**(suppl ii):ii18–28.

Deschamps C, Allen MS, Miller DL, et al. Management of postpneumonectomy empyema and bronchopleural fistula. *Semin Thorac Cardiovasc Surg* 2001;**13**:13–19.

Di Salvo G, Habib G, Pergola V, et al. Echocardiography predicts embolic events in infective endocarditis. *J Am Coll Cardiol* 2001;**37**:1069–76.

Diacon AH, Theron J, Schuurmans MM, et al. Intrapleural streptokinase for empyema and complicated parapneumonic effusions. *Am J Respir Crit Care Med* 2004;**170**:49–53.

El Oakley RM, Wright JE. Postoperative mediastinitis: classification and management. *Ann Thorac Surg* 1996;**61**:1030–6.

Engelman R, Shahian D, Shemin R, et al. The Society of Thoracic Surgeons practice guidelines series: antibiotic prophylaxis in cardiac surgery, Part II: antibiotic choice. *Ann Thorac Surg* 2007;**83**:1569–76.

Estrera AS, Landay MJ, Grisham JM, et al. Descending necrotizing mediastinitis. *Surg Gynecol Obstet* 1983;**157**:545–52.

Falguera M, Carratalà J, Bielsa S, et al. Predictive factors, microbiology and outcome of patients with parapneumonic effusion. *Eur Respir J* 2011;**38**:1173–9.

Filsoufi F, Castillo JG, Rahmanian PB, et al. Epidemiology of deep sternal wound infection in cardiac surgery. *J Cardiothorac Vasc Anesth* 2009;**23**:488–44.

Fowler VG Jr, Miro JM, Hoen B, et al., ICE Investigators. *Staphylococcus aureus* endocarditis: a consequence of medical progress. *JAMA* 2005a;**293**:3012–21 [published correction appears in *JAMA* 2005;**294**:900].

Fowler VG, O'Brien SM, Muhlbaier LH, et al. Clinical predictors of major infections after cardiac surgery. *Circulation* 2005b;**112** (suppl. I):I-358–65.

Freeman RK, Vallières E, Verrier ED, et al. Descending necrotizing mediastinitis: An analysis of the effects of serial surgical débridement on patient mortality. *J Thorac Cardiovasc Surg* 2000;**119**:26067

Freeman RK, Van Woerkom JM, Vyverberg A, et al. Esophageal stent placement for the treatment of spontaneous esophageal perforations. *Ann Thorac Surg* 2009;**88**:194–8.

Friedman ND, Bull AL, Russo PL, et al. An alternative scoring system to predict risk for surgical site infection complicating coronary artery bypass graft surgery. *Infect Control Hosp Epidemiol* 2007;**28**:1162–8.

Fry DE. Surgical site infections and the Surgical Care Improvement Project (SCIP): evolution of national quality measures. *Surg Infect* 2008;**9**:579–84.

Furnary AP, Gao G, Grunkemeier GL, et al. Continuous insulin infusion reduces mortality in patients with diabetes undergoing coronary artery bypass grafting. *J Thorac Cardiovasc Surg* 2003;**125**:1007–21.

Gårdlund B, Bitkover CY, Vaage J. Postoperative mediastinitis in cardiac surgery: microbiology and pathogenesis. *Eur J Cardiothorac Surg* 2002;**21**:825–30.

Gopalakrishnan, Shukla SK, Tak T. Infective endocarditis: Rationale for revised guidelines for antibiotic prophylaxis. *Clin Med Res* 2009;**7**:63–8

Gouge TH, Depan HJ, Spencer FC. Experience with the Grillo pleural wrap procedure in 18 patients with perforation of thoracic esophagus. *Ann Surg* 1989;**209**:612.

Grijalva CG, Zhu Y, Pekka Nuorti J, Griffin MR. Emergence of parapneumonic empyema in the USA. *Thorax* 2011;**66**:663–8.

Grillo HC, Wilkins EW Jr. Esophageal repair following late diagnosis of intrathoracic perforation. *Ann Thorac Surg* 1975;**20**:387–99.

Gummert JF, Barten MJ, Hans C, et al. Mediastinitis and cardiac surgery: an updated risk factor analysis in 10,373 consecutive adult patients. *Thorac Cardiovasc Surg* 2002;**50**:87–91.

Habib G, Hoen B, Tornos P, et al. ESC Committee for Practice Guidelines: Guidelines on the prevention, diagnosis, and treatment of infective endocarditis (new version 2009): The Task Force on the Prevention, Diagnosis, and Treatment of Infective Endocarditis of the European Society of Cardiology (ESC). *Eur Heart J* 2009;**19**:2369–413.

Han SY, McElvein RB, Aldrete JS, Tishler JM. Perforation of the esophagus: correlation of site and cause with plain film findings. *Am J Roentgenol* 1985;**145**:537–40.

Heffner JE, Klein JS, Hampson C. Diagnostic utility and clinical application of imaging for pleural space infections. *Chest* 2010;**137**:467–79.

Ishiguro T, Takayanagi N, Ikeya T, et al. Isolation of *Candida* species is an important clue for suspecting gastrointestinal tract perforation as a cause of empyema. *Intern Med* 2010;**49**:1957–64.

Jones WG, Ginsberg R. Esophageal perforation: A continuing challenge. *Ann Thorac Surg* 1992;**53**:534–43.

Kobayashi T, Mikamo A, Kurazumi H, et al. Secondary omental and pectoralis major double flap reconstruction following aggressive sternectomy for deep sternal wound infections after cardiac surgery. *J Cardiothorac Surg* 2011;**6**:56.

Koegelenberg CFN, Diacon AH, Bolliger CT. Parapneumonic pleural effusion and empyema. *Respiration* 2008;**75**:241–50.

Kuppusamy M, Hubka M, Felisky CD, et al. Evolving management strategies in esophageal perforation: surgeons using nonoperative techniques to improve outcomes. *J Am Coll Surg* 2011;**213**:164–71.

Lardinois D, Gock M, Pezzetta E, et al. Delayed referral and Gram-negative organisms increase the conversion thoracotomy rate in patients undergoing video-assisted thoracoscopic surgery for empyema. *Ann Thorac Surg* 2005;**79**:1851–6.

Lee SF, Lawrence D, Booth H, et al. Thoracic empyema: current opinions in medical and surgical management. *Curr Opin Pulm Med* 2010;**16**:194–200.

Li JS, Sexton DJ, Mick N, et al. Proposed modifications to the Duke criteria for the diagnosis of infective endocarditis. *Clin Infect Dis* 2000;**30**:633–8.

Linden PA, Bueno R, Mentzer SJ, et al. Modified T-tube repair of delayed esophageal perforation results in a low mortality rate similar to that seen with acute perforations. *Ann Thorac Surg* 2007;**83**:1129–33.

Lu JC, Grayson AD, Jha P, et al. Risk factors for sternal wound infection and mid-term survival following coronary artery bypass surgery. *Eur J Cardiothorac Surg* 2003;**23**:943–9.

Mackinlay TAA, Lyons GA, Chimondeguy DJ, et al. VATS debridement versus thoracotomy in the treatment of loculated postpneumonia empyema. *Ann Thorac Surg* 1996;**61**:1626–30.

Manniën J, Wille JC, Kloek JJ, van Benthem BH. Surveillance and epidemiology of surgical site infections after cardiothoracic surgery in The Netherlands, 2002–2007. *J Thorac Cardiovasc Surg* 2011;**141**:899–904.

Martinez-Selles M, Munoz P, Estevez A, et al. Long-term outcome of infective endocarditis in non-intravenous drug users. *Mayo Clin Proc* 2008;**83**:1213–17.

Maskell NA, Davies CWH, Nunn AJ, et al. U.K. controlled trial of intrapleural streptokinase for pleural infection. *N Engl J Med* 2005;**352**:865–874.

Mathisen DJ, Grillo HC. Clinical manifestations of mediastinal fibrosis and histoplasmosis. *Ann Thorac Surg* 1992;**54**:1053

Matros E, Aranki SF, Bayer LR, et al. Reduction in incidence of deep sternal wound infections: random or real?. *J Thorac Cardiovasc Surg* 2010;**139**:680–5.

Misthos P, Sepsas E, Konstantinou M, et al. Early use of intrapleural fibrinolytics in the management of postpneumonic empyema: a prospective study. *Eur J Cardiothorac Surg* 2005;**28**:599–603.

Modrau IS, Ejlertsen T, Rasmussen BS. Emerging role of *Candida* in deep sternal wound infection. *Ann Thorac Surg* 2009;**88**:1905–9.

Moghissi K, Pender D. Instrumental perforations of the oesophagus and their management. *Thorax* 1988;**43**:642–6.

Moss R, Munt B. Injection drug use and right side endocarditis. *Heart* 2003;**89**:577–81

Mugge A, Daniel WG, Frank G, et al. Echocardiography in infective endocarditis: reassessment of prognostic implications of vegetation size determined by the transthoracic and the transesophageal approach. *J Am Coll Cardiol* 1989;**14**:631–8.

Mylonakis E, Calderwood SB. Infective endocarditis in adults. *N Engl J Med* 2001;**345**:1318–30.

Nishimura RA, Carabello BA, Faxon DP, et al. ACC/AHA 2008 Guideline update on valvular heart disease: Focused update on infective endocarditis. *J Am Coll Cardiol* 2008;**52**:676–85.

Olsen MA, Krauss M, Agniel D, et al. Mortality associated with bloodstream infection after coronary artery bypass surgery. *Clin Infect Dis* 2008;**46**:1537–46.

Orringer MB, Stirling MC. Esophagectomy for esophageal disruption. *Ann Thorac Surg* 1990;**49**:35–43.

Pate JW, Walker WA, Cole FH, et al. Spontaneous rupture of the esophagus: A 30-year experience. *Ann Thorac Surg* 1989;**47**:689–92.

Pearse HE Jr. Mediastinitis following cervical suppuration. *Ann Surg* 1938;**107**:588–611

Porcel JM. Pleural fluid tests to identify complicated parapneumonic effusions. *Curr Opin Pulmon Med* 2010;**16**:357–61.

Prandini N, Lazzeri E, Rossi B, et al. Nuclear medicine imaging of bone infections. *Nucl Med Commun* 2006;**27**:633–44.

Rahman NM, Maskell NA, Davies CWH, et al. The relationship between chest tube size and clinical outcome in pleural infection. *Chest* 2010;**137**:536–543.

Rahman NM, Maskell NA, West A, et al. Intrapleural use of tissue plasminogen and DNase in pleural infection. *N Engl J Med* 2011;**365**:518–26.

Richardson JD. Management of esophageal perforations: the value of aggressive surgical treatment. *Am J Surg* 2005;**190**:161–5.

Roh TS, Lee WJ, Lew DH, Tark KC. Pectoralis major-rectus abdominis bipedicled muscle flap in the treatment of poststernotomy mediastinitis. *J Thorac Cardiovasc Surg* 2008;**136**:618–22.

Santos GH, Frater RWM. Transesophageal irrigation for the treatment of mediastinitis produced by esophageal rupture. *J Thorac Cardiovasc Surg* 1986;**91**:57–62.

Scholl L, Chang E, Reitz B, Chang J. Sternal osteomyelitis: use of vacuum-assisted closure device as an adjunct to definitive closure with sternectomy and muscle flap reconstruction. *J Cardiovasc Surg* 2004;**19**:453–61.

Sepesi B, Raymond DP, Peters JH. Esophageal perforation: surgical, endoscopic and medical management strategies. *Curr Opin Gastroenterol* 2010;**26**:379–83.

Sila CA. Neurological complications of bacterial endocarditis. *Handbk Clin Neurol* 2010: 221–9.

Silvis SE, Nebel O, Rogers G, et al. Endoscopic complications: Result of the 1974 American Society of Gastrointestinal Endoscopy survey. *JAMA* 1976;**235**:928–30.

Skinner DB, Little AG, DeMeester TR. Management of esophageal perforation. *Am J Surg* 1980;**139**:760–4.

Stokes T, Richey R, Wray D. Guideline Development Group. Prophylaxis against infective endocarditis: summary of NICE guidance. *Heart* 2008;**94**:930–1.

Strauss C, Mal F, Perniceni T, et al. Computed tomography versus water-soluble contrast swallow in the detection of intrathoracic anastomotic leak complicating esophagogastrectomy (Ivor Lewis):a prospective study in 97 patients. *Ann Surg* 2010;**251**:647–51.

Stulberg JJ, Delaney CP, Neuhauser DV, et al. Adherence to Surgical Care Improvement Project measures and the association with postoperative infections. *JAMA* 2010;**303**:2479–85.

Tammelin A, Hambraeus A, Ståhle E. Mediastinitis after cardiac surgery: improvement of bacteriological diagnosis by use of multiple tissue samples and strain typing. *J Clin Microbiol* 2002;**40**:2936–41.

Temes RT, Crowell RE, Mapel DW, et al. Mediastinitis without antecedent surgery. *Thorac Cardiovasc Surg* 1998;**46**:84–8.

Termaat MF, Raijmakers PG, Scholten HJ, et al. The accuracy of diagnostic imaging for the assessment of chronic osteomyelitis: a systematic review and meta-analysis. *J Bone Joint Surg Am* 2005;**87**:2464–71.

Thourani VH, Lancaster RT, Mansour KA, Miller JI. Twenty-six years of experience with the modified Eloesser flap. *Ann Thorac Surg* 2003;**76**:401–6.

Thuny F, Avierinos JF, Tribouilloy C, et al. Impact of cerebrovascular complications on mortality and neurologic outcome during infective endocarditis: a prospective multicentre study. *Eur Heart J* 2007, 28:1155–61.

Thuny F, Beurtheret S, Mancini J, et al: The timing of surgery influences mortality and morbidity in adults with severe complicated infective endocarditis: A propensity analysis. *Eur Heart J* 2011;**32**:2027–33.

Trussell J, Gerkin R, Coates B, et al. Impact of a patient care pathway protocol on surgical site infection rates in cardiothoracic surgery patients. *Am J Surg* 2008;**196**:883–9.

Urbani M, Mathisen DJ. Repair of esophageal perforation after treatment for achalasia. *Ann Thorac Surg* 2000;**69**:1609–11.

Urschel HC Jr, Razzuk MA, Wood RE, et al. Improved management of esophageal perforation: exclusion and diversion in continuity. *Ann Surg* 1974;**179**:587–91.

van Heel NC, Haringsma J, Spaander MC, et al. Short-term esophageal stenting in the management of benign perforations. *Am J Gastroenterol* 2010;**05**:1515–20.

Van Wingerden JJ, Lapid O, Boonstra PW, de Mol BAJM. Muscle flaps or omental flap in the management of deep sternal wound infection. *Interact Cardiovasc Thorac Surg* 2011;**13**:179–88.

Vogel SB, Rout WR, Martin TD, Abbitt PL. Esophageal perforation in adults: aggressive, conservative treatment lowers morbidity and mortality. *Ann Surg* 2005;**241**:1016–21.

Wait MA, Sharma S, Hohn J, Dal Nogare A. A randomized trial of empyema therapy. *Chest* 1997;**111**:1548–51.

Wang N, Razzouk AJ, Safavi A, et al. Delayed primary repair of intrathoracic esophageal perforation: is it safe? *J Thorac Cardiovasc Surg* 1996;**111**: 114–21.

White RK, Morris DM. Diagnosis and management of esophageal perforations. *Am Surg* 1992;**58**:112–19.

Wilson W, Taibert KA, Gewitz M, et al. Prevention of Infective Endocarditis: Guidelines From the American Heart Association: A Guideline From the American Heart Association Rheumatic Fever, Endocarditis, and Kawasaki Disease Committee, Council on Cardiovascular Disease in the Young, and the Council on Clinical Cardiology, Council on Cardiovascular Surgery and Anesthesia, and the Quality of Care and Outcomes Research Interdisciplinary Working Group *Circulation* 2007;**116**:1736–54

Wozniak CJ, Paull DE, Moezzi JE, et al. Choice of first intervention is related to outcomes in the management of empyema. *Ann Thorac Surg* 2009;**87**: 1525–30.

Wright CD, Mathisen DJ, Wain JC, et al. Reinforced primary repair of thoracic esophageal perforation. *Ann Thorac Surg* 1995;**60**:245–8.

Wu JT, Mattox KL, Wall MJ Jr. Esophageal perforations: new perspectives and treatment paradigms. *J Trauma* 2007;**63**:1173–84.

Yamashiro T, Kamiya H, Murayama S, et al. Infectious mediastinitis after cardiovascular surgery: role of computed tomography. *Radiat Med* 2008;**26**:343–7.

Francisco O. M. Vieira, Mitchell Challis, Shawn M. Allen

CERVICAL SPACE INFECTION

Anatomy

Complex head and neck anatomy often makes early recognition of cervical space infection challenging and delay in treatment poses a potential for severe complications. Multiple layers of cervical fascia encase anatomic contents to form superficial and deep cervical spaces. These fascial planes constitute barriers for the spread of infection or serve to direct infectious spread once their natural resistance has been overcome. Aggressive monitoring and management of the airway is the most critical aspect of care, followed by appropriate antibiotic coverage and surgical drainage. A growing number of patients with immune dysfunction are at risk for atypical and more complicated cases of deep cervical space infections.

Superficial and deep cervical fascial planes

The *superficial cervical fascia* underlies the skin of the head and neck in a continuous plane from the zygoma and muscles of facial expression down to the shoulders and thorax (**Figure 16.1a**). Although the area contained within this fascial plane is not considered a deep neck space, it may serve as an additional barrier for containing edema and pressure caused by infections in the underlying compartments of the neck.

The *deep cervical fascia* is divided into three layers – superficial, middle, and deep. These envelope the contents of the head and neck and form the potential deep neck spaces. The *superficial layer* encloses the inferior aspect of the skull base to the face and completely surrounds the neck. It is traditionally called "investing fascia" (**Figure 16.1b**). Above the hyoid bone level it encloses two muscles (anterior belly of the digastric and masseter), two salivary glands (parotid and submandibular), and two fascial compartments (parotid and masticator spaces). The *middle layer* encloses the anterior neck contents and has two divisions: The muscular division surrounds the infrahyoid strap muscles and extends from the thyroid cartilage and hyoid bone down to the sternum, clavicle, and scapulae (**Figure 16.1c, division M**); the visceral division envelops the trachea, larynx, pharynx, esophagus, and thyroid gland (**Figure 16.1c, division V**), and posteriorly the anterior wall of the retropharyngeal space. The carotid sheath receives connective tissue contributions from all three layers of deep cervical fascia, forming an anatomically independent com-

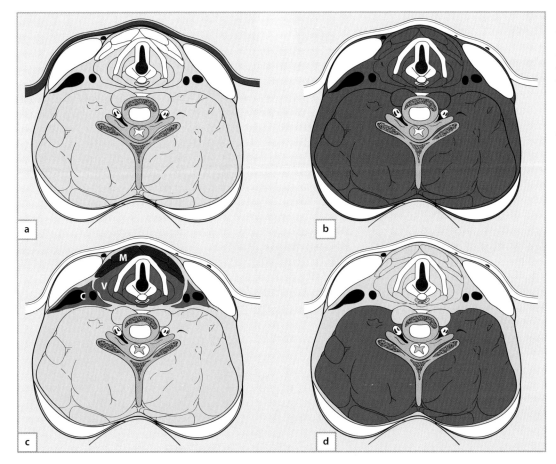

Figure 16.1 (a) The superficial cervical fascia. (b) The superficial layer of deep cervical fascia 'investing fascia'. (c) **M** represents the muscular division and **V** the visceral division of the middle layer of deep cervical fascia. **C** Represents the carotid sheath. (d) The deep layer of deep cervical fascia.

partment (**Figure 16.1c, division C**). The *deep layer* originates from vertebral spinous processes and encloses the posterior neck (**Figure 16.1d**). It also divides and forms the prevertebral fascia and the alar fascia. The alar fascia forms the posterior wall of the retropharyngeal space. The alar fascia also serves as the anterior boundary of the danger space, which extends inferiorly into the posterior mediastinum. The prevertebral fascia forms the posterior wall of the danger space.

Deep neck spaces are formed by cervical fascial planes and they functionally contain the infectious processes. Anteriorly, strong fascial attachments to the hyoid bone restrict downward infectious spread (**Figure 16.2**). Consequently, the deep neck spaces are classified into three anatomic groups: Suprahyoid, length of the neck, and infrahyoid.

Suprahyoid spaces

The *peritonsillar space* lies between the palatine tonsil and superior pharyngeal constrictor, and is also bounded by the tonsillar pillars. It is contiguous with the parapharyngeal and retropharyngeal spaces. Infections often present with fever, sore throat, dysphagia, odynophagia, muffled voice, and cervical adenopathy. A contrast computed tomography (CT) scan can define the presence of abscess. Cooperative patients can usually have these abscesses drained at the bedside with local anesthesia. Uncomplicated infections without airway compromise can be treated with an initial course of intravenous antibiotics for 12–36 h.

The *mandibular space* extends from the mandible to the hyoid bone. It is divided horizontally by the mylohyoid muscle into two compartments: Supramylohyoid and inframylohyoid. These two compartments communicate at the posterior end of the mylohyoid muscle insertion. The roots of the second and third molars lie below the attachment of the mylohyoid muscle and in the inframylohyoid compartment. The *supramylohyoid compartment* contains loose areolar tissue, sublingual glands, the Wharton's duct, geniohyoid muscles, and lingual and hypoglossal nerves. Anterior dental infections above the mylohyoid level can potentially spread directly into

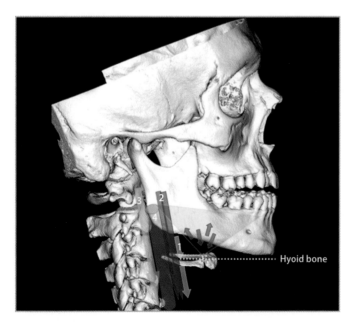

the parapharyngeal space, anterior visceral space, or carotid space. Infections often present with induration, swelling, and tenderness of the floor of the mouth. Protrusion and elevation of the tongue may occur as the swelling progresses, causing airway obstruction. The *inframylohyoid compartment* contains submandibular glands, lymph nodes, and digastric muscles. The central segment between the anterior bellies of the digastric muscles forms a subdivision known as submental space. Inframylohyoid infections cause induration, swelling, and tenderness below the mandible. They can also lead to elevation and protrusion of the tongue, causing respiratory obstruction. Posterior dental infections can spread directly into this compartment.

The *parapharyngeal space* approximates an inverted pyramid extending superiorly from the base of the skull down to the hyoid bone. It is divided into two compartments by the styloid process. Prestyloid compartment infections result from dental and pharyngeal infections. Clinically they present with fever, chills, neck pain, trismus, and bulging of the palatine tonsil. To avoid complications from rapid spread into adjacent neck spaces, prompt surgical drainage is required. An external approach along the anterosuperior border of sternocleidomastoid is used to gain adequate exposure, and avoid injury to the carotid sheath contents and spinal accessory nerve. Poststyloid compartment infections commonly cause no obvious pain or swelling. However, involvement of the carotid sheath can lead to septicemia, Lemierre syndrome, carotid artery aneurysm or rupture, Horner syndrome, and palsies of cranial nerves IX–XII. Management begins with imaging to determine the extent of spread, and proximity to the carotid sheath. Abscesses of the poststyloid compartment require external drainage.

The *masticator space* lies between the medial pterygoid and masseter muscles. It includes the temporalis muscle, parotid gland, divisions of the mandibular nerve (V3), and the internal maxillary artery. Most infections originate from the posterior mandibular molars. The initial presentation is usually trismus, sore throat, dysphagia, and pain surrounding the mandible or preauricular region. An extraoral approach avoids the facial nerve and the internal maxillary artery. An intraoral approach at the retromolar trigone may be attempted for draining abscesses medial to the mandible.

The *parotid space* is formed by the superficial layer of deep cervical fascia. The fascia on the medial aspect of the gland is thin and provides little resistance to spread into the adjacent parapharyngeal space. Infections often result from parotid duct obstruction and occasionally from odontogenic sources. They present with severe pain and swelling at the angle of the mandible, but little or no trismus. An external, parotidectomy-like approach is used to drain a parotid space abscess.

The *buccal space* contains the buccal fat pad, parotid duct, and facial artery. Most buccal space infections are odontogenic in origin and present with a warm and tender swelling within the cheek. Trismus may be present if the infection spreads posteriorly to the masticator space.

Entire length-of-neck spaces

The *retropharyngeal space* lies between the posterior pharynx and the alar fascia. Laterally, it is bounded by the carotid sheaths (see **Figure 16.2, arrow 1**). Retropharyngeal infection can result from trauma or as an extension from parapharyngeal space infection. It presents with neck pain, fever, anorexia, snoring, and dyspnea. The most feared complications of retropharyngeal infection are airway obstruction and rupture of abscess with aspiration. Patients with airway compromise should be intubated with the patient in the Trendelenburg position. Needle aspiration should be attempted preceding intraoral incision and drainage.

Figure 16.2 The freeway spaces to mediastinum and the hyoid bone level, which oppose as an anatomic barrier to the mediastinum represented by the pink upside-down triangle and the infectious process by the red short arrows. (1) The retropharyngeal space, (2) the carotid or vascular space, (3) the prevertebral space, and (4) the danger space.

The *danger space* lies between the alar and prevertebral fascias. It extends from the skull base into the posterior mediastinum to the level of the diaphragm. Involvement of this space may result from the spread of retropharyngeal, parapharyngeal, or prevertebral space infections. Infection has the tendency to spread inferiorly into the thorax resulting in mediastinitis, empyema, and sepsis (see **Figure 16.2, arrow 4**).

The *prevertebral space* is between the prevertebral fascia and the vertebral bodies (see **Figure 16.2, arrow 3**). Sources of infection include trauma to the posterior pharynx, and secondary spread from infectious discitis, retropharyngeal, or danger space infections. Complications include spinal osteomyelitis and spinal instability. Staphylococci are the most frequent bacteria. Once identified by a CT scan, prevertebral space abscesses should be drained externally to avoid a persistent draining fistula in the posterior pharynx.

The *carotid space* lies within the carotid sheath and encases the carotid artery, internal jugular vein, cervical sympathetic chain, and cranial nerves IX, X, XI, and XII (see **Figure 16.2, arrow 2**). The carotid sheath can potentially serve as a "highway" for infectious spread. Infections present with stiffness, swelling neck, fever, chills, Horner syndrome, or vocal fold paralysis. An external approach is used for incision and drainage.

Infrahyoid space

The anterior visceral space lies between the infrahyoid strap muscles and the esophagus. It contains the thyroid gland, trachea, and anterior esophageal wall. It extends from the thyroid cartilage into the superior mediastinum. Infections of this space often originate from traumatic perforation of the anterior esophageal wall. Clinically, they present with neck swelling, sore throat, dysphagia, odynophagia, hoarseness, and dyspnea. Perforation of visceral contents may cause crepitus in the neck, mediastinitis, or pneumothorax.

■ Risk factors

Diabetes mellitus is the most common risk factor in cervical space infection. Uncontrolled hyperglycemia causes changes in immunological responses and decreases the ability to confine infection. Older patients with diabetes respond poorly to conservative medical therapy and develop frequent complications (Huang at al. 2005). Other sources of immunosuppression – such as HIV infection, intravenous drug use, chemotherapy, chronic renal failure, hepatic disease, and chronic steroid therapy – also increase risk for severe and atypical infections. Cervical space infections can present as the initial manifestation of HIV infection.

Congenital lesions should be considered in immunocompetent patients with recurrent cervical space infections. Contrast CT can be useful to identify infected cystic lesions and help with surgical planning. Infected congenital cysts may respond well to antibiotic therapy. However, progression of the infection may require needle aspiration or incision and drainage. Once the infection has resolved complete surgical excision will prevent recurrent infections.

Head and neck malignancy can initially present as cervical space infection. Patients with such infections can present with lymphadenopathy refractory to treatment. Workup should include fine needle aspiration of the lymph nodes and panendoscopy.

■ Diagnosis

In the initial assessment of cervical space infection the airway is the first priority. Early identification of immunocompromised patients is also important to minimize potential complications. The most common symptoms are dysphagia, odynophagia, trismus, dysphonia, and dyspnea. A discriminating manual physical examination is vitally important to identify the severity of the process and to make sure that the airway is secure. Aspirates for culture of aerobes, anaerobes, fungus, and acid-fast bacilli should be obtained before antibiotics are instituted if possible. Negative cultures, despite the presence of organisms on Gram stain, may suggest an anaerobic infection or atypical sources.

Imaging studies

Management of cervical space infection is highly dependent on the location and extent of deep neck involvement. Appropriate diagnostic imaging is essential in many cases. The imaging method of choice is dependent on availability, operator skill, anatomic locations, and patient conditions. Choice of imaging modality will also depend on whether image-guided needle drainage or open surgical drainage is considered. Plain radiography is of limited utility for the evaluation of deep cervical space infections.

Ultrasonography can identify mainly superficially localized masses and fluid collections. It is readily available and has relatively low operational costs. It is also portable and does not expose patients to radiation. Ultrasonography is more accurate than CT in differentiating a drainable abscess from cellulitis, and should be used to supplement CT or MRI when deep neck abscess is uncertain. It is also useful for image-guided diagnostic and therapeutic needle aspiration. Ultrasonography is limited by its inability to penetrate bone or air-filled structures, and it may not visualize deeper lesions. It can be difficult to interpret, and is subject to operator skill level with variable reproducibility. It does not provide the anatomic detail of a contrast CT scan which is necessary for planning surgical approaches to deep space collections.

A *contrast CT scan* is the imaging modality of choice and the standard for the diagnosis and management of deep cervical space infections. CT scans are fast, relatively inexpensive, and widely available. A contrast CT scan can reliably localize a process and define its extent. It is particularly superior when evaluating cellulitis or abscess within the mediastinum (Stalfors et al. 2004). When combined with physical examination, CT has a reported accuracy of 89% in differentiating a drainable abscess from cellulites. Abscesses are seen as low-density lesions with rim enhancement, occasional air–fluid levels, and loculations. A discrete hypodensity >2 ml in volume on CT is more predictive of a deep neck abscess than just the presence of a ring-enhancing lesion.

MRI provides better resolution of soft tissues than CT. It is useful for assessing the extent of soft-tissue involvement and for delineating vascular complications. It also avoids radiation exposure, has less interference from dental fillings, and uses less allergenic contrast material. However, it requires a lengthy scan time, is limited in emergency settings, and is more expensive.

■ Microbiology

Cultures of aspirates from deep neck abscesses are commonly polymicrobial and reflect the oropharyngeal and odontogenic bacterial flora. Frequently isolated aerobes include *Streptococcus viridans* and *Staphylococcus aureus*. Less frequently, *Strep. pneumoniae, Strep. pyogenes, Klebsiella pneumoniae, Neisseria* spp., and *Hemophilus influenzae* are isolated. Common anaerobic isolates include peptostreptococci, *Bacteroides fragilis*, and *Fusobacterium* spp. *Eikenella corrodens* is a resistant anaerobe frequently isolated from intravenous drug abusers. In addition, meticillin-resistant *Staph. aureus* (MRSA), once considered a nosocomial infection, is seen with increasing prevalence as a community-acquired cause of cervical space infections especially in intravenous drug abusers and immunocompromised patients. *K. pneumoniae* is the most common cause of cervical space infections in patients who have poorly controlled diabetes mellitus.

Treatment

Airway management

Careful monitoring of the airway is the first priority when initiating management of a cervical space infection. The supine position in a patient may precipitate complete airway obstruction and should be considered when sending a patient for CT or MRI. Airway obstruction occurs most often in cases with multiple space involvement, Ludwig's angina, retropharyngeal, parapharyngeal, or anterior visceral space abscesses. Indications for airway control include dyspnea, stridor, retractions, or expected airway compromise. Monitoring of the airway should continue for at least 48 h after surgical intervention for swelling.

Endotracheal intubation is difficult with distorted airway anatomy, immobility of the soft tissues, or trismus. In less severe infections, trismus may be overcome with the use of general anesthesia. However, general anesthesia in more advanced infections can precipitate complete airway obstruction, resulting in an emergency surgical airway. Fiberoptic nasotracheal intubation is especially useful in patients who have severe trismus. In a study of fiberoptic-assisted nasotracheal intubation in patients with cervical space infection, titration of intravenous diazepam or midazolam with or without fentanyl was shown to reduce laryngeal spasm before the application of topical anesthesia (Ovassapian et al. 2005).

Tracheotomy under local anesthesia is indicated for impending airway obstruction when trismus or massive soft-tissue edema precludes endotracheal intubation, or when repeated attempts at intubation have failed. Separate incisions for tracheotomy and drainage procedures of the anterior neck should be used. The advantages of tracheotomy include airway security, less sedation, and earlier transfer to a non-critical care unit. The disadvantages of tracheotomy include bleeding, pneumothorax, and the potential for causing tracheal stenosis.

Cricothyrotomy can provide urgent airway access under emergency circumstances. Potential complications include trauma to the posterior wall of the trachea, esophagus, or subglottic stenosis. Cricothyrotomy should be converted to a standard tracheotomy within 12–36 h.

Antibiotic management

Once aspirates have been collected empirical antibiotic therapy should be started until culture and sensitivity results are available. Antibiotic therapy should be started against aerobic and anaerobic bacteria that are more commonly involved (polymicrobial organisms and streptococci). Either a b-lactamase penicillin inhibitor (such as amoxicillin or ticarcillin with clavulanic acid) or a b-lactamase-resistant antibiotic (such as cefoxitin, cefuroxime, imipenem, or meropenem) in combination with a drug that is highly effective against most anaerobes (such as clindamycin or metronidazole) is recommended for optimal empirical coverage. Vancomycin should be considered for empirical therapy in intravenous drug abusers at risk for infection with MRSA and in patients who have profound neutropenia or immune dysfunction. Ceftriaxone and clindamycin have been recommended as empirical therapy against community-acquired MRSA to ensure adequate coverage and avoid resistance to vancomycin (Naidu et al. 2005). Once available, the results of the culture and sensitivity tests should guide further antibiotic therapy.

In selected cases, an uncomplicated deep neck abscess or cellulitis can be effectively treated with antibiotics and careful monitoring,

without surgical drainage. It has been found that conservative treatment does not increase mortality or length of hospitalization in these patients. Steroids with antibiotic treatment may reduce the need for surgical intervention by minimizing airway edema, inflammation, and the progression of cellulitis into an abscess (Mayor et al. 2001). Parenteral antibiotic therapy should be continued until the patient has been afebrile for at least 48 h and then switched to oral therapy. Patients on intravenous antibiotic without improvement in 24–36 h will require surgical drainage.

Surgical management

Surgical intervention remains the mainstay of treatment for more severe or complicated cases of deep cervical space infections. Aggressive management of blood pressure, fluid resuscitation, and treatment of associated comorbidities is necessary before a surgical approach when possible.

Minimally invasive techniques such as image-guided needle aspiration and indwelling catheter placement have been used for well-defined, unilocular abscesses in patients without airway compromise. Multilocular abscesses usually require incision and drainage. Ultrasound guidance is effective for locating and draining abscesses. CT guidance is helpful for needle aspiration of deep fluid collections. Unilocular abscesses <3 cm have been successfully treated using ultrasound-guided percutaneous needle drainage (Yeow et al. 2001). Failure of improvement by percutaneous treatment requires conversion to open drainage

Surgical indications for open drainage are in **Box 16.1**. The external cervical approach is most often used when draining the anterior visceral, submandibular, parapharyngeal, prevertebral, and carotid spaces, and for complicated retropharyngeal abscesses that cannot be fully drained using an intraoral approach. Wounds requiring extensive debridement of necrotic tissue should be left open and packed with antimicrobial dressings. In cases involving descending infections,

---

Box 16.1 Indications for surgical management of cervical space infections.

- Emergency airway compromise
- Cervical space necrotizing fasciitis
- Uncontrolled diabetes mellitus
- Septicemia, bacteremia, or systemic inflammatory response syndrome
- Descending infection to mediastinum from the retropharyngeal, carotid, danger, prevertebral or anterior visceral spaces
- Failure of clinical improvement within 36–48 h of the initiation of conservative treatment
- Abscesses >3 cm in diameter that involve the prevertebral, anterior visceral, or carotid spaces
- Pre-existing congenital anomaly
- Abscesses that involve more than two spaces
- Failure of previous minimally invasive techniques

---

cervical drainage is sufficient as long as the infection remains above the carina. Transthoracic drainage is necessary when infection spreads below that level to the mediastinum.

Complications

Mediastinitis results from extension of infection from spaces that extend the length of the neck or the anterior visceral space. The causative organisms are mostly combined aerobes and anaerobes. Patients will have increasing chest pain or dyspnea, and chest radiography or CT may demonstrate a widened mediastinum or pneumomediastinum. Transthoracic drainage is necessary for infection below the carina. Mortality rates for patients who have mediastinitis are 40% (Huang et al. 2004).

Lemierre syndrome is suppurative thrombophlebitis of the internal jugular vein from extension of infection into the carotid space. Findings include swelling and tenderness at the angle of the jaw and sternocleidomastoid, signs of sepsis, and evidence of septic pulmonary emboli. Confirmation is obtained by use of high-resolution ultrasonography, CT scan, or MRI/MR angiography (MRA). Treatment involves prolonged antimicrobial therapy directed by culture and sensitivity, and anticoagulation for 3 months. Most cases resolve with medical management and do not require surgical ligation or resection of the internal jugular vein. Fibrinolytic agents may be used if jugular thrombosis is recognized within 4 days of onset, but have a higher risk of hemorrhage than anticoagulation.

Carotid artery aneurysm can present as a pulsatile neck mass with four cardinal signs:
1. Recurrent sentinel hemorrhages from the pharynx, nose or ear
2. Protracted clinical course (7–14 days)
3. Hematoma of the surrounding neck tissues
4. Hemodynamic collapse.

Endovascular stenting or vessel occlusion is an option in less urgent cases.

Ludwig's angina is the result of rapidly progressive bacterial infection in the supramylohyoid and inframylohyoid spaces. It is caused by firm indurated cellulites rather than abscess formation. Patients present with odynophagia, dysphagia, drooling, and displacement of the tongue superiorly and posteriorly, which may lead to airway compromise. If the airway is stable at presentation, intravenous broad-spectrum antibiotic coverage should be initiated. If the patient develops airway compromise, then an oropharyngeal airway (oral airway or Guedel cannula), nasopharyngeal airway (trumpet), nasotracheal fiberoptic intubation (if anatomic conditions are favorable), or trachesotomy or cricothyrotomy should be considered. These procedures should be attempted with the patient in a sitting-up position under close pulse oximetry monitoring. If conservative measures fail, a surgical tracheotomy is required. Ludwig's angina may invade the retropharyngeal or danger space. This can result in mediastinitis, pleural effusion, empyema, and infection of carotid sheath structures. Surgical debridement of necrotic tissue is necessary for compartment decompression. Currently Ludwig's angina with aggressive airway management, intravenous antibiotics, and surgical decompression carries a mortality rate of <10%.

Necrotizing cervical fasciitis is a fulminant infection that spreads along fascial planes. Patients are acutely ill with high fevers, and the skin overlying the necrosis may be tender, edematous, and erythematous, with indistinct transition to normal skin. Soft-tissue crepitus may be present. In more advanced cases, the skin becomes pale, anesthetic, and dusky, with blistering and sloughing. CT may demonstrate diffuse cellulitis with infiltration of the skin and subcutaneous tissues, myositis, compartmental fluid, and gas (Palacios and Rojas 2006). Managing necrotizing fasciitis is best accomplished in an intensive care unit (ICU) and involves parenteral antibiotics, along with early and frequent surgical debridement of any devitalized tissue. The wound should be left open and packed with antimicrobial dressings until the infection has subsided. Hyperbaric oxygen has been used as an adjunctive treatment in hemodynamically stable patients. The condition is often accompanied by mediastinitis and sepsis, which increase mortality rates.

Recurrent infections are commonly found with pre-existing congenital abnormality or head–neck cancer. Imaging is useful in making the diagnosis when recurrent infections occur in the same cervical spaces. The second branchial cleft cyst is the most common congenital neck abnormality (Nusbaum et al. 1999).

NOSOCOMIAL SINUSITIS

Nosocomial sinusitis (NS) is an important hospital-acquired infection. In contrast to community-acquired sinusitis, NS may be difficult to diagnose. Often these patients are intubated, unconscious, and do not complain of sinus symptoms. However, NS can be associated with serious complications including the development of ventilator-associated pneumonia and septicemia. Thus, timely diagnosis and treatment of this condition are important.

Anatomy

The paranasal sinuses are mucosa-lined cavities that are contiguous with the nasal cavity. They have several proposed roles including providing the brain protection from trauma, acting as resonating chambers for voice production, humidifying inspired air, and reducing the weight of the facial skeleton. The maxillary and ethmoid sinuses are present at birth, whereas the sphenoid sinus begins to form at about 3 years of age and the frontal sinus at 5–6 years.

The sinuses drain into the nasal cavity through several ostia. The frontal, maxillary, and anterior ethmoid sinuses drain into the area underneath the middle turbinate known as the middle meatus. The area where these ostia open is known as the osteomeatal complex. This is a bottleneck area for sinus drainage and obstruction can lead to mucus stasis, which predisposes to bacterial growth. The posterior ethmoids and sphenoid sinuses drain into the superior meatus. Sinus drainage can be blocked by a variety of abnormalities such as a deviated septum, inflammatory processes such as allergic rhinitis, and foreign bodies in the nose.

The sinuses and nasal cavity are lined with ciliated pseudostratified columnar epithelia. The cilia play an essential role in mucus clearance by beating the mucus blanket toward the ostia of the sinus. There is very little passive drainage from the sinuses. The function of the cilia can be impaired by factors including tobacco smoke, infection (viral and bacterial), and low humidity.

Knowledge of the close anatomic relationship of the paranasal sinuses to the orbits and brain is paramount, because of related major complications of sinusitis. The lamina papyracea is a paper-thin portion of the lateral ethmoid bone that separates the sinuses from the orbit and may serve as a route for the spread of infection. The roof of the nasal cavity is formed by the cribriform plate of the ethmoid bone, which also serves as the floor of the anterior cranial fossa and is another potential route for the spread of infection.

Risk factors, pathogenesis, and bacteriology

Nasal foreign bodies including nasoendotracheal tubes, nasogastric tubes, and nasal packing are thought to be the most important risk factor in the development of NS. Multiple studies have shown that NS rarely develops without a foreign body in the nose (Rouby and Laurent 1994). Several studies have attempted to further elucidate risk factors associated with development of NS. In a large study of 2368 trauma patients NS was identified in 32 (1.4%) of these patients. Predisposing risk factors were mechanical ventilation, nasogastric tubes, corticosteroid therapy, prior antibiotic use, facial trauma, nasoendotracheal tubes, and nasal packing (Caplan and Hoyt 1982). Most of these infections occurred during the second week of hospitalization. In a prospective study of 366 patients in an ICU for at least 48 h, risk factors were sedative use, nasoenteric feeding tube, Glasgow Coma Scale (GCS) score ≤7, and nasal colonization with enteric Gram-negative bacteria (George et al. 1998).

The pathogenesis of NS relates to a decrease in nasal patency with osteomeatal complex obstruction. The aforementioned foreign bodies in the nasal cavity can apply pressure against the osteomeatal complex, cause inflammation of the nasal mucosa, and lead to occlusion of the sinus ostia. Increases in central venous pressure, positive pressure ventilation, and supine position also play a role in inducing nasal congestion by increasing jugular venous pressure.

Occlusion of the sinus ostia predisposes the patient to NS. Mucus stasis, hypoxia, and bacterial toxins all play a role in disrupting cilia function, further complicating sinus drainage. In addition, tubes and the damaged mucosa surrounding them provide a surface for bacterial adhesion. This leads to the formation of biofilms which promote bacterial resistance to host defenses and antibiotic therapy.

Colonization of the paranasal sinuses occurs from endogenous flora or exogenous pathogens acquired from the hospital environment. *S. pneumoniae, H. influenzae,* and *M. catarrhalis* are the most common causes of community-acquired sinusitis. In contrast, these organisms are rare in NS. NS has a polymicrobial etiology that is often ICU specific. *P. aeruginosa, S. aureus, Acinetobacter* spp., *E. coli, Proteus mirabilis,* and streptococci are the most common isolates (Riga et al. 2010). Mixed anaerobes and fungal pathogens are less commonly isolated.

The normal sinus flora in critically ill patients is rapidly replaced by enteric Gram-negative bacilli. Colonization of the nasopharynx, oropharynx, and oral cavity (especially gingival plague) plays an important role in the colonization of the sinuses. Some contend that gastroesophageal reflux may lead to gastric colonization of the sinuses (Korinek et al. 1993).

■ Diagnosis

NS presents with a wide range of signs and symptoms, including face pain or pressure, nasal obstruction, rhinorrhea, postnasal drip, and fever. On physical examination the sinuses may be tender to palpation, the nasal mucosa may be erythematous and edematous, and there will likely be purulent drainage. Most commonly this is found in the middle meatus. Anterior rhinoscopy should be performed in patients with suspected NS. In many patients with NS, only fever may be present. Thus, a high index of suspicion and further studies may be required in order to make the diagnosis.

Historically, plain films were the most common radiographic study used for diagnosis of NS. However, they have low sensitivity and a high false-positive rate. CT has replaced conventional radiographs, and is particularly useful in diagnosis of NS in the unresponsive patient. CT also has the advantage of delineating sinus anatomy, and can identify any abnormalities or variants that may be important in surgical planning.

Diseased sinuses will show mucosal thickening or opacification (**Figure 16.3**). It is important to identify the osteomeatal complex and evaluate its patency. Isolated mucus retention cysts may be identified within the sinuses but these rarely have clinical significance. A prospective study evaluated ultrasonography in detecting NS. The authors examined 120 maxillary sinuses in ICU patients who had been nasotracheally intubated for ≥48 h and had clinical signs of sinus

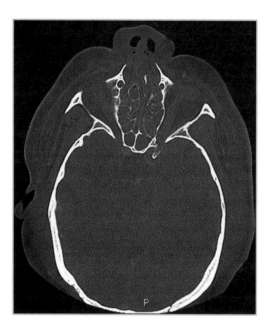

Figure 16.3 CT scan showing complete opacification of the ethmoid sinuses.

infection. They identified 84 sinuses that were positive for disease. Transantral punctures were then performed and confirmed sinus disease in 78 (93%) of the sinuses. Using these criteria, a sensitivity of 100% and a specificity of 86% were achieved in detecting NS with ultrasonography (Vargas and Bui 2006).

Imaging studies have limitations. Radiographic sinusitis does not always correlate with microbiological sinusitis. Imagining cannot differentiate purulent secretions, blood, mucus, or serous effusions. Furthermore, imaging studies do not provide information for antibiotic therapy.

Performing a sinus puncture by intranasal approach is more invasive and limited to the maxillary sinuses, but it does have advantages. First, in adults this can usually be performed at the bedside with local anesthesia, which saves transportation to the CT scanner. Second, sinus irrigation can be therapeutic as well as diagnostic. Importantly, it provides a microbiological specimen for cultures and sensitivities.

Vandenbussche and De Moor (2000) performed a retrospective review of 53 patients who underwent a total of 105 punctures. They noted no complications from these procedures other than minor bleeding, which required no further intervention. They diagnosed 21 (39.6%) patients with NS. They conclude that sinus puncture is safe, inexpensive, and effective for the immediate diagnosis of NS in ICU patients.

■ Prevention and treatment

Prevention of NS begins with removal of unnecessary nasotracheal and nasogastric tubes, semi-recumbent positioning, and strict adherence to hand washing and oral hygiene. Pharmacological prevention of NS was studied in a randomized placebo-controlled trial to evaluate a topically applied α-adrenergic agonist and corticosteroids in 79 polytrauma ICU patients who were anticipated to be intubated for at least 3 days. The treatment group received two drops of xylometazoline twice daily and 100 µg budesonide nasal spray. CT-diagnosed NS was detected in 54% of the treatment group compared with 84% of the control group. NS diagnosed by transnasal puncture and culture was found in 8% of the treatment group and 20% of the control group. This was not a statistically significant result, but results may suffer from an inadequate sample size (Pneumatikos et al. 2006).

Treatment of NS requires removal of any foreign bodies from the nose if possible. Management of blood glucose levels in patients with diabetes, repair of facial fractures, and early mobilization of the patient are also important.

Antibiotics remain the first-line treatment for NS. Empirical choice of antibiotic depends on probable infecting pathogen and bacterial antibiotic resistance patterns. Broad-spectrum coverage should be started initially and then tailored to cultures and sensitivity results.

Adjunctive treatments include nasal saline irrigations, mucolytics, and topical/oral decongestants. Topical decongestants should be used sparingly and for no longer than 72 h in order to prevent the rebound effects of rhinitis medicamentosa. Nasal steroid sprays can also be used as local anti-inflammatory agents in severe NS. Although their role in the acute setting is somewhat controversial, some studies have shown that they are beneficial in reducing acute NS symptoms (Meltzer et al. 2005).

Failure to improve with medical management is an indication for surgical intervention. Sinus puncture with irrigation is the first-line surgical intervention. However, puncture is limited to the maxillary sinuses. Endoscopic sinus surgery allows complete access to the paranasal sinuses. Endoscopic surgery permits direct visualization of the sinus ostia and removal of obstruction. Furthermore, the ostia can be widened to permit further drainage.

Complications

Complications of NS are similar to those of acute rhinosinusitis. Infection can penetrate the thin lamina papyracea to involve the orbit. This extension leads to pre- and postseptal orbital cellulitis (**Figure 16.4**). Left untreated this infection will progress to formation of a subperiosteal abscess and eventually an orbital abscess. A patient with orbital extension may present with proptosis, chemosis, pain with extraocular movement, and decreased visual acuity. Patients with loss of extraocular movement or decreased visual acuity should have emergency drainage of the sinuses and involved orbit.

Infection that spreads posteriorly can lead to intracranial complications, including epidural abscesses, cavernous sinus thrombosis, and brain abscesses. All these complications require surgical drainage of the affected sinus.

To evaluate the relationship between NS and ventilator-associated pneumonia, a randomized controlled trial was conducted with 399

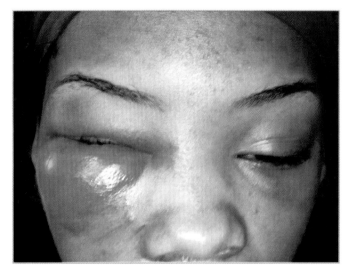

Figure 16.4 Orbital cellulitis.

nasotracheally intubated patients. The treatment group received CT sinus scans if the temperature was >38°C. The control group received standard fever workup without CT scan. NS in the treatment group was treated with intravenous antibiotics and sinus lavage without removal of the nasotracheal tube. Ventilator-associated pneumonia was identified in 34% of the treatment group and 47% of the control group ($p = 0.02$). It was concluded that early diagnosis and treatment of NS decreases the risk of ventilator-associated pneumonia (Holzapfel et al. 1999).

PAROTITIS

In 1881 US President, James Garfield, suffered an abdominal gunshot wound and subsequently died of complications related to suppurative parotitis. The parotid is the salivary gland most affected by inflammation. Acute parotitis (AP) usually afflicts very young children, the elderly or immunocompromised or otherwise debilitated patients. Historically, AP has been associated with significant morbidity and mortality. However, contemporary medical and surgical treatments have improved results. The incidence of AP has been estimated at 0.01–0.02% of all hospital admissions and 0.002–0.04% of postoperative patients (Fattahi et al. 2002). Understanding AP and the importance of timely diagnosis and treatment is important for favorable outcomes.

Anatomy

The parotid is the largest of the major salivary glands. It is located in the preauricular region deep to the skin and subcutaneous tissue. Anteriorly, it is located lateral to the masseter muscle and it extends posteriorly over the sternocleidomastoid muscle and behind the angle of the mandible. The gland is artificially divided into deep and superficial lobes by branches of the facial nerve. Stensen's duct courses anteriorly from the gland over the masseter muscle. It pierces the buccinator muscle to enter the buccal mucosa, usually opposite to the second maxillary molar. The average length of the duct is 4–6 cm. The parotid secretes only a thin watery saliva, under the control of the parasympathetic nervous system via the glossopharyngeal nerve.

Risk factors

AP occurs most commonly in elderly patients associated with systemic illness or surgical procedures. Obstructed or altered salivary flow from dehydration or malnutrition predisposes to AP. No oral intake compromises the stimulatory effects of mastication on the salivary glands.

Diuretics, anticholinergics, and antihistamines can also reduce saliva production. Sialoliths, tumors, and trauma to the duct can lead to obstruction and salivary stasis. Radiation therapy, Sjögren syndrome, and other autoimmune disorders are all associated with reductions in salivary secretions. Poor oral hygiene and immunocompromise are also risks for AP.

Pathogenesis and microbiology

The current understanding of the pathogenesis of AP is that retrograde migration of bacteria in the Stensen duct leads to AP. The continuous flow of saliva normally prevents retrograde bacterial movement but decreased salivation with dehydration, starvation, or the postoperative state permits microbial movement.

Anaerobic bacteria predominate in the oral flora and it is not surprising when they are isolated in AP. The actual frequency of anaerobes may be obscured by inefficiency in anaerobic recovery

Table 16.1 Bacteria commonly isolated in acute suppurative parotitis.

Aerobic and facultative bacteria	Anaerobic bacteria
Staphylococcus aureus	Peptostreptococci
Hemophilus influenzae	Actinomyces israelii
a-Hemolytic streptococci	Propionibacterium acnes
Streptococcus pneumoniae	Eubacterium lentum
Streptococcus pyogenes	Fusobacterium ssp.
Escherichia coli	Bacteroides fragilis
Klebsiella pneumoniae	Bacteroides melaninogenica
Pseudomonas aeruginosa	Prevotella intermedia
	Porphyromonas assacharolytica

of these organisms (Brook 2003a). Bacteria commonly isolated in AP are listed in **Table 16.1**. *S. aureus* is the most common pathogen. Any ICU-associated pathogen can colonize the oral cavity and can be identified in AP. Viruses have been reported to cause parotid inflammation and include enteroviruses, Epstein–Barr virus, cytomegalovirus, parainfluenza, and influenza (Brill and Gilfillan 1977).

Diagnosis

AP will typically present with a unilateral, sudden-onset, indurated, warm, and erythematous swelling of the cheek that extends to the angle of the jaw. The gland will be extremely tender to palpation. In up to 20% of cases of infection may be bilateral. Patients may also have fever, delirium, and other non-specific signs of infection.

The opening of the parotid duct may also appear inflamed. Pus can often be expressed from the duct with gentle pressure applied to the gland. Expression of purulent material from the orifice of the Stensen's duct is diagnostic of AP parotitis. Rarely, occlusion of the duct may prevent pus expression. Fine-needle aspiration of the gland may be performed with Gram stain, culture, and sensitivities of the specimens.

Imaging studies can be useful to determine if a sialolith or stricture is causing ductal obstruction. They can also rule out other unusual causes of acute parotid swelling such as neoplastic processes. CT or ultrasonography can also be used to determine if an abscess has formed that may require surgical drainage. Sialography is generally contraindicated in acute infection due to increased risk of rupture of an ectatic duct from the pressure of the injected dye (Graham et al. 1998).

Treatment

The first line of treatment consists of adequate hydration, systemic antibiotics, and pain control. Sialogogues and parotid massage are also useful adjuncts. Good oral hygiene should be practiced, and in many cases will help prevent infection. When started early, medical therapy alone may be sufficient. Most patients will improve significantly within the first 24–48 h of treatment.

Empirical antibiotics should be tailored to treat suspected organisms. Initially, broad-spectrum antibiotics are indicated to cover *S. aureus*, hemolytic streptococci, and other anaerobic and Gram-negative bacteria (see Table 16.1). Sensitivities will allow tailoring of antibiotic choices. A semisynthetic penicillin (e.g., nafcillin) or first-generation cephalosporin may be sufficient for meticillin-sensitive *S. aureus*. However, in patients with penicillin allergy or MRSA, vancomycin is appropriate. Clindamycin, cefoxitin, imipenem, meropenem, amoxicillin clavulanate, or a combination of macrolide and metronidazole may be necessary for other anaerobic and aerobic bacteria (Brook 2003a).

Occasionally, medical therapy fails or AP may progress to an abscess in the gland or adjacent lymph node. Patients with diabetes are at increased risk of abscess formation. In some cases facial nerve palsy has been associated with parotid abscess (Tan and Goh 2007). Once an abscess has formed surgical incision and drainage are usually indicated. Surgical drainage should also be considered if the patient fails to improve after 3–5 days of antibiotic therapy, the facial nerve is involved, or adjacent structures such as the deep fascial planes become involved.

Repeated episodes of AP may lead to damage of the duct and acini of the gland. This can result in chronic parotitis, which is characterized by recurrent, painful swelling of the gland. Initially, management of this condition should be conservative but may ultimately require surgical intervention including injection of sclerosing agents, ductoplasty, tympanic neuronectomy, or partotidectomy (Motamed et al. 2003).

MIDFACIAL CELLULITIS

Midfacial cellulitis encompasses a spectrum of disease including both primary and secondary infections of the skin and underlying soft tissues. The midface is uniquely prone to the development of dangerous complications due to venous communication with the cavernous sinuses. Several important etiologies of midfacial cellulitis are highlighted, followed by a brief discussion of its treatment, risk factors, and complications.

Primary cellulitic infections

Primary cellulitis of the midface includes infections that arise in otherwise healthy and intact skin. Such infections generally involve a single microbial species, and the exact entry point of the pathogen is often uncertain. The usual risk factors of immunosuppression, uncontrolled diabetes, corticosteroid therapy, and others (Figtree et al. 2010) are associated with all of the cellulitis conditions discussed.

Erysipelas refers to an acute, superficially spreading infection with 90% of cases occurring on the extremities and 10% on the face (Buckland et al. 2007). Facial erysipelas presents with an erythematous, indurated, and painful lesion with raised borders extending over the nasal dorsum and malar areas, with irregularly advancing margins. Systemic symptoms include fever, chills, and malaise. Extensive lymphatic involvement may lead to lymphedema and tender cervical lymphadenopathy. The most common bacterial isolate is group A b-hemolytic streptococci, although several others including groups B, C, and G streptococci and *S. aureus* have been observed. Most cases occur in very young, elderly, or immunocompromised patients. Infections in immunocompromised patients may involve atypical pathogens such as *Strep. pneumoniae, K. pneumoniae, Yersinia enterocolitica*, and *H. influenzae* and have a recurrence rate of up to 20%. When instituted early, antibiotics are generally curative with a mortality rate of <1%. Steroids or anti-inflammatory therapies have been shown to hasten the resolution of symptoms and decrease the duration of hospital stay (Celestin et al. 2007). Bacteremia has been noted in up to 5% of cases, and potential complications include sepsis, meningitis, endocarditis, necrotizing fasciitis, toxic shock syndrome, and chronic lymphedema (Buckland et al. 2007, Celestin et al. 2007).

Impetigo refers to a superficial infection of the epidermis resulting in non-follicular pustules with honey-colored crusting. It is the most common skin infection affecting children. The incidence is highest at age <5 years, and decreases to become rare in adulthood. *S. aureus* has surpassed streptococci as the most common microbial etiology of impetigo. Bullous impetigo is nearly always caused by *S. aureus*, and is characterized by blistering of the epidermis from exfoliative toxins associated with staphylococci (Bernard 2008). Initial treatment consists of cleansing regularly with soap and water, and application of topical antibiotic ointment effective against *S. aureus*, such as mupirocin. Widespread infections and those not responding to topical therapy require oral or parenteral antibiotic therapy.

Buccal cellulitis resulting from *H. influenzae* type b (Hib) infection is a disappearing disease that immunization has virtually eliminated. Before immunization, it represented the second most common etiology of facial cellulitis among children. Buccal cellulitis typically presented between the ages of 3 and 24 months with a history of mild upper respiratory infection followed by the development of high fever, irritability, and facial swelling. Bacteremia was frequently noted, with blood cultures positive in nearly 75% of cases. Complications resulted from hematogenous spread, and included meningitis. One study failed to identify a single case of buccal cellulitis over a 10-year period following the institution of Hib immunization.

Another primary cellulitis infection is group B streptococcal (GBS) infection after the first week of life. The infection typically presents in the buccal, submental, and submandibular areas of the face, and is complicated by GBS sepsis and meningitis in up to 25% of affected infants. Lumbar puncture is an essential component to the initial workup when GBS infection is suspected in the neonate, and broad-spectrum parenteral antibiotic therapy should be administered (Pickett and Gallaher 2004).

Secondary cellulitic infections

Secondary cellulitis of the midface arises from direct spread from an adjacent infectious entity or from inoculation of a pathogen with breach of the cutaneous barrier. The microbiology of secondary infections is variable, and polymicrobial infections are frequently observed. Successful treatment may require identification and resolution of the inciting factors.

Secondary bacterial infections may occur during viral illnesses such as chickenpox or shingles in otherwise healthy individuals. As in most skin infections, group A b-hemolytic streptococci and S aureus are the most frequent microbial isolates. The potential complications of pediatric chickenpox reportedly include impetigo, skin abscess, cellulitis, necrotizing fasciitis, myositis, osteomyelitis, and severe systemic processes such as sepsis and toxic shock-like syndrome (Santos-Juanes et al. 2001).

Odontogenic infection is one of the most common etiologies of facial cellulitis and deep cervical space infections. A history suggesting frequent toothache before the onset of facial edema and tenderness often identifies the source of infection. Fever and trismus arise as the infection progresses. Treatment includes antibiotic therapy followed by dental or surgical intervention to address the odontogenic source of infection. Potential complications vary according to the location of the infection. Maxillary infections spread to the paranasal sinuses and the upper face, and potential complications arise from orbital involvement, cavernous sinus thrombosis, and intracranial spread. In contrast, mandibular infections spread to the lower face and the deep cervical spaces with the potential for deep cervical abscess or Ludwig's angina with airway compromise.

Furuncles of the nasal vestibule result from the spread of *S. aureus* along hair follicles into the deep dermis where an abscess subsequently develops. Chronic carriers of *S. aureus* in the anterior nares have higher recurrence rates. In addition, MRSA and the presence of virulence factor Panton–Valentine leukocidin have been associated with epidemic outbreaks of more severe furunculosis (Bernard 2008). Treatment of furunculosis involves the evacuation of purulent debris and application of topical antimicrobial therapy to prevent recurrence. Oral antibiotics should be considered for refractory or severe infections. Epidemic furunculosis should be controlled using aggressive nasal hygiene with disinfecting washes, along with application of mupirocin ointment twice daily for 5 days for patients and their close contacts (El-Gilany and Fathy 2009). Complications such as alar stenosis and MRSA endocarditis have been reported (Bernard 2008).

Ethmoid sinusitis is classically associated with the potential for orbital complications, including preseptal or periorbital cellulitis. In addition, acute maxillary sinusitis in the absence of odontogenic disease has been reported as a cause of midfacial bullous cellulitis in an otherwise healthy patient. Successful treatment included functional endoscopic sinus surgery with maxillary antrostomy and removal of purulent material from the affected sinuses along with parenteral antibiotic therapy (Yemison et al. 2009).

Surgical site infection of the well-vascularized facial skin is uncommon when appropriate perioperative antiseptic and prophylactic practices are employed. Postoperative infection is more common after procedures involving the nose (6.5%) and ears (5%) than the face (1.5%). In addition, oncological surgery and complex procedures involving grafts and local flaps increase the risk of postoperative infection significantly when compared with non-oncological interventions with primary wound closure (Sylaidis et al. 1997).

Traumatic abrasions and lacerations of the facial skin are low risk for infectious complications, and local wound care is usually sufficient. Inoculation of debris such as soil into a deeper wound is, however, rarely associated with invasive soft tissue infection involving environmental pathogens such as the Zygomycetes class of fungi. Aggressive angioinvasion with hematogenous dissemination and rapidly progressing necrosis make early recognition of zygomycosis, treatment with surgical debridement, and parenteral amphotericin essential management (Kindo et al. 2007). Blunt trauma often results in facial fractures that allow for direct communication between the paranasal sinuses and the adjacent orbit. Once identified, the patient should be advised against nose blowing or straining. Treatment includes decongestants, humidification, and antibiotic therapy for clinical infection. Periorbital edema, ophthalmoplegia, and proptosis should prompt urgent CT evaluation to guide further management of orbital complications.

Treatment

β-Lactam or broad-spectrum quinolone antibiotics covering both streptococcal and staphylococcal infections are the mainstay of treatment for superficial infections of the midface. Community-associated MRSA infections are commonly treated with trimethoprim–sulfamethoxazole, doxycycline, or clindamycin. Inpatient MRSA infection is treated with vancomycin. Linezolid provides a costly yet effective means of either single-agent oral or parenteral therapy. Appropriate antibiotic therapy results in symptomatic improvement within 24–48 h. Continued advancement of the margins of erythema and induration suggests microbial resistance to therapy (O'Connor and Paauw 2010).

Complications

Sepsis is a potential complication of midface cellulitis regardless of the etiology, and should be suspected in the presence of the systemic inflammatory response, and treated accordingly with broad-spectrum parenteral antibiotic therapy, and surgical drainage and debridement when appropriate. Blood cultures should be obtained before initiating antibiotic therapy to validate the putative pathogen.

Necrotizing fasciitis involves the spread of infection along fascial planes with progressive thrombosis and necrosis of the dermis, subcutaneous fat, fascia, and underlying soft tissues (see Chapter 5). The clinical presentation may initially mimic cellulitis with unrelenting pain disproportionate to exam findings, bullae and discoloration of the overlying skin, subcutaneous emphysema, cutaneous anesthesia, woody induration of the subcutaneous tissue extending beyond the margins of erythema, rapid spread, and systemic toxicity (fever, leukocytosis, mental status changes, and renal failure). Imaging studies may suggest edema extending along fascial planes. Surgical exploration is required to define the extent and to provide early, aggressive surgical debridement with parenteral antibiotic therapy.

Meningitis presents clinically with rapid onset of fever, headache, mental status changes, photophobia, and meningismus. MRI is the imaging study of choice to evaluate intracranial pathology, because meningitis may have a normal appearance on CT scan. Treatment consists of broad-spectrum parenteral antibiotic coverage. Long-term neurological sequelae may include seizures and sensorineural deficits such as hearing loss in up to 25% of cases (Epstein and Kern 2008).

Cavernous sinus thrombosis is the feared complication of midfacial cellulitis. Venous outflow from the midface communicates directly with the cavernous sinuses through the valveless ophthalmic veins. Subsequent thrombosis and intracranial spread of infection results in headache, fever, altered consciousness, ophthalmoplegia secondary to deficits of cranial nerves III, IV, and VI, and paraesthesiae of the ophthalmic and maxillary branches of the trigeminal nerve. Involvement of the superior ophthalmic vein may lead to complications such as visual disturbances, orbital pain, and orbital cellulitis or abscess (Dhariwal et al. 2003). Contrast-enhanced CT of the skull base and CT venography are useful to detect cavernous sinus thrombus or filling defects, whereas MRI of the brain with contrast may demonstrate dural enhancement adjacent to the cavernous sinuses (Rana and Moonis 2011). Treatment consists of long-term, culture-directed, parenteral antibiotic therapy (up to 8 weeks) with or without the use of anticoagulation. The use of steroid therapy is not recommended (Epstein and Kern 2008). The mortality rate approaches 30–40% despite aggressive treatment (Oliver and Gillespie 2010).

ODONTOGENIC INFECTIONS

Odontogenic infections are widespread and represent the most common cause of deep cervical space abscesses in adults. Appropriate management requires a thorough understanding of the cervical spaces of head and neck anatomy, as well as the potentially severe complications that may accompany these infections. Dental expertise is also needed to address the source and prevent recurrence of the infection. Hospitalizations for acute dental infections have an incidence of approximately 1 in 2600 annually in the USA, and last an average of 8 days (Wang et al. 2005). Most severe or spreading odontogenic infections affect patients in their 20s and 30s (Boffano et al. 2011). Children have a much higher rate of maxillary odontogenic infection with associated buccal space infections, whereas adults are more prone to infections arising from the posterior mandible (Wang et al. 2005).

Pathogenesis

Odontogenic infection initially requires a compromise in the natural barriers that protect the dentoalveolar structures. The pathogenesis of these infections occurs in several different patterns. Breach of the dental enamel allows for entry of bacteria into the pulp chamber and subsequent endodontal spread to the root apex, where continued erosion and bone resorption accompany the formation of an apical abscess. Gingivitis is another route of bacterial spread along the periodontal ligaments resulting in bone resorption and subsequent periodontal pocket formation (Rana and Moonis 2011). Regardless of the pathway, the end result is infection within the mandibular or maxillary bone surrounding the diseased tooth. The infection progresses along the pathways of least resistance until the inner or outer cortex is penetrated and invasion of soft tissue ensues.

Maxillary odontogenic infections involving the incisors, premolars, and first molars are most likely to spread to the buccal space. Maxillary canine infections spread to the canine space resulting in blunting of the nasolabial fold. Second maxillary molar infections more often spread to the masticator space, and third maxillary molar infections usually spread to the parapharyngeal space.

Mandibular odontogenic infections involving the incisors occasionally spread to the submental space, whereas infected mandibular canines and first premolars are most likely to spread to the sublingual space above the mylohyoid muscle. Mandibular infections arising in the second and third molars exit the cortex below the attachment of the mylohyoid muscle and into the submandibular space (Christian 2010).

Odontogenic infections have the potential to invade the deep cervical spaces discussed above. Involvement of the deep cervical space increases the life-threatening potential of complications such as mediastinitis.

Risk factors

Odontogenic infection is primarily associated with dental caries and poor oral hygiene. Systemic diseases, particularly the hyperglycemia of diabetes, have been shown to increase the risk for cervical space infection and its associated complications. One prospective study recently found that spreading odontogenic infections were associated with tobacco smoking in 80% and social deprivation in 72% of their study population. Other comorbidities associated with odontogenic infection include alcohol abuse, intravenous drug abuse, immunosuppression, and other medical illnesses such as hypertension, asthma, malnutrition, and iron-deficiency anemia (Wang et al. 2005, Bakathir et al. 2009).

Microbiology

The mouth is colonized by at least 350 distinct bacterial species, many of which have the potential to cause odontogenic infection. Infections are polymicrobial. Cultures from odontogenic abscesses typically reveal four to seven separate bacterial isolates (Robertson and Smith 2009). Obligate anaerobes outnumber aerobic or facultative flora, and are essentially universal in odontogenic infections. Peptostreptococci, and Fusobacterium, Prevotella, Bacteroides, and Porphyromonas spp. comprise the strict anaerobes (Kuriyama et al. 2000, Robertson and Smith 2009). Facultative anaerobes are also present in more than 50% of cases (Kuriyama et al. 2000). Viridans group streptococci and b-hemolytic streptococci represent the most common facultatives observed, followed by Fusobacterium and Prevotella spp. in frequency (Robertson and Smith 2009).

Diagnosis

History and physical examination usually identify the source of infection, and special attention is given to evaluation of the airway.

Rapid airway compromise may develop in the setting of Ludwig's angina or an enlarging posterior deep cervical space abscess. Depending on the degree of airway compromise, either awake fiberoptic nasotracheal intubation or emergency tracheostomy or cricothyroidotomy may be necessary. Once the airway has been stabilized, appropriate antibiotic therapy should be initiated as described below. Any suspicion for deep cervical space involvement is an indication for CT of the neck to accurately identify the extent of infection before any surgical intervention. Ultrasonography has been found to accurately assess the more superficial cervical spaces (buccal, submandibular, canine, submasseteric, submental, and infraorbital spaces), but should not be relied on for assessment of the deeper spaces (masticator, parapharyngeal, and sublingual spaces) (Bassiony et al. 2009).

Treatment

Dental care, incision, and drainage, and appropriate antibiotic therapy, comprise the approach to managing odontogenic infections. The dentition responsible for inciting the odontogenic infection must be extracted at the time of surgical drainage. Any cervical space that appears to be involved with infection on CT should be incised, cleared of any purulent or necrotic debris, and a drain or irrigation catheter left in place. Needle drainage is not recommended in the setting of anaerobic infection with the potential for significant tissue destruction. Most of the spaces should be approached extraorally; however, the retropharyngeal, canine, and some isolated buccal and sublingual space infections can be safely incised and drained using a transoral approach. Appropriate empirical antibiotic therapy must take into account the susceptibilities of the common odontogenic pathogens. Anaerobes with significant b-lactamase activity, such as Prevotella and Bacteroides spp., often necessitate the use of b-lactamase-resistant therapies. Polymicrobial odontogenic abscesses require broad-spectrum coverage. Culture results have not been found to alter antibiotic management in the setting of adequate coverage; rather, changes in therapy are indicated when clinical indicators such as persistent fever or leukocytosis suggest therapeutic failure (Wang et al. 2005).

First-line treatment of uncomplicated odontogenic infections should consist of penicillin in combination with metronidazole, or monotherapy consisting of a formulation that includes a b-lactamase inhibitor such as amoxicillin–clavulanate (co-amoxiclav) or ampicillin–sulbactam. The addition of metronidazole provides coverage for most of the clinically important anaerobes, with the notable exception of Actinomyces spp. It should not, however, be used as monotherapy because it lacks aerobic activity. Clindamycin is an effective alternative to penicillin with adequate coverage of streptococci, most penicillin-resistant staphylococci, and clinically significant anaerobes. It is the recommended treatment for patients allergic to penicillin (Levi and Eusterman 2011).

Cephalosporins generally provide adequate microbial coverage with fewer potential side effects than clindamycin, but should be avoided in penicillin-allergic patients. b-Lactamase-resistant cephalosporins are particularly useful in severe infections (Kuriyama et al. 2000). Carbapenems possess excellent activity against most Gram-positive, Gram-negative, and anaerobic bacteria, and should be considered when other treatments fail (Levi and Eusterman 2011). Moxifloxacin provides adequate coverage for most odontogenic infections and was found to be superior to clindamycin with more rapid clinical resolution and fewer side effects (Cachovan et al. 2011). Finally, macrolides have been recommended in the past for treatment of odontogenic infection; however, emerging microbial resistance now limits their usefulness in moderate-to-severe infections (Kuriyama et al. 2000).

Complications

Cervical space infection (CSI) represents a complex spectrum of disease governed by the spread of infection along pathways of least resistance. Tonsillitis is the most frequent etiology of CSI in children, but odontogenic disease represents the most common cause in adults. Treatment consists of broad-spectrum antibiotic administration, and surgical interventions aimed at draining the involved cervical spaces and removing the odontogenic source of infection. Airway compromise, descending infection, and vascular sequelae may complicate severe cases of CSI.

Cervical necrotizing fasciitis (see above and Chapter 5), *mediastinitis* (Kinzer et al. 2009), and *Lemierre syndrome* (see above) are additional complications of invasive odontogenic infection. Lemierre cases with *Fusobacterium* spp. have been reported in the past decade, arising from pharyngeal and odontogenic infections that breach the retrostyloid compartment of the parapharyngeal space or spread directly from thrombophlebitis of the adjacent facial venous plexus. Septic emboli potentially give rise to microabscesses within the lungs, liver, kidneys, and central nervous system, and may lead to septic shock.

Intracranial infections from odontogenic bacterial infection can occur either by direct extension through the cribriform plate, hematogenous seeding, or retrograde thrombosis in the setting of odontogenic sinusitis. Intracranial pathology may include cavernous sinus thrombosis, abscess, or meningitis. Polymicrobial (primarily anaerobic) flora mirror those observed in odontogenic infections (Brook 2006).

As many as 86% of refractory *maxillary sinusitis* cases may actually be related to odontogenic infections, especially in the setting of radiographic evidence of oroantral fistula, periapical abscess, periodontal disease, projecting tooth root, and dental caries. Empirical antibiotic coverage in the setting of odontogenic origin (anaerobic infection) differs from that of non-odontogenic sinusitis. Dental pathology is addressed before consideration of functional endoscopic sinus surgery (Bomeli et al. 2009).

Oroantral fistula refers to an osteomucosal communication between the oral cavity and either the nose or one of the maxillary sinuses. It usually represents an iatrogenic complication of dental extraction, maxillary cyst removal, or the Caldwell–Luc approach to maxillary sinus surgery; however, it has been linked to odontogenic infection as well. Fistulas <5 mm in diameter can be expected to resolve with antibiotic therapy. Fistulas >5 mm require primary closure using local advancement or pedicle flaps. Closure should be deferred until any signs of ongoing maxillary sinusitis have responded to antibiotic or surgical therapy (Hajiioanou et al. 2010).

An *orocutaneous fistula* forms when periapical infection causes gradual erosion through alveolar bone with subsequent development of a sinus tract to the overlying skin. The resulting lesion can be mistaken for local trauma, furuncle, carcinoma, and several other entities, which may lead to >50% of patients undergoing unnecessary rounds of antibiotic therapy and dermatological procedures. Mandibular dentition is involved in 80% of cases. Radiographs reveal bone loss at the apex of the affected dentition. Orocutaneous fistulas generally resolve within 5–14 days of root canal or dental extraction as indicated (Pasternak-Junior et al. 2009).

Osteomyelitis related to odontogenic infection can lead to bony erosion of the mandible or maxilla. Dental implants, in particular, carry up to a 15% risk of localized osteomyelitis (Pigrau et al. 2009). Alveolar osteitis refers to focal osteomyelitis within a tooth socket after dental extraction, and occurs in about 3% of cases (Younis and Hantash 2011). These are often chronic polymicrobial infections, and are frequently resistant to clindamycin but remain sensitive to penicillin and fluoroquinolones. Prolonged antibiotic therapy in addition to surgical interventions, including debridement, marginal resection, and sequestrectomy, may be necessary. Hyperbaric oxygen therapy has also been used as adjunctive therapy (Pigrau et al. 2009).

Orbital complications are rare in association with odontogenic infection, whereas 80% of orbital infections are believed to arise from paranasal sinus disease. Infection anterior to the orbital septum presents as preseptal cellulitis with periorbital edema in the absence of orbital involvement. Infectious spread posterior to the orbital septum is further divided into intra- versus extraconal disease by the extraocular muscles. Signs of an orbital abscess include pain, swelling, chemosis, limitation of eye movements, proptosis, and decreased visual acuity. Optic neuritis, atrophy, and blindness may result from elevated intraorbital pressure in severe infections. Posterior infectious spread may lead to intracranial abscess, meningitis, and death. Treatment involves aggressive parenteral antibiotic therapy and surgical drainage for any suspected abscess, as well as emergency lateral canthotomy when necessary to relieve intraorbital pressure and prevent vascular insult to the orbital contents (Kim et al. 2007).

■ REFERENCES

Bakathir AA, Moos KF, Ayoub AF, et al. Factors contributing to the spread of odontogenic infections – a prospective pilot study. *Sultan Qaboos Univ Med J* 2009;**9**:296–304.

Bassiony M, Yang J, Abdel-Monem TM, et al. Exploration of ultrasonography in assessment of fascial space spread of odontogenic infections. *Oral Surg Oral Med Oral Pathol Oral Radiol Endod* 2009;**107**:861–9.

Bernard P. Management of common bacterial infections of the skin. *Curr Opin Infect Dis* 2008;**21**:122–8.

Boffano P, Roccia F, Pittoni D, et al. Management of 112 hospitalized patients with spreading odontogenic infections: correlation with DMFT and oral health impact profile 14 indexes. *Oral Surg Oral Med Oral Pathol Oral Radiol Endod* 2012;**113**:207–13.

Bomeli SR, Branstetter BF, Ferguson BJ. Frequency of a dental source for acute maxillary sinusitis. *Laryngoscope* 2009;**119**:580–4.

Boscolo-Rizzo P, Marchiori C, Zanetti F, et al. Conservative management of deep neck abscesses in adults: the importance of CECT findings. *Otolaryngol Head Neck Surg* 2006;**135**:894–9.

Brill SJ, Gilfillan RF. Acute parotitis associated with influenza type A. *N Engl J Med* 1977;**296**:1391.

Brook I. Acute bacterial suppurative bacterial parotitis: microbiology and management. *J Craniofacial Surg* 2003a;**14**:37–40.

Brook I. Microbiology and management of deep facial infections and Lemierre syndrome. *ORL J Otorhinolaryngol Relat Spec* 2003b;**65**:117–20.

Brook I. Microbiology of intracranial abscesses associated with sinusitis of odontogenic origin. *Ann Otol Rhinol Laryngol* 2006;**115**:917–20.

Bross-Soriano D, Arrieta-Gomez J, Prado-Calleros H, et al. Management of Ludwig's angina with small neck incisions: 18 years experience. *Otolaryngol Head Neck Surg* 2004;**130**:712–7.

Buckland GT, Carlson JA, Meyer DR. Persistent periorbital and facial lymphedema associated with Group A β-hemolytic streptococcal infection (erysipelas). *Ophthal Plast Reconstr Surg* 2007;**23**:161–3.

Cachovan G, Boger RH, Giersdorf I, et al. Comparative efficacy and safety of moxifloxacin and clindamycin in the treatment of odontogenic abscesses and inflammatory infiltrates: a phase II, double-blind, randomized trial. *Antimicrob Agents Chemother* 2011;**55**:1142–7.

Caplan ES, Hoyt NJ. Nosocomial sinusitis. *JAMA* 1982;**247**:639–641.

Celestin R, Brown J, Kihiczak G, et al. Erysipelas: a common potentially dangerous infection. Acta Dermatovenerol *Alp Panonica Adriat* 2007;**16**:123–7.

Christian JM. Odontogenic infections. In: Flint PW (ed.), *Otolaryngology: Head and neck surgery*, 5th edn. Amsterdam: Elsevier, 2010: 177–90.

Dhariwal DK, Kittur MA, Farrier JN, et al. Post-traumatic orbital cellulitis. *Br J Oral Maxillofac Surg* 2003;**41**:21–8.

El-Gilany AH, Fathy H. Risk factors of recurrent furunculosis. *Dermatol Online J* 2009;**15**:16.

Epstein VA, Kern RC. Invasive fungal sinusitis and complications of rhinosinusitis. *Otolaryngol Clin N Am* 2008;**41**:497–524.

Fattahi TT, Lyu PE, Van Sickels JE. Management of acute suppurative parotitis. *J Oral Maxillofac Surg* 2002;**60**:446–8

Figtree M, Konecny P, Jennings Z, et al. Risk stratification and outcome of cellulitis admitted to hospital. *J Infect* 2010;**60**:431–9.

George DL, Falk PS, Meduri GU, et al. Nosocomial sinusitis in patients in the medical intensive care unit: a prospective epidemiological study. *Clin Infect Dis* 1998;**27**:463–70.

Graham SM, Hoffman HT, McCulloch TM, et al. Intra-operative ultrasound-guided drainage of parotid abscess. *J Laryngol Otol* 1998;**112**:1098.

Hajiioannou J, Koudounarakis E, Alexopoulos K, et al. Maxillary sinusitis of dental origin due to oroantral fistula, treated by endoscopic sinus surgery and primary fistula closure. *J Laryngol Otol* 2010;**124**:986–9.

Holzapfel L, Chastang C, Demingeon G, et al. A randomized study assessing the systematic search for maxillary sinusitis in nasotracheally mechanically ventilated patients. Influence of nosocomial maxillary sinusitis on the occurrence of ventilator-associated pneumonia. *Am J Respir Crit Care Med* 1999;**159**:695–701.

Huang T, Liu T, Chen P, et al. Deep neck infection: analysis of 185 cases. *Head Neck* 2004;**26**:854–60.

Huang T, Tseng F, Liu C, et al. Deep neck infection in diabetic patients: comparison of clinical picture and outcomes with nondiabetic patients. *Otolaryngol Head Neck Surg* 2005;**132**:943–7.

Kim IK, Kim JR, Jang KS, et al. Orbital abscess from an odontogenic infection. *Oral Surg Oral Med Oral Pathol Oral Riol Endod* 2007;**103**:e1–6.

Kindo AJ, Shams NR, Kumar K, et al. Fatal cellulitis caused by Apophysomyces elegans. *Indian J Med Microbiol* 2007;**25**:285–7.

Kinzer S, Pfeiffer J, Becker S, Ridder GJ. Severe deep neck space infections and mediastinitis of odontogenic origin: clinical relevance and implications for diagnosis and treatment. *Acta Otolaryngol* 2009;**129**:62–70.

Korinek AM, Laisne MJ, Nicolas MH, et al. Selective decontaminationof the digestive tract in neurosurgical intensive care unit patients: a double-blind, randomized, placebo-controlled study. *Crit Care Med* 1993;**21**:1466–73.

Kuriyama T, Karasawa T, Nakagawa K, et al. Bacteriologic features and antimicrobial susceptibility in isolates from orofacial odontogenic infections. *Oral Surg Oral Med Oral pathol Oral Radiol Endod* 2000;**90**:600–8.

Levi ME, Eusterman VD. Oral infections and antibiotic therapy. *Otolaryngol Clin North Am* 2011;**44**:57–78.

Mayor G, Millan J, Martinez-Vidal A. Is conservative treatment of deep neck space infections appropriate? *Head Neck* 2001;**23**:126–33.

Meltzer EO, Bachert C, Staudinger H. Treating acute rhinosinusitis: comparing efficacy and safety of ometasone furoate nasal spray,amoxicillin and placebo. *J Allergy Clin Immunol* 2005;**116**:1289–95.

Motamed M, Laugharne D, Bradley PJ. Management of chronic parotitis: a review. *J Laryngol Otol* 2003;**117**:521–6.

Naidu S, Donepudi S, Stocks R, et al. Methicillin-resistant *Staphylococcus aureus* as a pathogen in deep neck abscesses: a pediatric case series. *Int J Pediatr Otorhinolaryngol* 2005;**69**:1367–71.

Nusbaum A, Som P, Rothschild M, et al. Recurrence of a deep neck infection: a clinical indication of an underlying congenital lesion. *Arch Otolaryngol Head Neck Surg* 1999;**125**:1379–82.

O'Connor K, Paauw D. Erysipelas: rare but important cause of malar rash. *Am J Med* 2010;**123**:414–16.

Oliver ER, Gillespie MB. Deep neck space infections. . In: Flint PW (ed.), *Otolaryngology: Head and neck surgery*, 5th edn. Amsterdam: Elsevier, 2010: 201–28.

Ovassapian A, TuncbilekM, Weitzel E, et al. Airway management in adult patients with deep neck infections: a case series and review of the literature. *Anesth Analg* 2005;**100**:585–9.

Palacios E, Rojas R. Necrotizing fasciitis of the neck. *Ear Nose Throat J* 2006;**85**:638.

Pasternak-Junior B, Teixeira CS, Silva-Sousa YT, Sousa-Neto MD. Diagnosis and treatment of odontogenic cutaneous sinus tracts of endodontic origin: three case studies. *Int Endod J* 2009;**42**:271–6.

Pickett KC, Gallaher KJ. Facial submandibular cellulitis associated with late-onset Group B streptococcal infection. *Adv Neonatal Care* 2004;**4**:20–5.

Pigrau C, Almirante B, Rodriguez D, et al. Osteomyelitis of the jaw: resistance to clindamycin in patients with prior antibiotics exposure. *Eur J Clin Microbiol Infect Dis* 2009;**28**:317–23.

Pneumatikos L, Konstantonis D,Tsagaris I, et al. Prevention of nosocomial maxillary sinusitis in the ICU: the effects of topically applied α-adrenergic agonists and corticosteroids. *Intensive Care Med* 2006;**32**:532–7

Rana RS, Moonis G. Head and neck infection and inflammation. *Radiol Clin N Am* 2011;**49**:165–82.

Rega A, Aziz S, Ziccardi V. Microbiology and antibiotic sensitivities of head and neck space infections of odontogenic origin. *J Oral Maxillofac Surg* 2006;**64**:1377–80.

Riga M, Danielidis V. Pneumatikos I. Rhinosinusitis in the intensive care unit patients: A review of the possible underlying mechanisms and proposals for the investigation of their potential role in functional treatment interventions. *J Crit Care* 2010;**25**:171.e9–14.

Robertson D, Smith AJ. The microbiology of the acute dental abscess. *J Med Microbiol* 2009;**58**(Pt 2):155–62.

Rouby J, Laurent P. Risk factors and clinical relevance of nosocomial maxillary sinusitis in the critically ill. *Am J Respir Crit Care Med* 1994;**150**:776–83.

Santos-Juanes J, Medina A, Concha A, et al. Varicella complicated by Group A streptococcal facial cellulitis. *J Am Acad Dermatol* 2001;**45**:770–2.

Sichel J, Attal P, Hocwald E, et al. Redefining parapharyngeal space infections. *Ann Otol Rhinol Laryngol* 2006;**115**:117–23.

Smith J, Hsu J, Chang J. Predicting deep neck space abscess using computed tomography. *Am J Otolaryngol* 2006;**27**:244–7.

Stalfors J, Adielsson A, Ebenfelt A, et al. Deep neck space infections remain a surgical challenge: a study of 72 patients. *Acta Otolaryngol* 2004;**124**:1191–6.

Sylaidis P, Wood S, Murray DS. Postoperative infection following clean facial surgery. *Ann Plast Surg* 1997;**39**:342–6.

Tan VES, Goh BS. Parotid abscess: a five year review clinical presentation diagnosis and management. *J Laryngol Otol* 2007;**121**:872–9.

Vandenbussche T, De Moor S. Value of antral puncture in the intensive care patient with fever of unknown origin. *Laryngoscope* 2000;**110**:1702–6

Vargas F, Bui H. Transnasal puncture based on echographic sinusitis evidence in mechanically ventilated patients with suspicion of nosocomial maxillary sinusitis. *Intensive Care Med* 2006;**32**:858–66.

Wang J, Ahani A, Pogrel MA. A five-year retrospective study of odontogenic maxillofacial infections in a large urban public hospital. *Int J Oral Maxillofac Surg* 2005;**34**:646–9.

Weed HG, Forest LA. Deep neck infection. In: Cummings CW, Flint PW, Harker LA, et al. (eds), *Otolaryngology: Head and neck surgery*, 4th edn, vol. 3. Philadelphia, PA: Elsevier Mosby, 2005: 2515–24.

Yemison M, Sagit M, Karakas O. Facial bullous cellulitis caused by acute sinusitis. *Int J Infect Dis* 2009;**13**:e525–6.

Yeow K, Liao C, Hao S. US-guided needle aspiration and catheter drainage as an alternative to open surgical drainage for uniloculated neck abscesses. *J Vasc Interv Radiol* 2001;**12**:589–94.

Younis A, Hantash A. Dry socket: frequency, clinical picture, and risk factors in a Palestinian dental teaching center. *Open Dent J* 2011;**5**:7–12.

Chapter 17 Vascular surgical site infection

Kelley D. Hodgkiss-Harlow, Dennis F. Bandyk

Surgical site infection (SSI) after vascular intervention, an important cause of postoperative morbidity, requires patient-specific treatment and an accurate microbiological diagnosis. Based on the clinical presentation, microbiology of the infectious process, and extent of graft involvement, multiple surgical options are appropriate, including graft excision alone, graft preservation, *in situ* graft replacement, or graft excision proceeded by *ex situ* bypass via uninvolved tissue planes. As most patients present with low virulence infection, the preferred approach is *in situ* revascularization, using autologous conduit (femoral or saphenous vein), cryopreserved allograft, or an antibiotic (rifampin)-impregnated prosthesis. Antibiotic therapy is essential and should utilize bactericidal drugs that penetrate bacteria biofilms. Antibiotic delivery to the infected surgical site is conventionally done with parenteral drugs, but antibiotic-impregnated beads may be used for local administration. Prevention of vascular infection requires the surgeon to be cognizant of its changing epidemiology, the known patient risk factors, and application of effective measures to reduce its incidence. The majority of vascular SSIs are caused by Gram-positive bacteria. Meticillin-resistant *Staphylococcus aureus* (MRSA) is the most common pathogen and is identified in more than a third of cases. Nasal colonization by *S. aureus*, recent hospitalization, a failed arterial reconstruction, and the presence of a groin incision are major risk factors for developing a vascular SSI. Preoperative measures to decolonize the nares and surgical site of *S. aureus*, together with appropriate, bactericidal antibiotic prophylaxis, meticulous wound closure, and postoperative care to optimize patient host defense regulation mechanisms (temperature, oxygenation, blood sugar), can minimize vascular infection occurrence.

Vascular infection occurs as a result of perioperative events leading to bacterial colonization of the wound and frequently the underlying prosthetic graft when present. The vascular patient requiring arterial reconstruction has an increased SSI risk with an overall incidence in the range of 5–10%. This rate of infection is significantly higher than the 1.5–5% rate predicted by the Centers for Disease National Nosocomial Infections Surveillance System for "clean" procedures in risk index categories 1 and 2 (Culver et al. 1991, Vogel et al. 2008, 2010). The increased likelihood of SSI is due to both procedure- and patient-specific risk factors – highest after lower limb bypass for critical limb ischemia, lowest after carotid endarterectomy or endovascular aortic aneurysm repair. Implantation of a vascular prosthesis increases SSI risk by producing a microenvironment conducive to bacterial attachment and biofilm formation which sustains bacterial colonization and protects encased organisms from host defenses and antimicrobial therapy. Injured skin/skin structures and soft-tissue edema are common sequelae after femoral and lower limb arterial revascularizations and impede wound healing. In addition to intraoperative contamination, postoperative skin separation of the incision with underlying hematoma and serous wound drainage extend the time available for bacterial invasion from external sources.

Bacteremia from remote sources or bacterial transport via lymphatic channels in the reconstructed extremity can be sources of secondary infection of the surgical site and arterial graft. The non-healing wound facilitates colonization by bacterial strains with the virulence factor of biofilm formation, and if not addressed can progress to an SSI with predictable increased morbidity. Healthcare costs are then increased from an extended hospitalization, return to the operating room for wound debridement/closure procedures, and necessary home healthcare and outpatient visits for wound management. Prevention of SSI should be of paramount concern but reducing the incidence requires knowledge of its changing epidemiology and the use of effective patient-care strategies. An implanted vascular graft or endovascular stent graft is most susceptible to colonization during the early (<1 month) postoperative period from either bacteremia or, more commonly, the adherence of pathogenic strains to the device with the development of a bacterial biofilm – an organism-produced microenvironment protective against host defenses and antibiotics. Understanding the implications of a biofilm infection, especially the concept of selective antibiotic resistance, is essential for clinical success in treatment of vascular SSIs (Frei et al. 2011).

EPIDEMIOLOGY OF VASCULAR SITE INFECTION

Infection involving a vascular wound may be *superficial*, i.e., cellulitis, *deep incisional* involving the subcutaneous tissue/fascia, or involving other areas than the incision itself, i.e., *organ/space*, such as along the length of an implanted vascular prosthesis or as an intracavitary aortic graft infection. For autogenous arterial revascularizations, only infections occurring within 30 days should be classified as an SSI, but when a prosthetic graft or endovascular device is implanted the incidence of SSIs is calculated for 1 year. The diagnostic criteria for SSIs should include signs/symptoms of infection (pain, tenderness, erythema, swelling), purulent drainage for the wound, and organisms isolated from aseptically obtained cultures of fluid or tissue.

Although virtually any microorganism can produce an SSI or infect a vascular prosthesis, Gram-positive bacteria, especially *S. aureus*, are the prevalent pathogens involved in approximately 80% of all cases (Reifsnyder et al. 1992, Cowie et al. 2005, Armstong et al. 2007, Vogel et al. 2010, Frei et al. 2011). As in other surgical disciplines, the microbiology of vascular SSIs has changed since 2000 with an increased prevalence of antibiotic-resistant organisms, including staphylococcal strains. An audit of prosthetic arterial graft infections treated by our vascular surgery group demonstrated a fourfold increase in MRSA infection from 10% in the 1990s to 40% since 2000 (Perl et al. 2002, Pounds et al. 2005). In a series of complex vascular SSIs treated by aggressively staged surgical debridement, antibiotic bead therapy, and selective sartorius muscle flap coverage, MRSA accounted for 20% of all infections and 50% of reinfections (Frei et al. 2011). This trend has been verified from other vascular centers in the USA and Europe, including a 2005 report from the University of Texas Galveston documenting a SSI rate of 11% after lower bypass grafting with *S. aureus* involved in 64% of cases of which half were caused by MRSA (Cowie et al. 2005). MRSA should be suspected in any vascular patient presenting with an SSI, including patients with a non-healing lower limb amputation performed for ischemia. The changing microbiology of SSIs, especially the increase in MRSA infection, has implications for initial treatment of SSIs, as well as antibiotic prophylaxis in vascular patients with multiple risk factors for postoperative infection, especially MRSA nasal and skin colonization (Armstrong et al. 2007). Patient outcomes are less favorable with an MRSA versus meticillin-sensitive *S. aureus* (MSSA) SSIs with an increase in both 30-day mortality (odds ratio of 3.4) and morbidity (median of 5 days additional hospitalization) (Armstrong et al. 2007).

The appearance time for vascular SSIs depends on procedure type and whether a prosthetic graft has been implanted. Although wound infections typically are clinically demonstrated within 30 days of surgery, infection involving a lower limb prosthetic arterial bypass usually presents beyond 4 months (mean of 7 months), and after aortic grafting, clinical signs of infection may appear years later (mean of 3.5 years) (Bandyk 2002, Perl et al. 2002, Pounds et al. 2005). The late presentation of vascular graft infection is attributed to the bacteria biofilm nature of the infectious process caused by low virulence *S. epidermidis* strains. Once the graft is colonized by bacterial biofilm, the infection can evolve to a more virulent, invasive process by superinfection with other bacterial species, such as MSSA, MRSA, or Gram-negative bacteria. The likelihood of this is increased if graft erosion progresses through the skin (graft cutaneous sinus tract) or into the gastrointestinal (GI) tract (graft enteric erosion). When the presentation of aortic graft infection includes Gram-negative bacteria, graft enteric erosion should be suspected. Overall, Gram-negative bacteria account for approximately 20–25% of vascular SSIs with the most common strains being *Escherichia coli*, *Pseudomonas aeruginosa*, *Proteus* spp., and *Klebsiella pneumoniae*. When confronted with a vascular SSI, initial antibiotic therapy should be guided by Gram stain of wound or aspirated perigraft fluid. Identification of Gram-positive organisms should prompt antibiotic therapy with bactericidal killing properties to MRSA (Perl et al. 2002).

RISK FACTORS FOR VASCULAR INFECTION

Most arterial surgery procedures are classified as "clean" class I by the National Research Council because the surgical exposure and revascularization are performed in uninfected tissues without inflammation. Furthermore, the respiratory, alimentary, or infected urinary tract is not entered. These wounds are closed primarily with suction drainage if necessary (Culver et al. 1991). Although diseased arteries may harbor bacteria, most commonly *S. epidermidis* strains that are within atherosclerotic plaque or mural thrombus, the inoculum and virulence are considered low. This observation is an important rationale for routine antibiotic prophylaxis. Arterial revascularization is not recommended in patients with invasive remote infection or bacteremia except when the intervention is judged life saving. In patients with critical limb ischemia and a clinical presentation of foot sepsis or wet gangrene, initial management should be surgical debridement of infected tissues together with antibiotic therapy. Debridement and antibiotic therapy are followed by open or endovascular revascularization when the invasive infectious process has been controlled.

Vascular SSI involves a complex interaction of the bacterial inoculum, host defense mechanisms, and surgical site healing. Audits performed in US hospitals of SSIs have identified patient, procedure, and environmental risk factors that increase the risk for postoperative infection for the vascular reconstruction patient (**Box 17.1**). For the

---

Box 17.1 Patient, procedure, and environmental risk factors for surgical site infection.

Patient-related risk factors
Nasal carriage of *Staphylococcus aureus*
Prolonged preoperative length of stay
Postoperative bacteremia
End-stage renal disease
Obesity
Malnutrition/low serum albumin
Older age
Smoking/Nicotine use
Diabetes mellitus
Prior incision site irradiation
Malnutrition/low serum albumin
Autoimmune disease/corticosteriod therapy
Malignancy/chemotherapy

Procedure-related risk factors
Femoral/groin incision
Remote infection
Biomaterial implant
Emergency/reoperative procedure
American Society of Anesthesiology (ASA) score >2
Extended operative time
Hypothermia
Shock
Hyperglycemia

Environmental risk factors
Operating suite ventilation – environmental surface cleaning
Instrument and vascular implant sterility
Surgical attire and sterile operative technique

---

vascular patient, the most significant risk factors are: nasal colonization with MSSA/MRSA, presence of a groin incision, prosthetic grafting or patch angioplasty, lower limb arterial bypass grafting, postoperative bacteremia, and end-stage renal disease (ESRD). Characteristics such as obesity, advanced age, smoking, and diabetes are known risk factors for SSIs in all surgical patients and are present in most vascular patients.

Numerous studies have confirmed increased SSI rates in people with *S. aureus* nasal carriage. Approximately 6–35% of vascular patients harbor *S. aureus* in their nares with the prevalence highest in patients with ESRD, active skin infection, immunodeficiency states such as infection with HIV, or residence in a long-term care facility. Preoperative *S. aureus* carriage has been shown to the risk of SSI by four- to eightfold in patients undergoing cardiothoracic, neurosurgical, and orthopedic procedures. The "cause–effect" mechanism is felt to be patient transmission of bacteria from the nares to the surgical site(s) via their hands. Nasal colonization with MRSA versus MSSA further increases the likelihood of SSI to approximately eight- to tenfold compared with an *S. aureus* carrier, and has been linked to MRSA SSI outbreaks in hospital wards (Cowie et al. 2005). In vascular patients, MRSA colonization has been shown to increase the frequency (odds ratio of 4.5) of any nosocomial (wound, blood, urine, lung) infection (44% incidence). MRSA infection increases hospital stay when compared with similar MSSA infections. These epidemiological observations prompted a randomized clinical trial of decolonizing therapy with application of intranasal antibiotic ointment (mupirocin calcium) before and after surgical procedures. Mupirocin, a topical anti-staphylococcal agent that inhibits RNA and protein synthesis, eliminated *S. aureus* carriage in 83% of colonized patients (23% of study population) compared with no effect in the placebo group. However, no decrease in SSI rates was observed (7.9% vs 8.5%) (Cowie et al. 2005).

Of note, this study demonstrated that the odds of a *S. aureus* carrier developing SSI was 4.5 times that of a non-carrier (*p* <0.001). There was a trend to reduced *S. aureus* SSIs (38% reduction) but the differences between the treatment and placebo groups were not significant. These data confirm the increased SSI risk in MSSA and MRSA nasal carriers, but reduction in postoperative infection rate requires a treatment strategy beyond intranasal decolonization alone. Of note, prolonged use of topical mupirocin has been associated with the development of resistant strains. Audits of patients admitted for elective arterial revascularization procedures or abdominal aortic aneurysm (AAA) repair have documented an 4–8% incidence of MRSA nasal colonization; but much higher rates of nasal colonization (30–40%) in dialysis-dependent patients (Bandyk 2008).

Procedure-specific risk factors for vascular SSIs include 'open' versus endovascular intervention, the presence of a femoral groin incision, and prosthetic graft/patch usage. If a procedure lasts >3 h, is associated with shock or hypothermia, or requires blood transfusion, then the likelihood of postoperative infection is increased. Intraoperative hypothermia of 1–1.5°C increases the relative risk of postoperative infection twofold. SSI risk is lowest after AAA repair with a similar incidence after open (0.2%) and stent-graft (0.16%) repair. There is an increased incidence of SSIs in patients who developed any nosocomial infection during hospitalization (Cowie et al. 2005). Similarly, carotid endarterectomy and endovascular interventions involving stent angioplasty (carotid, visceral, iliac, femoropopliteal) are also associated with low (<1%) SSI rates.

By contrast, open arterial reconstructions for peripheral arterial disease are associated with overall wound and graft infection rates of 8–10%. These rates are significantly higher after infrainguinal prosthetic (10–29%) or *in situ* saphenous vein (18–22%) bypass grafting procedures (Perl et al. 2002, Vogel et al. 2008, Frei et al. 2011). The increased rates of SSIs in lower limb arterial procedures is related to tissue injury/ischemia of critical ischemia, secondary lymphedema produced by surgical trauma and revascularization edema, and failure of the femoral/groin incision to heal. The development of wound hematoma or incision separation caused by dermal or fat necrosis reduces the bacteria inoculum required to produce an invasive infection. These wound problems occur more frequently in the groin incision, especially in the clinical setting of a repeat arterial construction or in patients who are obese or diabetic. Extensive utilization of electrocautery and extended application of wound retractors can produce skin and soft tissue trauma, which results in large volumes of necrotic tissue that become evident in the early postoperative period by cyanotic incision skin margins.

TREATMENT OF VASCULAR GRAFT INFECTIONS

The management of vascular SSIs, especially abdominal aorta graft enteric erosions, fistulas, or mycotic aneurysms, require adherence to the guidelines based on clinical presentation, and microbiology that are presented in **Table 17.1** and **Figure 17.1** (Bandyk et al. 2001, Oderich et al. 2001, 2006, Armstrong et al. 2005, Stone et al. 2006, Bandyk 2008, Vogel et al. 2008, Reifsnyder et al. 1992). The diagnostic process begins with *computed tomography* (CT) to assess extent of graft/artery involvement (presence of perigraft fluid–air). This is followed by *surgical exploration* in selected patients to confirm the infectious process and its microbiology. In most patients, sterilization of the surgical site with parenteral antibiotics and antibiotic bead placement is possible leading to "staged" *in situ* graft replacement using either autologous vein or an antibiotic-impregnated vascular prosthesis (Bandyk et al. 2001, Oderich et al. 2001, 2006, Stone et al.

Table 17.1 Reported outcome for treatment of aortic and peripheral graft infections (Bandyk et al 2001, Oderich et al 2001, 2006, Armstrong et al 2005, Stone et al 2006, Bandyk 2008, Vogel et al 2008, Frei et al 2011).

Aortic graft infection					
Procedure	Operative mortality rate (%)	Amputation rate (%)	Reinfection rate (%)	Survival rate >1 year (%)	Comments
Ex-situ bypass and total graft excision	11–24	5–25	3–13	73–86	Previously considered the "gold standard" treatment
In situ replacement and total graft excision					
Deep vein	7–10	5	0–1	82–85	Complicated procedure, some patients are not candidates
Allograft	12–24	5	10–15	70–80	Graft deterioration can occur
Rifampin–PTFE graft	0–15	<5	10–20	80–90	Bridge graft or *in situ* reconstruction or biofilm infection

Peripheral graft infections			
Graft site	Operative mortality rate (%)	Amputation or stroke rate (%)	Comments
Infrainguinal bypass	0–9	5–33	Low (<5%) infection rate with autogenous bypass
Thoracic aorta	10–12	0	Life-long antibiotic suppression
Carotid–subclavian	10–20	10	High morbidity associated with carotid ligation
Carotid patch	5	5–10	Autogenous vein reconstruction recommended

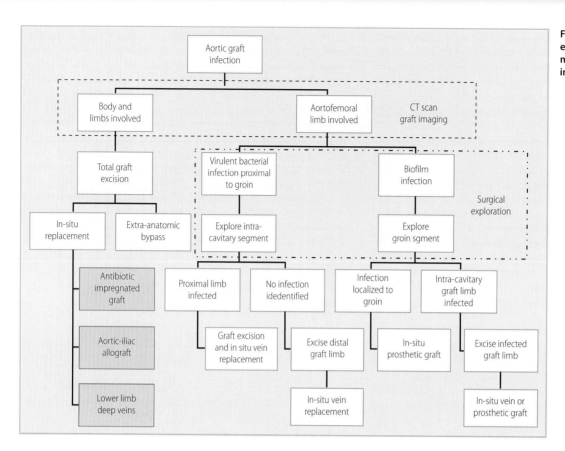

2006, Bandyk 2008). Accurate anatomic assessment of the infection extent is critical because *in situ* prosthetic replacement should be considered only in the presence of bacterial biofilm infection with no signs of mycotic aneurysm formation. CT, magnetic resonance imaging (MRI), and indium-111-labeled white blood cell scans are helpful in assessment of graft involvement, but surgical exploration remains the most reliable method of confirming or excluding infection. The presence of hydronephrosis after aortofemoral bypass indicates advanced perigraft inflammation and denotes diffuse graft involvement by a biofilm infection.

Antibiotic therapy

Broad-spectrum bactericidal, parenteral antibiotic therapy should be started on clinical suspicion of a vascular SSI. The most common infecting organisms (in decreasing order of prevalence) are staphylococcal strains (*S. aureus*, *S. epidermidis*), streptococci, *E. coli*, *Klebsiella* and *Pseudomonas* spp., and *Candida albicans*. MRSA now accounts for 50% of early and 25% of late aortofemoral graft infections. If *S. aureus* or *S. epidermidis* is the proven or suspected pathogen, parenteral antibiotic therapy with a first- or second-generation cephalosporin is employed for MSSA. A preferred antibiotic for Gram-positive infection where MRSA is suspected or documented is daptomycin (6 mg//kg with dosing based in renal function) because of rapid, concentration-dependent bactericidal activity to all Gram-positive bacteria, including MRSA. Daptomycin has also been demonstrated to penetrate bacteria biofilms and kill bacteria in stationary phase growth. Vancomycin and linezolid are also be used to treat MRSA infections but these antibiotics have time-dependent bacteriostatic activity and do not penetrate bacteria biofilms. In patients allergic to penicillin, administration of an

aminoglycoside or a fluoroquinolone is recommended for extended Gram-negative bacteria coverage. Once the infecting organism has been isolated (e.g., by needle aspiration of perigraft fluid or surgical exploration), antibiotic coverage should be modified based on antibiotic susceptibility testing of the recovered strains. Antibiotic therapy, including both parenteral administration and local delivery via antibiotic-impregnated beads, is an adjunct to surgical management which includes drainage of perigraft abscesses, debridement of infected tissues, and excision of the infected graft (Stone et al. 2006, Armstrong et al. 2007).

Patient selection for in situ graft replacement

The option of *in situ* replacement therapy depends on the clinical presentation, extent of graft infection, and clinical microbiology as determined by surgical exploration of the involved graft segment (see Figure 17.1) (Bandyk et al. 2001, Oderich et al. 2001, 2006). The intent of the evaluation process is to accurately establish whether the infection involves the entire aortic graft or is localized to a graft segment. This initial assessment is followed by a determination of whether a graft biofilm is present (amenable to *in situ* prosthetic grafting) or there is a more virulent infectious process. If surgical exploration demonstrates an invasive, virulent graft infection (organisms present on intraoperative Gram stain, positive perigraft tissue cultures), an autogenous vein *in situ* reconstruction should be considered. Preliminary implantation of antibiotic-impregnated beads in the perigraft space is recommended to aid in surgical site sterilization (Stone et al. 2006). For Gram-positive infection, implantation of daptomycin (1.5 g/40 g bone cement powder) beads is recommended; for Gram-negative infections, tobramycin bone cement should be used. When possible, autogenous vein reconstruction of the excised graft segment should be performed in all cases except when a "localized" biofilm infection is present. When an aortic graft infection is associated with a graft–enteric fistula, extra-anatomic (axillofemoral) reconstruction together with graft excision and aortic stump closure is still considered the "safest" option when an adequate length of infrarenal aorta is present for ligation. Infection involving the pararenal aorta should be managed by *in situ* replacement therapy combined with adjunctive antibiotic bead implantation.

If the infectious process is isolated to an aortofemoral graft limb or peripheral bypass, a staged surgical approach is recommended. In the presence of extensive inguinal inflammation or abscess, a combined inguinal and lower abdominal oblique ("transplantation") retroperitoneal incision can be used for surgical exposure. At the initial operation, the perigraft abscess is drained, necrotic tissue excised, and the cavity is locally irrigated with a solution composed of half strength hydrogen peroxide and 10 ml Betadine (povidone–iodine)/500 ml. This solution disrupts bacterial biofilms, and aids in surgical site debridement and tissue sterilization. Antibiotic beads fabricated within a plastic bead mold are then placed adjacent to the infected graft and the wound closed. The second stage is performed 3–5 days later after culture results are available (Stone et al. 2006). Exploration of the proximal aortofemoral graft limb is performed to assess for the presence of graft incorporation. If found to be uninvolved with infection (i.e., no perigraft fluid), with graft incorporated with surrounding tissue, the proximal graft limb is clamped and transected. The distal graft is then excised to the femoral anastomosis and the graft bed irrigated with an antibacterial solution (clorpactin 3 g/l) using a pulsed wound irrigation system. Depending on the prior culture results, either deep vein or a rifampin-bonded PTFE (polytetrafluoroethylene) graft is implanted.

Before wound closure, all surgical fields are pulse lavaged again with the clorpactin solution and, if a rifampin graft is used, the external graft surface re-soaked with the rifampin (60 mg/ml) solution (Oderich et al. 2011). If The Gram stain indicates a Gram-negative infection or presence of a graft–enteric erosion, tobramycin powder is spread along the arterial reconstruction and at anastomotic sites. Perigraft fluid cavities and empty grafts tunnels are drained using flat, closed-suction drain systems. Closed-suction drains are also placed in beds of the excised femoral vein and the sartorius muscle is used to cover the extracavitary segment of the in situ graft reconstruction. Antibiotic-impregnated beads are placed in the superficial portion of the groin wound for 7–10 days to prevent bacterial biofilm formation. The beads are attached to a 2/0 polypropylene suture brought through the skin and attached to a button for extraction at the bedside.

Parenteral antibiotic therapy administration is modified based on the explanted graft cultures with the intent to maintain bactericidal serum levels for 4–6 weeks after the in situ grafting procedure. Before discharge from the hospital a baseline CT scan of the abdomen and femoral regions is obtained. This scan is repeated at 3 months and then every 6–12 months depending on the type of in situ reconstruction. In general, prolonged oral antibiotic therapy is not prescribed after femoropopliteal vein (FPV) reconstruction, but used for at least 3 months after in situ prosthetic reconstruction. The oral antibiotic prescribed is selected based on graft culture results and antibiotic susceptibility testing. Reported outcomes for treating aortic and peripheral graft infections are shown in **Table 17.2**.

▮ PREVENTIVE MEASURES

A multipronged approach is required to minimize the occurrence of vascular SSI, including attention to pre-, intra-, and postoperative preventive measures published by the Centers for Disease Control in 1999 (Mangram et al. 1999). The guidelines address aspects of patient preparation, sterile surgical technique, surgical team antisepsis, hand disinfection, incision care, and antimicrobial prophylaxis. Surveillance of patients for nasal carriage of *S. aureus*, especially MRSA, as well as review in each patient of the inventory of SSI risk factors, can identify the "high-risk" cases and prompt an individualized prevention strategy. The increasing incidence of drug-resistant Gram-positive infections after arterial surgery is a concern and serves to re-emphasize the importance of preventive strategies. Surgeon should recognize that expanding the coverage of antibiotic prophylaxis is not a primary solution. Instead prevention strategies to decolonize the *S. aureus* carrier in combination with meticulous wound care and thoughtful antibiotic prophylaxis is recommended. There is accumulating evidence that regulation of host defense factors – body temperature, oxygenation, and blood sugar – are important in determining the SSI risk in an individual patient. Care measures to maintain normal temperature during and after surgical procedures, use of insulin therapy to keep blood sugar levels <180 mg/dl, and pulse oximetry monitoring to ensure 100% hemoglobin saturation are associated with reductions in SSI rates. Supplemental oxygen in the immediate postoperative period improves incisional oxygen tension and decreases wound-healing complications (Greif et al. 2000).

Antimicrobial prophylaxis in vascular patients should include therapy directed at *S. aureus* nasal colonization, parenteral anti-

Table 17.2 Patient selection criteria for treatment of a prosthetic graft infection by excision alone, *in situ* replacement, or ex situ bypass and graft excision.

Treatment option	Clinical presentation	Microbiology
Excision alone	Thrombosed graft and adequate collateral flow	+ cultures
In situ replacement Autogenous vein Allograft Rifampin-bonded graft	 Invasive graft infection Invasive graft infection and no suitable autogenous conduit Bacterial biofilm graft infection	 + cultures + cultures *S. epidermidis*/*S. aureus* *Salmonella* sp.
Excision and *ex situ* bypass Simultanous procedure Staged procedure	 Unstable patient with GEE or GEF Stable patient +/- GEE or GEF	 No exclusion criteria No exclusion criteria
GEE, graft enteric erosion; GEF, graft enteric fistula		

biotic therapy to ensure that adequate tissue levels are achieved before the procedure is begun and throughout the procedure, and surgical site care to impend bacteria colonization of injured skin and soft tissue is provided (**Box 17.2**). For effective antibiotic prophylaxis, a first- or second-generation cephalosporin is administered 30–60 min before the procedure. Daptomycin has been used when MRSA is suspected but this is not a Food and Drug Administration (FDA)-approved indication. Daptomycin cannot be used alone for vascular procedure prophylaxis because it does not have activity against Gram-negative bacteria known to produce vascular SSIs. If vancomycin is used for prevention then the infusion should be initiated 120 min before incision to reduce complications of drug administration. The author recommends cephalosporin antibiotics should be re-dosed if the procedure takes longer than 3 h or if blood loss exceeds 1.5 l. Preventive antibiotics are administered for 24 h.

CONCLUSION

Antimicrobial-resistant pathogens are an increasing threat in prevention and treatment of vascular SSIs. A program of patient surveillance for nasal carriage for MRSA, decolonization, preventing transmission to other patients, and thoughtful antibiotic prophylaxis usage, combined with local antiseptic measures (preoperative skin cleansing, antimicrobial sutures, silver eluting dressings), is an effective strategy to reduce SSIs. The entire surgical team must participate in institutional efforts to control nosocomial infections, antimicrobial resistance in bacteria, and SSI rates.

Box 17.2 Preventive strategies to prevent vascular surgical site infection.

Patient screening for nasal carriage of *S. aureus*, including MRSA
Preoperative intranasal mupirocin (applied to both nares for 3 days before and 2 days after surgery)
Hibiclens wipes to decolonize skin surface at planned incision site(s)
Antibiotic prophylaxis
Cefazolin, weight based, intravenous (IV) 1–3 g slowly 60 min before procedure, and repeated 1–2 g if procedure >3 h or blood loss >1.5 l. Dosing repeated every 8 h for 24 h, or IV cefuroxime 1.5 g 60 min before surgery and every 12 h for total of 6 g
For "high-risk" patient based on surgical site infection (SSI) risk factors, including MRSA nasal carriage or history of MRSA infection – add IV daptomycin 6 mg/kg (single dose) over 2 min before procedure, or IV vancomycin 15 mg/kg slowly over 1 h, 120 min before the procedure.
If patient has a cephalosporin allergy, give IV aztreonam 1 g 60 min before procedure and every 8 h for 24 h
If patient has vancomycin allergy, give IV daptomycin 6 mg/kg (single dose) before procedure
Soaking vascular prosthesis in a rifampin (30–60 mg/ml) solution for 15 min
Use of silver-impregnated wound dressing for 24–48 h, followed by topical mupirocin ointment to incision if wound drainage or injured skin edges present

---

REFERENCES

Armstrong PA, Back MR, Wilson JF, et al. Improved outcomes in the recent management of secondary aortoenteric fistula. *J Vasc Surg* 2005;**42**:660–6.

Armstrong PA, Back MR, Bandyk DF, et al. Selective application of sartorius muscle flap and aggressive staged surgical debridement can influence long-term outcomes of complex graft infections. *J Vasc Surg* 2007;**46**:71–8.

Bandyk DF. Antibiotics – Why so many and when should we use them? *Semin Vasc Surg* 2002;**15**:268–274.

Bandyk DF. Vascular surgical site infection – risk factors and preventive measures. *Semin Vasc Surg* 2008;**21**:119–123.

Bandyk DF, Novotney M, Johnson BL, Back, MR, et al. Expanded application of in situ replacement for infected vascular grafts. *J Vasc Surg* 2001;**34**:411–20.

Cowie SE, Ma I, Lee SK, et al. Nosocomial MRSA infection in vascular patients: Impact on patient outcome. *Vasc Endovasc Surg* 2005;**39**:327–34.

Culver DH, Horan TC, Gaynes RP, et al. Surgical wound infection rates by wound class, operative procedure, and patient risk index. *Am J Med* 1991;**91**:S152–7.

Frei E, Hodgkiss-Harlow KD, Rossi PJ, et al. Microbial pathogenesis of bacterial biofilms: A causative factor of vascular surgical site infection. *Vasc Endovasc Surg* 2011;**45**:688–96.

Grief R, Akca O, Horn EP, et al. for the Outcomes Research Group. Supplemental perioperative oxygen to reduce of surgical-wound infection. *N Eng J Med* 2000;**342**:161–7.

Mangram AJ, Horan TC, Pearson ML, et al. Hospital Infection Control Practices Advisory Committee. Guideline for prevention of surgical site infection, 1999. *Infect Control Hosp Epidemiol* 1999;**20**:250–61.

Oderich DS, Panneton JM, Bower TC, et al. Infected aortic aneurysms: aggressive presentation, complicated early outcome, but durable results. *J Vasc Surg* 2001;**34**:900–8.

Oderich GS, Bower TC, Cherry KJ, et al. Evolution from axillofemoral to *in situ* prosthetic reconstruction of the treatment of aortic graft infection at a single center. *J Vasc Surg* 2006;**43**:1166–74.

Oderich GS, Bower TC, Hofer J, et al. In situ rifampin-soaked grafts with omental coverage and antibiotic suppression are durable with low infection rates in patients with aortic graft enteric erosion or fistula. *J Vasc Surg* 2011;**53**:99–107.

Perl TM, Cullen JJ, Wenzel RP, et al. The mupirocin and the risk of *Staphylococcus aureus* study team: intranasal mupirocin to prevent postoperative *Staphylococcus aureus* infections. *N Engl J Med* 2002;**346**:1987–90.

Pounds LL, Montes-Walters M, Mayhall CG, et al. A changing pattern of infection after major vascular reconstructions. *Vasc Endovasc Surg* 2005;**39**:511–15.

Reifsnyder TR, Bandyk DF, Seabrook G, et al. Wound complications of the in situ saphenous vein bypass technique. *J Vasc Surg* 1992;**15**:843–50.

Stone PA, Armstrong PA, Bandyk DF, et al. Use of antibiotic-loaded polymethylmethacrylate beads for the treatment of extracavitary prosthetic graft infections. *J Vasc Surg* 2006;**44**:757–61.

Vogel TR, Symons R, Flum DR. The incidence and factors associated with graft infection after aortic aneurysm repair. *J Vasc Surg* 2008;**47**:264–9.

Vogel TR, Dombrovsky VY, Carson JL, et al. Infectious complications after elective vascular surgical procedures. *J Vasc Surg* 2010;**51**:122–30.

Chapter 18 | Urological infections

Mathew C. Raynor, Ian Udell, Raj Kurpad, Culley C. Carson

Urological infections are one of the most common reasons people seek medical attention and the urinary tract is the most common entry point for bacteria causing nosocomial infections, bacteremia, and sepsis. Over half of women will have at least one urinary tract infection during their lifetime and most of these will require a physician visit and antibiotic treatment. The high prevalence continues to the inpatient setting where genitourinary infections are the most common nosocomial infection. The efficient diagnosis and effective treatment of urological infections is a major healthcare concern. Factors such as economic efficiency and emerging resistance are increasingly becoming more important considerations in providing patient care. Urological infections are among the most likely to be multi-antibiotic resistant and are often difficult to treat without combined medical and surgical approaches.

PYELONEPHRITIS

Pyelonephritis refers to inflammation of the kidney and renal pelvis and is considered an upper urinary tract infection (UTI). Acute pyelonephritis is a clinical diagnosis based on the classic presentation of fever (>100°F), chills, and flank or costovertebral angle pain. These signs and symptoms may be associated with urinary urgency, frequency, and dysuria. However, patients do not always present with classic symptoms. Gastrointestinal symptoms, such as nausea and emesis may be present. Patients usually have a history of a previous UTI.

Diagnosis of acute pyelonephritis is based mainly on clinical symptoms. Laboratory diagnosis consists of urinalysis, urine culture, complete blood count (CBC), and serum chemistries. Urinalysis usually demonstrates evidence of inflammation and infection with hematuria, pyuria, and bacteriuria. Leukocytosis is usually present with a predominance of neutrophils. Serum creatinine is usually normal. However, an elevated creatinine could indicate the presence of obstruction or severe infection. Blood cultures are not routinely drawn, unless the patient exhibits signs of significant illness (sepsis) or has risk factors for a complicated UTI, including previous urological instrumentation, indwelling catheter, urinary tract anatomic abnormality, or pregnancy. Blood cultures have been shown to be positive in about a quarter of patients, with uncomplicated pyelonephritis in women (Velasco et al. 2003). However, this finding does not alter management decisions about therapy, so blood cultures can be omitted in cases of uncomplicated pyelonephritis.

The use of imaging studies in the diagnosis of acute pyelonephritis is a difficult clinical decision. The presence of a urinary tract obstruction or stone in the setting of acute infection would certainly alter treatment strategies. However, most cases of uncomplicated pyelonephritis do not result from a stone or obstruction. Imaging options include plain radiograph, intravenous urogram (IVU), renal ultrasonography, or computed tomography (CT). The use of plain radiographs has a very limited role in the management of the urinary tract. It may be useful to investigate other causes of abdominal pain. Likewise, IVU has fallen out of favor, given the routine availability and better anatomic detail with other modalities. Renal ultrasonography is a useful screening tool

to rule out the presence of hydronephrosis. CT can be performed with or without intravenous contrast agents to assess for hydronephrosis or calculus disease. There are no specific radiological findings on CT to diagnose pyelonephritis. Some subtle findings to suggest the diagnosis include renal enlargement and perinephric fat stranding. In reality, if a patient presents with acute fever and flank or abdominal pain, most patients will undergo cross-sectional abdominal imaging to evaluate for other causes, such as appendicitis, diverticulitis, or urolithiasis. Imaging should be strongly considered in a patient with clinical signs and symptoms of pyelonephritis and risk factors for a complicated UTI. These include known functional or anatomic abnormalities in the urinary tract, recent instrumentation, recent antibiotic use, immunosuppression, pregnancy, or history of diabetes.

Escherichia coli accounts for about 80% of cases of pyelonephritis. Special virulence, including P pili, K antigens, and endotoxins contribute to the pathogenesis of infection. Patients with P blood group antigen receptors may be susceptible to recurrent bouts of pyelonephritis due to the ability of the bacteria to adhere to the receptor through P pili, and lead to repeated episodes of infection (Roberts 1991). Patients with a history of recurrent UTIs or those with recent hospitalization, instrumentation, or indwelling catheter may be prone to more resistant species of bacteria, including *Proteus, Klebsiella, Serratia, Enterobacter,* or *Citrobacter* spp. *Enterococcus faecalis, Staphylococcus epidermidis,* and *S. aureus* are the most common Gram-positive organisms to cause pyelonephritis.

Management of acute pyelonephritis depends on properly classifying patients into uncomplicated and complicated groups. Any patient with presumed acute pyelonephritis without complicating factors and minimal symptoms without significant nausea or emesis can be treated as an outpatient. Empirical oral antimicrobial therapy should be initiated until results of urine cultures are finalized. In the vast majority of cases, *E. coli* is the causative bacterium. A much smaller percentage of Gram-positive bacteria can cause pyelonephritis (*S. epidermidis, S. aureus,* and *E. faecalis*). Therefore, antimicrobial therapy can be chosen based on the presumed causative bacteria. Typically, a fluoroquinolone for 10–14 days is sufficient in an otherwise healthy non-pregnant patient with a normal urinary tract. Alternatively, trimethoprim–sulfamethoxazole can be used for 10–14 days. If a Gram-positive organism is suspected, then amoxicillin or amoxicillin–clavulanic acid can be used.

Patients who are severely ill or have complicating factors require hospital admission. These patients should undergo abdominal imaging to evaluate for obstruction or other causes of illness. Broad-spectrum parenteral antibiotics should be instituted, including a fluoroquinolone, aminoglycoside with or without ampicillin, or extended-spectrum cephalosporin with or without an aminoglycoside (Warren et al. 1999). If there is any evidence of urinary tract abnormality or obstruction, urgent urological consultation is needed because drainage of the urinary tract may be required with either a ureteral stent or percutaneous nephrostomy. Parenteral antibiotic therapy should be continued until susceptibilities are returned and the patient demonstrates clinical improvement. Once improved and afebrile for more than 24 h, oral antibiotics can be started and continued for a total of 14 days. If a patient remains febrile with or without persistent leukocytosis after 72 h of therapy, then repeat abdominal imaging is warranted to evaluate for possible renal or perinephric abscess. In addition, repeat cultures from urine and blood should be obtained.

Follow-up urine culture should be obtained before completion of therapy and again several weeks after completion of therapy to ensure sterility. Relapse of infection can occur and usually requires a repeat 14-day course of culture-specific therapy.

RENAL ABSCESS/PERINEPHRIC ABSCESS

Renal abscess refers to an abscess confined to the renal parenchyma, whereas a perinephric abscess refers to an abscess cavity extending into or involving the perinephric space. Perinephric abscesses can result from extension of a renal abscess into the perinephric space or extension from another source, such as a psoas abscess, perforated appendicitis, or diverticulititis. Renal abscesses usually arise from ascending urinary tract infections and can often be associated with obstruction or calculus disease. Gram-negative bacteria account for most renal abscesses. Gram-positive organisms can spread hematogenously and should be suspected in patients with symptoms of pyelonephritis and coexisting skin infections, endocarditis, or intravenous drug use. On the other hand, perinephric abscesses can often be polymicrobial.

Diagnosis of a renal or perinephric abscess is suspected in patients with fever and abdominal or flank pain. In addition, renal or perinephric abscess should be suspected in patients with clinical pyelonephritis who have remained febrile for >72 h despite appropriate antimicrobial therapy. A marked leukocytosis is usually present. Urinalysis and urine culture can be misleading. These tests can often be negative in a patient in whom the abscess cavity does not communicate with the collecting system. This situation most commonly occurs where there has been hematogenous spread of an infection. Blood cultures are usually positive in these cases.

Unlike cases of uncomplicated pyelonephritis, imaging is diagnostic for renal or perinephric abscess. Ultrasonography is a very reliable and inexpensive method of diagnosis. However, CT is the imaging procedure of choice, given its excellent anatomic delineation (**Figure 18.1**).

Management involves broad-spectrum antibiotics. In cases of small (<3 cm) renal abscesses, these can be managed similar to complicated pyelonephritis, with parenteral antibiotics and conversion to oral antibiotics. Follow-up imaging is needed to document improvement or resolution of the abscess. In cases of larger renal abscesses (>3–5 cm), smaller abscesses that do not respond to antimicrobial therapy, patients with diabetes, or in immunosuppressed patients, percutaneous aspiration and drainage of the abscess are indicated. Antibiotic regimens can be tailored to culture results. Urological consultation is recommended in these cases, because follow-up imaging will be necessary. With today's improvements in imaging and image-guided therapy, surgical drainage is rarely necessary (Shu et al. 2004).

Management of perinephric abscesses requires drainage. These abscesses do not respond to antimicrobial therapy alone. Most of these cases can be aspirated and drained percutaneously. Surgical drainage is, again, usually not required. However, in cases of large abscess cavities or poorly functioning kidneys, open drainage or nephrectomy may be necessitated. In addition, the presence of a perinephric abscess usually indicates an underlying problem. This could include an obstructed and infected kidney or a possible enteric communication. Further treatment directed at the underlying cause is needed once the abscess has been appropriately managed.

EMPHYSEMATOUS PYELONEPHRITIS/PYELITIS

Emphysematous pyelonephritis is a rare and very serious infection involving gas-forming bacteria, which results in renal parenchymal necrosis. This condition usually occurs in patients with diabetes and has a high mortality rate, ranging from 19% to 60% (Somani et al. 2008). In addition to diabetes, many patients may have underlying poor renal function, urolithiasis, or urinary tract obstruction.

Diagnosis is made on the basis of clinical findings and, primarily, on imaging studies. Most patients have diabetes and present with high fever, flank pain, and vomiting. Laboratory studies show a significant leukocytosis and may demonstrate elevated serum creatinine, resulting

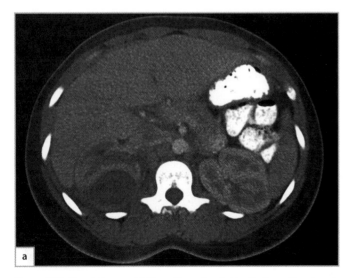
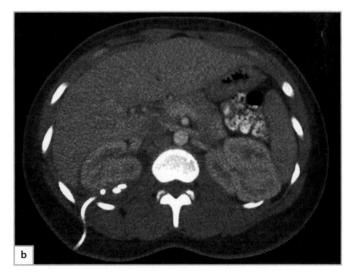

Figure 18.1 Renal abscess. (a) Hypoattenuating fluid collection with enhancing rim confined to the renal parenchyma. (b) Imaging after antibiotics and percutaneous drainage demonstrates resolution.

from parenchymal necrosis and destruction. Urinalysis and urine culture usually demonstrate bacteriuria. The most common causative organism is *E. coli*, followed by *Proteus* and *Klebsiella* spp. These patients are generally severely ill, with sepsis and hypotension common.

Imaging is diagnostic of emphysematous pyelonephritis. Plain radiograph or IVU is rarely used, but can demonstrate a collection of gas around the location of the kidney. This can be confused with bowel gas. CT is the imaging modality of choice, and demonstrates significant loculated gas throughout the renal parenchyma, even extending into the perinephric space. In severe cases, there can be complete destruction of the renal parenchyma. Emphysematous pyelonephritis must be differentiated from emphysematous pyelitis. This entity refers to the finding of gas within the collecting system of the kidney and not in the renal parenchyma. This condition is usually caused by a gas-forming bacterial UTI and does not require any special intervention unless urinary tract obstruction is present. In cases of emphysematous pyelonephritis, a renal scan is recommended to assess split renal function.

Emphysematous pyelonephritis should be treated as an emergency. Patients are generally severely ill and require aggressive hydration, broad-spectrum antimicrobial therapy, and management of sepsis. Urological consultation should be promptly obtained. Historically, emphysematous pyelonephritis was considered a surgical emergency and usually resulted in emergent nephrectomy. However, recent evidence suggests that medical management may actually improve outcomes and renal salvage (Pontin and Barnes 2009). In a recent systematic review, mortality rates were 50% with medical management alone, 25% with medical management and emergent nephrectomy, and 13.5% with medical management and percutaneous nephrostomy drainage (Somani et al. 2008).

In general, management usually involves emergent percutaneous drainage of the affected kidney with a percutaneous nephrostomy. If conservative management fails, surgical therapy may be considered, but mortality rates after failure of conservative therapy are extremely high. Risk factors for mortality with emphysematous pyelonephritis include altered mental status, thrombocytopenia, hyponatremia, and bilateral renal involvement. Surgical therapy after successful conservative management may still be required if significant renal parenchymal destruction has occurred.

■ MANAGEMENT OF URINARY INFECTION WITH OBSTRUCTION

In patients with evidence of UTI and imaging demonstrating obstruction of the urinary tract, urological consultation is warranted. Obstruction causing hydronephrosis in the setting of an infection can lead to serious complications, including sepsis and death. The causes of obstruction include urolithiasis, ureteral stricture or scar, extrinsic compression, or significant bladder outlet obstruction resulting in urinary retention (**Figure 18.2**). In the setting of obstruction and infection, pyonephrosis can occur. This term refers to a collection of purulent material in the collecting system proximal to the site of obstruction. This is essentially equivalent to an abscess in the urinary tract. Prompt intervention and drainage of the urinary tract are needed, usually including Foley catheter placement, ureteral stent placement, or nephrostomy drainage. Culture-specific antibiotics should be continued for at least 14 days and management of the underlying cause will be needed. In general, in cases of urinary tract obstruction and coexisting infection, antibiotics and urinary tract drainage are necessitated.

Xanthogranulomatous pyelonephritis (XGP) represents a rare and severe form of renal deterioration secondary to obstruction and infection. Most patients present with flank pain, fever, and recurrent UTI with persistent bacteriuria. CT is the imaging modality of choice and usually demonstrates an enlarged, poorly functioning kidney with dilated calyces and thinning of the renal parenchyma. In most cases, the condition affects the entire kidney. The classic radiological finding is a severely enlarged, hydronephrotic kidney with a thin rim of parenchyma and a centrally obstructing stone in the renal pelvis. Multiple renal or perinephric abscesses can occur (**Figure 18.3**). *Proteus* spp. and *E. coli* are the most common causative bacteria (Korkes et al. 2008). Nuclear medicine renal function studies usually demonstrate severely diminished or no function in the affected kidney.

Management of XGP depends on the initial presentation and renal function of the affected kidney. Patients presenting acutely ill need medical stabilization and imaging to investigate for abscess and/or obstruction. Acute management of these patients usually involves broad-spectrum antibiotics and percutaneous drainage of the kidney. Once stabilized and treated with appropriate antibiotics,

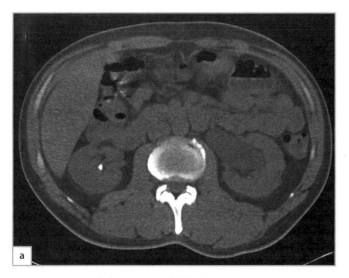

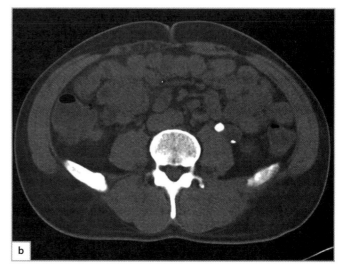

Figure 18.2 Ureteral obstruction and infection. (a) Cross-sectional imaging demonstrates hydronephrosis and perinephric fat stranding. (b) A mid-ureteral obstructing stone was identified with proximal hydroureter.

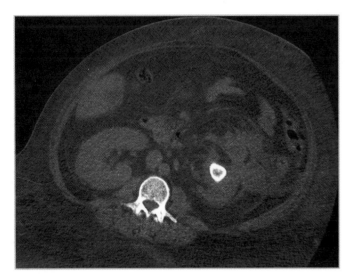

Figure 18.3 Xanthogranulomatous pyelonephritis. Imaging shows a large centrally obstructing stone with complete obliteration of renal parenchyma and perinephric abscesses.

treatment then depends on renal function. If the kidney still maintains decent function, management of the obstructing stone and UTI can be pursued. Segmental involvement of XGP may be amenable to partial nephrectomy. If the kidney has little or no function, delayed nephrectomy is usually recommended.

EPIDIDYMO-ORCHITIS

Epididymitis and orchitis refer to inflammation of the epididymis and testis, respectively. These conditions manifest clinically with pain, swelling, and inflammation. Epididymo-orchitis can be divided into several classifications, including acute bacterial, non-bacterial infectious, non-infectious, and chronic epididymo-orchitis. This section focuses on the acute infectious and non-infectious causes, because these types would be most common in the surgical patient.

Acute infectious epididymo-orchitis is most commonly caused by urinary pathogens reaching the epididymis and testis from the urethra, prostate, or bladder through the ejaculatory ducts and vasa deferentia. In boys and elderly men, coliform organisms that are common causes of bacteriuria are the most frequent causative agents (*E. coli*). In young, sexually active men, sexually transmitted infections are the most common cause (*Neisseria gonorrheae, Chlamydia trachomatis*) (Berger et al. 1979).

Acute non-bacterial causes of infection include viral, fungal, and parasitic organisms. Mycobacterial organisms have also been implicated, including granulomatous inflammation seen after bacillus Calmette–Guérin (BCG) bladder instillations for the treatment of bladder cancer. In rare cases of isolated orchitis without epididymitis, a viral cause is found, most commonly mumps and mononucleosis.

Clinical presentation of acute epididymo-orchitis is usually acute-onset scrotal pain and swelling. Patients may experience fever and other symptoms suggestive of a coexisting UTI, along with abdominal pain, nausea, and emesis. Sexually active men may complain of concomitant urethral discharge, suggestive of a sexually transmitted infection. Physical examination typically demonstrates a tender, erythematous, and/or edematous scrotum. The affected testis and epididymis are usually exquisitely tender to palpation. Pain may be improved with scrotal elevation.

Diagnostic evaluation of any acute onset scrotal pain should include scrotal ultrasonography with Doppler flow studies to evaluate for testicular torsion. Further evaluation usually involves urinalysis and urine culture, especially in patients with indwelling urinary catheters or recent urinary instrumentation. In men at risk for a sexually transmitted infection, urethral swabs should also be obtained. In young boys with epididymo-orchitis, evaluation should also include abdominal ultrasonography and voiding cystourethrography, because these patients may have an underlying urinary tract anatomic abnormality (Tracy et al. 2008).

In most cases of postoperative epididymo-orchitis, the underlying cause is urinary tract instrumentation or urinary catheterization, and subsequent UTI. Indwelling urinary catheters are commonly left in critically ill patients for volume monitoring, after urological procedures for healing, secondary to mobility issues after surgery or injury, in spinal cord injury patients, or in patients with urinary retention. These patients are at higher risk of developing a catheter-associated UTI and are at risk for development of acute epidiymo-orchitis.

Treatment is usually directed at the underlying cause, if identified. Scrotal elevation and anti-inflammatory medications are helpful in managing discomfort. Antibiotics are tailored to the specific pathogen and are usually continued for 14 days. However, urine cultures are frequently non-diagnostic and treatment is started empirically. The Centers for Disease Control recommends that men aged <35 receive ceftriaxone or doxycycline and men >35 receive a fluoroquinolone (Workowski and Berman 2011).

PROSTATITIS/PROSTATE ABSCESS

Prostatitis represents one of the most common urological complaints among men, affecting up to 16% of men in their lifetime (Sharp et al. 2010). Prostatitis can be subdivided into several classifications, ranging from acute bacterial prostatitis to chronic pelvic pain syndrome and asymptomatic prostatitis. This section focuses only on infectious causes because as these would be most prevalent in the surgical patient.

Acute bacterial prostatitis refers to acute infection of the prostate and usually requires urgent treatment. Often, these patients are acutely ill with symptoms of a UTI. High fever, significant suprapubic pain, dysuria, urinary urgency, and even urinary retention from prostate inflammation can be present. Patients may exhibit signs of sepsis in advanced cases. Physical examination usually demonstrates lower abdominal tenderness to palpation. Examination of the scrotum may demonstrate epididymal or testicular pain on palpation, if concomitant epididymo-orchitis is present. Digital rectal examination can confirm the suspected diagnosis because the prostate is exquisitely tender to gentle touch, although prostate massage must be avoided as this may cause florid bacteremia or sepsis. Imaging is usually not necessary in the initial diagnostic evaluation. Bladder ultrasonography may be useful to evaluate for urinary retention. Indwelling urethral catheters are also a significant risk factor for acute prostatitis and UTI.

Laboratory studies likely show a leukocytosis. Urinalysis and mid-stream urine culture should be obtained and identify a causative pathogen in most cases. *E. coli* is the most common bacterial cause of acute prostatitis. Other causative organisms include *Klebsiella* and *Pseudomonas* spp., and enterococci. Younger sexually active men should also be screened for *N. gonorrhea* and *C. trachomatis* with a urethral swab.

Treatment of acute prostatitis involves antibiotics. Typically, acutely ill patients require admission and parenteral broad-spectrum antibiotics, usually with a penicillin derivative and an aminoglycoside (ampicillin and gentamicin). For patients with acute urinary retention, urinary catheter drainage may be needed. Treatment is continued until the patient is afebrile and then antibiotics are tailored to urine culture sensitivities. Antibiotics should be continued for 4–6 weeks. If no clinical improvement is seen or if fever persists, pelvic imaging should be obtained to evaluate for prostatic abscess (pelvic CT with/without intravenous contrast). Mildly ill patients may be treated as an outpatient with oral antibiotics for 4–6 weeks (trimethoprim–sulfamethoxazole or a fluoroquinolone).

Chronic bacterial prostatitis refers to a persistent bacterial infection of the prostate. Chronic bacterial prostatitis is the most common cause of recurrent UTI in men. *E. coli* and enterococci are the most common causes. Etiologies as to the cause of chronic bacterial prostatitis range from persistent untreated bacteria after acute prostatitis, BPH with urinary obstruction, urethral stricture, to urinary catheterization or instrumentation.

Diagnosis is usually made on history and physical examination. In contrast to acute bacterial prostatitis, men with chronic bacterial prostatitis do not usually appear ill. Urinary urgency, frequency, and dysuria are common, suggestive of an underlying UTI. Perineal and scrotal pain may also be present. Fevers are uncommon. Physical examination findings often vary and may demonstrate a tender prostate, but this is not a universal finding.

Diagnosis involves examination of the urine. A modified two-glass voiding test can be used to identify bacterial prostatitis. This test involves a mid-stream urine specimen collected and examined for WBCs and bacteria and an additional urine specimen obtained after vigorous prostate massage via digital rectal examination. In addition, expressed prostatic secretions (EPSs) obtained at the time of prostate massage may be examined and sent for culture. Theoretically, the initial urine specimen represents bladder flora. The post-prostate massage specimen represents a mixture of prostatic and bladder flora. An increase in WBCs or bacteria of the post-prostate massage or EPSs is indicative of bacterial prostatitis. Serum prostate-specific antigen (PSA) is rarely indicated in the diagnosis of prostatitis and is likely to be markedly elevated.

Treatment for chronic bacterial prostatitis involves antibiotics. Fluoroquinolones are the preferred treatment, due to their ability to concentrate in the prostate. Doxycycline or trimethoprim–sulfamethoxazole is considered a second-line treatment alternative. Treatment should be continued for a minimum of 4 weeks. Recurrence is relatively common (Benway and Moon 2008).

Prostate abscess represents a rare infectious condition, although it is more prevalent in immunocompromised patients and should be considered (Lebovitch and Mydlo 2008). Prostate abscesses may arise from a concomitant UTI or acute prostatitis, hematogenous spread (especially Gram-positive bacteria), or iatrogenic (prostate biopsy). *E. coli* is the most common cause, followed by enterococci.

Diagnosis of prostate abscess is suspected based on history and physical examination. Urine culture should be obtained and is usually positive. Patients may present similar to acute prostatitis, appearing quite ill with fever and suprapubic pain. Dysuria is common. Urethral discharge may be present if the abscess cavity communicates with the urethra. Digital rectal examination should be performed gently and usually demonstrates an exquisitely tender prostate with possible fluctuance. Urinary retention is common. Imaging should be performed in patients where prostate abscess is suspected. A pelvic CT with and without intravenous contrast is the procedure of choice. Transrectal ultrasonography may also be useful.

Treatment is usually multimodal. Small abscesses (<1 cm) in patients who are not severely ill or immunocompromised may be treated with bladder drainage and parenteral antibiotics. Repeat imaging is necessary to ensure response to treatment. However, most patients require intervention to drain the abscess. Broad-spectrum parenteral antibiotics are initiated and tailored to culture results. Drainage of the abscess can be performed via transrectal or transperineal ultrasound-guided aspiration and drainage or via transurethral unroofing and drainage. Transurethral drainage is considered the gold standard procedure but requires general or spinal anesthesia. Worsening of sepsis is possible with drainage. Suprapubic catheter placement may be necessary in cases of large prostate abscesses, but urethral catheterization usually suffices. Catheter drainage should continue for 1–2 weeks and antibiotic therapy should be continued for 4–6 weeks. Repeat imaging is recommended to ensure resolution.

■ NECROTIZING FASCIITIS (FOURNIER GANGRENE)

Necrotizing fasciitis of the male genitalia represents a urological emergency. It is a life-threatening infection with a mortality rate of up to 40% (Morpurgo and Galandiuk 2002). Immunocompromised patients, including patients with diabetes or alcohol dependence, may be at higher risk due to atypical presentation or delayed diagnosis. In the vast majority of cases, mixed bacterial flora are isolated, including Gram-positive, Gram-negative, and anaerobic bacteria. Group A streptococcal infections of the soft tissue can also occur, even in healthy immunocompetent patients. The source of infection can arise from the skin, urethra or rectum. Local skin infections, such as balanitis (cellulitis of glans penis), posthitis (cellulitis of prepucial skin), or scrotal/perineal abscess can lead to necrotizing infections. Perirectal abscesses and urethritis, especially associated with urethral stricture disease, can lead to perineal spread of infection. Necrotizing fasciitis can also be seen postoperatively after circumcision, hernia repair, orchiectomy, or any other inguinal, perineal, or scrotal surgery. Necrotizing fasciitis can spread rapidly along fascial planes and extend along the abdominal wall to the chest in advanced cases.

Patients usually present acutely ill with fevers and significant pain out of proportion to the visible extent of infection. Physical examination usually reveals significant erythema suggestive of cellulitis. Necrotic appearing skin may be visible as the subcutaneous infection progresses, leading to vascular congestion, thrombosis, and ischemia of small vessels to the skin. Crepitus ("popping" or cracking sound with palpation) may be present and represents collection of gas in the subcutaneous tissues (**Figure 18.4**). The penis should be examined for extent of disease and potential causative infectious sources. Likewise, rectal examination should be performed to evaluate for abscess.

Laboratory evaluation usually demonstrates leukocytosis and anemia. Elevated serum creatinine, hyponatremia, and hypercalcemia are common. Imaging can be obtained in cases where the diagnosis is in doubt. However, imaging should not delay surgical exploration when the index of suspicion is high. CT is the imaging modality of choice and can demonstrate subcutaneous air and/or abscess. Plain radiography may also show pockets of subcutaneous gas (**Figure 18.5**) (Levenson et al. 2008).

The mainstay of treatment is surgical intervention. Broad-spectrum parenteral antibiotics are started but removal of the involved soft tissue is paramount to patient survival. Aggressive wide debridement of involved skin and soft tissue is undertaken. Removal of all visibly necrotic skin with debridement back to healthy bleeding tissue is necessitated. Usually, the testes are not involved and can be spared. In cases where scrotal skin is excised, the testes can be wrapped with saline gauze and preserved. Historically, thigh pouches were created to protect the testes, but this practice is rarely performed today. Urinary diversion with suprapubic catheter drainage and bowel diversion with diverting colostomy may be required in advanced cases. After debridement, a large tissue defect is usually present. Wound packing

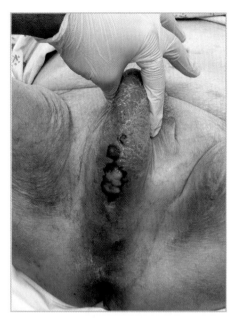

Figure 18.4 Fournier gangrene. Examination reveals necrotic tissue at the base of scrotum extending inferiorly to perineum.

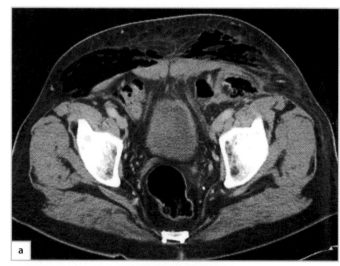

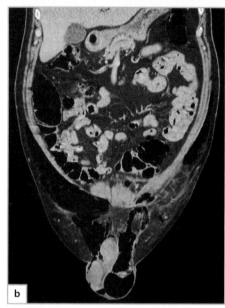

Figure 18.5 Fournier gangrene. (a) Cross-sectional and (b) coronal imaging demonstrate massive subcutaneous gas present within the perineum, scrotum, and anterior abdominal wall. Surgical exploration identified the source as a ruptured sigmoid diverticulum.

or a negative-pressure wound device (wound vac) is usually required. Patients routinely return to the operating room in 24–48 h after initial debridement for re-evaluation and excision of unhealthy tissue. In most cases, multiple debridement procedures are required. Hyperbaric oxygen therapy has been shown in some studies to be beneficial in improving wound healing after excision.

After debridement, most patients require extensive skin grafting to cover large tissue defects. Primary closure of scrotal defects can be performed even when up to 50% of scrotal skin has been removed. Otherwise, meshed split-thickness skin grafts are used. The testes are sewn together in approximation before grafting to prevent formation of a bifid neoscrotum. Non-meshed skin grafts are used to cover penile skin defects (Chen et al. 2010).

Necrotizing fasciitis is a true surgical emergency and requires a team approach. These patients are usually acutely ill and require critical care expertise in addition to urologists, general surgeons, and plastic surgeons to appropriately treat this potentially rapidly progressive condition.

■ REFERENCES

Benway BM, Moon TD. Bacterial prostatitis. *Urol Clin North Am* 2008;**35**:23–32, v.

Berger RE, Alexander ER, Harnisch JP, et al. Etiology, manifestations and therapy of acute epididymitis: prospective study of 50 cases. *J Urol* 1979;**121**:750–4.

Chen SY, Fu JP, Wang CH, et al. Reconstruction of scrotal and perineal defects in Fournier's gangrene. *J Plast Reconstr Aesthet Surg* 2010;**64**:528–34.

Korkes F, Favoretto RL, Broglio M, et al. Xanthogranulomatous pyelonephritis: clinical experience with 41 cases. *Urology* 2008;**71**:178–80.

Lebovitch S, Mydlo JH. HIV-AIDS: urologic considerations. *Urol Clin North Am* 2008;**35**:59–68; vi.

Levenson RB, Singh AK, Novelline RA. Fournier gangrene: role of imaging. *Radiographics* 2008;**28**:519–28.

Morpurgo E, Galandiuk S. Fournier's gangrene. *Surg Clin North Am* 2002;**82**:1213–24.

Pontin AR, Barnes RD. Current management of emphysematous pyelonephritis. *Nat Rev Urol* 2009;**6**:272–9.

Roberts JA. Etiology and pathophysiology of pyelonephritis. *Am J Kidney Dis* 1991;**17**:1–9.

Sharp VJ, Takacs EB, Powell CR. Prostatitis: diagnosis and treatment. *Am Fam Physician* 2010;**82**:397–406.

Shu T, Green JM, Orihuela E. Renal and perirenal abscesses in patients with otherwise anatomically normal urinary tracts. *J Urol* 2004;**172**:148–50.

Somani BK, Nabi G, Thorpe P, et al. Is percutaneous drainage the new gold standard in the management of emphysematous pyelonephritis? Evidence from a systematic review. *J Urol* 2008;**179**:1844–9.

Tracy CR, Steers WD, Costabile R. Diagnosis and management of epididymitis. *Urol Clin North Am* 2008;**35**:101–8; vii.

Velasco M, Martinez JA, Moreno-Martinez A, et al. Blood cultures for women with uncomplicated acute pyelonephritis: are they necessary? *Clin Infect Dis* 2003;**37**:1127–30.

Warren JW, Abrutyn E, Hebel JR, et al. Guidelines for antimicrobial treatment of uncomplicated acute bacterial cystitis and acute pyelonephritis in women. Infectious Diseases Society of America (IDSA). *Clin Infect Dis* 1999;**29**:745–58.

Workowski KA, Berman SM. Centers for Disease Control and Prevention Sexually Transmitted Disease Treatment Guidelines. *Clin Infect Dis* 2011;**53**(suppl 3):S59–63.

Chapter 19 Bone and joint infections

Charalampos G. Zalavras, Michael J. Patzakis

INTRODUCTION

Bone and joint infections are challenging to treat, lead to morbidity and even mortality, and have a considerable socioeconomic impact. Infections after orthopedic procedures prolong hospitalization, increase healthcare costs, create physical limitations, and reduce quality of life for patients (Whitehouse et al. 2002, Lee et al. 2006, Poultsides et al. 2010). Orthopedic surgical site infections significantly increase the median duration of hospitalization (19 days with infection versus 5 days without) and median direct cost of hospitalization ($24 344 vs $6636 in 1997 and 1998 prices) (Whitehouse et al. 2002). Infection after orthopedic surgery in elderly patients is an independent risk factor for mortality (Lee et al. 2006).

Therefore, the importance of prevention, prompt diagnosis, and effective treatment cannot be overemphasized. The treatment goals are control of infection and restoration of function. Pathogen resistance and tissue loss resulting from infection or surgical debridement often complicate achievement of these goals. The treatment principles include aggressive surgical debridement, appropriate antibiotic administration, and, if needed, bone stabilization, soft-tissue coverage, and bone defect reconstruction (Patzakis and Zalavras 2005). This chapter discusses the pathogenesis, diagnosis, and management of the common bone and joint infections.

PATHOGENESIS

The pathogenesis of musculoskeletal infections involves, first, inoculation of microorganisms into musculoskeletal tissues and, second, interaction of these microorganisms with the host. When the host is unable to eradicate or control the inoculated microorganisms, they proliferate and result in an inflammatory response and host tissue damage, with the resultant clinical picture of infection.

Microorganisms may gain access to musculoskeletal tissues through three principal mechanisms: hematogenous spread after bacteremia (e.g., acute pediatric osteomyelitis), spread from a contiguous source of infection (e.g., adjacent osteomyelitis in cases of septic arthritis), or direct inoculation during trauma (e.g., infections after open fractures) or surgical procedures (e.g., periprosthetic joint infections) (Lazzarini et al. 2004). The interaction of inoculated microorganisms with the host will determine the occurrence and severity of infection.

Microorganism factors

Virulence is the ability of a microorganism to overcome the host defenses and cause infection. Virulence varies among and within organism species. *Staphylococcus aureus* is the most common pathogen in musculoskeletal infections and employs distinct mechanisms in order to cause infection (Gordon and Lowry 2008, Fry and Barie 2011).

Staph. aureus initially expresses surface proteins, called "microbial surface components recognizing adhesive matrix molecules," which bind molecules such as fibronectin and facilitate adhesion of the organism on host tissues as well as prosthetic devices. The organism evades host defenses by several strategies: Protein A inactivates immunoglobulins, chemotaxis inhibitory protein interferes with leukocyte chemotaxis, capsular polysaccharide reduces opsonization and phagocytosis of the organism, and leukocidins damage leukocytes. *Staph. aureus* releases enzymes that destroy host tissues and produces toxins that lead to a systemic inflammatory reaction.

Infections with *Staph. aureus* may persist because of slow growing subpopulations that may persist intracellularly (small colony variants) and/or biofilm formation. Biofilm formation is a key pathogenic mechanism of chronic musculoskeletal infections (Costerton et al. 1999, Costerton 2005, Zalavras and Costerton 2009). A biofilm is a highly structured multicellular community of microorganisms that adhere to an inert or living surface, and are embedded within a self-produced polymeric matrix mainly composed by polysaccharides. Biofilm microorganisms demonstrate decreased susceptibility to antibiotics and host immune responses compared with individual or planktonic organisms. Protective mechanisms include incomplete biofilm penetration by antibiotics and antibodies, altered chemical microenvironment, slow-growing or starved state of biofilm cells, and development of resistant phenotypes as an adaptive response to stress. As a result, formation of biofilm leads to persistence and chronicity of infection (Costerton et al. 1999, Costerton 2005). Radical debridement with removal of foreign bodies and nonviable bone and soft tissue is essential for control of infection (Patzakis and Zalavras 2005, Zalavras and Costerton 2009).

Local and systemic host factors

Local host factors that facilitate infection include compromised vascularity (resulting from arterial disease, venous stasis, irradiation, scarring, and smoking) and trauma. Trauma reduces tissue perfusion, devitalizes tissues, creates a dead space filled by hematoma, and results in exposure and contamination of the underlying bone.

Systemic host factors that reduce the ability of the host's immune system to respond to the pathogen include systemic diseases (such as diabetes mellitus, renal and liver disease, malignancy, rheumatological disease, acquired immune deficiency syndrome, alcoholism, malnutrition) and medications (e.g., anti-rheumatic drugs, glucocorticoids, and others).

Host status is a key part of the Cierny–Mader classification of osteomyelitis and refers to the patient's physiological capacity to overcome infection and withstand treatment (Cierny et al. 1985). An otherwise healthy patient is classified as an A host, a B host has comorbidities with a detrimental effect on immune response and wound healing, and a C host is so compromised that surgical intervention poses a greater risk than the infection itself, and qualifies for only palliative treatment. Host status has important management and prognostic implications. Compromised hosts demonstrate increased infection rates after open fractures and increased recurrence rates after surgical management of osteomyelitis.

DIAGNOSIS OF BONE AND JOINT INFECTIONS: AN OVERVIEW

Diagnosis of bone and joint infections is based on clinical findings, laboratory tests, imaging modalities, histopathology, and microbiological methods. New molecular diagnostic methods appear to be promising.

Clinical findings

Local clinical findings of inflammation (pain, edema, erythema, increased temperature) as well as systemic findings (fever, chills) may be present in acute infections but are usually absent in chronic musculoskeletal infections. Drainage from a sinus tract may be present in chronic infections.

Laboratory tests

An elevated peripheral blood white blood cell (WBC) count with increased polymorphonuclear cells is indicative of infection, but has low sensitivity. The erythrocyte sedimentation rate (ESR) and C-reactive protein (CRP) are markers of the acute phase response secondary to inflammatory processes of infectious or noninfectious etiology. Although these inflammatory markers have high sensitivity, their specificity is relatively low and false positives may occur in patients with systemic inflammatory diseases or neoplasms. Also they may be elevated in the postoperative period as a response to surgery. Interleukin-6 is another inflammatory marker that appears to be promising in the diagnosis of infection. Analysis of joint fluid is discussed below.

Imaging modalities

Radiographs should be evaluated for bone changes (presence of sequestrum, resorption, periosteal new bone formation). In posttraumatic infections the status of bone healing and the integrity of any implants should be assessed. In infections following fracture fixation, radiographs may show lucency around the implants; however, this may also result from aseptic loosening.

Computed tomography (CT) demonstrates subtle changes of cortical bone, such as erosion and periosteal reaction, but is not helpful for evaluation of surrounding soft tissue.

Magnetic resonance imaging (MRI) can detect early changes secondary to infection. Increased water content secondary to edema and hyperemia results in decreased marrow signal in T1-weighted images and increased signal in T2-weighted images. MRI has 98% sensitivity for detecting osteomyelitis with a specificity of 75% (Erdman et al. 1991). MRI provides details of the extent of involvement of the medullary canal and adjacent soft tissues.

Bone scintigraphy using technetium-99m evaluates perfusion and osteoblastic activity of the skeleton and helps identify multiple anatomic areas of infection, but has low specificity. Indium-111-labeled leukocyte scintigraphy has 83% sensitivity and 86% specificity for musculoskeletal infection but is labor intensive and produces low-resolution images (Merkel et al. 1985). Positron emission tomography (PET) with [18F]fluorodeoxyglucose is a new and promising modality.

Histopathology

Identification of organisms after a Gram stain of specimens from the involved area has low sensitivity but is very specific. Evaluation of frozen sections of tissue for polymorphonuclear leukocytes can help establish the diagnosis of infection intraoperatively.

Microbiological methods

Cultures have been considered the gold standard for the diagnosis of infection; however, there are clinical problems with their use. False-positive results may occur due to contamination, so culture swabs should be opened immediately before use and each tissue sample should be taken with separate, sterile instruments. False-negative results may be due to prior administration of antibiotics, inadequate specimen sampling, improper specimen handling and transportation, or short incubation time. Biofilm formation is another reason for negative cultures in chronic bone and joint infections.

Molecular methods

Molecular diagnostic methods may improve diagnostic efficacy. Polymerase chain reaction (PCR) can amplify and detect bacterial DNA, leading to increased sensitivity but concerns exist about false-positive results secondary to contamination (Costerton et al. 2011). A novel method with mass spectrometric technology appears promising for detection of musculoskeletal infection in the presence of negative cultures (Gallo et al. 2011).

PEDIATRIC SEPTIC ARTHRITIS AND OSTEOMYELITIS

Epidemiology and pathogenesis

Septic arthritis and osteomyelitis are more common in children aged <5 years, usually involve the larges joints of the lower extremity, and are most commonly caused by *Staph. aureus* (Ross 2005). Other organisms include coagulase-negative staphylococci, group A β-hemolytic streptococci, *Streptococcus pneumoniae*, group B streptococci, and *Kingella kingae*. Children with sickle cell disease are more prone to infections from *Salmonella* spp. *Hemophilus influenzae* type b used to be a common pathogen in children aged between 1 and 3 years, but routine immunization has almost eliminated its role in pediatric infections.

Septic arthritis and osteomyelitis are usually hematogenous in origin. Septic arthritis may also result from contiguous spread of adjacent infection or from direct inoculation of microorganisms after a penetrating injury. Pediatric acute hematogenous osteomyelitis has a predilection for the metaphysis of long bones. The sluggish circulation and relative absence of tissue macrophages in the metaphyseal bone allow bacterial proliferation. Purulent exudate may spread through the metaphyseal bone to the subperiosteal region, resulting in a subperiosteal abscess. Elevation of the periosteum by the abscess may devitalize cortical bone, which then becomes a sequestrum. The periosteum forms new bone, called the involucrum, which surrounds the sequestrum. Infants have a distinct vascular pattern with metaphyseal vessels traversing into the epiphyseal area, which allows osteomyelitis to spread to the epiphysis.

It should be noted that septic involvement of the adjacent joint occurs in 33% of patients with metaphyseal osteomyelitis (Perlman et al. 2000). Joint involvement is facilitated if the metaphysis is intra-articular. Therefore, careful evaluation of the adjacent joint should be an important part of the evaluation of any child with osteomyelitis. The infectious process may also spread to the surrounding soft tissues and rarely to the medullary canal. Acute hematogenous osteomyelitis in older children usually involves a single site but in neonates may involve multiple bones.

Diagnosis

The clinical picture of musculoskeletal infection in children usually consists of pain and inability to use the extremity. In septic arthritis the range of motion of the involved joint is markedly decreased and painful. Fever may not always be present. A history of local trauma is often reported and the treating physician needs to consider both infection and trauma in the differential diagnosis. Diagnosis can be challenging in neonates because the clinical picture is often subtle and a high index of suspicion is needed.

The ESR and CRP are elevated in 90% and 95% of children with septic arthritis, respectively, and reach a peak in 5 and 2 days, respectively (Kallio et al. 1997). The ESR and CRP are elevated in 92% and 98% of children with osteomyelitis, respectively. The ESR rises within 2 days from the onset of infection, reaches a peak in 3–5 days and returns to normal after approximately 3 weeks, whereas the CRP begins rising within 6 h, reaches a peak in 2 days, and returns to normal approximately 1 week after successful therapy (Unkila-Kallio et al. 1994). Combining these two markers results in increased sensitivity in pediatric osteoarticular infections. Surgical treatment prolongs the peak and normalization times of both markers (Khachatourians et al. 2003). The CRP demonstrates a closer temporal relationship to the course of infection and is preferable for monitoring recovery. Only 35% of children with acute hematogenous osteomyelitis had a WBC count >12 000/mm^3 at the time of admission (Unkila-Kallio et al. 1994), so values within normal limits should be interpreted with caution.

Radiographs show soft-tissue swelling during the early stages of acute hematogenous osteomyelitis but do not demonstrate osseous changes until 7–14 days later. MRI shows joint effusion in septic arthritis, evaluates adjacent bone for osteomyelitis, and identifies soft-tissue abscesses. Bone scanning is helpful when the pathology location is uncertain or involvement of multiple locations is suspected.

In septic arthritis aspiration of the involved joint should be performed to establish the diagnosis and identify the pathogen. The joint aspirate should be sent for Gram stain, cultures and sensitivity testing, WBC count, and differential. WBC count >50 000/mm^3 and neutrophil percentage >75% suggest septic arthritis but lower values may be seen. Bone cultures and blood cultures are essential in the management of osteomyelitis. Bone cultures can be obtained by needle aspiration or intraoperatively.

The differential diagnosis of septic arthritis includes transient synovitis of the hip, juvenile rheumatoid arthritis, poststreptococcal reactive arthritis, and rheumatic fever. Trauma and neoplasms may present with a clinical picture resembling osteomyelitis. Distinguishing septic arthritis from transient synovitis of the hip in a young child with an acutely irritable hip may be difficult. Fever, inability to weight bear, ESR >40 mm/h, and peripheral WBC count >12 000 cells/mm^3 are independent variables that can help differentiate the two conditions. The probability of septic arthritis was found to be 99.6% for children with all four factors, 93.1% for those with three factors, 40% for those with two factors, and 3% for those with one factor only (Kocher et al. 1999). However, a subsequent study reported a 59% predicted probability of septic arthritis in a child with all four factors (Luhmann et al. 2004).

Treatment

Treatment modalities include antibiotics and surgery. Empirical antibiotic therapy should be started immediately after appropriate cultures have been collected and should always target *Staph. aureus*. Coverage for other pathogens should be provided based on the child's age and the clinical setting (**Table 19.1**). Septic arthritis and/or osteomyelitis in neonates may also be caused by group B streptococci and Gram-negative organisms. Children younger than 3 years of age may have *Kingella kingae* or *Hemophilus influenzae* type b infections if non-immunized. Children older than 3 years may have *Streptococcus pneumoniae* or group A *S. pyogenes* infections. In sexually active adolescents with septic arthritis *Neisseria gonorrhoeae* should be considered as a pathogen. Children with sickle cell disease may have salmonella infections. Systemic administration of antibiotics can be converted to oral therapy if the patient is afebrile with considerable clinical improvement and considerably decreased CRP levels. The optimal duration of antibiotic therapy has not been defined. For uncomplicated cases that respond rapidly to treatment, 3 weeks of antibiotic therapy may be sufficient in septic arthritis and 4 weeks in acute osteomyelitis.

Table 19.1 Common pathogens and empirical antibiotic therapy in pediatric bone and joint infections.

Clinical setting	Common pathogens	Empirical antibiotic therapy
Neonate	*Staphylococcus aureus* *Streptococcus pyogenes* group B Gram-negative organisms	Penicillinase-resistant penicillin (oxacillin) and aminoglycoside (gentamicin) or Third-generation cephalosporin (ceftriaxone)
Child <3 years	*Staph. aureus* *Hemophilus influenzae* (if nonimmunized) *Kingella kingae*	Third-generation cephalosporin (ceftriaxone)
Older child	*Staph. aureus* *Strep. pneumoniae* *Strep. pyogenes* group B	Penicillinase-resistant penicillin (oxacillin)
Child with sickle cell disease	*Staph. aureus* *Salmonella* species	Third-generation cephalosporin (ceftriaxone)
Risk factors for MRSA	Meticillin-resistant *Staph. aureus* (MRSA)	Vancomycin or clindamycin
Immunocompromised patient	Gram-positive organisms Gram-negative organisms	Penicillinase-resistant penicillin (oxacillin) and aminoglycoside (gentamicin)
Sexually active patient	*Staph. aureus* *Neisseria gonorrhoeae*	Third-generation cephalosporin (ceftriaxone)

Surgical intervention in septic arthritis consists of decompression and irrigation by open arthrotomy or arthroscopy. Joint aspiration may be an alternative in easily accessible joints but careful monitoring is necessary. If there is no improvement within 24 h, then surgical decompression is warranted. Prompt intervention is especially important in septic arthritis of the hip because delayed or incomplete decompression impairs perfusion of the femoral head and may result in osteonecrosis, hip dislocation, and osteomyelitis. Surgical intervention in acute hematogenous osteomyelitis is warranted when an abscess is present. However, early antibiotic therapy may contain the infectious process and prevent abscess formation. Surgery is also indicated when septic arthritis of an adjacent joint is present.

SEPTIC ARTHRITIS IN ADULTS
Epidemiology and pathogenesis

In adults the knee joint is most often involved by septic arthritis. *Staphylococcus aureus* is the most common pathogen (Ross 2005). Immunocompromised patients may also have infections with Gram-negative organisms or unusual pathogens, such as mycobacteria or fungi (Zalavras et al. 2006a). Intravenous drug users and elderly patients in addition to *Staph. aureus* may have infections with Gram-negative organisms. Young, otherwise healthy, sexually active adults may have infections with *Neisseria gonorrhoeae*.

The portals of pathogen entry in septic arthritis include hematogenous inoculation, spread from adjacent infection, or inoculation by a penetrating or surgical wound. Immunocompromised patient status, pre-existing joint pathology such as rheumatoid arthritis, and loss of skin integrity or skin infections are important risk factors for development of septic arthritis. Microorganisms in the joint cavity trigger an inflammatory response that recruits polymorphonuclear cells to the involved area. Both the bacterial invasion and the inflammatory response contribute to cartilage damage. Enzymes and toxins released by bacteria, as well as enzymes and cytokines released by inflammatory cells, result in loss of glycosaminoglycans and collagen.

Diagnosis

Septic arthritis usually presents as monoarthritis. The involved joint is painful, swollen, with limited range of motion, and may be erythematous. Fever is present in approximately half the patients and other systemic symptoms and signs may be absent. Gonococcal arthritis may present as monoarthritis or migratory polyarthritis with rash and tenosynovitis of the dorsal aspect of the wrist and hand.

CRP and ESR are elevated in >90% of cases (Mehta et al. 2006). Ultrasonography is useful in detecting a joint effusion. MRI shows intra-articular fluid and detects potential spread of infection into adjacent bone or soft tissues.

Aspiration of the involved joint helps establish the diagnosis and identify the pathogen. The joint aspirate should be sent for Gram stain, cultures, and sensitivity testing, WBC count and differential, and polarizing microscopy to detect crystals. WBC count >50 000/mm^3 and neutrophil percentage >75% indicate but do not confirm the diagnosis of septic arthritis. Blood cultures also detect the pathogen.

Treatment

Empirical antibiotic therapy should be started immediately after aspiration and collection of joint fluid for culture. It should cover the most likely pathogens based on the clinical setting. In otherwise healthy adults, antibiotic therapy should cover both *N. gonorrhoeae* and *Staph. aureus*. Immunocompromised hosts and intravenous drug users should receive coverage for both *Staph. aureus* and Gram-negative organisms including *Pseudomonas aeruginosa*. The duration of antibiotic therapy for an uncomplicated case septic arthritis that responds well to treatment is 3 weeks. In gonococcal arthritis 1 week of antibiotic therapy is sufficient.

Surgical decompression and irrigation of the septic joint by arthrotomy or arthroscopy relieve pressure and evacuate enzymes, toxins, inflammatory mediators, and bacteria from the joint, thereby preventing further cartilage damage. Repeated joint aspirations may be sufficient in an easily accessible joint such as the knee. Synovial biopsy for culture and histology may be useful in recurrent cases or when the diagnosis is uncertain. Persistence of clinical signs of infection after surgical management of septic arthritis should raise the suspicion of adjacent osteomyelitis, especially in patients with comorbidities, and MRI helps detect residual infection (Zalavras et al. 2006b).

ADULT OSTEOMYELITIS

Osteomyelitis in adults usually results from either trauma (infections after open fractures) or surgical procedures (postoperative infections). Postoperative infections may develop after joint arthroplasty procedures (periprosthetic joint infections) or fixation of closed fractures. Contiguous spread from adjacent infections and hematogenous spread are uncommon pathogenic mechanisms. The most common organisms causing adult osteomyelitis are *Staph. aureus* and other Gram-positive cocci. *P. aeruginosa* or other Gram-negative organisms, mycobacteria, or fungi may cause infection in immunocompromised patients.

PREVENTION OF INFECTION IN OPEN FRACTURES

Open fractures are complex injuries that involve not only the bone but also the surrounding soft tissue envelope, and may lead to considerable morbidity or amputation of the extremity (Zalavras and Patzakis 2003). The soft-tissue injury results in communication of the open fracture with the outside environment and contamination of the wound with microorganisms, which increases the risk of infection. Infection complicates management and leads to further morbidity. Therefore, prevention is an important management principle.

The risk of clinical infection depends on the severity of the injury, host status, and treatment factors. The severity of the injury is described by the Gustilo and Anderson classification system, subse-

Table 19.2 Open fracture classification by Gustilo and Anderson, modified by Gustilo, Mendoza, and Williams.

Type I	Puncture wound of ≥1 cm, with minimal contamination or muscle crushing
Type II	Laceration >1 cm long with moderate soft-tissue damage and crushing; bone coverage is adequate and comminution minimal
Type IIIA	Extensive soft-tissue damage, often due to a high-energy injury, with severe comminution and/or contamination
Type IIIB	Extensive soft-tissue damage with periosteal stripping and bone exposure requiring flap coverage
Type IIIC	Associated arterial injury requiring repair

quently modified by Gustilo et al. (1984) (**Table 19.2**). Classification of the open fracture should be done only in the operating room after wound exploration and debridement. Infection rates are in the range 0–2% for type I, 2–10% for type II, and 10–50% for type III (Zalavras and Patzakis 2003).

Host status, such as presence of medical comorbidities and smoking, are important. Presence of one or two comorbidities is associated with an approximately threefold increased risk of infection, and three or more comorbidities with an approximately sixfold increased risk (Bowen and Widmaier 2005).

Treatment factors that help prevent infection after open fractures include early administration of appropriate antibiotic therapy, wound debridement, soft-tissue coverage, and fracture stabilization (Patzakis and Wilkins 1989). The length of antibiotic therapy, elapsed time from injury to surgery, and type of wound closure do not have a significant association with infection (Patzakis and Wilkins 1989, Skaggs et al. 2005).

■ Antibiotic therapy in open fractures

Antibiotic therapy plays an important role in prevention of infection in open fractures. This was established in a study by Patzakis et al. (1974), which demonstrated that administration of a cephalosporin decreased the infection rate (2/84 fractures, 2%) compared with no antibiotics (11/79 fractures, 14%).

A commonly used antibiotic therapy protocol consists of a first-generation cephalosporin (e.g., cefazolin), which is active against Gram-positive organisms, combined with an aminoglycoside (e.g., gentamicin or tobramycin), which is active against Gram-negative organisms. Antibiotics should be effective against both Gram-positive and Gram-negative organisms, because contamination with both types of pathogens occurs in open fractures. Anaerobic coverage (e.g., ampicillin or penicillin) is needed in farm injuries and vascular injuries to prevent clostridial myonecrosis (gas gangrene). Antibiotics should be started upon patient presentation because a delay >3 h has been shown to increase the risk of infection (Patzakis and Wilkins 1989). The recommended duration of therapy is 3 days with an additional 3 days for subsequent surgical procedures (Patzakis and Wilkins 1989, Zalavras and Patzakis 2003).

Local antibiotic delivery with the antibiotic-impregnated polymethylmethacrylate cement bead pouch technique has been used in open fractures to achieve high local concentration of antibiotics, minimal systemic toxicity, and prevention of secondary contamination (**Figures 19.1–19.4**) (Zalavras et al. 2004). Aminoglycosides are common choices because of their broad spectrum of activity and heat stability. Vancomycin is not recommended as an initial agent because of potential development of resistance. The antibiotic bead pouch technique has been shown to significantly reduce the overall infection rate from 12% when only intravenous (IV) antibiotics were used to 3.7% when IV antibiotics were combined with antibiotic beads (Ostermann et al. 1995).

Wound cultures in open fractures often fail to identify the organism, subsequently causing an infection. Pre-debridement wound cultures are not recommended. Post-debridement cultures are controversial but help select empirical antibiotic therapy if an early infection occurs.

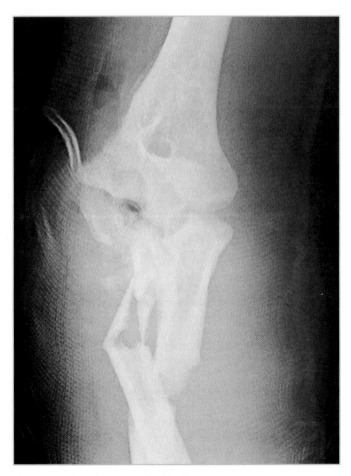

Figure 19.1 Open fracture of the distal humerus.

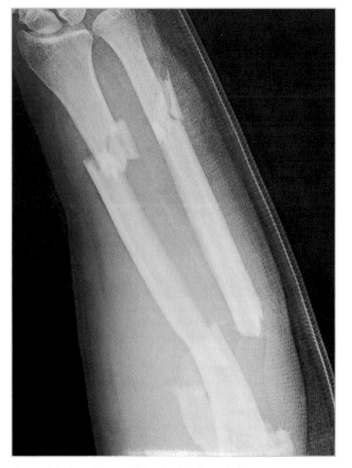

Figure 19.2 Open fracture of the distal radius and ulna.

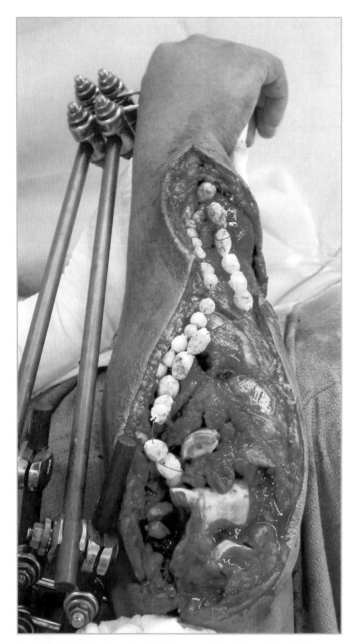

Figure 19.3 Application of antibiotic cement beads to achieve high local concentration of antibiotics.

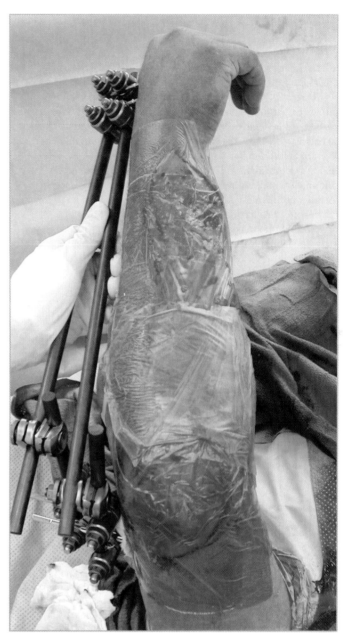

Figure 19.4 Coverage of the open fracture wound with a semipermeable membrane to prevent secondary contamination.

■ Debridement

Surgical debridement is an important management principle. Retained nonviable tissue and foreign material facilitate biofilm formation and development of a persistent infection. All nonviable bone and soft tissue should be resected. Bone fragments without any soft tissue attachments should not be retained unless they contain a considerable articular fragment. The injury wound should be surgically extended to allow assessment of tissue viability and execution of debridement. Debridement performed within or after 6 h from the injury does not appear to be associated with the infection rate. Open fractures in children treated within 6 h from the injury had an infection rate of 3% (12/344) compared with 2% (4/210) for those treated 6 h after the injury (Skaggs et al. 2005). If necessary, a repeat debridement may be performed after 48 h based on the degree of contamination and soft-tissue damage.

The wound should also be copiously irrigated. The optimal volume, delivery method, and irrigation solution remain controversial. High-pressure pulsatile irrigation may create bone damage and propagate bacteria into soft tissue and low-pressure pulsatile or gravity flow may be preferable (Petrisor et al. 2011). No significant differences in infection rates were reported when irrigation was performed with soap solution versus saline (Petrisor et al. 2011).

■ Wound management

Primary wound closure, after a thorough debridement, does not increase the infection rate and may prevent secondary contamination. However, it may lead to gas gangrene if debridement is inadequate. The partial closure technique, in which the surgical extension of the wound is closed but the traumatic wound is left open, is recommended for type I and type II open fractures. Type III open fracture wounds should be left open.

Reconstruction of the soft-tissue envelope is necessary in type IIIB open fractures to cover the wound, prevent secondary contamination, and improve local vascularity, thereby enhancing local host defenses and delivery of antibiotics at the fracture site. Soft-tissue coverage is of particular concern in open fractures of the tibia, and may be accomplished by local or free muscle flaps depending on the location and size of the defect. The muscle gastrocnemius is useful for coverage of proximal third defects of the tibia, and the soleus for middle third defects. Local muscle that has been compromised by the injury (direct trauma, ischemia, compartment syndrome) should not be transferred. A free muscle flap is necessary in these cases as well as in defects involving the distal third of the tibia. Soft-tissue reconstruction should be performed early, within the first 3–7 days.

◼ Fracture stabilization

Stabilization of the open fracture prevents further soft-tissue injury and helps reduce the infection rate. Fixation can be definitive or provisional and techniques include intramedullary nailing, external fixation, and plate fixation. The selection of technique for a specific injury depends on the fractured bone, the location of the fracture (intra-articular, metaphyseal, diaphyseal), the extent of soft-tissue injury, degree of contamination, and patient's physiological status.

◼ Specialized procedures

Bone defects >6 cm require specialized reconstructive procedures, such as vascularized bone grafts (fibula, iliac crest) or distraction osteogenesis. The free vascularized fibular graft provides structural support and new blood supply to the defect site can be used in defects up to 26 cm, and is a versatile graft that can include bone, muscle, skin, and fascia (Malizos et al. 2004). The Ilizarov technique, based on the principle of distraction osteogenesis, can reconstruct large bone defects and correct malalignment (Paley and Maar 2000).

◼ POST-TRAUMATIC OSTEOMYELITIS

The tibia is the most common site of adult post-traumatic osteomyelitis. Adult osteomyelitis is staged with the Cierny–Mader classification system, which evaluates the anatomic type of bone involvement (medullary, superficial, localized, diffuse) and the physiological class of the host (A: normal; B: compromised, systemic, local, or both; C: treatment is worse than disease) (Cierny et al. 1985) (**Table 19.3**).

Diagnosis is based on clinical findings (pain, erythema, draining sinuses, systemic symptoms), laboratory tests (elevated CRP, ESR), and imaging modalities (radiographs, MRI, scintigraphy). Cultures and sensitivity testing help identify the responsible organism and determine antibiotic therapy. The clinical picture may be subtle and laboratory tests may be normal in chronic infections, so a high index of suspicion is necessary in nonunions after an open fracture or internal fixation of a closed fracture.

Management of the patient with post-traumatic osteomyelitis is usually complex and prolonged. Amputation is an option in some cases and should be discussed with the patient. Management of adult post-traumatic osteomyelitis with limb salvage is based on a staged protocol that includes debridement, systemic and local antibiotic treatment, skeletal stabilization, soft-tissue coverage, and management of bone defects and ununited fractures (Patzakis and Zalavras 2005). Management is optimized by the presence of a multidisciplinary team consisting of an orthopedic surgeon, an infectious disease specialist, and a microvascular surgeon.

Debridement needs to be radical and achieve resection of all nonviable tissues (including skin, other soft tissues, and bone) and removal of implants. Specimens of purulent fluid, soft tissue, and bone are sent for aerobic, anaerobic, mycobacterial, and fungal cultures. The goal of debridement is to have only bleeding, viable tissue present at the wound. Inadequate debridement fails to remove the biofilm that has formed on local tissues and implants, thereby leading to recurrence of infection. However, fracture fixation implants may be retained in the early postoperative period if they are intact and providing stability to a healing fracture. In this case, the goal is not eradication but suppression of infection until the fracture heals.

Local antibiotic delivery via methylmethacrylate beads or spacers impregnated with antibiotics results in high local concentration and low systemic side effects of antibiotics, and eliminates dead space after debridement (Zalavras et al. 2004). The area is sealed with a semipermeable membrane to keep eluted antibiotics at the involved area. A potential disadvantage of nonabsorbable antibiotic delivery vehicles is the need for reoperation and removal, so that the vehicle does not act as a foreign body. However, reoperation is usually planned to manage the dead space and reconstruct the existing bone or soft-tissue defect. Biodegradable delivery systems appear promising (McKee et al. 2010). Systemic antibiotic administration is based on culture and sensitivity results and the recommended duration is 4–6

Table 19.3 Cierny–Mader classification system.

Anatomic type of bone involvement (increasing order of complexity)	
Medullary	Infection involves the endosteal bone and the medullary canal. Association with intramedullary implants in healed fractures without presence of a sequestrum Hematogenous mechanism rare in adults
Superficial	Infection involves the superficial part of an otherwise healthy bone. Association with soft-tissue defects
Localized	Infection involves the full thickness of the cortex but bone is stable Association with healed fractures in the presence of a cortical sequestrum
Diffuse	Infection involves the full thickness of the cortex but bone is unstable or will become unstable after debridement Association with infected acute healing fractures and infected nonunions
Physiological class of the host (increasing order of compromised physiology)	
A: Normal	Otherwise healthy patient with normal response to infection, wound healing, and treatment
B: Compromised	Patient with comorbidities (local, systemic, or both) that compromise response to infection, wound healing, and treatment
C: Treatment worse than disease	Morbidity associated with treatment exceeds the impact of infection on the patient

weeks in localized or diffuse osteomyelitis. Antibiotic therapy is not a substitute for inadequate debridement.

Skeletal stabilization is necessary for infection control in the presence of anatomic type IV osteomyelitis, as in infected healing fractures or infected nonunions. Different techniques may be applicable for each anatomic location but our preference is to stabilize the tibia with an external fixator, the femur with an intramedullary rod, and the humerus and forearm with plates and screws.

Wound management and soft-tissue coverage are performed, if needed, at a second stage usually 3–7 days after the initial debridement. Muscle flaps eliminate dead space, prevent secondary contamination, enhance vascularity, improve local host defenses, and facilitate the healing process. Soft-tissue coverage is of particular concern in osteomyelitis of the tibia and may be accomplished by local or free muscle flaps, depending on the location and size of the defect.

Management of bone defects and ununited fractures by bone grafting is performed at a third stage, usually 6–8 weeks after the muscle transfer to ensure viability of the flap and initial control of infection. Autogenous iliac crest bone graft is the gold standard for management of bone defects and can be harvested from the anterior or posterior iliac crest (Ahlmann et al. 2002). In nonunions of the tibia, bone graft can be placed either directly at the nonunion site or posterolaterally to achieve tibiofibular synostosis. Bone defects >6 cm require specialized reconstructive procedures, such as vascularized bone grafts or distraction osteogenesis.

The described limb salvage protocol can achieve a satisfactory outcome. An outcomes study of 46 patients with chronic osteomyelitis of the tibia with a mean follow-up of 5 years showed that limb salvage was accomplished in all patients, infection control in 98% (45/46), and union in 95% (44/46) (Siegel et al. 2000). In this study 85% (39/46) were able to ambulate independently without pain.

PERIPROSTHETIC JOINT INFECTIONS

Epidemiology and pathogenesis

Periprosthetic joint infection (PJI) is a challenging complication that occurs in approximately 1–2% of primary arthroplasty cases. The most common pathogens are *Staph. aureus* and *Staph. epidermidis*. The pathogenesis of infection involves direct inoculation of microorganisms (contamination during the procedure), hematogenous spread (at any point postoperatively as a result of infection at a remote location and bacteremia), or contiguous spread from adjacent infection.

Diagnosis

The clinical picture of PJI is often subtle and pain may be the only symptom. Decreased range of motion, drainage, and systemic symptoms may be present.

Inflammatory markers are helpful. In patients without connective tissue disorders, elevated ESR (>30 mm/h) has 82% sensitivity and 85% specificity, elevated CRP (>10 mg/l) has 96% sensitivity and 92% specificity, and elevated WBC count has 20% sensitivity and 96% specificity (Spangehl et al. 1999). Interleukin-6 has 97% sensitivity, 91% specificity, and the advantage of returning to normal values a few days after surgery (Berbari et al. 2010).

Aspiration at the site of a prosthetic hip or knee joint provides useful information. In chronic PJIs a synovial leukocyte count >1760 cells/mm^3 has 90% sensitivity and 99% specificity for the diagnosis and a neutrophil percentage >73% has a sensitivity and specificity of 93% and 95%, respectively (Parvizi et al. 2006). In PJI developing within 6 weeks of surgery, a synovial leukocyte count >27 800 cells/mm^3 has 84% sensitivity and 99% specificity for the diagnosis and a neutrophil percentage >89% has a sensitivity and specificity of 84% and 69%, respectively (Bedair et al. 2011).

Plain radiographs may reveal loosening of the implant, osteolysis, or periosteal reaction but cannot differentiate septic from aseptic loosening. Technetium-99m bone scan has low sensitivity for detection of PJI and may be positive up to 2 years postoperatively in a well-fixed prosthesis. ^{111}In-labeled leukocyte scan has 77% sensitivity and 86% specificity in the diagnosis of PJI (Scher et al. 2000). PET with [^{18}F] fluorodeoxyglucose is a promising new modality with 95% sensitivity and 93% specificity for PJI (Parvizi et al. 2006).

Intraoperative tests can be helpful in equivocal cases. Gram stain has 19% sensitivity and 98% specificity, whereas frozen sections with more than five stromal polymorphonuclear leukocytes per high power field have 80% sensitivity and 94% specificity (Spangehl et al. 1999). Cultures obtained intraoperatively have 94% sensitivity and 97% specificity (Spangehl et al. 1999). Another study reported that the culture sensitivity decreases from 77% with an antibiotic-free interval >14 days to 48% with an interval of 4–14 days (Trampuz et al. 2007). Sonication of explanted prosthesis has been shown to improve sensitivity of cultures. In hip and knee PJs the sensitivity of tissue cultures was 61% whereas that of sonicate fluid cultures was 78% (Trampuz et al. 2007). Recently, a definition of PJI was proposed by the Workgroup of the Musculoskeletal Infection Society (**Box 19.1**) (Parvizi et al. 2011).

Box 19.1 Definition of periprosthetic joint infection proposed by the workgroup of the Musculoskeletal Infection Society.

Major criteria
1. Sinus tract communicating with the prosthesis
2. Pathogen isolated by culture from at least two separate tissue or fluid samples obtained from the affected prosthetic joint

Minor criteria
1. Presence of purulence in the affected joint
2. Elevated erythrocyte sedimentation rate (ESR) and C-reactive protein (CRP) concentration
3. Elevated synovial leukocyte count
4. Elevated synovial neutrophil percentage
5. More than five neutrophils per high-power field in five high-power fields observed from histological analysis of periprosthetic tissue at × 400 magnification
6. Isolation of a microorganism in one culture of periprosthetic tissue or fluid

Definite periprosthetic joint infection exists in the presence of one of the two major criteria or in the presence of four of the six minor criteria. Periprosthetic joint infection may be present even if fewer than four of the six minor criteria are met.

Treatment

Management of PJI depends on the timing and duration of infection, the medical condition of the patient, the susceptibility of the pathogen to antibiotics, and the status of the surrounding soft-tissue envelope and the implant. Surgical management options for PJI include debridement with retention of components, exchange arthroplasty (one-stage vs two-stage), arthrodesis, permanent resection arthroplasty, and amputation (McPherson et al. 1999). Surgical management is complemented by systemic antibiotic administration for a period of usually 6 weeks. Nonsurgical management with chronic antibiotic suppression may be considered in selected patients.

Debridement with exchange of the polyethylene liner and retention of the components is an option in early infections (<3 weeks postoperatively) or acute hematogenous infections (acute onset with symptom duration <3 weeks in a previously well-functioning patient) by the presence of well-fixed implants (Zimmerli et al. 1998).

Exchange arthroplasty is the preferred option in late chronic infections (developing more than 3 weeks postoperatively with indolent course and duration >3 weeks) and when loosening of the implants is present. Flap coverage may be necessary if the soft-tissue envelope is compromised. Exchange arthroplasty can be performed with either a one-stage protocol (reimplantation at the same surgical procedure as debridement and component removal) or a two-stage protocol (reim-

plantation at a subsequent procedure with an interval of 6–12 weeks). One-stage exchange arthroplasty avoids an additional procedure and expedites patient management, if successful. Optimal indications for one-stage exchange arthroplasty include an otherwise healthy patient with good soft-tissue envelope and infection by a susceptible pathogen.

Two-stage exchange arthroplasty requires an additional procedure but allows for repeat debridement and local antibiotic delivery during the reimplantation interval via antibiotic-impregnated spacers.

Exchange arthroplasty may not be feasible due to patient comorbidities, poor soft-tissue envelope, deficient bone stock, or presence of resistant organisms. Other management options include arthrodesis, resection arthroplasty (in patients with limited functional demands), chronic antibiotic suppression (in severely compromised patients with low-grade infections by organisms sensitive to oral antibiotics), or amputation (in severely compromised patients with severe or uncontrollable infections).

■ REFERENCES

Ahlmann E, Patzakis M, Roidis N, et al. Comparison of anterior and posterior iliac crest bone grafts in terms of harvest-site morbidity and functional outcomes. *J Bone Joint Surg* 2002;**84A**:716–20.

Bedair H, Ting N, Jacovides C, et al. The Mark Coventry Award: diagnosis of early postoperative TKA infection using synovial fluid analysis. *Clin Orthop Rel Res* 2011;**469**:34–40.

Berbari E, Mabry T, Tsaras G, et al. Inflammatory blood laboratory levels as markers of prosthetic joint infection: a systematic review and meta-analysis. *J Bone Joint Surg* 2010;**92A**:2102–9.

Bowen TR and Widmaier JC. Host classification predicts infection after open fracture. *Clin Orthop Rel Res* 2005;**433**:205–11.

Cierny G 3rd, Mader JT, Penninck JJ. A clinical staging system for adult osteomyelitis. *Contemp Orthop* 1985;**10**:17–37.

Costerton JW. Biofilm theory can guide the treatment of device-related orthopaedic infections. *Clin Orthop Relat Res* 2005;**437**:7–11.

Costerton JW, Stewart PS, Greenberg EP. Bacterial biofilms: a common cause of persistent infections. *Science* 1999;**284**:1318–22.

Costerton JW, Post JC, Ehrlich GD, et al. New methods for the detection of orthopedic and other biofilm infections. *FEMS* 2011;**61**:133–40.

Erdman WA, Tamburro F, Jayson HT, et al. Osteomyelitis: characteristics and pitfalls of diagnosis with MR imaging. *Radiology* 1991;**180**:533–9.

Fry DE, Barie PS. The changing face of *Staphylococcus aureus*: a continuing surgical challenge. *Surg Infect* 2011;**12**:191–203.

Gallo PH, Melton-Kreft R, Nistico L, et al. Demonstration of *Bacillus cereus* in orthopaedic-implant-related infection with use of a multi-primer polymerase chain reaction-mass spectrometric assay: report of two cases. *J Bone Joint Surg* 2011;**93A**:e851–6.

Gordon RJ, Lowy FD. Pathogenesis of methicillin-resistant *Staphylococcus aureus* infection. *Clin Infect Dis* 2008;**46**(suppl 5):S350–9.

Gustilo RB, Mendoza RM, Williams DN. Problems in the management of type III (severe) open fractures: a new classification of type III open fractures. *J Trauma* 1984;**24**:742–6.

Kallio MJ, Unkila-Kallio L, Aalto K, Peltola H. Serum C-reactive protein, erythrocyte sedimentation rate and white blood cell count in septic arthritis of children. *Pediatr Infect Dis J* 1997;**16**:411–13.

Khachatourians AG, Patzakis MJ, Roidis N, Holtom PD. Laboratory monitoring in pediatric acute osteomyelitis and septic arthritis. *Clin Orthop Relat Res* 2003;**409**:186–94.

Kocher MS, Zurakowski D, Kasser JR. Differentiating between septic arthritis and transient synovitis of the hip in children: an evidence-based clinical prediction algorithm. *J Bone Joint Surg* 1999;**81A**:1662–70.

Lazzarini L, Mader JT, Calhoun JH. Osteomyelitis in long bones. *J Bone Joint Surg* 2004;**86A**:2305–18.

Lee J, Singletary R, Schmader K, et al. Surgical site infection in the elderly following orthopaedic surgery. Risk factors and outcomes. *J Bone Joint Surg* 2006;**88A**:1705–12.

Luhmann SJ, Jones A, Schootman M, et al. Differentiation between septic arthritis and transient synovitis of the hip in children with clinical prediction algorithms. *J Bone Joint Surg* 2004;**86A**:956–962.

McKee MD, Li-Bland EA, Wild LM, Schemitsch EH. A prospective, randomized clinical trial comparing an antibiotic-impregnated bioabsorbable bone substitute with standard antibiotic-impregnated cement beads in the treatment of chronic osteomyelitis and infected nonunion. *J Orthop Trauma* 2010;**24**:483–90.

McPherson EJ, Tontz W Jr, Patzakis M, et al. Outcome of infected total knee utilizing a staging system for prosthetic joint infection. *Am J Orthop* 1999;**28**:161–5.

Malizos KN, Zalavras CG, Soucacos PN, et al. Free vascularized fibular grafts for reconstruction of skeletal defects. *J Am Acad Orthop Surg* 2004;**12**:360–369.

Mehta P, Schnall SB, Zalavras CG. Septic arthritis of the shoulder, elbow, and wrist. *Clin Orthop Relat Res* 2006;**451**:42–5.

Merkel KD, Brown ML, Dewanjee MK, Fitzgerald RH Jr. Comparison of indium-labeled-leukocyte imaging with sequential technetium-gallium scanning in the diagnosis of low-grade musculoskeletal sepsis. A prospective study. *J Bone Joint Surg* 1985;**67A**:465–476.

Ostermann PA, Seligson D, Henry SL. Local antibiotic therapy for severe open fractures. A review of 1085 consecutive cases. *J Bone Joint Surg* 1995;**77B**:93–7.

Paley D, Maar DC. Ilizarov bone transport treatment for tibial defects. *J Orthop Trauma* 2000;**14**:76–85.

Parvizi J, Ghanem E, Menashe S, et al. Periprosthetic infection: what are the diagnostic challenges? *J Bone Joint Surg* 2006;**88A**(suppl 4):138–47.

Parvizi J, Zmistowski B, Berbari EF, et al. New definition for periprosthetic joint infection. *Clin Orthop Relat Res*. 2011;**469**:2992–4.

Patzakis MJ, Wilkins J. Factors influencing infection rate in open fracture wounds. *Clin Orthop Relat Res* 1989;**243**:36–40.

Patzakis MJ, Zalavras CG. Chronic posttraumatic osteomyelitis and infected nonunion of the tibia: current management concepts. *J Am Acad Orthop Surg* 2005;**13**:417–27.

Patzakis MJ, Harvey JP Jr, Ivler D. The role of antibiotics in the management of open fractures. *J Bone Joint Surg* 1974;**56A**:532–41.

Perlman MH, Patzakis MJ, Kumar PJ, Holtom P. The incidence of joint involvement with adjacent osteomyelitis in pediatric patients. *J Pediatr Orthop* 2000;**20**:40–3.

Petrisor B, Sun X, Bhandari M, et al. Fluid lavage of open wounds (FLOW): a multicenter, blinded, factorial pilot trial comparing alternative irrigating solutions and pressures in patients with open fractures. *J Trauma* 2011;**71**:596–606.

Poultsides LA, Liaropoulos LL, Malizos KN. The socioeconomic impact of musculoskeletal infections. *J Bone Joint Surg* 2010;**92A**:e13.

Ross JJ. Septic arthritis. *Infect Dis Clin N Am* 2005;**19**:799–817.

Scher DM, Pak K, Lonner JH, et al. The predictive value of indium-111 leukocyte scans in the diagnosis of infected total hip, knee, or resection arthroplasties. *J Arthroplasty* 2000;**15**:295–300.

Siegel HJ, Patzakis MJ, Holtom PD, et al. Limb salvage for chronic tibial osteomyelitis: an outcomes study. *J Trauma* 2000;**48**:484–9.

Skaggs DL, Friend L, Alman B, et al. The effect of surgical delay on acute infection following 554 open fractures in children. *J Bone Joint Surg* 2005;**87A**:8–12.

Spangehl MJ, Masri BA, O'Connell JX, Duncan CP. Prospective analysis of preoperative and intraoperative investigations for the diagnosis of infection at the sites of two hundred and two revision total hip arthroplasties. *J Bone Joint Surg* 1999;**81A**:672–83.

Trampuz A, Piper KE, Jacobson MJ, et al. Sonication of removed hip and knee prostheses for diagnosis of infection. *N Engl J Med* 2007;**357**:654–63.

Unkila-Kallio L, Kallio MJ, Eskola J, Peltola H. Serum C-reactive protein, erythrocyte sedimentation rate, and white blood cell count in acute hematogenous osteomyelitis of children. *Pediatrics* 1994;**93**:59–62.

Whitehouse JD, Friedman ND, Kirkland KB, et al. The impact of surgical-site infections following orthopedic surgery at a community hospital and a university hospital: adverse quality of life, excess length of stay, and extra cost. *Infect Control Hosp Epidemiol* 2002;**23**:183–9.

Zalavras CG, Costerton JW. Biofilm, biomaterials, and bacterial adherence. In: Cierny G 3rd, McLaren AC, Wongworawat MD (eds), *Orthopaedic Knowledge Update: Musculoskeletal Infection*. Rosemont, IL, American Academy of Orthopaedic Surgeons, 2009: 33–41.

Zalavras CG, Patzakis MJ. Open fractures: evaluation and management. *J Am Acad Orthop Surg* 2003;**11**:212–19.

Zalavras CG, Patzakis MJ, Holtom P. Local antibiotic therapy in the treatment of open fractures and osteomyelitis. *Clin Orthop Relat Res* 2004;**427**:86–93.

Zalavras CG, Dellamaggiora R, Patzakis MJ, et al. Septic arthritis in patients with human immunodeficiency virus. *Clin Orthop Relat Res* 2006a;**451**:46–9.

Zalavras CG, Dellamaggiora R, Patzakis MJ, et al. Recalcitrant septic knee arthritis due to adjacent osteomyelitis in adults. *Clin Orthop Relat Res* 2006b;**451**:38–41.

Zimmerli W, Widmer AF, Blatter M, et al. Role of rifampin for treatment of orthopedic implant-related staphylococcal infections: a randomized controlled trial. *JAMA* 1998;**279**:1537–41.

Chapter 20 Obstetric and gynecological infections

Sebastian Faro, Jonathan Faro, Constance Faro

Infection associated with the obstetric and gynecological patients has a long history. This chapter deals with the current available information and foregoes the historical information pertaining to this subject. Suffice it to state that the first real association among healthcare givers, bacteriology, and nosocomial infection was brought to light by the publications of Semmelweis and Holmes describing the transmission of *Streptococcus pyogenes* from infected patients to non-infected patients via healthcare providers.

Infectious diseases in obstetrics and gynecology slowly gained interest before 1980 and reached a zenith from 1980 to the early 1990s. Interest has since waned but has not dissipated. Modern technology has resurrected interest and is leading to a better understanding of the infectious diseases associated with obstetric and gynecological patients. This treatment of the subject will be limited to those infections requiring not only antimicrobial therapy but also surgical intervention. The key to applying both therapies is recognizing the opportune time for surgical intervention. Delaying surgical intervention results in increased morbidity and mortality.

VULVAL INFECTIONS

Although there are many infections that afflict the vulva, those that may require surgical intervention are mainly of a bacterial etiology. They can be divided into the following categories: (1) Cellulitis, (2) furuncle, (3) carbuncle, (4) abscess, (5) hidradenitis suppurativa, and (5) Fournier gangrene (necrotizing fasciitis). These infections can all involve *Staphylococcus aureus* but can also involve the microflora commonly found in the vagina and rectum. Therefore, although furuncles and carbuncles are most commonly caused by *Staph. aureus* the others listed above may indeed involve *Staph. aureus* but can also be polymicrobial. Location of the infection, characteristic changes in the skin at the point of infection, presence of fever, and pain are all important clinical findings, but not pathognomonic of bacterial infections and must be differentiated from viral and fungal infections.

Cellulitis

Cellulitis is a condition that is not uncommon, occurring mainly in the labia majora. However, cellulitis must be differentiated from other skin conditions such as erysipelas and impetigo. *Erysipelas* is a superficial skin and soft-tissue infection involving the dermal lymphatic system. Erysipelas presents as a tender, well-demarcated, bright-red edematous area with raised borders. The borders are indurated and progressive (Bisno and Stevens 1996, Rogers and Perkins 2006). Erysipelas is most commonly caused by *Strep. pyogenes* but other species of *Streptococcus* can also cause it. The infection is treated by antibiotics. Other bacteria can cause an erysipelas-like picture but this is very uncommon. Erysipelas is managed by medical therapy only. *Impetigo* is a superficial infection involving the epidermis and is a highly contagious infection. It is caused by *Staph. aureus*, meticillin-resistant *Staph. aureus* (MRSA), and *Strep. pyogenes*. Impetigo is typically treated with antibiotics.

Cellulitis can present as a blanching erythematous cutaneous infection, or may be associated with other conditions such as the Bartholin or Skene gland abscess, surgical site abscess, furuncles, and carbuncles. Cellulitis is an infection of the deeper dermis and may extend to the subcutaneous tissues (King et al. 2006, Sachdeva and Tomecki 2008). Cellulitis usually presents with the four cardinal signs of inflammation: Rubor (erythema), calor (heat), dolor (pain), and tumor (swelling). Cellulitis commonly follows cutaneous trauma but can occur from folliculitis or even from remote hematogenous seeding of the skin.

Cellulitis associated with an abscess (e.g., Bartholin or Skene gland abscess or surgical site infection) requires both antibiotic therapy and surgical intervention. Antibiotics alone will not suffice in the treatment of these conditions, in contrast to cellulitis without abscess. If the treatment requires the administration of antibiotics and surgical intervention, the antibiotics should be administered before making the incision. Preferably the antibiotics should be administered 1 hour before making the incision and continued until the clinical cellulitis has resolved, the patient's white blood cell count (WBC) has returned to normal, and the fever has resolved.

The principles involved for treating cellulitis associated with an abscess are based on a logical approach to evaluating the etiology, diagnosis, and management of any abscess. The first step is to identify its location, the second step is having a strong inclination as to which bacteria are likely to be involved, the third step is to obtain a specimen for Gram stain, culture, and antibiotic sensitivities, and the fourth step is management.

Individuals who have pure cellulitis seldom have culture information. Therefore, antibiotic selection is based on knowledge gained from the literature and realizing that the bacteria involved are most likely from the patient's own endogenous vaginal microflora.

Furuncles

A furuncle is an acute inflammatory infection involving a hair follicle. Initially, it appears as a round, firm, or nodular, erythematous lesion. These perifollicular lesions are most commonly caused by *Staph. aureus*. The evolution of the lesion is characterized by it becoming firm and painful, with the development of central suppuration. The furuncle will frequently drain spontaneously and resolve. However, it can become quite large and have a significant amount of surrounding cellulitis.

Furuncles and carbuncles should be viewed as potentially serious infections. Initially these infections start as a folliculitis and can proceed to abscess, bacteremia, and necrotizing fasciitis. Infections such as folliculitis, furuncles and carbuncles have become significant infections because they are commonly caused by community-acquired MRSA (King et al. 2006, Moran et al. 2006).

Carbuncles

A carbuncle is made up of two or more confluent furuncles in close proximity, with invasion of the subcutaneous tissue. Multiple abscesses are separated by connective tissue septations. A carbuncle is a more serious infection, accompanied by pain, fever, and malaise. In common with furuncles, patients often attempt to express the contents of a furuncle and carbuncle, which often leads to deeper invasion of the infection and the potential for bacteremia.

Treatment of furuncles and carbuncles includes antibiotics, application of hot compresses to encourage spontaneous drainage, and, ultimately, incision and drainage. Frequently, the pus within the furuncle or carbuncle becomes very viscous and is not easily removed. The purulent content forms an almost solid core and requires surgical intervention to remove the contents of the abscess. As the most likely cause is community-acquired MRSA and, therefore, b-lactam antibiotics, e.g., cephalosporin, and broad-spectrum penicillins (piperacillin/tazobactam, ampicillin/sulbactam) are not effective. Recommended antibiotics are listed in **Table 20.1** (Stevens et al. 2005).

Patients requiring incision and drainage should be given intravenous (IV) antibiotics. A blood urea nitrogen (BUN) and creatinine should be obtained because if the patient has renal impairment adjustment in the antibiotic dose may be necessary. Incision of a carbuncle will require the disruption of septa because the lesion is made up of closely oppressed or coalesced abscesses or furuncles. As these infections are extremely inflamed and very painful, incision and drainage will require anesthesia.

Surgical management begins with providing anesthesia, thus allowing cleansing of the area with an antiseptic, draping the area with sterile towels, and obtaining a specimen for Gram stain, culture of bacteria, and identification of the infecting organism, as well as determining the antibiotics to which the isolate is sensitive and resistant. An incision is made that is long enough to allow for good exploration to disrupt any septa that may be present. The wound should be well irrigated with sterile 0.9% saline. The abscess cavity that remains should be packed with iodoform gauze, which is removed within 24–48 h. The area should be bandaged until the lesion has healed.

Table 20.1 Antibiotic choices for cellulitis, furuncles, and carbuncles.

Oral therapy	Dosage
Doxycycline	100 mg twice daily for 10 days
Minocycline	100 mg twice daily day for 10 days
Clindamycin	300–450 mg three times per day for 10 days
Trimethoprim–sulfamethoxazole	One tablet (400 mg trimethoprim/80 mg sulfa) twice daily for 10 days
Dicloxacillin	250 mg four times daily for 10 days (not for MRSA)
Intravenous therapy	**Dosage (continued until switch to oral treatment)**
Vancomycin	30 mg/kg every 12 h
Linezolid	600 mg every 12 h
Daptomycin	4 mg/kg every 24 h
Clindamycin	600 mg every 8 h

Abscesses

Vulval abscesses, aside from pyodermatous lesions such as folliculitis, furuncles, and carbuncles, can occur in the labia majora, Bartholin glands, Skene glands, and urethral diverticulum. The most common vulva abscesses are the Bartholin gland abscess and a true labial abscess. A labial abscess must be distinguished from a Bartholin gland abscess because the two are treated very differently. The goal of treating a Bartholin gland abscess is to maintain a functioning draining gland.

The approach to treating a labial abscess is to first establish that the mass is an abscess (**Table 20.2**). This holds true for a true labial mass, a mass in the area of the Bartholin gland, or a mass in the area of the vaginal introitus.

Before initiating an invasive procedure, ultrasonography of the mass and surrounding area could be performed. This will allow the determination of whether the mass is cystic or solid, and whether it contains septations or is uniloculated. Ultrasonography will also allow the examiner to determine the distance from the epithelial surface to the inner aspect of the cyst. This information will help in determining the depth of penetration that is needed to enter the cyst or abscess to obtain a specimen via aspiration, as well as for incision and drainage. This approach can also be used in the management of a Bartholin cyst, although the tissue depth in the true labia majora is thicker than that of a Bartholin abscess or cyst.

Labial abscess

The involved labia should be prepped with an antiseptic solution and local anesthetic (e.g., 1% xylocaine) is injected into the skin overlying the mass where the incision is to be made. Large masses may require the operating room and either general anesthesia or IV sedation plus local anesthetic. A 20-gauge needle is used to obtain an aspirate of 2–5 ml fluid. Part of the specimen should be used for a Gram stain and the remainder processed for the isolation, identification, and antibiotic sensitivities of facultative and obligate anaerobic bacteria. The incision should be made in either the lateral fold or the medial aspect of the labial majora, but not on the anterior surface. Incising the anterior surface of the labia majora typically results in penetrating a thicker layer of tissue and the healing often results in a depression of the healed incised area. The incision should be large enough to allow for adequate drainage, disruption of any septations, and packing the area with iodoform gauze.

Bartholin gland abscess

The initial approach is much the same as in the initial approach in a labial abscess. The incision is made extending from the superior to the

Table 20.2 Differential diagnosis of a labial mass.

Vulval mass	Vaginal mass
Sebaceous cyst	Inclusion cyst
Dysontogenetic cyst	Endometriosis
Hematoma	Adenosis
Syringoma	Gartner duct cyst
Endometriosis	Leiomyoma
Myoblastoma	Inguinal hernia
Accessory breast tissue	
Von Recklinghausen tumor	
Adenocarcinoma	

inferior border of the abscess. Typically, if this is the first episode in a woman of reproductive age, a simple incision is made through the epithelium and the abscess capsule. If this is a recurrent abscess or the first episode in a postmenopausal woman elliptically shaped tissue is excised, including the epithelium and the abscess wall, and this tissue is sent to pathology for histological examination. Carcinomas of Bartholin gland are rare tumors and account for approximately 1% of all gynecological cancers (Barclay et al. 1964, Copeland et al. 1986, Felix et al. 1993, Lelle et al. 1994, DiSaia and Creasman 1997). The majority, 80–90%, are squamous cell carcinomas and adenocarcinomas (Felix et al. 1993). Most of these carcinomas occur in postmenopausal women aged >65 years.

Before aspirating or incising the abscess, antibiotics should be administered. The microbiology of a Bartholin gland abscess is varied and can involve sexually transmitted bacteria and bacteria from the lower genital tract or rectum. Therefore, empirical therapy is initially with a combination of antibiotics until bacteria have been isolated, identified, and the antibiotic sensitivities are known. *Chlamydia trachomatis*, *Neisseria gonorrhoeae*, Gram-negative and Gram-positive facultative, and obligate anaerobic bacteria are common causes of Bartholin gland abscess and a combination of antibiotics is necessary (**Box 20.1**).

> **Box 20.1 Antibiotic choices for treatment of a Bartholin gland abscess (intravenous therapy).**
>
> Combination antibiotic choices and dosing
> Clindamycin 900 mg every 8 h + ampicillin 2 g every 6 h + gentamicin 5 mg/kg body weight every 24 h
> Metronidazole 500 mg every 8 h + ampicillin 2 g every 6 h + gentamicin 5 mg/kg body weight every 24 h
> Metronidazole 500 mg every 8 h or clindamycin 900 mg every 8 h + levofloxacin 500 mg every 24 h
> Metronidazole 500 mg every 8 h or clindamycin 900 mg every 8 h + doxycyline 100 mg every 12 h

Broad-spectrum antibiotic administration is indicated because there is usually a significant inflammatory response surrounding the Bartholin gland abscess and this may indicate an associated cellulitis. In addition, the surgical procedure may cause bacteremia. Once the Gram stain results are known adjustment in antibiotic therapy can be made (**Table 20.3**). Although the identity of the bacteria present cannot be determined from the Gram stain, it is possible to choose appropriate antibiotic coverage.

If the contents of the Bartholin gland abscess had a foul odor and the Gram stain revealed large Gram-positive cocci in clusters, this would suggest anaerobic bacteria, peptococci, or if in chains peptostreptococci to be present. The presence of intracellular Gram-negative diplococci indicates the presence of *N. gonorrhoeae*. *C. trachomatis* lacks a cell wall and therefore does not stain with Gram reagents; if present it will be undetected by the Gram stain.

The abscess cavity should be explored with a hemostat to disrupt any septations present and copiously irrigate the cavity with sterile saline until the contents issuing forth are clear. The abscess wall is sutured to the epithelium with interrupted suture (marsupialization). The cavity is packed with half-inch (1.25-cm) iodoform gauze and left in place for 24–48 h. Repacking is not necessary; the cavity will fairly rapidly collapse and the diameter of the opening will be reduced to a small opening and leave the gland functioning.

An alternative to marsupialization is placement of a Word catheter into the abscess cavity, which is indicated in patients experiencing their first Bartholin cyst or a simple abscess. The patient treated with a Word catheter should not have signs or symptoms of a systemic response to infection. In treatment of a Bartholin abscess with a Word catheter, if septations are present within the abscess are and are not disrupted, the patient will likely experience a recurrence.

A Word catheter is approximately 6 cm long, diameter is equal to 10 French (Fr), and there is a 1-ml inflatable balloon at the tip (Word 1968). The Word catheter is typically used to drain a Bartholin cyst or abscess in an office setting or emergency room. The procedure is performed by cleansing the surface epithelium overlying the enlarged Bartholin gland with an antiseptic, such as povidone iodine. Insert a sterile 20-G needle into the abscess and withdraw approximately 2 ml purulent fluid. Send the fluid in a capped syringe or instill the fluid into an appropriate transport system for Gram stain, and culture of *C. trachomatis*, *N. gonorrhoeae*, and facultative and obligate anaerobic bacteria. A stab incision is then made into the Bartholin gland abscess. Aspirate all fluid, and insert a hemostat into the cavity to disrupt any adhesions or septations that may be present. Irrigate the abscess cavity with copious amounts of sterile saline. Insert the Word catheter and inflate the balloon with sterile saline; do not use air because this will not permit the balloon to remain inflated. The catheter should be left in place for 4–6 weeks, at which time it can be removed. Patients who develop a recurrent Bartholin abscess should undergo marsupialization of the abscess and this procedure should also be used for such patients. Individuals who develop recurrent Bartholin abscesses or cysts should have the gland removed.

Empirical antibiotic administration should include antimicrobial activity against *C. trachomatis*, *N. gonorrhoeae*, and facultative and obligate anaerobic bacteria. A combination of metronidazole 500 mg every 8 h and levofloxacin 500 mg daily will provide such coverage. When collecting specimens, a specimen for culture of *N. gonorrhoeae* should be obtained in case the polymerase chain reaction (PCR) test for gonorrhea is positive. An alternative antibiotic regimen is a single dose of metronidazole and ceftriaxone followed by doxycyline (100 mg) twice daily for 7 days.

Hidradenitis suppurativa

Hidradenitis suppurativa, also known as acne inversa or acne tetrad, is a skin disorder of unknown etiology. The current theory is that hyperkeratosis of the follicular epithelium results in occlusion of the follicle and associated apocrine gland with subsequent follicular rupture (Slade et al. 2003, Wiseman 2004). Once the follicular canal and apocrine gland become obstructed, the bacterial infection leads to abscess formation. It occurs two to five times more often in women, and in 1–4% of the population (Von der Werth and Jemec 2001).

Table 20.3 Interpretation of the Gram stain based on microbial morphology.

Bacterial species	Microscopic morphology
Staphylococci	Gram-positive cocci in clusters
Streptococci	Gram-positive cocci in chains
Enterobacteriaceae	Gram-negative rods, morphological similar
Bacteroides or *Prevotella* spp.	Pleomorphic Gram-negative rods
Fusobacterium spp.	Fusiform Gram-negative rods
Clostridium spp.	Gram-positive rods with endospores

The disease has multiple components: first there is the obstructive phase in which the follicular canal becomes blocked; second is the infection phase in which bacteria trapped below the obstruction initiate the infection, eventually forming abscesses; third is development of fistulae or sinus tracts emanating from the abscess and granulating inflammation – these sinus tracts extend into the dermis in a leaf-like pattern – and fourth is progression to new lesions (Kurzen et al. 1999). The disease can invade the subcutaneous tissue and this is usually seen in patients with long-standing chronic disease. Hydradenitis suppurativa may appear similar to many other perineal conditions (**Box 20.2**). It requires a careful history, detailed inspection, and may even require biopsy to differentiate it from other conditions.

Box 20.2 Differential diagnosis for anogenital hidradenitis suppurativa (acne inversa).

Furuncle
Carbuncle
Labial abscess
Bartholin abscess
Lymphadenitis
Infected sebaceous cyst
Epidermoid or dermoid cyst
Granuloma inguinale
Lymphogranuloma venereum
Crohn disease
Cryptoglandular fistula
Steatocytoma multiplex
Pilonidal cyst
Actinomycosis
Scrofuloderma

Treatment of hidradenitis suppurativa consists of medical and surgical therapy. Although medical therapy has been and continues to be used it has met with limited success. Various medical treatments have been administered, including antibiotic regimens, monoclonal antibody therapy directed against tumor necrosis factor (TNF)-α (infliximab, etanercept, adalimonab), and antiandrogens (Van der Zee et al. 2011). Isotretinoin has also been used, but is of questionable value and is known to be teratogenic.

Decisions to pursue surgical management of hidradenitis suppurative are commonly made by using the Hurley (1989) staging system. Stage 1 disease is single or multiple abscesses but without sinus tracts and scarring. Stage 2 represents recurrent abscesses with sinus tract formation and scarring. There may be a single or multiple lesions. Stage 3 is multiple areas of involvement with multiple interconnected sinus tracts, abscesses, and scarring.

Disease that has advanced to stages 2 and 3 usually requires surgical intervention. The surgical approaches that have been used have been incision and drainage, excision of the lesion with a narrow margin, excision of the lesion with a wide margin, and wide excision with excision of the sinus tracts (Matuziak et al. 2009).

Skene gland abscess

Skene glands are the homolog to the male prostate and are subject to the same diseases although their occurrence is much rarer. However, Skene glands are subject to infection by *C. trachomatis*, *N. gonorrhoeae*, and *Trichomonas vaginalis*, as well as facultative and obligate anaerobic bacteria. Skene glands can abscess and the approach to management can be either incision and drainage or marsupialization.

Simple incision and drainage could result in the gland developing an adhesion between oppressing walls and render the gland relatively non-functional, depending on how much of the gland becomes obliterated. An alternative treatment, marsupialization, would leave the gland open with a small duct and, thus, leave a functioning gland.

In 1880 Skene published a report describing two ducts that drain the distal apart of the gland through two openings which are adjacent to the urethral meatus (Skene 1880, Gittes and Nakamura 1996). Huffman in two publications (1948, 1951) described Skene glands as branching paraurethral structures originating from the urethral lumen into the adjacent soft tissues, traveling along the distal two-thirds of the urethra. Clinical symptoms characteristic of Skene gland abscess is vulvar pain, dysuria, urinary obstruction, and dyspareunia.

Therefore, the first step in managing an abscess in this region is to determine if the abscess is in a urethral diverticulum or in the Skene gland. A Skene gland abscess usually appears as a fluctuant mass lateral or inferolateral to the urethral meatus. Typically, unlike a urethral diverticulum, a Skene gland abscess does not communicate with the urethra. However, during the evaluation of the patient with a suspected Skene gland abscess, it should be documented that the abscess does not communicate with the urethra.

■ POSTOPERATIVE INFECTIONS

Postoperative infections occurring in the obstetric and gynecological patient are typically due to the patient's own endogenous vaginal bacteriology. Interestingly, the bacteriology of the vagina impacts not only the patient's potential risk of developing a postoperative infection but also the effectiveness of antibiotic prophylaxis. *Staph. aureus*, including MRSA, is a common cause of abdominal SSI.

The number of surgical sites varies depending on the operation being performed. Patients undergoing an abdominal hysterectomy will have at least two surgical sites that are at risk for infection: The abdominal incision and the vaginal apical incision. Patients undergoing a vaginal hysterectomy with anterior and posterior repair will have at least three surgical incisions. Therefore, the gynecological surgeon must be aware of the potential of each surgical site to be contaminated by the bacteria of the vagina. Once the vagina has been opened the operation is classified as a clean-contaminated case and the pelvic floor is potentially contaminated. Bringing instruments and the gloved hands of the surgeon and assistants, repeatedly, from the pelvic floor through the abdominal incision can contaminate the abdominal incision. Care must be taken to minimize this potential for contamination.

A vaginal hysterectomy is conducted through this contaminated field from start to finish. If reconstructive procedures are performed vaginally and the rectum is not covered adequately, in addition to the vaginal bacteriology, the rectal microflora can also contaminate the surgical field. The use of synthetic and biologic adjuncts in vaginal reconstructive surgery adds a potential risk for infection. These adjuncts are foreign bodies and as such can become colonized by these bacteria and thus add another dimension to postoperative infection.

The patient undergoing a cesarean delivery poses a significant risk for developing an abdominal SSI as well as a the potential for developing postpartum endometritis. The patient who labors with ruptured amniotic membranes for >6 h is at significant risk for developing a postoperative infection. Labor in the presence of ruptured amniotic membranes provides time for bacteria to ascend into the uterine cavity, colonize the decidual layer of the uterus, and invade the myometrium, allowing for infection to begin during labor. During manual delivery of the fetal head, copious amounts of vaginal fluid are brought up into the uterine cavity as well as over the uterine and abdominal incisions.

Thus in both the obstetric and the gynecological patient, the risk for infection is considerable because most surgical procedures are clean-contaminated operations, and the potential sources of infection are numerous (**Table 20.4**). Therefore, preventive measures begin well before the operations by assessing the endogenous vaginal microflora. One it has been decided that the patient is in need of surgery, evaluation of the vaginal microflora should be performed and corrected if it is altered.

Vaginal microflora

Managing both the obstetric and the gynecological patient who develops an SSI requires an understanding of the endogenous bacteriology of the lower genital tract. The lower genital tract is a complex ecologic niche consisting of metabolic products from both the host and microbes, breakdown products of cellular components from the host and the microbes, and introduced compounds via douching, feminine hygiene products, or foreign bodies (e.g., sexual toys) and sexual practices. Any exogenous factor as well as endogenous factors that can alter the pH of the vagina will result in a change in the microbial composition of the vagina.

Thus, this environment exists in a dynamic and fragile state, and is constantly challenged. The status of the bacteriology of the lower genital tract depends on which bacteria are dominant. A healthy endogenous vaginal ecosystem is characterized by having a pH of 3.8–4.5, the dominant bacterium is *Lactobacillus* spp., squamous epithelial cells that are well estrogenized, and the number of white blood cells (WBCs) is ≥5 per field at 40 × magnification (Lin et al. 1999, Burrows et al. 2004). The species of *Lactobacillus* that are present in the vagina are important, because they must produce sufficient quantities of organic acids, hydrogen peroxide (H_2O_2), and bacteriocin. The endogenous vaginal bacteriology is complex and consists of Gram-positive and Gram-negative facultative and obligate anaerobic bacteria. It is through the ability of *Lactobacillus* spp., e.g., *L. crispatus*, to produce lactic acid keeping the pH of the vagina <4.5, and the production of H_2O_2 and bacteriocin (lactocin) that the pathogenic bacteria are suppressed to low numbers. In a healthy state the concentration of lactobacilli is ≥10^6 bacteria/ml vaginal fluid and the pathogenic bacteria numbers are ≤10^3 bacteria/ml vaginal fluid or a ratio of approximately 1000 lactobacilli:1 pathogen. Therefore, patients undergoing an obstetric or gynecological operation where the vagina is entered have their pelvic cavity and pelvic organs exposed to potential bacterial contamination. This places the patient at significant risk for the development of a postoperative infection.

However, when the vaginal pH is between 4.5 and 5, lactobacilli are in danger of losing dominance and one or more of the pathogenic bacteria will gain dominance. Which bacterium or bacteria gain dominance depends on several factors that are not well understood. The events that initiate a change in pH are not always known. However, once the vaginal pH ≥5 lactobacilli do not grow well and cannot compete with the pathogenic bacteria. The inhibition of lactobacilli result in a significant decrease in the concentration of lactobacilli in the vagina. The concentration of lactobacilli declines from ≥10^6 bacteria/ml to ≤10^3 bacteria/ml vaginal fluid.

The administration of antibiotics for surgical prophylaxis is not sufficient to overcome this concentration of pathogenic bacteria and failure to prevent postoperative infection is likely to result. Lin et al. (1999) found that women with bacterial vaginosis undergoing hysterectomy were statistically more likely to develop a postoperative pelvic infection than women with a *Lactobacillus* or group B streptococcus-dominant vaginal microflora. Therefore, two preventive measures that can be taken to reduce the risk of the patient developing a postoperative pelvic infection are: (1) Evaluation of the vaginal microflora and (2) the administration of antibiotic for surgical prophylaxis. The vaginal pH should be determined at least 1 week before the surgery date, and if the pH ≥5 it should be corrected. This can be achieved, in most cases, by the intravaginal administration of boric acid, 600 mg twice a day for 7 days. Patients not evaluated the week before surgery can be evaluated in the operating room by determining the vaginal pH. If the pH ≥5 and there is a fish-like odor associated with the discharge, then metronidazole can be administered in addition to cefazolin or other antibiotic that is routinely administered for surgical prophylaxis. This combination will provide antimicrobial activity against obligate anaerobes (metronidazole) and Gram-positive and Gram-negative facultative bacteria (cefazolin).

Surgical site infection

There are multiple surgical incision sites in obstetric and gynecological patients. The most visible surgical incision sites are those made in the abdominal wall and the perineum. Infections occurring in either of these sites that require surgical intervention are abscess, necrotizing cellulitis, and necrotizing fasciitis. Most SSIs are uncomplicated and respond to antibiotic therapy; however, some may require incision and drainage.

Indication that an SSI is developing typically begins with a slight increase in the patient's temperature, e.g., in the late afternoon or early evening a temperature >38°C but <38.5°C may be noted on one or two occasions. In addition there may be a slight rise in the patient's pulse rate (>90) and erythema that extends >1 cm around the incision. There may be an associated induration of the erythematous area. These can all be very early findings of a surgical site that is developing an infection. The wound may begin to drain within the next day or two. Once these conditions have developed the infection may progress in one of three directions (**Figure 20.1**).

A logical approach to evaluating the surgical incision and to determining if there is a fluid collection (seroma, infected seroma, hematoma, infected hematoma, or abscess), cellulitis, or necrotizing infection is to perform imaging studies, either ultrasonography or computed tomography (CT) of the area. The appearance of cellulitis

Table 20.4 Postoperative infections in the obstetric and gynecological patient.

Obstetrics	Gynecology
Abdominal incision	Abdominal incisions
Postpartum endometritis	Endometritis
Myometrial microabscesses	Pelvic cellulitis
Myometrial necrosis	Tubo-ovarian abscess
Episiotomy	Pelvic abscess
Infected pelvic hematoma	Infected pelvic hematoma
Necrotizing fasciitis	Necrotizing fasciitis
Bacteremia	Bacteremia
Pneumonia	Pneumonia
Pyelonephritis	Pyelonephritis
Cystitis	Cystitis
Sepsis/septic shock	Sepsis/septic shock

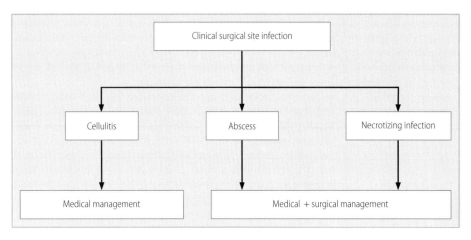

Figure 20.1 Progression of surgical site infections.

does not preclude presence of infection in the deeper tissues. Therefore, a thorough evaluation of the suspicious site must be undertaken to avoid unnecessary delay in institution of appropriate management, including both medical and surgical management.

Postpartum endometritis
Risk factors

Postpartum endometritis is more likely to occur in women delivered by cesarean section compared with those delivered by the vaginal route. Burrows et al. (2004) reported that women who went into labor and subsequently delivered by primary cesarean section had a 21-fold increased risk of developing endometritis compared with women who delivered vaginally. Women delivered by primary cesarean section who did not go into labor had a 10-fold risk of developing endometritis compared with women delivering vaginally. Additional risk factors are listed in **Box 20.3**.

Box 20.3 Risk factors for the development of postpartum endometritis.

Cesarean section
Prolonged rupture of amniotic membranes
Prolonged rupture of amniotic membranes and labor
Lack of prenatal care
Altered vaginal microflora (bacterial vaginosis, dominant colonization by group B streptococci or facultative Gram-negative rod)
Presence of bacteriuria
Nasal carriage of *Staphylococcus aureus*
Multiple vaginal examinations
Use of intrauterine monitoring devices
Obesity (body mass index $\geq$30 kg/m^2)

Patients with ruptured amniotic membranes are at risk, and this risk is enhanced if the patient is in labor for a prolonged period of time because bacteria from the vagina can ascend into the uterus (Faro et al. 1990, Pinell et al. 1993). Once in the uterus and amniotic fluid, these bacteria can multiply and achieve concentrations >10^6 bacteria/ml amniotic fluid. The longer the patient is in labor the greater the risk that bacteria can colonize the decidual layer of the uterus and invade the myometrium, thus setting the stage for endometritis.

Asymptomatic bacteriuria has been linked to early postpartum endometritis. The Gram-negative facultative bacteria are the most common bacteria isolated from blood in the immediate postpartum period (Monif and Baer 1976, Ledger et al. 1975, Monif 1982). Monif (1991) demonstrated that asymptomatic bacteriuria was associated with postpartum endometritis, in that the same bacterium was isolated from the urine and endometrium of postpartum women with endometritis.

Aside from the risk factors listed in Box 20.3, the endogenous vaginal microflora contributes to bacteriuria and therefore plays a role in early postpartum endometritis. *Strep. agalactiae* colonization of the vagina also is a significant risk factor in the development of early postpartum endometritis and sepsis (Faro 1980, 1981).

Clinical presentation and diagnosis

Patients with postpartum endometritis present with a cluster of findings that establish the diagnosis clinically. It is the rare patient who will present with a purulent lochia. Postpartum endometritis can be divided into two categories with regard to presentation; early postpartum endometritis, occurs within the first 48 h of delivery, and late postpartum endometritis, occurs 72 h and beyond delivery. Early postpartum endometritis tends to be unimicrobial and due mainly to facultative anaerobic bacteria, e.g., *Strep. agalactiae* (a group B streptococcus), *Strep. pyogenes*, and members of the *Enterobacteriaceae*, especially *Escherichia coli*. Patients who develop late-onset postpartum endometritis typically have a polymicrobial infection characterized by facultative and obligate anaerobic Gram-positive and Gram-negative bacteria.

The clinical onset of postpartum endometritis is indicated by a significant change in the patient's vital signs, notably fever and tachycardia. Fever as a sole indicator for the presence of infection is a poor indicator. Fever in the postoperative patient can be secondary to the tissue trauma associated with the surgical procedure or perioperative medications. The bacteria responsible for endometritis are likely the result of contamination during some point in labor. There is no doubt that bacteria endogenous to the lower genital tract migrate to the uterine cavity during labor (Pinell et al. 1993). Once in the uterine cavity these bacteria multiply and the longer the labor the greater the numbers of bacteria. Thus, the microbiology of postpartum endometritis originates from the patient's own endogenous lower genital tract bacteriology. When the patient's lower genital tract microbiology shifts from a lactobacilli-dominant microflora to an altered microflora or bacterial vaginosis (e.g., dominated by *E. coli* or *Strep. agalactiae*), the threat of postpartum endometritis is significant.

Postpartum endometritis can be mild and easily treated, or it can be more severe with the development of myometrial microabscesses, leading to necrosis of the myometrium. Postpartum endometritis can be associated with bacteremia. Depending on the virulence of the bacteria causing postpartum endometritis, sepsis and septic shock can occur.

Patients with postpartum endometritis typically present with fever, defined as a temperature ≥38°C measured on two occasions and taken at least 6 h apart, or a temperature ≥38.5°C occurring at any time with a corresponding pulse rate >90 beats/min. A pulse rate that parallels the fever is indicative of a patient with a significant postoperative infection. In addition, the patient's WBC count ≥12 000 and/or a differential with ≥10% band forms is consistent with postpartum endometritis. In addition the pelvic examination should reveal a uterus that is not involuting appropriately, uterine tenderness to palpation and motion, adnexal or parametrial tenderness, and the lochia may be purulent with or without a foul odor. The presence of a foul-smelling lochia is indicative of the presence of anaerobic bacteria. Typically patients treated for postpartum endometritis with broad-spectrum antibiotics who do not show significant improvement within 48–72 h should be considered to have failed initial treatment. These patients require re-evaluation for having a resident bacterium, an abscess, necrosis of the uterine incision, or myometrial microabscesses and microthrombosis of the uterine vasculature.

Management

Pelvic examination reveals that the vaginal discharge may resemble the color of port wine, contain particulate matter, or be purulent. The cervix is usually dilated admitting one to two fingers, allowing palpation of the lower uterine segment, which is often necrotic and not intact. The uterus is subinvoluted and boggy on palpation.

The antibiotic regimen can be maintained and the patient should undergo an exploratory laparotomy. The antibiotic regimen most commonly administered is clindamycin or metronidazole plus ampicillin and gentamicin. Individuals who are allergic to ampicillin should receive vancomycin, daptomycin, or linezolid. This complication is not because a resistant bacterium has assumed dominance but because the uterine tissue cannot be adequately perfused. Typically the uterus cannot be salvaged and a total hysterectomy is indicated. The ovaries are usually not involved in the infection nor is there any evidence of ovarian thrombosis. Therefore, the ovaries do not need to be removed at the time of hysterectomy (**Figure 20.2**).

Postoperatively these patients do well. However, as a result of having had postpartum endometritis and two major operations in a relatively short period of time, there is the possibility of the patient developing an ileus or bowel obstruction.

Patients whose uterus is involuting and cervix is closing, but still exhibit signs of postpartum endometritis, should undergo ultrasonography to determine whether there are any retained products of conception. This is unlikely if the uterus is involuting, firm, but tender and the cervix is not dilated. It is very likely that a resistant bacterium has been selected, most likely a Gram-negative facultative anaerobe. A specimen obtained from the endometrium as well as venous blood

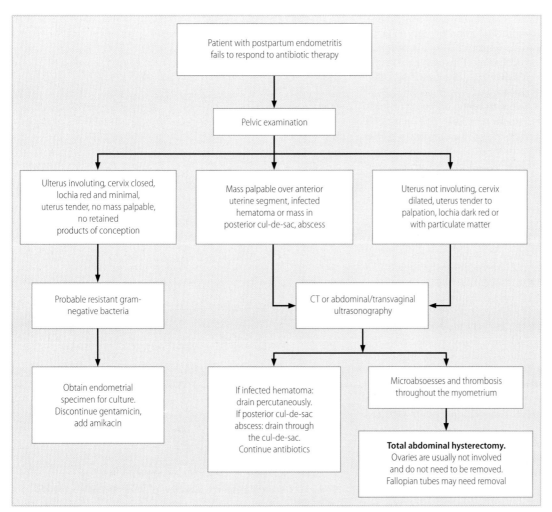

Figure 20.2 Treatment strategies for the patient with endometritis who fails to respond to antibiotic therapy.

cultures should be obtained. Discontinuing the gentamicin and instituting amikacin would be appropriate because Gram-negative bacteria resistant to gentamicin tend to be sensitive to amikacin. Once the culture and sensitivity are known, appropriate antibiotic changes can be made.

Episiotomy infections

Episiotomy continues to be a procedure that is still performed and the frequency varies from 13% to 85% depending on a variety of circumstances (Hartmann et al. 2005). There are basically two types of episiotomies that are performed: A midline, where the incision is made directly through the body of the perineum, and a mediolateral, where the incision is made beginning at the 7 o'clock position at a 45° angle avoiding the anal sphincter. The incision is carried through the bulbospongiosus, the deep and superficial transverse perineal muscles. The perineal body or central perineal tendon consists of a fibromuscular structure formed by the conglomeration of the deep and superficial transverse and bulbospongiosus muscles.

Infection rates for episiotomy range from 0.2% to 1.9% (Yokoe et al. 2001). Infection of the episiotomy site has been categorized as: (1) Simple, midline involving the skin, mediolateral involving the skin and subcutaneous tissue; (2) superficial fascial; (3) superficial fascial necrosis; and (4) myonecrosis (Shy and Eschenbach 1972). The microbiology of episiotomy infection can be monomicrobial or polymicrobial, involving bacteria such as *Staph. aureus, Strep. agalactiae, Strep. pyogenes, Clostridium sordellii,* and *C. perfringens,* as well as Gram-negative and Gram-positive facultative and obligate anaerobes.

Infection of the episiotomy should be handled aggressively. Typically the episiotomy will undergo dehiscence when it becomes infected. If the episiotomy is surrounded by erythema and induration, and there is no evidence of fluctulancy, this may indicate that there is cellulitis. The difficulty is determining which patient has an uncomplicated cellulitis versus a complex infection (i.e., abscess plus necrotizing infection). The patient who develops increasing pain or erythema should be considered to have a complex infection and undergo imaging studies. Time is of the essence and, therefore, the physician should not delay in either obtaining imaging studies or exploring the episiotomy site.

Imaging of the area with ultrasonography or a CT can be used to determine if there is a fluid collection and/or gas within the tissues. If there is a fluid collection the surgical site can be aspirated and the fluid sent for Gram stain, bacterial culture, and antibiotic sensitivity testing of the bacteria isolated. The incision should be opened and all necrotic tissue debrided. The wound should be left opened and packed with gauze moistened with an appropriate antiseptic solution (e.g., 0.025% acetic acid). The packing should be removed and replaced with a fresh moistened packing at least three times a day. Another approach is to cleanse the wound, after debridement of necrotic tissue, with 10% povidone–iodine solution, hydrogen peroxide, and 0.9% saline. Once a fine layer of granulation tissue has formed the wound can be sutured close (Hauth et al. 1986, Hankins et al. 1990, Ramin et al. 1992, Uygur et al. 2004). The patient should be started on broad-spectrum antibiotics (see Box 20.1). If the Gram stain results are available then the antibiotic regimen can be guided by the Gram stain results (see Table 20.3).

The wound should not be closed until there is a fine layer of granulation tissue; this indicates that there is no infection present. Closing an infected wound can lead to the development of serious complications, such as recurrent abscess formation, recurrent dehiscence, and necrotizing fasciitis.

Postoperative pelvic infection

Patients undergoing pelvic surgery where the vagina was involved in the surgical procedure are at risk for the development of a postoperative pelvic infection. The infection can be a relatively uncomplicated infection such as pelvic cellulitis or a more complex infection such as an abscess. Again, any time that the vagina is involved in the surgical procedure post-surgical infection will most likely involve the endogenous vaginal microflora. In the gynecological patient the infection is typically polymicrobial, involving both Gram-negative and Gram-positive facultative as well as obligate anaerobic bacteria. Therefore, knowledge about the status of the endogenous vaginal bacterial flora before performing surgery can be of assistance in managing a postoperative infection.

Pelvic cellulitis is the most frequent postoperative infection that occurs after a hysterectomy. This is an SSI because there is an incision in the vaginal epithelium and associated tissues. Typically there is no adipose tissue present in the area where the vagina is incised in close proximity to the cervix. The vaginal epithelium, vaginal fascia and connective tissue, muscle, and peritoneum can easily become infected. The cellulitis can easily be treated with broad-spectrum antibiotics and patients usually respond within 48–72 h.

The more complicated postoperative pelvic infection is the pelvic abscess or infected pelvic hematoma (**Figure 20.3**). The latter is more frequently encountered than the former condition. The hematoma typically forms at the vaginal apex because of blood oozing from the dissection accompanying excision of the cervix from the vagina. Complete hemostasis is sometimes difficult to achieve in this area. Postoperative bleeding leads to formation of a hematoma at the vaginal

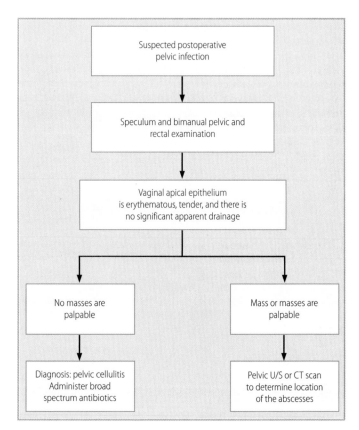

Figure 20.3 Algorithm for the diagnosis of suspected postoperative pelvic infection.

cuff, sited between the proximal side of the vaginal epithelium and distal to the pelvic peritoneum, if the pelvic peritoneum is closed. If the peritoneum is not closed then the hematoma will form in the floor of the pelvic cavity.

Closing the vaginal cuff and pelvic peritoneum creates a space between the vaginal epithelium and the pelvic peritoneum (retroperitoneal space). It has been demonstrated that an average of 40 ml (range 10–200 ml) of serosanguineous fluid can accumulate in this retroperitoneal fluid. This serves as an excellent incubator and culture medium. The bacteria found to inhabit the lower genital tract, especially when this flora is altered, contain combinations of bacteria that are abscessogenic.

Management of a vaginal cuff-infected hematoma or abscess depends on the exact location, whether or not it is uniloculated or multiloculated, and whether or not it extends to the deep pelvis or into the abdominal cavity. Simple abscesses that are confined to the vaginal cuff can be managed by opening the vaginal cuff, draining the abscess thoroughly, and irrigating copiously with sterile 0.9% saline. A drain such as a Foley catheter can be placed into the abscess area; inflate the balloon and attach the Foley catheter to a suction device. Ultrasonography at the time of drainage can be of significant assistance by delineating the abscess and determining its course. Care must be taken when draining the abscess and suctioning the abscess not to injure bowel that will be adjacent to the abscess. A pelvic abscess is typically surrounded by both large and small bowel and the bowel is usually inflamed and edematous. Use of even dull instruments can easily penetrate this fragile and edematous bowel, thus complicating the patient's condition.

A pelvic abscess that is not located adjacent to the vaginal apex can be managed in one of two ways: Via either laparotomy or percutaneous drainage. The choice of procedure is based on location and complexity of the abscess (Johnson et al. 1981). The success rate for percutaneous drainage of abdominal and pelvic abscesses is 80–90% (Lambiase et al. 1992). The recurrence rate is between 5 and 10% (Von Sonnenberg et al. 1984). Corsi et al. (1999) reported a success rate of 93% employing transvaginally guided drainage of tubo-ovarian and postoperative pelvic abscesses.

These criteria have been modified to include multiloculated abscesses as well as abscesses that cannot be approached transabdominally. Abscesses that are deep in the pelvis and in close proximity to the bladder, large and/or small bowel, and uterus may be approached transvaginally or transrectally (Von Sonnenberg et al. 1991). Laparotomy still remains as an acceptable approach; even when percutaneous drainage is attempted a surgeon must stand by to intervene if there are complications.

Approaching a pelvic abscess via laparotomy requires that a vertical incision be made to allow for adequate exposure to the pelvis and abdomen. Many gynecologists continue to use a transverse lower abdominal incision; however, performing an incision for cosmetic reasons is not in the best interest of the patient. A vertical incision placed in the midline of the lower abdomen allows for less dissection of the anterior abdominal wall, less risk of anterior abdominal wall hematoma formation, less risk of infection, and better exposure. If there is a need to extend the incision to the upper abdomen this can be easily accomplished.

The dilemma occurs when the patient has a transverse lower abdominal incision and subsequently requires a laparotomy for a postoperative pelvic or lower abdominal abscess. These abscesses are often surrounded by small and large bowel and therefore are not easily accessible. Abscesses located in the posterior cul de sac are typically densely adherent to the rectum, rectosigmoid, cecum, and omentum. There may even be interloop abscesses of the small bowel. Approaching these abscesses through a transverse incision can be difficult but can be accomplished safely. However, if the upper abdomen is involved, this approach may not be feasible and a vertical incision may have to be performed to allow for complete inspection of the entire abdominal cavity. Once the abscess have been located and drained, the abdomen and pelvic should be irrigated with copious amounts of sterile saline. Enough saline should be used to completely cleanse the entire abdomen and pelvis of all purulent fluid and floating debris. The saline irrigation should return clear when aspirated out of the peritoneal cavity.

Drains can be placed in the right colonic gutters as well as the pelvis. Patients who have had a hysterectomy can have a drain placed in the pelvis and exit through the vagina. This drain should be attached to a closed drainage system. Drains that are placed in the right and left colonic gutters should exit through the right and left lower abdomen. They should be attached to suction devices to actively remove any fluid that has accumulated. If the fluid is serous but cloudy, a specimen should be aspirated from the tubing, and sent for Gram stain and culture. If the fluid is bloody, serial specimens can be obtained and sent for a hematocrit; if the hematocrit is rising then a diagnosis of intra-abdominal or pelvic bleeding can be made. In this case an exploratory laparotomy is indicated to determine the source of bleeding and correct it.

Whether or not percutaneous drainage is employed depends on the skill of the interventional radiologist and the location of the abscesses. Abscesses that are surrounded by bowel and do not permit direct access to the abscess should not be approached via percutaneous drainage. Penetration of the bowel, especially the large bowel, will contribute to the development of intra-abdominal sepsis.

The patient who has a well-contained or walled-off abscess, is afebrile, pulse rate <90 beats/min, and whose WBC count is within the normal range or slightly elevated is the best candidate for percutaneous drainage. The patient who is significantly febrile and has a markedly elevated WBC count is probably not a good candidate for percutaneous drainage, and is best served by exploratory laparotomy. Once the abscess has been successfully removed, the patient should defervesce and the WBC count should return to normal with 48–72 h. Drains should be removed when there is <30 ml fluid accumulated in the drains over a 24-hour period.

■ REFERENCES

Barclay DL, Collins CG, Macey HB. Cancer of the Bartholin gland. A review and report of 8 cases. *Obstet Gynecol* 1964;**24**:329–35.

Bisno AL, Stevens DL. Streptococcal infections of skin and soft tissues. *N Engl J Med* 1996;**334**:240–5.

Burrows LJ, Meyn LA, Weber AW. Maternal morbidity associated with vaginal versus cesarean delivery. *Obstet Gynecol* 2004;**103**:907–12.

Copeland LJ, Sneige N, Gerghenson DM, McGuffee VB, Abdul-Kareem F, Rutledge FN. Batholin gland carcinoma. *Obstet Gynecol* 1986;**67**:794–801.

Corsi PJ, Johnson SC, Gonik B, Hendrix SL, McNeeley Jr, Diamond MP. Transvaginal ultrasound-guided aspiration of pelvic abscesses. *Infect Dis Obstet Gynecol* 1999;**7**:216–21.

DiSaia P, Creasman WT. *Clinical Gynecologic Oncology. Invasive cancer of the vulva.* New York: Mosby, 1997: 228–9.

Faro S. Group B streptococcus and puerperal sepsis. *Am J Obstet Gynecol* 1980;**138**:1219–20.

Faro S. Group B beta-hemolytic streptococci and puerperal infections. *Am J Obstet Gynecol* 1981;**139**:686–9.

Faro S, Martens MG, Hammill HA, et al. Antibiotic prophylaxis: is there a difference? *Am J Obstet Gynecol* 1990;**162**:900–7.

Felix JC, Cote RJ, Kramer EEW, Saigo P, Goldman GH. Carcinomas of Bartholin's gland. Histogenesis and the etiological role of human papillomavirus. *Am J Pathol* 1993;**142**:925 – 933.

Gittes RF, Nakamura RM. Female urethral syndrome: A female prostatis? *Western J Med* 1996;**164**:435–8.

Hankins GDV, Hauth JC, Gilstrap LC, Hammond TL, Yemons ER, Snyder RR. Early repair of episiotomy dehiscence. *Obstet Gynecol* 1990;**75**:48–51.

Hartmann K, Viswanathan M, Palmieri R, Gartlehmer G, Thorp J Jr, Lohr KN. Outcomes of routine episiotomy. A systematic review. *JAMA* 2005;**293**:2141–8.

Hauth JC, Gilstrap LC III, Ward SC, Hankins GDV. Early repair of an external sphincter ani muscle and rectal mucosal dehiscence. *Obstet Gynecol* 1986;**67**:806 – 9.

Huffman JW. The detailed anatomy of the paraurethral ducts in the human female. *Am J Obstet* 1948;**55**:86–100.

Huffman JW. Clinical significance of the paraurethral ducts and glands. *Arch Surg* 1951;**62**:615–26.

Hurley HJ. Axillary hyperhidrosis, apocrine bromhidrosis, hidradenitis suppurativa, and familial benign pemphigus: surgical approach. In: Roenigk RK, Roenigk HH (eds), *Dermatologic Surgery*. New York: Marcel Dekker, 1989: 729–739.

Johnson WC, Gerzof SG, Robbins AH, Nabseth DC. Treatment of abdominal abscesses. *Ann Surg* 1981;**194**: 510–19.

King MD, Humphrey BJ, Wang YF, Kourbatova EV, Ray SM, Blumberg HM. Emergence of community-acquired methicillin-resistant *Staphylococcus aureus* infections among patients USA 300 clone as the predominant cause of skin and soft-tissue infections. *Ann Intern Med* 2006;**144**:309–17.

Kurzen H, Jung EG, Hartschuh, Moll I, Franke WW, Molls R. Forms of epithelial differentiation of draining sinus in acne inversa (hidradenitis suppurativa). *Br J Dermatol* 1999;**141**:231–9.

Lambiase RE, Deyoe L, Cronan JJ, Dorfman GS. Percutaneous drainage of 335 consecutive abscesses: results of primary drainage with 1 year follow-up. *Radiology* 1992;**184**:167–79.

Ledger WF, Norman M, Gee C, Lewis W. Bacteremia on an obstetric gynecologic service. *Am J Obstet Gynecol* 1975;**121**:205–12.

Lelle RJ, Davis KP, Roberts JA. Adenoid cystic carcinoma of the Bartholin's gland: the University of Michigan experience. *Int J Gynecol Cancer* 1994;**4**:145–9.

Lin L. Song J, Kimber N, et al. The role of bacterial vaginosis in infection after major gynecologic surgery. *Infect Dis Obstet Gynecol* 1999;**7**:169–74.

Matusiak L, Bieniek A, Szepietowski JC. Increased serum tumour necrosis factor-alpha in hidradenitis suppurativa patients;is there a basis for treatment with anti-tumour necrosis factor-alpha agents? *Acta Dermatol Venerol (Stockh)* 2009;**89**:601–3.

Monif GRC. Association of Enterobacteriaceae septicemia in the immediate postpartum period and asymptomatic bacteriuria. *Obstet Gynecol* 1982;**60**:184–7.

Monif GRC. Intrapartum bacteriuria and postpartum endometritis. *Obstet Gynecol* 1991;**78**:245–8.

Monif GRC, Baer H. Polymicrobial bacteremia in obstetric patients. *Obstet Gynecol* 1976;**48**:167–9.

Moran GJ, Krishnadasan A, Gorwitz RJ, et al. Methicillin-resistant *Staphylococcus aureus* infections among patients in the emergency department. *N Engl J Med* 2006;**355**:666–74.

Pinell P, Faro S, Roberts S, et al. Intrauterine pressure catheter in labor: associated microbiology. *Infect Dis Obstet Gynecol* 1993;**1**:60–4.

Ramin SM, Ramus RM, Little BB, Gilstrap LC III. Early repair of episiotomy dehiscence associated with infection. *Am J Obstet Gynecol* 1992;**167**:1104–7.

Rogers RL, Perkins J. Skin and soft tissues infections. *Prim Care* 2006;**33**:697–710.

Sacheva MP, Tomecki KJ. Cellulitis and erysipelas. In: Schlossberg D (ed.), *Clinical Infectious Diseases*. New York: Cambridge University Press, 2008: 151–6

Skene AJC. The anatomy and pathology of 2 important glands of the female urethra. *Am J Obstet* 1880;**13**:265.

Slade DEM, Powell BW, Mortimer PS. Hidradenitis suppurativa: pathogenesis and management. *Br J Plast Surg* 2003;**56**:451–61

Stevens DL, Bisno AL, Chambers HF, et al. Practice guidelines for the diagnosis and management of skin and soft –tissue infections. *Clin Infect Dis* 2005;**41**:1373–406.

Shy KK, Eschenbach DA. Fatal perineal cellulitis from an episiotomy site. *Obstet Gynecol* 1972;**54**:292–8.

Uygur D, Yesildaglar N, Kis S, Sipahi. Early repair of episiotomy dehiscence. *Aust N Z J Obstet Gynecol* 2004;**44**:244–6.

Van der Zee HH, de Ruiter L, van den Broecke DG, Dik WA, Laman JD, Prens EP. Elevated levels of tumpr necrosis factor (TNF)-α, interleukin (IL)-1β and IL-10 in hidradenitis suppurativa skin: a rationale for targeting TNF-α and IL-1β. *Br J Dermatol* 2011;**164**:1292–8.

Von der Werth JM, Jemec GBE. Morbidity in patients with hiodradenitis suppurativa. *Br J Dermatol* 2001;**144**:809–13.

Von Sonnenberg E, Mueller PR, Ferrucci JT Jr. Percutaneous drainage of 250 abdominal abscesses and fluid collections. I. Results, failures, and complications. *Radiology* 1984;**151**:337–41.

Von Sonnenberg E, D'Agostino HB, Casola G, Halasz NA, Sanchez RB, Goodacre BW. Percutaneous abscess drainage: Current concepts. *Radiology* 1991;**181**:617–26.

Wiseman MC. Hidradenitis suppurativa:a review. *Dermatol Ther* 2004;**17**:50–4.

Word B. Office treatment of cyst and abscess of Bartholin's gland duct. *South Med J* 1968;**61**:514 – 18.

Yokoe DS, Christiansen CL, Johnson R, et al. Epidemiology of and surveillance for postpartum infections. *Emerg Infect Dis* 2001;**7**:837–41.

Chapter 21 Necrotizing enterocolitis

Shannon L. Castle, Henri R. Ford

Necrotizing enterocolitis (NEC) is the most common medical and surgical emergency affecting the gastrointestinal tract of newborn infants. Approximately 1–5% of all preterm infants develop NEC (Stoll 1994, Llanos et al. 2002). Up to 50% of neonates who develop NEC eventually require surgical intervention (Guillet et al. 2006, Holman et al. 2006), with the mortality rate for these patients varying from 20% to 50% (Rowe et al. 1994, McElhinney et al. 2000). The mortality rate approaches 100% for infants with panintestinal NEC. Although most infants who develop NEC are premature with extremely low birthweight, NEC can also affect term infants, especially those with cyanotic heart disease. As advances in neonatal medicine have resulted in increased survival of both preterm infants and those with complex medical problems, the incidence of NEC continues to rise.

Risk factors that have been implicated in the development of NEC include prematurity, hypoxia, initiation of enteral feeding, congenital heart disease, and bacterial infection. NEC is characterized by intestinal inflammation and mucosal destruction, leading to gut barrier failure. Infants with the most severe form of NEC typically develop full-thickness destruction of the intestinal wall, leading to intestinal perforation, peritonitis, sepsis, and death. Those who survive may experience additional morbidity such as stricture formation or adhesions, which may result in intestinal obstruction, or they may require long-term parenteral nutrition due to intestinal failure (Horwitz et al. 1995, Holman et al. 1997, Blakely et al. 2005).

PATHOPHYSIOLOGY
Immature intestinal barrier

The intestinal epithelial barrier consists of a single layer of polarized epithelial cells (enterocytes) that serve to protect the host from invasion by pathogenic organisms while tolerating commensal bacteria (Muller et al. 2005, Neu et al. 2005). Maintenance of gut barrier function depends on both structural and biochemical elements which prevent the translocation of bacteria across the intestinal epithelium. Structural barriers include epithelial tight junctions, intestinal mucin production, fluid secretion, and peristalsis, all of which serve to limit adhesion of bacteria to the cell surface, the first step in the process of translocation (Berseth 1989, Kelly et al. 1993, Hecht 1999, Lin et al. 2008). In the proximal intestine, gastric acidity serves as a first line of defense against bacterial passage beyond the stomach. Biochemical barriers to the entry of pathogenic bacteria include a- and b-defensins, which are specialized antimicrobial peptides secreted by Paneth cells and intestinal epithelial cells, respectively, as well as secretory IgA, which serves as an antiseptic paint to bind bacteria and prevent their adhesion to the intestinal epithelium. Paneth cells, specialized enterocytes at the base of intestinal crypts, further contribute to the biochemical defense by producing phospholipase A_2 and lysozyme. In neonates, particularly premature infants, both the structural and biochemical components that are responsible for maintaining gut barrier integrity are immature, thus predisposing them to the development of NEC.

Role of enteral feeding

Initiation of enteral feeds, particularly rapid advancement of feeding, is a known risk factor for NEC. However, long-term hospitalization without feeds carries the risk of intestinal atrophy and inflammation, which also increases the risk of NEC. In fact, previous studies have shown that trophic feeds are beneficial in the preterm population. Multiple trials have shown that low-volume feeding (2–24 ml/kg per day) does not increase the risk of NEC (Berseth 1992, Tyson and Kennedy 2000). Optimal volume and rate of advancement of enteral feeding in very-low-birthweight infants remain controversial (Bombell and McGuire 2008, Hay 2008).

Compared with formula, breast milk has been shown to protect against the development of NEC in both human and animal studies (Lucas and Cole 1990, Schanler et al. 1993). The exact mechanism by which breast milk protects against NEC is unknown and remains an active field of study. Breast milk contains a number of factors believed to be protective against the development of NEC, including the immunoglobulins IgM, IgG, secretory IgA, lysozyme, lactoferrin, epidermal growth factor, and complement proteins, to name a few.

Immunoglobulins

Human breast milk contains IgM, IgG, and secretory IgA. IgA is the predominant immunoglobulin in breast milk. Its linkage with the secretory component renders IgA resistant to proteolysis in the stomach and intestine. This allows passive transfer of immunity from the mother to the infant against a variety of bacterial and viral pathogens. However, oral or intravenous administration of immunoglobulins has not been shown to be protective against NEC (Foster and Cole 2004); in fact, the use of intravenous immunoglobulin in newborns with hemolytic disease has been linked to the subsequent development of NEC (Figueras-Aloy et al. 2010).

Abnormal bacterial colonization

At birth, the neonate's intestine is sterile but it becomes rapidly colonized by bacteria from the environment. *Escherichia coli* and streptococci rapidly colonize most infants, followed by enterobacters, and colonization with other bacteria such as enterococci, lactobacilli, clostridia, and *Bacteroides* spp. (Mackie et al. 1999, Enck et al. 2009). The specific colonization pattern may be influenced by the route of delivery, whether vaginal or via cesarean section, the type of feeding, whether breast milk or formula, and the environment during and after birth. Bacterial colonization in preterm infants is heavily influenced by the hospital environment (Sharma et al. 2007). Abnormal bacterial colonization patterns in neonates admitted to the neonatal intensive care unit (ICU) or other hospital environment may further increase susceptibility to NEC (Stoll et al. 1996). Although most cases of NEC are sporadic in nature and no specific bacteria or viruses have been consistently isolated in infants with NEC, the occurrence of occasional outbreaks suggests a role for a transmissible agent in the pathogenesis of the disease (Emami et al. 2009).

Inflammatory mediators and NEC

The current hypothesis regarding the pathogenesis of NEC is that a hypoxic or infectious insult further compromises the already immature intestinal barrier of the neonate, thereby allowing pathogenic bacteria to translocate across the damaged epithelium and incite an inflammatory cascade that exacerbates the mucosal injury, and ultimately leads to full-blown gut barrier failure (Hsueh et al. 2003, Emami et al. 2009). Multiple inflammatory mediators have been implicated in the development of NEC, including tumor necrosis factor (TNF)-a, platelet-activating factor, interleukins IL-1, IL-6, IL-18, endothelin-1, thromboxanes, and oxygen free radicals, to name a few (Caplan et al. 2005, Markel et al. 2006, Lugo et al. 2007, Chokshi et al. 2008). Nitric oxide (NO), the product of nitric oxide synthase (NOS), has also been implicated as a key inflammatory mediator in the pathogenesis of intestinal barrier failure in NEC. NOS exists in three isoforms, two of which, endothelial NOS and neuronal NOS, are expressed constitutively at low levels. The third, inducible NOS, is expressed at high levels during inflammation. The resultant overproduction of NO during inflammation contributes to intestinal barrier damage by reacting with superoxide to form the potent toxic intermediate, peroxynitrite (Potoka et al. 2003, Chokshi et al. 2008).

Prostanoids are inflammatory mediators formed by the conversion of the membrane lipid arachidonic acid to prostaglandin G_2 by cyclooxygenase (COX). Prostaglandin G_2 is then converted to multiple biologically active prostanoids by specific synthases (Park et al. 2006). Prostanoid production by the COX enzymes is critical for maintenance of the intestinal barrier. COX-1 is produced at constitutively low levels and exerts a protective effect on mucosal barrier function, whereas COX-2 is upregulated during inflammation and may contribute to epithelial injury. In NEC, increased activity of the COX enzymes, in particular the COX-2 isoform, may exacerbate the level of inflammation (Grishin et al. 2004).

DIAGNOSIS

Clinical

Infants with NEC may present with both gastrointestinal and systemic signs including abdominal distension, feeding intolerance, bloody stools, hypoxia, respiratory distress, and hypoperfusion. In preterm infants, NEC tends to occur within the first few weeks of life, whereas in full-term infants, it may present in the first few days of life (Wiswell et al. 1988, Andrews et al. 1990).

Before 1978, no standardized system existed to diagnose and study NEC. The grading system introduced by Bell et al. (1978), which relies on clinical and radiographic criteria, has been widely adopted since its publication. A single modification was made to distinguish between perforated and non-perforated NEC (**Box 21.1**) (Kliegman and Walsh 1987). Recently, however, the utility of the Bell staging has been questioned because the increased viability of infants at lower gestational ages due to improved critical care and surfactant therapy has significantly changed the population of infants in the neonatal ICU (NICU). Some authors have also argued that infants who are now better classified as having focal intestinal perforation were grouped with NEC under the old system for purposes of research and treatment, and therefore the Bell classification needs to be re-evaluated and revised (Gordon et al. 2007).

Box 21.1 Modified Bell stages of necrotizing enterocolitis.

I Suspected disease
IA
Mild systemic signs (apnea, bradycardia, temperature instability)
Mild intestinal signs (abdominal distension, gastric residuals, occult blood in stool)
IB
Mild systemic signs (apnea, bradycardia, temperature instability)
Mild intestinal signs (abdominal distension, gastric residuals, occult blood in stool)
Non-specific or normal radiological findings

II Definite disease
IIA
Mild systemic signs (apnea, bradycardia, temperature instability)
Additional intestinal signs (absent bowel sounds, abdominal tenderness)
Specific radiographic signs (pneumatosis intestinalis or portal venous air)
Laboratory changes (metabolic acidosis, thrombocytopenia)
IIB
Moderate systemic signs (apnea, bradycardia, temperature instability, mild metabolic acidosis, mild thrombocytopenia)
Additional intestinal signs (absent bowel sounds, abdominal tenderness, abdominal mass)

III Advanced disease
IIIA
Severe systemic illness (same as IIB with additional hypotension and shock)
Intestinal signs (severe abdominal distension, abdominal wall discoloration, peritonitis, intestine intact)
Severe radiographic signs (definite ascites)
Progressive laboratory derangements (metabolic acidosis, disseminated intravascular coagulopathy)
IIIB
Severe systemic illness (same as IIIA)
Intestinal signs (large abdominal abscess, abdominal wall discoloration, peritonitis, intestinal perforation)
Severe radiographic signs (definite ascites and pneumoperitoneum)
Worsening laboratory derangements (metabolic acidosis, disseminated intravascular coagulopathy)

Laboratory findings

Infants with NEC may have a variety of derangements in laboratory values. Hematological abnormalities commonly include neutropenia and thrombocytopenia, with roughly 37% of severe cases having a WBC $<1.5 \times 10^9$ (Hutter et al. 1976, Ragazzi et al. 2003). Metabolic abnormalities include acidemia, hypercapnia, and hypoxemia (Hallstrom et al. 2006). Although an elevated C-reactive protein (CRP) value is not specific for NEC, it has been shown to predict the likelihood of complications, such as abscess or stricture formation, or the need for surgical management (Pourcyrous et al. 2005). Gram stain and cultures will show bacteremia in up to 50% of patients (Sharma et al. 2007).

During the recovery phase, thrombocytopenia will often persist even after other parameters have normalized because the megakaryocytes are typically the last cells to recover from the generalized bone marrow suppression that characterizes severe NEC.

Radiographic

Radiographic signs pathognomonic for NEC include intramural gas on abdominal radiographs (pneumatosis intestinalis), portal venous gas, and free intraperitoneal air in the case of perforation (Epelman et al. 2007). Dilated loops of bowel may be present. Although it may not be specific for NEC, the presence of a loop of bowel that remains unchanged in position on multiple serial abdominal radiographs, referred to as a "fixed loop," is associated with full-thickness necrosis.

An anteroposterior and a left lateral decubitus abdominal radiograph are the diagnostic tests of choice in infants suspected of having NEC. The use of abdominal ultrasonography may also be helpful because it may show increased bowel wall thickness and fluid collections with greater sensitivity than plain films. It is subject to operator experience, however, and thus has not replaced plain films as the standard of care.

Contrast studies are not indicated in the initial evaluation of an infant with NEC, but patients who recover should be evaluated for intestinal strictures with contrast studies should they develop signs and symptoms of bowel obstruction (Radhakrishnan et al. 1991).

Differential diagnosis

The differential diagnosis for NEC includes infectious enterocolitis, milk or formula allergy, sepsis, and ileus (Engum and Grosfeld 1998, Gordon et al. 2007). Obstruction due to a number of causes, including atresias, intussusception, and Hirschsprung disease, may also present with feeding intolerance and abdominal distension. Focal intestinal perforation (FIP) is now recognized as a distinct disease entity from NEC, with different pathological and morphological characteristics (Aschner et al. 1988, Pumberger et al. 2002). FIP is more commonly seen in very premature infants (fewer than 26 weeks' gestation) and seems to be related to inhibition of mucosal blood flow regulation in the distal ileum due, at least in part, to the use of COX inhibitors such as indometacin, which is frequently used to accelerate closure of a patent ductus arteriosus (PDA). As a result, FIP tends to be truly focal and more common in very premature babies with chronic lung disease and symptomatic PDA.

PATHOLOGY

Histopathological examination of the intestine affected by NEC typically shows neutrophilic infiltration, epithelial sloughing, submucosal gas, and edema (**Figure 21.1**) (Balance et al. 1990). Advanced NEC is characterized by transmural necrosis and perforation. NEC may occur anywhere in the bowel, but the terminal ileum is most commonly affected. In very severe cases, the entire bowel may be affected, causing pan-necrosis of the intestine (**Figure 21.2**).

TREATMENT

Medical management

Initial management of suspected or confirmed NEC consists of cessation of oral feeds, placement of an orogastric tube for gastric decompression, intravenous fluid resuscitation, and administration of broad-spectrum antibiotics. In more severe cases characterized by

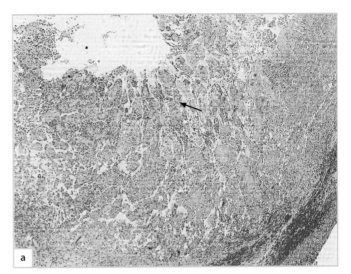
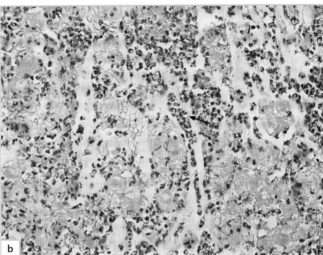

Figure 21.1 Hematoxylin and eosin-stained permanent section of ileum with severe necrotizing enterocolitis (NEC). (a) Pan-necrosis, loss of villous architecture, and neutrophil infiltration in the mucosa (× 40). Arrow indicates area of necrosis. (b) The mucosa in severe NEC shows neutrophil infiltration (arrow) and massive sloughing of necrotic epithelium (× 200).

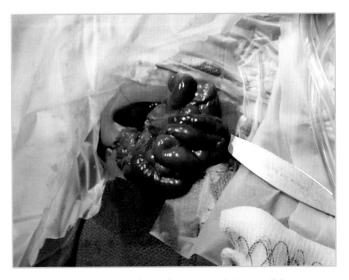

Figure 21.2 Intraoperative photo of pan-necrosis in necrotizing enterocolitis.

systemic sepsis or the neonatal form of the systemic inflammatory response syndrome, endotracheal intubation, and/or pressors may be required for ventilatory and hemodynamic support respectively. Coagulopathy or thrombocytopenia should be treated with appropriate blood products.

Antibiotics with broad activity against both Gram-negative and Gram-positive organisms should be administered at the first signs of disease. There is insufficient evidence to support a single antibiotic regimen, but the high rate of bacteremia supports the use of broad coverage, and evidence from multiple animal models show improved survival with antibiotic treatment (Bell et al. 1978, Brook 2008, Lin et al. 2008). Appropriate combinations include ampicillin with gentamicin or a third-generation cephalosporin (i.e., cefotaxime) plus metronidazole or clindamycin. An alternative treatment widely used in some NICUs consists of piperacillin–tazobactam with the addition of tobramycin for double Gram-negative coverage. In cases complicated by suspected meticillin-resistant *S. aureus* (MRSA) or ampicillin-resistant enterococci, vancomycin should be added to the antibiotic treatment. Vancomycin levels should be measured to ensure the therapeutic plasma concentration. Antibiotic choices can then be tailored based on intraoperative or blood culture results, and guided by an institution-specific antibiogram. If cultures indicate a fungal infection, fluconazole or amphotericin B should be added for antifungal coverage. Antibiotics should be continued for at least 7 days or until the patient recovers, as evidenced by hemodynamic stability, return of gastrointestinal (GI) function and normalization of laboratory values, although the thrombocytopenia may persist for weeks.

EXPERIMENTAL AND EMERGING SCIENCE ON TREATMENT

Probiotics

Probiotics are non-pathogenic microbial organisms that colonize the intestinal tract and modulate the gut immune response (Caplan 2009). The adult intestine normally includes a variety of commensal anaerobes and facultative aerobes. There is an increasing body of evidence to support the immunomodulatory effects of these bacteria in inflammatory disorders of the intestine. Given the hypothesis that altered bacterial colonization predisposes to NEC, administration of several non-pathogenic bacteria, including lactobacilli and *Bifidobacterium* spp., have been studied as a preventive strategy for NEC. These studies show a decrease in the rate of development of severe NEC, mortality, and sepsis in premature infants given prophylactic probiotics (Deshpande et al. 2010, Alfaleh et al. 2011). Although there have been isolated case reports of systemic infections (bacteremia) caused by the administration of probiotics to some infants, large clinical trials or meta-analyses have failed to consistently document this complication.

Growth factor receptors

Epidermal growth factor (EGF) is one of several components of breast milk that may confer protection from NEC. EGF and another member of the family of EGF-related peptides, heparin-binding EGF-like growth factor (HB-EGF), are present in breast milk, although EGF is two to three times more abundant than HB-EGF. Their actions on the EGF receptor play a critical role in intestinal epithelial cell proliferation, maturation, and restitution. The fetal intestine is exposed to EGF in the amniotic fluid and, in the neonatal gut, breast milk is a major source of EGF for the intestine. However, neither EGF nor HB-EGF is present in commercially available infant formula. Both EGF and HB-EGF have shown promise as a preventive and therapeutic strategy in NEC. Research in a neonatal rat model of NEC has shown that oral administration of EGF (Dvorak et al. 2002) or HB-EGF (Feng et al. 2006) can decrease the incidence and severity of experimental NEC.

Surgical management
Indications for surgery

The only absolute indication for surgical intervention in NEC is the presence of pneumoperitoneum, which indicates transmural intestinal necrosis that has progressed to perforation. However, extensive necrosis can occur without evidence of free air on an abdominal radiograph. Surgery may also be indicated in the following settings: Significant abdominal wall erythema or cellulitis, which suggests the presence of a contained perforation; a fixed intestinal loop on serial plain abdominal radiographs; a palpable abdominal pass; a positive paracentesis; or clinical deterioration despite aggressive medical therapy.

Surgical options for the management of advanced or perforated NEC vary and are generally determined by the extent of intestinal involvement and the clinical condition or hemodynamic stability of the infant. The primary goal of surgery is to control the source of infection while preserving the maximum amount of viable intestine.

Surgical approaches

Surgical management of NEC remains a subject of ongoing controversy. Ein et al. (1977) introduced the concept of peritoneal drainage (PD) as a temporizing measure before definitive laparotomy in hemodynamically unstable infants with perforated NEC. Since then, several studies have advocated PD as definitive treatment, rather than simply as a temporizing measure for some unstable infants, and this approach has gained popularity over the last three decades. Multiple retrospective studies have advocated primary PD as definitive therapy in all extremely low-birthweight infants with Bell stage III NEC (Lessin et al. 1998, Rovin et al. 1999), but others report that most of these infants eventually require laparotomy, and that in patients with birthweight >1000 g, the overall outcome is unchanged (Ahmed et al. 1998). In an effort to determine the best strategy, Moss et al. (2001) performed a meta-analysis of 10 studies from 1978 to 1999, which failed to show any superiority of PD over laparotomy. A similar retrospective analysis by Baird et al. (2006) showed improved outcome in very-low-birthweight (VLBW) infants treated with primary laparotomy or rescue laparotomy after PD. A subsequent prospective, non-randomized, multi-institutional study by Demestre et al. (2002) of 44 neonates showed improvement in 86% of infants after PD; 54% required surgery after PD. Overall survival rate was 95% for infants >1000 g.

Blakely et al. (2006) prospectively studied the long-term outcome in VLBW infants (<1000 g) undergoing primary PD versus laparotomy for perforated NEC. They did not find a significant survival difference between infants treated with primary laparotomy versus PD; 23% of patients required subsequent laparotomy after initial PD. Notably, this study included patients with FIP as well as NEC. PD was more likely to be used for FIP, whereas laparotomy was more likely to be employed for the surgical treatment of NEC. When the NEC cohort was analyzed separately, the survival rate after PD without laparotomy was only 32% in NEC compared with 57% in the cohort treated with initial laparotomy. Moss et al. (2006) subsequently conducted a prospective, multi-institutional, randomized controlled trial of PD versus laparotomy in 177 patients weighing <1500 g and >34 weeks' gestational age with perforated NEC. This study found a similar mortality in the groups treated with PD and laparotomy (34.5% vs 35.5%) and no difference in length of hospitalization or need for parenteral nutrition. However, roughly 38% of those randomized to PD needed subsequent laparotomy for deteriorating status. In non-enrolled infants, those who underwent PD had a 41% mortality rate compared with 15% for those undergoing initial laparotomy.

Rees et al. (2008) also published a randomized multicenter study in 31 countries, with 69 infants with birthweight <1000 g and a diagnosis of NEC or FIP enrolled. The authors found a trend toward increased survival in those treated with primary laparotomy. Laparotomy was ultimately required in 26/35 (74%) of those randomized to PD, and thus only 11% of the infants received PD as definitive treatment. More recently, Sola et al. (2010) conducted a meta-analysis, which showed an increased mortality rate of 55% in patients treated with PD for NEC and FIP compared with those treated with laparotomy. Thus it is possible that better outcomes can be achieved with careful patient selection for laparotomy.

Based on these studies, we conclude that infants weighing >1500 g and requiring surgical intervention for perforated NEC are probably best managed with laparotomy and resection of the necrotic intestine, with the goal to limit the extent of resection to avoid the complication of short bowel syndrome.

In cases of NEC with segmental necrosis or isolated perforation, surgical options include resection and ostomy creation or primary repair. Proponents of ostomy creation and thus intestinal diversion cite a number of studies showing higher rates of survival with enterostomy compared with primary anastomosis. In a retrospective study of 173 patients over 14 years, Cooper et al. compared 27 infants treated with primary repair to those treated with resection and stoma formation. They reported a 48% survival rate in the primary repair group versus 72% in the enterostomy group (Cooper et al. 1988).

Proponents of primary repair argue that there is significant morbidity in ostomy creation and subsequent ostomy closure, particularly in VLBW infants (O'Connor and Sawin 1998). In a study of 18 infants with perforated NEC treated by resection and primary anastomosis (Ade-Ajayi et al. 1996). there was no anastomotic leaks and the mortality rate (N = 2, 18%) was comparable to published rates in infants treated with enterostomies. Although the mean weight of the infants undergoing primary anastomosis was 1494 g, a subsequent report from the same group demonstrated the efficacy of this approach in infants weighing <1000 g (Hall et al. 2005). Thus, the authors concluded that primary anastomosis, in selected patients, has comparable morbidity and mortality to stoma formation.

Pan-necrosis presents a major challenge for preserving intestinal length in the face of extensive involvement. Options include resection of diseased intestine with creation of multiple ostomies, proximal diversion with or without a "second-look" procedure, and the "clip and drop-back" technique introduced by Vaughn et al. (1996). Resection of necrotic intestine with creation of multiple enterostomies was once a popular approach, but it has been abandoned because the multiple ostomies invariably lead to the loss of viable intestine. Proximal diversion, without sacrificing intestinal segments with borderline viability, can limit the extent of resection without increasing morbidity and mortality (Luzzatto et al. 1996). The "clip and drop-back" technique resects all nonviable bowel, but avoids ostomy creation by closing the segments without anastomosis at the time of initial laparotomy (Ron et al. 2009). A second-look operation is then performed after 4–72 h. The ideal management remains controversial and further prospective studies are needed to determine the best approach in such situations.

COMPLICATIONS

Acute

Acute complications of NEC are due to infection and resultant inflammation. Infectious complications include sepsis, meningitis, peritonitis, and intra-abdominal abscess formation. Resultant inflammation may lead to coagulopathy and disseminated intravascular coagulation, respiratory and cardiovascular compromise, and metabolic derangements including acidosis and hypoglycemia.

Chronic

The most common long-term problem in NEC survivors is stricture formation. Strictures occur in >30% of patients with medically or surgically treated NEC (Schwartz et al. 1980, Lemelle et al. 1994). Strictures may occur anywhere in the affected bowel, but the most common location is in watershed areas of the colon (Schimpl et al. 1994). If a stricture is suspected based on clinical symptoms of obstruction such as abdominal distension, feeding intolerance, or bilious emesis, a water-soluble contrast enema should be obtained. Any stricture requires surgical resection. Short bowel syndrome is a problem that affects up to 10% of infants requiring surgical intervention for NEC (Horwitz et al. 1995). Short bowel syndrome occurs when the intestine remaining after resection of diseased segments is insufficient to support full enteral nutrition (O'Keefe et al. 2006). The resultant dependence on parenteral nutrition carries a risk of chronic cholestasis and recurrent central line infections (Cavicchi et al. 2000, Duro et al. 2008). The former may eventually lead to liver failure. Recent retrospective studies of fish-oil-based fat emulsions as opposed to soybean lipid emulsions as an adjunct to parenteral nutrition in these children show decreased cholestasis and liver injury (Gura et al. 2008, Diamond et al. 2009). Prospective studies of this emerging therapy are ongoing. Surgical treatment of short bowel syndrome includes intestinal lengthening procedures and small bowel transplantation (Kaufman et al. 2001).

Infants who survive NEC have a particularly increased risk of neurodevelopmental impairment, which is seen in 43% of those with severe NEC and 15% of those with mild-to-moderate disease (Vohr et al. 2000). The incidence is higher in patients requiring surgical intervention, presumably due to more severe disease, and in VLBW infants, likely due to the increased comorbidities of prematurity (Hintz et al. 2005). Treatment strategies to minimize the neurodevelopmental impact of NEC are a subject of ongoing research.

■ REFERENCES

Ade-Ajayi N, Kiely E, Drake D, Wheeler R, Spitz L. Resection and primary anastomosis in necrotizing enterocolitis. *J R Soc Med* 1996;**89**:385–8.

Ahmed T, Ein S, Moore A. The role of peritoneal drains in treatment of perforated necrotizing enterocolitis: recommendations from recent experience. *J Pediatr Surg* 1998;**33**:1468–70.

Alfaleh K, Anabrees J, Bassler D, Al-Kharfi T. Probiotics for prevention of necrotizing enterocolitis in preterm infants. *Cochrane Database Syst Rev* 2011;(**3**):CD005496.

Andrews DA, Sawin RS, Ledbetter DJ, Schaller RT, Hatch EI. Necrotizing enterocolitis in term neonates. *Am J Surg* 1990;**159**:507–9.

Aschner JL, Deluga KS, Metlay LA, Emmens RW, Hendricks-Munoz KD. Spontaneous focal gastrointestinal perforation in very low birth weight infants. *J Pediatr* 1988;**113**:364–7.

Baird R, Puligandla PS, St Vil D, Dube S, Laberge JM. The role of laparotomy for intestinal perforation in very low birth weight infants. *J Pediatr Surg* 2006;**41**:1522–5.

Ballance WA, Dahms BB, Shenker N, Kliegman RM. Pathology of neonatal necrotizing enterocolitis: a ten-year experience. *J Pediatr* 1990;**117**(1 Pt 2):S6–13.

Bell MJ, Ternberg JL, Feigin RD, et al. Neonatal necrotizing enterocolitis. Therapeutic decisions based upon clinical staging. *Ann Surg* 1978;**187**:1–7.

Berseth CL. Gestational evolution of small intestine motility in preterm and term infants. *J Pediatr* 1989;**115**:646–51.

Berseth CL. Effect of early feeding on maturation of the preterm infant's small intestine. *J Pediatr.* 1992;**120**:947–53.

Blakely ML, Lally KP, McDonald S, et al. Postoperative outcomes of extremely low birth-weight infants with necrotizing enterocolitis or isolated intestinal perforation: a prospective cohort study by the NICHD Neonatal Research Network. *Ann Surg* 2005;**241**:984–9; discussion 989–94.

Blakely ML, Tyson JE, Lally KP, et al. Laparotomy versus peritoneal drainage for necrotizing enterocolitis or isolated intestinal perforation in extremely low birth weight infants: outcomes through 18 months adjusted age. *Pediatrics* 2006;**117**:e680–7.

Bombell S, McGuire W. Delayed introduction of progressive enteral feeds to prevent necrotising enterocolitis in very low birth weight infants. *Cochrane Database Syst Rev* 2008(**2**):CD001970.

Brook I. Microbiology and management of neonatal necrotizing enterocolitis. *Am J Perinatol* 2008;**25**:111–18.

Caplan MS, Simon D, Jilling T. The role of PAF, TLR, and the inflammatory response in neonatal necrotizing enterocolitis. *Semin Pediatr Surg* 2005;**14**:145–51.

Caplan MS. Probiotic and prebiotic supplementation for the prevention of neonatal necrotizing enterocolitis. *J Perinatol* 2009;**29**(suppl 2):S2–6.

Cavicchi M, Beau P, Crenn P, Degott C, Messing B. Prevalence of liver disease and contributing factors in patients receiving home parenteral nutrition for permanent intestinal failure. *Ann Intern Med* 2000;**132**:525–32.

Chokshi NK, Guner YS, Hunter CJ, Upperman JS, Grishin A, Ford HR. The role of nitric oxide in intestinal epithelial injury and restitution in neonatal necrotizing enterocolitis. *Semin Perinatol* 2008;**32**:92–9.

Cooper A, Ross AJ 3rd, O'Neill JA, Jr., Schnaufer L. Resection with primary anastomosis for necrotizing enterocolitis: a contrasting view. *J Pediatr Surg* 1988;**23**(1 Pt 2):64–8.

Demestre X, Ginovart G, Figueras-Aloy J, et al. Peritoneal drainage as primary management in necrotizing enterocolitis: a prospective study. *J Pediatr Surg* 2002;**37**:1534–9.

Deshpande G, Rao S, Patole S, Bulsara M. Updated meta-analysis of probiotics for preventing necrotizing enterocolitis in preterm neonates. *Pediatrics* 2010;**125**:921–30.

Diamond IR, Sterescu A, Pencharz PB, Kim JH, Wales PW. Changing the paradigm: omegaven for the treatment of liver failure in pediatric short bowel syndrome. *J Pediatr Gastroenterol Nutr* 2009;**48**:209–15.

Duro D, Kamin D, Duggan C. Overview of pediatric short bowel syndrome. *J Pediatr Gastroenterol Nutr* 2008;**47**(suppl 1):S33–6.

Dvorak B, Halpern MD, Holubec H, et al. Epidermal growth factor reduces the development of necrotizing enterocolitis in a neonatal rat model. *Am J Physiol Gastrointest Liver Physiol* 2002;**282**:G156–64.

Ein SH, Marshall DG, Girvan D. Peritoneal drainage under local anesthesia for perforations from necrotizing enterocolitis. *J Pediatr Surg* 1977;**12**:963–7.

Emami CN, Petrosyan M, Giuliani S, et al. Role of the host defense system and intestinal microbial flora in the pathogenesis of necrotizing enterocolitis. *Surg Infect (Larchmt)* 2009;**10**:407–17.

Enck P, Zimmermann K, Rusch K, Schwiertz A, Klosterhalfen S, Frick JS. The effects of maturation on the colonic microflora in infancy and childhood. *Gastroenterol Res Pract* 2009;**752**:401.

Engum SA, Grosfeld JL. Necrotizing enterocolitis. *Curr Opin Pediatr* 1998;**10**:123–30.

Epelman M, Daneman A, Navarro OM, et al. Necrotizing enterocolitis: review of state-of-the-art imaging findings with pathologic correlation. *Radiographics* 2007;**27**:285–305.

Feng J, El-Assal ON, Besner GE. Heparin-binding epidermal growth factor-like growth factor reduces intestinal apoptosis in neonatal rats with necrotizing enterocolitis. *J Pediatr Surg* 2006;**41**:742–7; discussion 742–747.

Figueras-Aloy J, Rodriguez-Miguelez JM, Iriondo-Sanz M, Salvia-Roiges MD, Botet-Mussons F, Carbonell-Estrany X. Intravenous immunoglobulin and necrotizing enterocolitis in newborns with hemolytic disease. *Pediatrics* 2010;**125**:139–44.

Foster J, Cole M. Oral immunoglobulin for preventing necrotizing enterocolitis in preterm and low birth-weight neonates. *Cochrane Database Syst Rev* 2004;(**1**):CD001816.

Gordon PV, Swanson JR, Attridge JT, Clark R. Emerging trends in acquired neonatal intestinal disease: is it time to abandon Bell's criteria? *J Perinatol* 2007;**27**:661–71.

Grishin A, Wang J, Hackam D, et al. p38 MAP kinase mediates endotoxin-induced expression of cyclooxygenase-2 in enterocytes. *Surgery* 2004;**136**:329–35.

Guillet R, Stoll BJ, Cotten CM, et al. Association of H2-blocker therapy and higher incidence of necrotizing enterocolitis in very low birth weight infants. *Pediatrics* 2006;**117**:e137–42.

Gura KM, Lee S, Valim C, et al. Safety and efficacy of a fish-oil-based fat emulsion in the treatment of parenteral nutrition-associated liver disease. *Pediatrics* 2008;**121**:e678–86.

Hall NJ, Curry J, Drake DP, Spitz L, Kiely EM, Pierro A. Resection and primary anastomosis is a valid surgical option for infants with necrotizing enterocolitis who weigh less than 1000 g. *Arch Surg* 2005;**140**:1149–51.

Hallstrom M, Koivisto AM, Janas M, Tammela O. Laboratory parameters predictive of developing necrotizing enterocolitis in infants born before 33 weeks of gestation. *J Pediatr Surg* 2006;**41**:792–8.

Hay WW Jr. Strategies for feeding the preterm infant. *Neonatology* 2008;**94**:245–54.

Hecht G. Innate mechanisms of epithelial host defense: spotlight on intestine. *Am J Physiol.* Sep 1999;**277**(3 Pt 1):C351–8.

Hintz SR, Kendrick DE, Stoll BJ, et al. Neurodevelopmental and growth outcomes of extremely low birth weight infants after necrotizing enterocolitis. *Pediatrics* 2005;**115**:696–703.

Holman RC, Stoll BJ, Clarke MJ, Glass RI. The epidemiology of necrotizing enterocolitis infant mortality in the United States. *Am J Public Health* 1997;**87**:2026–31.

Holman RC, Stoll BJ, Curns AT, Yorita KL, Steiner CA, Schonberger LB. Necrotising enterocolitis hospitalisations among neonates in the United States. *Paediatr Perinat Epidemiol* 2006;**20**:498–506.

Horwitz JR, Lally KP, Cheu HW, Vazquez WD, Grosfeld JL, Ziegler MM. Complications after surgical intervention for necrotizing enterocolitis: a multicenter review. *J Pediatr Surg* 1995;**30**:994–8; discussion 998–9.

Hsueh W, Caplan MS, Qu XW, Tan XD, De Plaen IG, Gonzalez-Crussi F. Neonatal necrotizing enterocolitis: clinical considerations and pathogenetic concepts. *Pediatr Dev Pathol* 2003;**6**:6–23.

Hutter JJ Jr, Hathaway WE, Wayne ER. Hematologic abnormalities in severe neonatal necrotizing enterocolitis. *J Pediatr* 1976;**88**:1026–31.

Kaufman SS, Atkinson JB, Bianchi A, et al. Indications for pediatric intestinal transplantation: a position paper of the American Society of Transplantation. *Pediatr Transplant* 2001;**5**:80–7.

Kelly EJ, Newell SJ, Brownlee KG, Primrose JN, Dear PR. Gastric acid secretion in preterm infants. *Early Hum Dev* 1993;**35**:215–20.

Kliegman RM, Walsh MC. Neonatal necrotizing enterocolitis: pathogenesis, classification, and spectrum of illness. *Curr Probl Pediatr* 1987;**17**:213–88.

Lemelle JL, Schmitt M, de Miscault G, Vert P, Hascoet JM. Neonatal necrotizing enterocolitis: a retrospective and multicentric review of 331 cases. *Acta Paediatr Suppl* 1994;**396**:70–3.

Lessin MS, Luks FI, Wesselhoeft CW Jr, Gilchrist BF, Iannitti D, DeLuca FG. Peritoneal drainage as definitive treatment for intestinal perforation in infants with extremely low birth weight (<750 g). *J Pediatr Surg* 1998;**33**:370–2.

Lin PW, Nasr TR, Stoll BJ. Necrotizing enterocolitis: recent scientific advances in pathophysiology and prevention. *Semin Perinatol* 2008;**32**:70–82.

Llanos AR, Moss ME, Pinzon MC, Dye T, Sinkin RA, Kendig JW. Epidemiology of neonatal necrotising enterocolitis: a population-based study. *Paediatr Perinat Epidemiol* 2002;**16**:342–9.

Lucas A, Cole TJ. Breast milk and neonatal necrotising enterocolitis. *Lancet* 1990;**336**:1519–23.

Luzzatto C, Previtera C, Boscolo R, Katende M, Orzali A, Guglielmi M. Necrotizing enterocolitis: late surgical results after enterostomy without resection. *Eur J Pediatr Surg* 1996;**6**:92–4.

Lugo B, Ford HR, Grishin A. Molecular signaling in necrotizing enterocolitis: regulation of intestinal COX-2 expression. *J Pediatr Surg* 2007;**42**:1165–71.

McElhinney DB, Hedrick HL, Bush DM, et al. Necrotizing enterocolitis in neonates with congenital heart disease: risk factors and outcomes. *Pediatrics* 2000;**106**:1080–7.

Mackie RI, Sghir A, Gaskins HR. Developmental microbial ecology of the neonatal gastrointestinal tract. *Am J Clin Nutr* 1999;**69**:1035S–45S.

Markel TA, Crisostomo PR, Wairiuko GM, Pitcher J, Tsai BM, Meldrum DR. Cytokines in necrotizing enterocolitis. *Shock* 2006;**25**:329–37.

Moss RL, Dimmitt RA, Henry MC, Geraghty N, Efron B. A meta-analysis of peritoneal drainage versus laparotomy for perforated necrotizing enterocolitis. *J Pediatr Surg* 2001;**36**:1210–13.

Moss RL, Dimmitt RA, Barnhart DC, et al. Laparotomy versus peritoneal drainage for necrotizing enterocolitis and perforation. *N Engl J Med* 2006;**354**:2225–34.

Muller CA, Autenrieth IB, Peschel A. Innate defenses of the intestinal epithelial barrier. *Cell Mol Life Sci* 2005;**62**:1297–307.

Neu J, Chen M, Beierle E. Intestinal innate immunity: how does it relate to the pathogenesis of necrotizing enterocolitis. *Semin Pediatr Surg* 2005;**14**:137–44.

O'Connor A, Sawin RS. High morbidity of enterostomy and its closure in premature infants with necrotizing enterocolitis. *Arch Surg* 1998;**133**:875–80.

O'Keefe SJ, Buchman AL, Fishbein TM, Jeejeebhoy KN, Jeppesen PB, Shaffer J. Short bowel syndrome and intestinal failure: consensus definitions and overview. *Clin Gastroenterol Hepatol* 2006;**4**:6–10.

Park JY, Pillinger MH, Abramson SB. Prostaglandin E2 synthesis and secretion: the role of PGE2 synthases. *Clin Immunol* 2006;**119**:229–40.

Potoka DA, Upperman JS, Zhang XR, et al. Peroxynitrite inhibits enterocyte proliferation and modulates Src kinase activity in vitro. *Am J Physiol Gastrointest Liver Physiol* 2003;**285**:G861–9.

Pourcyrous M, Korones SB, Yang W, Boulden TF, Bada HS. C-reactive protein in the diagnosis, management, and prognosis of neonatal necrotizing enterocolitis. *Pediatrics* 2005;**116**:1064–9.

Pumberger W, Mayr M, Kohlhauser C, Weninger M. Spontaneous localized intestinal perforation in very-low-birth-weight infants: a distinct clinical entity different from necrotizing enterocolitis. *J Am Coll Surg* 2002;**195**:796–803.

Radhakrishnan J, Blechman G, Shrader C, Patel MK, Mangurten HH, McFadden JC. Colonic strictures following successful medical management of necrotizing enterocolitis: a prospective study evaluating early gastrointestinal contrast studies. *J Pediatr Surg.* Sep 1991;**26**:1043–6.

Ragazzi S, Pierro A, Peters M, Fasoli L, Eaton S. Early full blood count and severity of disease in neonates with necrotizing enterocolitis. *Pediatr Surg Int* 2003;**19**:376–9.

Rees CM, Eaton S, Kiely EM, Wade AM, McHugh K, Pierro A. Peritoneal drainage or laparotomy for neonatal bowel perforation? A randomized controlled trial. *Ann Surg* 2008;**248**:44–51.

Ron O, Davenport M, Patel S, et al. Outcomes of the "clip and drop" technique for multifocal necrotizing enterocolitis. *J Pediatr Surg* 2009;**44**:749–54.

Rovin JD, Rodgers BM, Burns RC, McGahren ED. The role of peritoneal drainage for intestinal perforation in infants with and without necrotizing enterocolitis. *J Pediatr Surg* 1999;**34**:143–7.

Rowe MI, Reblock KK, Kurkchubasche AG, Healey PJ. Necrotizing enterocolitis in the extremely low birth weight infant. *J Pediatr Surg* 1994;**29**:987–90; discussion 990.

Schanler RJ, Shulman RJ, Lau C. Feeding strategies for premature infants: beneficial outcomes of feeding fortified human milk versus preterm formula. *Pediatrics* 1999;**103**(6 Pt 1):1150–7.

Schimpl G, Hollwarth ME, Fotter R, Becker H. Late intestinal strictures following successful treatment of necrotizing enterocolitis. *Acta Paediatr Suppl* 1994;**396**:80–3.

Schwartz MZ, Richardson CJ, Hayden CK, Swischuk LE, Tyson KR. Intestinal stenosis following successful medical management of necrotizing enterocolitis. *J Pediatr Surg* 1980;**15**:890–9.

Sharma R, Tepas JJ 3rd, Hudak ML, et al. Neonatal gut barrier and multiple organ failure: role of endotoxin and proinflammatory cytokines in sepsis and necrotizing enterocolitis. *J Pediatr Surg* 2007;**42**:454–61.

Sola JE, Tepas JJ 3rd, Koniaris LG. Peritoneal drainage versus laparotomy for necrotizing enterocolitis and intestinal perforation: a meta-analysis. *J Surg Res* 2010;**161**:95–100.

Stoll BJ. Epidemiology of necrotizing enterocolitis. *Clin Perinatol* 1994;**21**:205–18.

Stoll BJ, Gordon T, Korones SB, et al. Early-onset sepsis in very low birth weight neonates: a report from the National Institute of Child Health and Human Development Neonatal Research Network. *J Pediatr* 1996;**129**:72–80.

Tyson JE, Kennedy KA. Minimal enteral nutrition for promoting feeding tolerance and preventing morbidity in parenterally fed infants. *Cochrane Database Syst Rev* 2000;(**2**):CD000504.

Vaughan WG, Grosfeld JL, West K, Scherer LR, 3rd, Villamizar E, Rescorla FJ. Avoidance of stomas and delayed anastomosis for bowel necrosis: the "clip and drop-back" technique. *J Pediatr Surg* 1996;**31**:542–5.

Vohr BR, Wright LL, Dusick AM, et al. Neurodevelopmental and functional outcomes of extremely low birth weight infants in the National Institute of Child Health and Human Development Neonatal Research Network, 1993–1994. *Pediatrics* 2000;**105**:1216–26.

Wiswell TE, Robertson CF, Jones TA, Tuttle DJ. Necrotizing enterocolitis in full-term infants. A case-control study. *Am J Dis Child* 1988;**142**:532–5.

Chapter 22 Postoperative infections of the central nervous system

H. Richard Winn, Saadi Ghatan

The present chapter focuses on infections involving the central nervous system (CNS) after cranial and spinal surgery. With rare exception in a non-immunocompromised host, such infections are almost exclusively bacterial and, consequently, this review is primarily devoted to bacterial infections.

Common infectious disorders after craniotomy include meningitis, epidural and subdural empyema, osteomyelitis (bone flap infections), and brain abscess. Infections after ventriculoperitoneal shunts require special attention because of their high frequency. This chapter also highlights the factors associated with infections after simple and complex spine surgery. In most circumstances, postoperative spinal infections do not affect the CNS directly, but rather involve the bone and soft tissue surrounding the spinal cord and the cauda equina. Superficial incisional infections occurring after both cranial and spinal surgery are also discussed although this topic is covered extensively in earlier chapters.

■ SPECIAL CONSIDERATIONS OF CNS INFECTIONS

Postoperative evaluation and treatment of infections affecting the brain and spinal cord function are difficult because of two unique aspects of the anatomy of the CNS. First, the brain and spinal cord are surrounded by the boney skeleton of the cranium and vertebral spine. This protected position of the CNS makes the diagnosis of postoperative infections difficult. Rather than observing the direct manifestations of infection, the surgeon must establish the diagnosis based on the consequences of infection: The symptoms and signs of dysfunction of the CNS or surrounding structures. Second, the diagnosis of postoperative CNS infection is made more difficult by the pre-existing alteration of CNS function related to the patient's primary disease and/or the initial operation.

The other unique anatomic aspect of the CNS is the presence of barriers that are designed to isolate the CNS from constituents in blood and cerebral spinal fluid (CSF): The blood–brain barrier (BBB) and the CSF–brain barrier. These barriers are dependent on special anatomic and physiological features of the endothelial cells lining the inner surface of the blood vessels of the CNS, and the ependymal cells lining the walls of the brain ventricles. These barriers limit the entry of many drugs that are normally capable of perfusing and penetrating non-CNS organs. Chemotherapeutic agents under normal conditions thus have limited access to the CNS, making problematic routine treatment with antibiotics and other drugs. However, in the inflamed state, the integrity of the BBB and the CSF–brain barrier is altered and antibiotic entry is enhanced. As the infectious process responds to medical therapy, these barriers return to a more competent, less leaky state, decreasing antibiotic penetrance and increasing the likelihood of a persistent residual nidus of infection.

The spectrum of organisms involved in postoperative CNS infections is different from new infections of the brain and spine (McClelland and Hall 2007). Most of the organisms involved in postoperative infections are skin contaminants. The most common organism is *Staphylococcus aureus* with some studies finding >50% incidence of this organism (Gantz 2004). Coagulase-negative staphylococci are the next most frequent, followed by enterococci, streptococci, *Acinetobacter* spp., *Pseudomonas aeruginosa*, *Klebsiella pneumoniae*, *Citrobacter* spp., *Enterobacter* spp., and *Escherichia coli*. There is some degree of correlation between the type of infection and organisms cultured, e.g., Gram-negative bacilli are the most common organisms cultured with postoperative meningitis whereas Gram-negative bacilli and polymicrobial infections are the most frequent in brain abscess. There is recent growing awareness that an anaerobic Gram-positive bacillus and skin contaminant, *Propionibacterium acnes*, is involved in indolent postoperative CNS infections (Nisbet et al. 2007)

■ OVERVIEW OF RISK FACTORS FOR POSTOPERATIVE CNS INFECTIONS

Patient-related and technique specific factors have been described as being associated with the development of postoperative CNS infections in multiple studies (Korinek 1997, Olsen et al. 2003, McClelland and Hall 2007). These factors are displayed in **Tables 22.1–22.3** and can be summarized as:

- General surgery studies have identified a variety of factors such as diabetes, obesity, and age that correlate with the development of postoperative infections. All of these conditions affect host immunological status. In addition, neurosurgery patients have additional causes that will alter host immunological status such as CNS trauma, malignant brain tumors, stroke, steroid administration, and radiation.
- Presumably, many of the observations made in general surgery patients may be extrapolated to the neurosurgery patient. However, differences exist, e.g., low body temperature has been shown in general surgery patients undergoing abdominal surgery to correlate with postoperative infections (Kurz et al. 1996). In contrast, no differences in postoperative infections (e.g., meningitis, incisional, bone flap, pneumonia, or urinary) were found in patients undergoing craniotomy for aneurysm clipping who were randomized to normothermia versus moderate hypothermia (Todd et al. 2005). However, the incidence of bacteremia was higher in the hypothermic group.
- Prophylactic antibiotics have been demonstrated in randomized trials to lower the incidence of postoperative infections in clean craniotomies and spinal procedures (Horwitz and Curtin 1975, Young and Lawner 1987, Bullock et al. 1988, Dempsey et al. 1988, Barker 1994), and their use has been extended to other types (i.e.,

Table 22.1 Risk factors for postoperative infection after craniotomy.

PATIENT RISK FACTORS	Association
Immune state	H
Nutritional status	H
Steroids	M
Radiation	M
Chemotherapy	M
Trauma	H
Diabetes mellitus	L
Neurological status	M
SURGICAL RISK FACTORS	
Postoperative CSF leak	Very H
Duration >4 h	H
Contaminated	H
Emergency	H
Previous neurosurgery <4 months	H
Use of foreign material	H
Sinus entry	M
Placement of drains	L

CSF, cerebrospinal fluid; H, high; L, low; M, moderate; M-L, inconsistent.

Table 22.2 Risk factors for postoperative infection after ventriculoperitoneal shunt.

PATIENT RISK FACTORS	Association
Age: <6 months old	H
Diagnosis	M-L
Etiology of hydrocephalus	M-L
Concurrent infection (e.g., UTI)	M
Previous shunt	M
SURGICAL RISK FACTORS	
Postoperative CSF leak	Very H
Double gloving	L
Draping	L
Type of preoperative skin prep	L
Duration of operation	L
Surgical training	L
Type of shunt	L

CSF, cerebrospinal fluid; H, high; L, low; M, moderate; M-L, inconsistent; UTI, urinary tract infection.

Table 22.3 Risk factors for postoperative infection after spinal surgery.

PATIENT RISK FACTORS	Association
Prolonged preoperative hospitalization	H
Diabetes mellitus	H
Immune state	H
Malignancy	H
Nutritional state	H
Trauma	H
Obesity	H
Tobacco use	M
Steroid use	M
Concurrent infection	M-L
SURGICAL RISK FACTORS	
Postoperative CSF leak	H
Duration	H
Blood loss	H
Approach	H
Extent (e.g., levels)	H
Graft	M
Instrumentation	M

H, high; L, low; M, moderate; M-L, inconsistent.

be supplemented during prolonged surgeries, and should be discontinued within 24 h of surgery (Fry 2001).

- Intraoperative factors and conditions influence the development of postoperative infections. Obviously, sterile conditions must be followed throughout the case. The skin should be prepared with an antiseptic, but no agent appears to be superior to any other. In the past, hair shaving was a standard part of preoperative preparation, but no or minimal hair removal has not been shown to increase the risks of postoperative infections. The exception to leaving hair *in situ* may be shunt operations. If hair is to be removed, it should be accomplished immediately before surgery. An electric shaver or clipper should be used rather than a razor. The latter has the potential to cause small cuts and abrasions with consequent colonization by skin flora.

- Specific, well-defined risk factors for craniotomy (Table 22.1) have been identified as follows (Korinek 1997): CSF leak, re-operation, duration of surgery (3–4 h), emergency operations, clean-contaminated and contaminated operations. Of these risk factors, CSF has the most robust association (Korinek 1997) and thus, when closing a cranial wound, careful, meticulous closure is required. Other factors that may be associated with post-craniotomy infections include the use of drains, diabetes mellitus, opening paranasal sinuses, poor neurological status, and implantation of foreign material (e.g., shunts), to mention a few.

- Specific factors that correlate with postspinal infections (Table 22.3) include (Levi et al. 1997, Wimmer et al. 1998) site (posterior versus anterior), complexity (number of levels and approach), duration (may be an epiphenomenon reflecting complexity), trauma (may reflect duration and/or complexity), blood loss (correlates with trauma, surgical duration, complexity), and the implantation of hardware.

contaminated) of CNS operations. Some individual randomized studies, focusing on spinal operations, have failed to confirm the utility of prophylactic antibiotics. This failure may relate to the low incidence of postoperative spinal infections in control groups and the small numbers of patients studied. In contrast, utilizing pooled data and meta-analysis, Barker found that postoperative infections were significantly lowered to 2.2% from 5.9% (Barker 2002). To be effective and safe, the drug should be appropriate, must be administered 1 hour before incision, if short acting should

POSTOPERATIVE CRANIAL INFECTIONS

In this chapter and for the purposes of clarity, craniotomy and craniectomy are considered as the same technique because there are no definitive studies that document any differences in postoperative infection rates between these two operations. Furthermore, in most circumstances maintenance of vascular perfusion and drainage is viewed as an important component of infection prevention. Despite much debate about the relative merits of craniotomies performed with vascularized (i.e., muscle remaining intact) versus free bone flaps (muscle stripped off the skull before creation of the bone flap), no firm data demonstrate the superiority of either technique in decreasing or increasing postoperative infections.

Meningitis

Bacterial meningitis after cranial operations is fortunately uncommon, occurring in <1% of craniotomies (McClelland and Hall 2007, Zarrouk et al. 2007). However, undiagnosed and untreated, the mortality rate is high (>20%). The symptoms, as with most other CNS postoperative infections, are frequently more muted and subtle as compared with meningitis occurring anew. The prerequisite of findings with new infectious meningitis are fever, headache, alteration in mental or neurological status, and meningeal irritation (manifested by stiff neck and/or photophobia). In contrast, these findings are frequently incomplete, absent, or masked by the original entity that prompted craniotomy.

Many factors contribute to the difficulty in establishing the diagnosis of infectious post-craniotomy meningitis. Sterile (also called chemical or aseptic) meningitis occurs in a high frequency (50–70%) of patients undergoing craniotomy and thereby may add to the confusion in establishing the diagnosis of bacterial meningitis (Carmel and Greif 1993, Zarrouk et al. 2007). The etiology of this sterile meningitis is undoubtedly related to contamination of the CSF by blood (subarachnoid hemorrhage or SAH). Some degree of SAH is observed even after craniotomy for benign etiologies, and is always noted in the preoperative state after trauma, aneurysm rupture, and frequently late in the course of brain tumors. SAH evokes the same symptoms (fever, headache, alteration in mental or neurological status, and meningeal irritation) as that observed with bacterial meningitis.

Adding to the difficulty in establishing the diagnosis of postoperative septic meningitis is the routine use of steroids in a variety of brain (and spinal – see below) disorders. Steroids can mute the symptoms and signs of both aseptic and septic meningitis. The use of anticonvulsants in the post-craniotomy period is frequent and these drugs can evoke a drug fever, thereby further confusing the clinical picture and diagnosis of meningitis (Temkin et al. 1990).

Systemic markers of infection such as an elevation in the sedimentation rate (ESR) and C-reactive protein (CRP), useful in new meningitis and other infections, are non-specific because these parameters routinely rise after craniotomy: CRP peaks at approximately 1 week and ESR may remain elevated for 2–3 weeks.

A diagnosis of septic meningitis can be established only with a positive CSF culture. In contrast, the diagnosis of aseptic meningitis requires a sterile CSF culture (Carmel and Greif 1993, Zarrouk et al. 2007). Studies using Gram stains are sufficiently inconsistent to not be a reliable indicator of septic meningitis. In a similar fashion, the CSF cell count and CSF glucose are non-specific because both can be altered with aseptic meningitis. Analysis of CSF using molecular markers of infection has been suggested, but definitive studies remain to be done.

Treatment of postoperative meningitis begins by establishing the diagnosis as outlined above and instituting antibiotic therapy. Choice of antibiotic depends on isolating the causative agent by obtaining CSF by either lumbar puncture or ventricular sampling, and then determining the susceptibility of the agent to therapy. Initial broad-spectrum, multidrug regimens are utilized until a positive culture is established.

Subdural empyema

As with meningitis, symptoms of subdural empyema after craniotomy are different from those observed anew. In the former situation, the symptoms are more muted and headache and temperature elevation are usually absent (Post and Modesti 1981, Tunkel 2005). Masking of headache and fever may be related to the routine use of postoperative steroids. The most likely association with the presence of a postoperative empyema is the presence of a superficial wound infection (Tunkel 2005). Subdural empyema is frequently found several weeks to months after the initial craniotomy.

There are no definitive clinical, laboratory, and imaging findings. A high degree of suspicion is required to establish the diagnosis of subdural empyema. As already noted, a subdural empyema typically occurs in a delayed fashion when postoperative systemic markers of inflammation, such as white blood cell count (WBC), ESR, and CRP, have returned to normal ranges. Potentially, elevation of these systemic markers could be of assistance in establishing the diagnosis of a subdural empyema. However, ESR and CRP are rarely altered, e.g., in only 63% of cases of postoperative subdural empyema was the WBC elevated (Hlavin et al. 1994, Farrell et al. 2008). Lumbar CSF findings are non-diagnostic and performing a lumbar puncture in the setting of a subdural empyema may result in neurological deterioration.

Imagining studies (computed tomography [CT] or magnetic resonance imaging [MRI]) may reveal crescent-shaped, extra-parenchymal fluid collections, but such fluid collections are frequently seen on postoperative CT and MRI. Contrast enhancement of the pial surface can be indicative of a subdural empyema, but such changes are also observed in uninfected patients postoperatively. In 29% of patients with a subdural empyema, even diffusion changes in the brain parenchymal adjacent to the subdural empyema collection may be lacking (Farrell et al. 2008). The most reliable diagnostic finding to establishment of the presence of a subdural empyema is enlargement of fluid collection on sequential imaging or progressive edema adjacent to fluid collections.

The most likely organisms cultured from a subdural empyema cavity are skin flora and Gram-negative bacilli. Antibiotic penetration of the empyema cavity is poor and thus chemotherapeutics alone is unlikely to result in control of the infection. Moreover, the coexistent inflammatory reaction in the pial veins often results in a thrombophlebitis and resultant brain edema.

Surgical treatment of subdural empyemas remains the most effective treatment. However, treatment depends critically on early suspicion and rapid diagnosis. Unfortunately, definitive establishment of the presence of a subdural empyema is often delayed. Controversy exists as to whether evacuation of subdural collections is best achieved via burr holes or craniotomy. One advantage of craniotomy compared with burr hole drainage is that craniotomy provides greater access and therefore greater likelihood of achieving maximal removal of purulent material. Another advantage of craniotomy is that, in cases where significant brain edema exists, not replacing the bone flap allows decompression of the brain. In all cases, the surgical evacuation is combined with prolong (4–6 weeks) coverage with the appropriate intravenous antibiotic. Frequently, after cessation of intravenous antibiotics, the patient is maintained on oral chemotherapy for an additional 4–6 weeks.

EPIDURAL INFECTIONS AND OSTEOMYELITIS OF THE BONE FLAP

Superficial infections of the surgical incision site after craniotomy are similar to incisional site infections elsewhere in the body, but are unique because the possibilities that, untreated or inappropriately treated, the bone flap or the underlying brain can become involved. Therefore, any hint of incisional inflammation must be addressed in a prompt fashion. In most cases, culture of the wound, establishment of drainage, and placement on appropriate antibiotic will prevent deeper infection and involvement of the bone and brain.

The likelihood of developing an incisional superficial infection is increased by previous surgery at the same site, radiation in the area of the surgical bed, poor nutritional status, and the presence of foreign bodies (Hlavin et al. 1994, Korinek 1997, McClelland and Hall 2007). If a non-biological material is used as a cranioplasty, the incision must be designed to avoid placing the cranioplasty directly under the incision.

The signs of a local infection are tenderness, erythema, and swelling. Any wound breakdown must be assumed to be related to an underlying infection. Repetitive superficial infections may represent an epiphenomenon of an underlying osteomyelitis of the bone flap. The most common organisms cultured from superficial infections after craniotomy are Gram-positive cocci, including *Staphylococcus aureus*, coagulase-negative staphylococci, and *Propionibacterium acnes* (Post and Modesti 1981, Dempsey et al. 1988, Kurz et al. 1996, Mangram et al. 1999).

Infections of the bone flap, often associated with epidural empyema, may or may not coexist with superficial infections. In the vast majority of cases, the infection is located primarily within the free bone flap and does not involve the vascularized, surrounding intact bone of the skull. Bone flap infections can occur from a primary inoculation by skin flora at the time of surgery or as a result of a delayed incisional infection.

Even in the uninfected state, bone flaps may become demineralized and disintegrate over the long term (months to years) and the appearance on skull radiograph and CT may be difficult to distinguish from osteomyelitis. Bone flap infections are usually delayed and therefore systemic findings, such as persistent fever and elevation of WBC, ESR, and CRP, may aid in the establishment of a diagnosis of osteomyelitis.

The most effective treatment is removal of the bone flap, leaving a cosmetically displeasing bone deficit. The flap removal is then followed by appropriate and prolonged antibiotic therapy. In a delayed fashion, usually 3–6 months and after establishing compelling evidence that the infection has been eradicated, the bone defect is replaced using either a foreign substance (i.e., methylmethacrylate) or an autologous split-thickness bone graft obtained from the ribs or a second cranial site. The advantages of methylmethacrylate are the ease of molding the material to conform to the contour of the bone deficit and the simplicity of the procedure. The disadvantage is that, in an inadequately treated infection, the cranioplasty may serve as a nidus for a persistent infection. In contrast, split-thickness bone graft operations are more complex, requiring an additional donor site incision, but may have a lower risk of infection. Free bone also has a small risk of bony resorption.

Alternative to the multistaged treatment course outlined above is treatment with a prolonged course of antibiotics, assuming that a culture and sensitivity can be established. In most cases, prolonged antibiotic treatment only delays definitive surgical treatment. In contrast, Bruce and Bruce (2003) have proposed a one-step procedure with removal and debridement of the bone flap combined with immersion of the flap in a solution of povidine and antibiotics. The flap is then placed back into the skull avoiding a cosmetic defect. Bruce and Bruce were successful in the short term with such an approach in 85% (11 of 13) of cases.

Brain abscess

Brain abscess is a much-feared complication after craniotomy, but, fortunately, an uncommon event. The etiology is either direct intraoperative inoculation or spread from more superficial infected sites.

The initial step in the development of a brain abscess is localized cerebritis (Winn et al. 1979). Left untreated, this cerebritis will progress to an organized focal infection over the course of 5–10 days. Wall formation results from fibroblastic migration from the pial surface and collagen deposition which, in its most classic form, is thinnest toward the ventricle and thickest toward the surface of the brain (**Figure 22.1**).

In contrast to new brain abscesses, patients with post-craniotomy abscess formation do not present with the classic findings of headache, focal neurological findings, and fever (Yang et al. 2006, Carpenter et al. 2007). Fever is evident in 25%, neurological deterioration in 55%, and seizure in approximately 20%. These findings are therefore not specific.

The diagnosis is best established by changes on imaging studies by either CT or MRI. The characteristic location of new abscesses at the gray–white junction is unlikely to be present in the postoperative period; more likely, the abscess is located in the operative bed or along the access tract. The observable changes on imaging studies are related to the maturation of the abscess. Early on, the classic finding of cerebritis on CT is lucency whereas on MRI high T2-weighted signals with patchy enhancement may be seen. As the cerebritis progresses, the infection coalesces, wall formation occurs, and ring enhancement is observed. However, similar changes may be seen after intraparenchymal hemorrhage, tumor resection, and radiation. Moreover, the entire MRI profile and ring enhancement may be influenced by steroid use.

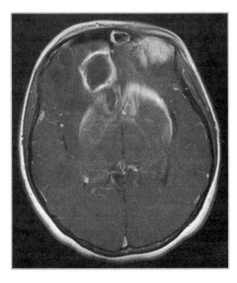

Figure 22.1 The typical computed tomography findings of a brain abscess.

Therefore, as with all other postoperative infections, with brain abscess there are no definitive diagnostic studies.

Treatment consists of surgery plus prolonged intravenous antibiotic therapy. As noted above, the first step is to have a high level of suspicion for the diagnosis. CSF sampling by lumbar puncture may be not only dangerous because of high intracranial pressure, but also unlikely to yield a positive culture. With the usual scenario of broad antibiotic treatment in a patient suspected to have a postoperative abscess, even ventricular CSF sampling may not be rewarding.

Direct surgery is the preferred approach with the recognition that the postoperative abscess is likely to be more complex in its configuration than the new disorder. The operating surgeon needs to carefully review the imaging studies and be familiar with the original operation and any distorted anatomy. The goal is to drain pus, debride necrotic tissue, and relieve increased intracranial pressure (ICP). In extreme conditions, the bone flap will be not replaced to lower ICP. Potentially, cranial decompression may require that the original skin and bone flap be enlarged. Moreover, the removed bone flap may be contaminated and therefore might need to be discarded.

An alternative to open craniotomy is aspiration using stereotactic assistance. Such an approach, although less invasive, may be less effective because of the distorted postoperative anatomy. Moreover, the multiloculated postoperative abscess may be less amendable to effective needle drainage and require multiple aspirations.

Once a specimen has been obtained, the usual preoperative broad-spectrum antibiotics can be narrowed and a targeted treatment tailored to the results of culture. However, in 30% of cases (Mampalam and Rosenblum 1988) the patient will have been on broad-spectrum antibiotics for a considerable time and, consequently, culture specimens may be sterile. In these cases, empirical broad antibiotic treatment will be utilized.

As in the treatment of subdural empyema and bone flap osteomyelitis, prolonged antibiotic treatment will be required. Consequently, the patient is at risk for the development of system complications and superinfections such as *Clostridium difficile*. In addition, steroids, frequently used in an attempt to ameliorate brain edema, have the potential for affecting wound healing and impairing systemic responses.

Serial CT and/or MRI is useful to determine the success or failure of treatment. Failure of the abscess to regress or, conversely, any suggestion of enlargement of the area of inflammation or brain edema over time (i.e., days to weeks) should be considered as indicating failure of treatment and should suggest the need to consider re-exploration and drainage and/or alteration in antibiotic therapy.

Lastly, brain abscess are highly epileptogenic. Whereas anticonvulsant therapy has not been proven to prevent epilepsy in the long term, such drugs should be routinely given during the acute period to prevent seizures. In a patient with high ICP, a seizure can be fatal. The downside of anticonvulsant therapy is that these drugs can cause fever and systemic responses, and therefore add confusion to the clinical picture of a patient being treated for a CNS infection (Temkin et al. 1990).

Shunt infections

Of all clean neurosurgical procedures, operations designed to permanently divert CSF, so-called "shunt" operations, have the highest (3–10%) postoperative infection rates (Kestle and Walker 2005). Shunt operations, although appearing to be not technically challenging, are nevertheless complex and fraught with difficulties. In patients over the long term, as measured in years, 40% of shunts fail or need revision, with infections being the primary cause (Casey et al. 1997, Gupta et al. 2007). Neurosurgeons have therefore intensively analyzed shunts, shunt surgery, and postoperative sequelae in both children and adult patients. However, most of the data concerning shunt infections stem from the former group.

Under normal conditions, CSF is mainly formed by the choroid plexus in the cerebral ventricles and then circulates through the ventricular system and the subarachnoid space. Egress of the CSF from the CNS occurs through the arachnoid villi, which are primarily located in the walls of the cerebral venous sinuses. Obstruction in any part of this pathway and process will result in hydrocephalus.

Shunt operations are designed to overcome obstruction of CSF flow, lower ICP, and decrease ventricular enlargement. Such operations involve the insertion of a catheter into the lateral cerebral ventricle, usually by means of a small frontal skin flap and burr hole. The ventricular catheter is then attached to a valve, which regulates CSF egress, and the valve is positioned subcutaneously under the skin flap. The distal end of the valve is in turn attached to a small catheter, which is tunneled subcutaneously from the frontal flap down the neck and chest and inserted into the abdomen. Multiple variations in approaches exist, each having advocates and detractors. In all cases, the location of the skin opening should be designed to avoid placement of the shunt valve and tubing directly under the surgical incision.

There are multiple factors (see Table 22.2) that have been identified as contributing to shunt infections (Casey et al. 1997). As with all surgical procedures, there are systemic factors, such as nutrition, diabetes, and immunological status, that will contribute to the likelihood of a postoperative shunt infection. The age of the patient has been shown to be related to the infection rate, with neonates and younger children having a higher risk than older children and adults (Casey et al. 1997). Prolonged preoperative hospitalizations, skin breakdown, and systemic infections (i.e., urinary tract infections) have also been suggested as being related to shunt infections.

As most post-shunt infections are recognized within several (1–3) months after surgery and involve skin organisms, inoculation and colonization during surgery appear to be the initiating event (Burke 1963, Casey et al. 1997). Therefore, avoidance of surgical contamination has been the main means of preventing postoperative shunt infection. Neurosurgeons have utilized a variety of intraoperative measures to decrease shunt infections, such as double gloving and a "no-touch" technique for handling the shunt valve and tubing. Generous removal of hair with clippers (but not shaving) in the operating room has been advocated to avoid potential contamination by a stray hair, especially in adults, has been advocated in contrast to minimal hair removal in most other cranial surgery. Only the use of perioperative antibiotics has been rigorously studied and, by meta-analysis, shown to be affected (Haines and Walters 1994).

Wound breakdown is highly associated with the development of a shunt infection and all incisions need to be carefully planned to avoid having the shunt valve and tubing located directly under the surgical site. Surgical technique plays an important role in complication avoidance in shunt surgery. Therefore, the surgeon needs to remain vigilant to tissue handling, avoidance of skin and subcutaneous injury, and careful wound closure.

The symptoms and signs of a shunt infection will be influenced by the age of the patient. Infants may present with a range of findings, from subtle fussiness to a catastrophic picture of fully developed meningitis and elevated ICP. Adult patients, usually treated for normal pressure hydrocephalus, may revert to their pre-shunt inability to ambulate, decreased mental capacity, and/or urinary incontinence. Local wound inflammation should always be considered as a postoperative shunt infection. Ventricular enlargement on imaging studies indicates a shunt failure that may be secondary to an infection. Repetitive shunt "failures" should always raise the concern of a low-grade, indolent infection, usually caused by skin flora such as *Staphylococcus epidermis* (Casey et al. 1997).

Confirmation of a shunt infection, in the absence of wound problems, is usually established by CSF culture. CSF profile alone (i.e., cell count, differential, glucose, and protein) may be misleading in both directions: Non-infected CSF may reveal altered cell count, glucose, and protein, whereas infected CSF, especially in the setting of an indolent organism, may appear benign or equivocal. CSF is usually obtained by percutaneous tapping of a reservoir that is in series with the valve. Lack of growth in the CSF does not rule out the presence of an infection – the absence of proof does not constitute the proof of absence. Prolonged culture of CSF might be required to establish an infection and isolate an organism, especially with an indolent organism. In some cases of distal infections (abdominal site), CSF culture may not reveal an infection, but abdominal ultrasonography will reveal cystic collections.

Multiple strategies have been proposed for the treatment of shunt infections (James et al. 1980). In all cases, appropriate antibiotics must be administered, usually for a protracted duration. The most successful approach requires two operations. In the first, the existing infected shunt is removed and replaced with a ventricular catheter that allows CSF drainage and frequent assessment of CSF profile and culture. After sterilization has been achieved, a second operation is performed and a new shunt placed. This multi-operation approach has been shown by series and randomized trial to achieve the highest cure rate (James et al. 1980).

An alternative surgical strategy involves only one operation. In this approach, antibiotics are continued with the existing shunt in place and CSF being sampled frequently from the shunt reservoir. When CSF sterilization is achieved, the old shunt is removed in its entirety and replaced with a new ventricular catheter, valve, and shunt tubing. This approach avoids a second procedure, but has a slightly lower success rate (90%) compared with the two-stage strategy (100%) (James et al. 1980).

Lastly, a non-surgical strategy involves treatment with antibiotics alone. This method of treatment has only a 30% likelihood of achieving success and the length of hospital stay is longer than with either surgical approach (James et al. 1980). A factor in the low rate of success for medical treatment alone may be the observation that many of the usual organisms (i.e., coagulase-negative staphylococci and *Staphylococcus aureus*) responsible for shunt infections have the capability to form a protective biofilm or slime around the shunt tubing (Tessier 2011). Antibiotics are less able to penetrate this slime matrix which is devoid of vascular supply. Moreover, organisms immersed in this slime become less metabolically active and enter into a stationary phase of growth, further impeding the effectiveness of antibiotics. Both of these factors contribute to the reduced cure rate with antibiotic therapy alone (Tessier 2011)

POSTOPERATIVE SPINE INFECTIONS

In contrast to post-craniotomy infections, infections after spinal operations are less common even though the frequency of spinal surgery is considerably higher on a population basis than cranial procedures (Davis 1994, McClelland and Hall 2007). Furthermore, postspinal surgical infections tend to be more superficial and less likely to result in primary CNS sequelae (McClelland and Hall 2007). The lesser rate of infection may be related to the fact that most spine operations do not violate the dural covering of the spinal cord or cauda equina. Thus the isolation and integrity of the CNS remain intact and infectious processes tend to be primarily located in the surrounding bone, disk, soft tissue, and muscle.

Risk factors for infections after spinal surgery

Patient risk factors for postspinal infections (see Table 22.3) are not dissimilar to those factors that have been noted earlier for infections after craniotomy, e.g., increased age, malnutrition, obesity, immunological compromise, diabetes mellitus, trauma, prolonged pre-surgical hospitalization, and excessive alcohol use have all been found to be associated with postoperative infections after spinal surgery (Weinstein et al. 2000, Olsen et al. 2003, Fang et al. 2005). The presence of malignancy has been demonstrated to increase the risk of postoperative spinal infections to >20% (McPhee et al. 1998, Weinstein et al. 2000).

The interactions and interdependency of these multiple factors for postspinal infections are unclear, e.g., malignancy is associated with an altered immunological response and, in some patients, malnutrition. Prolonged pre-surgical hospitalization may reflect a patient's concurrent diseases (i.e., cancer, diabetes, to mention a few) and/or nutritional status. Obesity may be an epiphenomenon related to length of surgery because surgical durations in obese individuals are frequently longer than in non-obese patients. Additional factors playing a role in the obese patient could be excessive retraction, larger deep space, and more complex and difficult closures. Obese patients are more likely to have diabetes and therefore the increased risks associated with obesity may reflect only the underlying metabolic and microvascular effects of glucose intolerance. Patients with diabetes undergoing spinal surgery have been reported to have a 24% chance of developing a postoperative infection (Simpson et al. 1993, Fang et al. 2005).

Prolonged tobacco use is associated with osteoporosis and an increased risk of degenerative spine change. In addition, smokers have an increased risk of having a postoperative infection after surgery (Sorensen et al. 2003, Fang et al. 2005). The mechanisms involved are unclear, but may be related to well-described neutrophil malfunction and/or decreased arterial levels of oxygen and resultant tissue hypoxia observed in smokers.

Surgical risk factors are similar to those observed with craniotomy, but are mainly correlated with the severity of the surgical procedure itself. Thus, the surgical length (>5 h), extent of exposure, and amount of blood loss (>1000 ml) have all been associated with increased chances of a patient developing a postoperative infection (Weinstein et al. 2000, Olsen et al. 2003, Fang et al. 2005). In addition, allografts and instrumentation have been shown to increase the postoperative infection risk (Weinstein et al. 2000, Fang et al. 2005).

Surgical approaches have been observed to be related to the risk of developing a postoperative infection (Weinstein et al. 2000, Olsen et al. 2003), e.g., the risks for posterior single level discectomy alone, lumbar laminectomy without fusion, and lumbar laminectomy with non-instrumented fusions are <1%, 2%, and >2%, respectively (Davis 1994, Fang et al. 2005). Instrumentation increases the risk for lumbar procedures to 3–8% (Levi et al. 1997, Weinstein et al. 2000). Anterior approaches in the lumbar spine, while having a higher complication rate, do not appear to have an increased infection rate, although most series are small in number (Levi et al. 1997). Combined posterior and anterior approaches appeared to have the highest infection rate which may reflect the length of surgery, blood loss and replacement, and other factors, rather than the complexity of the surgery itself (Olsen et al. 2003, Fang et al. 2005). The spinal level involved does not appear to influence the rate of postoperative infection, although the anterior approach to the cervical spine routinely reports very low infection rates. On the other hand, anterior cervical spinal surgery has the potential for an esophageal injury and the development of devastating mediastinitis. The recent development of endoscopic techniques may allow a reduction in postoperative spinal infections.

Prevention

Assuming that the patient and surgical factors listed above are causally related to the risks of developing a postoperative infection, the surgeon preoperatively should maximize the patient's nutritional status, encourage weight loss, and effectively treat any systemic or local infections. Cessation of smoking has been demonstrated to lower postoperative infections, but the duration of non-smoking is unclear.

Prophylactic antibiotics have been demonstrated by meta-analysis to lower postoperative infection rates, although individual studies have reported both non-supportive and supportive data (Horwitz and Curtin 1975, Bullock et al. 1988, Dempsey et al. 1988, Barker 2002). Nevertheless, perioperative antibiotic therapy has been considered the standard of care since the 1970s. Antibiotics ideally should be administered 30–60 min before skin incision to allow achievement of appropriate blood and tissue levels. Additional doses should be given every 4–6 h and with blood loss (>1500 ml), but discontinued after 24 h. Prolonged administration has been associated with the development of resistant organisms and superinfections.

Three are many other intraoperative measures that may decrease postoperative infections, e.g., during prolonged surgery, the surgeon can periodically release retractors to lessen tissue pressure and increase tissue blood flow. The use of copious irrigation and the addition of bacitracin to the irrigation fluid have been advocated in many studies. Chang et al. (2006) have demonstrated in a randomized trial that dilute (0.35%) povidone–iodine (Betadine) reduced post-bone grafting infections to 0% from 3.4%. On the other hand, prophylactic antibiotics for the duration of drain placement have not been shown to be effective in lowering the infection rate.

Diagnosis

The diagnosis of postoperative infections after spine surgery can be challenging. In comparison to the post-craniotomy state, the post-spinal surgery clinical picture is not as confusing, and without the overlay of neurological changes related to the initial surgical intervention into the brain. The baseline neurological status of the postoperative spinal patient should, in most cases, be unaffected by the surgery and be similar or improved compared with the preoperative clinical state. Delayed deterioration from this postoperative state should suggest the possible diagnosis of an infection, although there are other causes for neurological deterioration such as displacement of hardware or change in bony alignment. In many cases where the clinical and neurological status remain stable, the surgeon will be alerted to postoperative infection by systemic signs and radiological changes.

Unlike post-craniotomy infections, the timing of postspinal surgical infections is often more delayed. Consequently, the systemic changes related to surgical intervention, such as ESR, WBC, and CRP, have usually returned to or are tending toward normal by the time a post-surgical spinal infection is evident. As indicated earlier, in the postoperative period, CRP and ESR start to return to baseline by the first postoperative week and are usually in the normal range by the

second and third weeks, respectively. Consequently, persistent elevation or an increase in these parameters in the setting of an elevated fever suggests the diagnosis of a postoperative infection.

Radiological and imaging studies can be useful in assisting in the diagnosis, but postoperative expected changes on plain films, CT, and MRI may be difficult to separate from the findings with infection, especially in the early stages of an infection. Comparison of sequential postoperative studies will provide the best approach and should be evaluated in the context of systemic markers of infection as outlined above. Postoperative baseline imaging studies may also document alignment and instrument placement, but whether such studies are cost-effective is unclear.

In general, 2–3 weeks are required before an infectious process will sufficiently alter bone, disk elements, and/or the disk to be seen on plain radiographs. CT is more sensitive to these changes and is also more likely to diagnose paravertebral collections and other soft-tissue changes. Contrast-enhanced CT will increase the chances of imaging changes suggestive of a postoperative infection. CT can also assist in surgical planning.

However, among imaging techniques, MRI is the most useful in diagnosing a postoperative infection; specificity and sensitivity in this setting are >90%. Plain and contrast-enhanced studies on multiple sequences have a high probability of revealing changes in the bone marrow, end plate, disk and disk elements, and the development of paravertebral collections. The latter is the best indicator of a postoperative infection, but to document "change" requires a baseline postoperative study.

Treatment

Optimal treatment is critically dependent on early establishment of the diagnosis. Less clear among treatment options is the definitive treatment. With regard to chemotherapy, in most circumstances, the patient will already be on antibiotics effective against the most common responsible organism, *Staphylococcus aureus*. Not infrequently, these hospital-acquired infections are due to meticillin-resistant *S. aureus*. Delayed infections are more likely to be a result of low virulent skin contaminants. Therefore, antibiotic choice ideally depends on culture and sensitivity.

Surgical debridement is dictated by location and extent of the infection, but definitive clinical approach has not been clearly established in randomized trials. Superficial wound infections usually respond to antibiotics alone. Discitis likewise responds to antibiotic therapy alone, but the causative agent can usually be established by blood cultures or percutaneous biopsy. The latter usually involves intraoperative navigation or utilizing CT direction. Biopsies in the lumbar and cervical regions are less problematic than in the thoracic spine where endoscopic techniques may be beneficial. The duration of antibiotic therapy has not been established definitively, but 6 weeks of intravenous therapy followed by an addition 6 weeks of oral therapy is a frequent treatment paradigm.

Infections that do not respond to medical therapy and/or have caused wound dehiscence, significant bone or soft-tissue destruction, or fluid collection, especially in deep aspects of the surgical bed, should be treated with surgical debridement. Such an approach also allows reassessment by culture of the causative agent. Obviously, if stabilization has been affected by the infection, realignment should also be addressed with reoperation. Considering the complexities of the clinical scenario, thoughtful planning, consideration of all contingencies, and careful evaluation of imaging studies are required before reoperation. In general, all aspects of the previous surgical field should be exposed and necrotic and purulent tissue vigorously removed. Multiple specimens should be sent for culture at all levels of the wound. Various techniques for irrigation, both with and without antibiotics and during and after debridement, have been advocated, but none has been rigorously compared. Another area of controversy relates to whether stabilizing hardware should be removed in the setting of a postoperative infection. Older steel instrumentation has been associated with recurrent infections whereas more recent titanium constructs appear to have a lower likelihood of incurring a persistent infection. However, even with titanium implants, reoccurrence of infection can occur.

Multiple options exist for wound closure after surgery for postoperative infections. Drains of various types are routinely placed to facilitate decompression of residual fluctuancy. In some cases, secondary closure will be required, although every effort should be made to approximate the wound in a primary fashion. In severe cases, a planned staged "second-look" surgery may be necessary. In all cases, frequent monitoring of systemic parameters and imaging studies are required to document recovery.

■ REFERENCES

Barker FG 2nd. Efficacy of prophylactic antibiotics for craniotomy: a meta-analysis. *Neurosurgery* 1994;**35**:484–90; discussion 491.

Barker FG 2nd. Efficacy of prophylactic antibiotic therapy in spinal surgery: a meta-analysis. *Neurosurgery* 2002;**51**:391–400; discussion 400.

Bruce JN, Bruce SS. Preservation of bone flaps in patients with postcraniotomy infections. *J Neurosurg* 2003;**98**:1203–7.

Bullock R, van Dellen JR, Ketelbey W, et al. A double-blind placebo-controlled trial of perioperative prophylactic antibiotics for elective neurosurgery. *J Neurosurg* 1988;**69**:687–91.

Burke JF. Identification of the sources of staphylococci contaminating the surgical wound during operation. *Ann Surg* 1963;**158**: 898–904.

Carmel PW, Greif LK. The aseptic meningitis syndrome: a complication of posterior fossa surgery. *Pediatr Neurosurg* 1993;**19**: 276–280.

Carpenter J, Stapleton S, Holliman R. Retrospective analysis of 49 cases of brain abscess and review of the literature. *Eur J Clin Microbiol Infect Dis* 2007;**26**:1–11.

Casey AT, Kimmings EJ, Kleinlugtebeld AD, et al. The long-term outlook for hydrocephalus in childhood. A ten-year cohort study of 155 patients. *Pediatr Neurosurg* 1997;**27**:63–70.

Chang FY, Chang MC, Wang ST, et al. Can povidone-iodine solution be used safely in a spinal surgery? *Eur Spine J* 2006;**15**:1005–14.

Davis RA. A long-term outcome analysis of 984 surgically treated herniated lumbar discs. *J Neurosurg* 1994;**80**:415–21.

Dempsey R, Rapp RP, Young B, Johnston S, Tibbs P. Prophylactic parenteral antibiotics in clean neurosurgical procedures: a review. *J Neurosurg* 1988;**69**:52–7.

Fang A, Hu SS, Enders N, et al. Risk factors for infection after spinal surgery. *Spine* 2005;**30**:1460–5.

Farrell CJ, Hoh BL, isculli ML, Henson JW, Barker FG, Curry WT. Limitations of diffusion-weighted imaging in the diagnosis of postoperative infections. *Neurosurgery* 2008;**62**:577–83.

Fry DE. Basic aspects of and general problems in surgical infections. *Surg Infect (Larchmt)* 2001;**2**:(suppl 1):S3–11.

Gantz NM. Nosocomial central nervous system infections. In: Mayhall CG (ed.), *Hospital Epidemiology and Infection Control*. Philadelphia: Lippincott Williams & Wilkins, 2004: 415–39.

Gupta N, Park J, Solomon C, Kranz DA, Wrensch M, Wu YW. Long-term outcomes in patients with treated hydrocephalus. *J Neurosurg* 2007;**106**(5 suppl):334–9.

Haines SJ, Walters BC. Antibiotic prophylaxis for cerebrospinal fluid shunts: a metanalysis. *Neurosurgery* 1994;**34**:87–92.

Hlavin ML, Kaminski HJ, Fenstermaker RA, et al. Intracranial suppuration: a modern decade of postoperative subdural empyema and epidural abscess. *Neurosurgery* 1994;**34**:974–80; discussion 980.

Horwitz NH, Curtin JA. Prophylactic antibiotics and wound infections following laminectomy for lumber disc herniation. *J Neurosurg* 1975;**43**:727–31.

James HE, Walsh JW, Wilson HD. Prospective randomized study of therapy in cerebrospinal fluid shunt infection. *Neurosurgery* 1980;**7**:459–63.

Kestle JR, Walker ML. A multicenter prospective cohort study of the Strata valve for the management of hydrocephalus in pediatric patients. *J Neurosurg* 2005;**102**(2 suppl):141–5.

Korinek AM. Risk factors for neurosurgical site infections after craniotomy: a prospective multicenter study of 2944 patients. The French Study Group of Neurosurgical Infections, the SEHP, and the C-CLIN Paris-Nord. Service Epidemiologie Hygiene et Prevention. *Neurosurgery* 1997;**41**:1073–9; discussion 1079.*

Kurz A, Sessler DI, Lenhardt R. Perioperative normothermia to reduce the incidence of surgical-wound infection and shorten hospitalization. Study of Wound Infection and Temperature Group. *N Engl J Med* 1996;**334**:1209–15.

Levi AD, Dickman CA, Sonntag VK. Management of postoperative infections after spinal instrumentation. *J Neurosurg* 1997;**86**:975–80.

McClelland S 3rd, Hall WA. Postoperative central nervous system infection: incidence and associated factors in 2111 neurosurgical procedures. *Clin Infect Dis* 2007;**45**:55–9.

McPhee IB, Williams RP, Swanson CE. Factors influencing wound healing after surgery for metastatic disease of the spine. *Spine* 1998;**23**:726–32; discussion 732.

Mampalam TJ, Rosenblum ML. Trends in the management of bacterial brain abscesses: a review of 102 cases over 17 years. *Neurosurgery* 1988;**23**:451–8.

Mangram AJ, Horan TC, Pearson ML, et al. Guideline for prevention of surgical site infection, 1999. Hospital Infection Control Practices Advisory Committee. *Infect Control Hosp Epidemiol* 1999;**20**:250–78; quiz 279–80.

Nisbet M, Briggs S, Fresard A, et al. *Propionibacterium acnes*: an under-appreciated cause of post-neurosurgical infection. *J Antimicrob Chemother* 2007;**60**:1097–103.

Olsen MA, Mayfield J, Lauryssen C, et al. Risk factors for surgical site infection in spinal surgery. *J Neurosurg* 2003;**98**(2 suppl):149–55.

Post EM, Modesti LM. Subacute postoperative subdural empyema. *J Neurosurg* 1981;**55**:761–5.

Simpson JM, Silveri CP, Balderston RA, et al. The results of operations on the lumbar spine in patients who have diabetes mellitus. *J Bone Joint Surg Am* 1993;**75**:1823–9.

Sorensen LT, Karlsmark T, Gottrup F. Abstinence from smoking reduces incisional wound infection: a randomized controlled trial. *Ann Surg* 2003;**238**:1–5.

Temkin NR, Dikmen SS, Wilensky AJ, Keihm J, Chabal S, Winn HR. A randomized, double-blind study of phenytoin for the prevention of post-traumatic seizures. *N Engl J Med* 1990;**323**:497–502.

Tessier JM. Basic science of central nervous sytem infections. Winn HR (ed.), *Youmans' Textbook of Neurological Surgery*, 6th edn. Philadelphia, PA: Saunders/Elsevier, 2011: 544–58.

Todd MM, Hindman BJ, Clarke WR, Torner JC. Mild intraoperative hypothermia during surgery for intracranial aneurysm. *N Engl J Med* 2005;**352**:135–45.

Tunkel AR. Subdural empyema, epidural abscess, and suppurative intracranial thrombophlebitis. In: Douglas RG, Bennett JE et al. (eds), *Mandell, Douglas, and Bennett's Principles and Practice of Infectious Diseases*, 6th edn. Philadelphia, PA: Elsevier/Churchill Livingstone, 2005:1164–71.

Weinstein MA, McCabe JP, Cammisa FP. Postoperative spinal wound infection: a review of 2,391 consecutive index procedures. *J Spinal Disord* 2000;**13**:422–6.

Wimmer C, Gluch H, Franzreb M, Ogon M. Predisposing factors for infection in spine surgery: a survey of 850 spinal procedures. *J Spinal Disord* 1998;**11**:124–8.

Winn HR, Mendes M, Moore P, Wheeler C, Rodeheaver G. Production of experimental brain abscess in the rat. *J Neurosurg* 1979;**51**:685–90.

Yang, KY, Chang WN, Ho JT, et al. Postneurosurgical nosocomial bacterial brain abscess in adults. *Infection* 2006;**34**: 247–51.

Young RF, Lawner PM. Perioperative antibiotic prophylaxis for prevention of postoperative neurosurgical infections. A randomized clinical trial. *J Neurosurg* 1987;**66**:701–5.

Zarrouk V, Vassor I, Bert F, et al. Evaluation of the management of postoperative aseptic meningitis. *Clin Infect Dis* 2007;**44**:1555–9.

Chapter 23 Bioterrorism

Donald E. Fry

A reality of the current world is that microbes or microbial products may be used as weapons to inflict harm on civilian populations. In the last decade anthrax spores have been distributed through the mail service to political targets. In the current era of genetic engineering, the possibilities of manipulating microbes to have unusually virulent characteristics is a reality that makes bacteria and viruses potential weapons in military or civilian events.

Surgical care will be required for patients exposed to microbes used as weapons. Surgeons will be participants in disaster planning and implementation. They will be mobilized when disaster events occur and will need to be informed about potential agents and processes of microbial decontamination. As biological agents as weapons pose logistical challenges of delivery by the assailant, it would not be surprising to find biological payloads accompanying conventional explosive devices as a variant on the concept of the "dirty" bomb (Fry et al. 2005).

The disaster plan of communities must take into consideration the possibilities of biological weapons in civilian populations. The list of potential biological agents is extensive with the virulence of the putative pathogens being quite variable (**Table 23.1**) The full scope of planning, recognition, triage of patients, development of alternative patient care sites, and decontamination is beyond the scope of this presentation and is detailed elsewhere (Fry 2006). This chapter focuses on the reality of potential biological pathogens and their management.

ANTHRAX

Anthrax has been an infectious disease that has received the greatest amount of attention as a biological weapon. Anthrax infection is caused by *Bacillus anthracis,* a Gram-positive aerobic rod that exists as a spore when exposed to adverse environmental conditions (Sweeney et al. 2011). As is true of all spore-forming bacteria, *B. anthracis* transitions into the vegetative form if environment conditions exist to promote growth and replication. The spores are ubiquitous in soil and have traditionally posed problems for lethal infections of cattle and

Table 23.1 Categorization of the currently recognized bioterrorism threats (Centers for Disease Control 2012).

Potential agents of interest	Comments
Category A	**Category A agents are considered of greatest threat to be used in a bioterrorism attack**
Anthrax	Easily disseminated, airborne, fulminant inhalational disease
Botulinum toxin	Fine powder; extremely potent biological toxin
Bubonic plague	High mortality rate; human-to-human transmission
Smallpox	Vulnerable, unvaccinated population; human-to-human transmission
Tularemia	Incapacitating disease with a low death rate
Viral hemorrhagic fever	Fulminant and highly fatal illness
Category B	**Category B agents are easily disseminated but low mortality rates**
Brucellosis	Small inoculum for infection; protracted infection
Epsilon toxin of *Clostridium perfringens*	Airborne powder
Food poisoning (e.g., *Salmonella*)	Malicious contamination of fresh fruits and vegetables
Water poisoning (cholera)	Potential contaminant of drinking water supplies
Glanders/Melioidosis	Small inoculum and high mortality with acute infection
Psittacosis	Severe pulmonary infection by this natural avian pathogen
Q fever	Small inoculum for infection, protracted clinical course
Ricin	Easily produced castor bean product
Staphylococcal enterotoxin B	Potent airborne powder
Typhus	An intracellular parasitic rickettsial infection
Equine encephalitis	Easily grown and stored; very infectious to humans
Category C	**Emerging pathogens with potential for production and dissemination**
Nipah virus	Encephalitis or respiratory infection; human-to-human transmission
Hantavirus	Airborne pathogen with a hemorrhagic fever clinical picture
Influenza viruses	Selected influenza viruses (H1N1) are severe and contagious
Severe acute respiratory syndrome	An airborne transmitted coronavirus

sheep. Anthrax infection was a major focus of Robert Koch in proving the germ theory of disease, and anthrax was used by Pasteur in the development of a vaccine for prevention of infection in grazing animals.

Anthrax infection occurs in three separate scenarios. Cutaneous anthrax occurs when spores contaminate an open wound and cause a necrotizing local infection. The black eschar of cutaneous anthrax (Greek *anthracis* for coal) was the first recognized infection of this pathogen in humans, and was noted to be "wool sorters' disease" among workers handling spore-laden wool from contaminated sheep. The infection is painful, tends to spread progressively, and is fatal in about 20% of untreated cases. Effective treatment has reduced death rates to 1%.

Gastrointestinal anthrax follows the ingestion of a critical number of spores, which survive the acidity of the stomach and then result in invasive infection from the gut. This is an uncommon cause of infection in humans but extrapolation from animal observations indicates that the spore is likely transported to regional lymph nodes where the vegetative form of the bacteria results in invasive infection. This is likely to have a very high mortality rate (>50%) but epidemiological studies in humans are not available.

Inhalational anthrax is of greatest concern as a biological weapon. The spore is very small (1 μm) which escapes the normal mucociliary defense mechanisms of the lung. Inhalation of as few at 2500 spores is sufficient to cause pulmonary anthrax infection (Inglesby et al. 1999). The spores are transported by macrophage cells to regional lymph nodes, where they germinate and cause invasive infection. The bacteria produce exotoxins and have a capsule that retards phagocytosis of the vegetative form. Fulminate bacteremia occurs from the pulmonary lymph nodes with a resultant systemic infection that is uniformly fatal without prompt treatment. Thus, it must be understood that anthrax-infected patients have the lung as the entry site of the spore, but the infection originates within the regional lymph nodes. This is not a pulmonary infection. The established infection is not contagious to others because neither spores nor vegetative organisms are transmitted from the patient's lung to the environment. The risk to healthcare workers would be ineffective decontamination of the acute contaminated patients from spores in clothing and on the surface of the patient, and not bacteria transmitted from infected patients.

Clinical infection from anthrax is quite uncommon, and accordingly the diagnosis of the infection is difficult. The cutaneous infection has the initial appearance of a cutaneous abscess, which evolves into an umbilicated black eschar (**Figure 23.1**). This is a painless lesion that differentiates it from the cutaneous infection of community-associated meticillin-resistant *Staphylococcus aureus* or a brown recluse spider bite. The evolving local cutaneous infection becomes invasive with clinical lymphangitis and lymphadenitis. Lymphatic and vascular invasion can result in systemic infection. The anthrax bacilli are readily identified on blood agar cultures. The occurrence of cutaneous anthrax infection in the absence of exposure to livestock should trigger concern about malicious dissemination of the spores. Ingestion of the spores may result in the black eschar lesions in the oropharynx, but true gastrointestinal anthrax will have non-specific abdominal pain and tenderness and is difficult to recognize. The inhalational form of the disease begins as a flu-like syndrome with fever, leukocytosis, malaise, and rapidly evolves to a systemic inflammatory response syndrome (SIRS). The chest radiograph may demonstrate hilar adenopathy and characteristically evolves into the typical appearance of adult respiratory distress. Pneumonic infiltrates would be evidence against inhalational anthrax. Blood cultures are positive, but bacteremic patients have a natural history of infection that will likely be fatal before results are available. The massive bacteremia

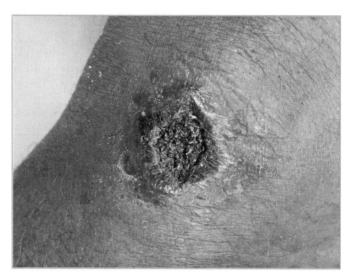

Figure 23.1 The black necrotic lesion of cutaneous anthrax infection. (From http://phil.cdc.gov/phil/details.asp, courtesy of CDC/James H. Steele. ID no.: 2033, 1962.)

from systemic anthrax infection is illustrated by positive Gram stains of blood that are positive for the Gram-positive rod. The reality is the inhalational form of anthrax will be diagnosed only *post mortem* and must trigger an investigation into the source of the spores.

Antibiotics and supportive care are the principal treatments for anthrax infection. Penicillin (12–24 MU/day) or doxycycline (200 mg initially; then 100 mg every 12 h) are the approved treatments. In vitro data would support the use of quinolones (e.g., ciprofloxacin 400 mg every 8–12 h). A theoretical case can be made for the addition of clindamycin as a second drug to any of the above choices to inhibit exotoxin production by the anthrax bacilli. Effective antibiotic therapy for cutaneous anthrax before systemic dissemination is effective with a 1% mortality rate. Inhalational anthrax will have mortality rates exceeding 90%.

Postexposure preventive antibiotic administration is recommended, although clinical effectiveness is unproven. Oral doxycycline or ciprofloxacin is associated with efficient bioavailability after oral administration and is a recommended choice. An anthrax vaccine has been developed, but requires six doses over 18 months for recommended effectiveness. Annual booster doses are required after full immunization. The vaccine is considered only for use in high-risk military personnel.

Infection control with a suspected anthrax exposure event is to effectively decontaminate the patients by standard methods. Clothing, hair, and cutaneous surface contamination are the risk of spores to healthcare personnel, and these risks are managed with standard decontamination procedures. It is likely that public exposure events may not be appreciated until infected patients are presented to the healthcare facility. Fear and panic among healthcare personnel require the repeated emphasis that the effectively decontaminated patient with inhalational anthrax infection is not infectious to others.

■ Plague infection

Yersinia pestis is the pathogen of bubonic plague that has ravaged Europe and Asia with pandemics in centuries past. This Gram-negative rod has been speculated as a biological weapon because it is an airborne pathogen, it requires a small inoculum of bacteria to cause clinical infection, the evolution of the pulmonary form is a fulminant infection with a high mortality rate, but most significant is the efficiency of human-to-human transmission (Inglesby et al. 2000). *Y. pestis* has virulence due to surface antigens that facilitate its binding to pulmonary epithelium, and its endotoxins and secreted exotoxin products. Amplification of virulence and enhancement of antimicrobial resistance can be engineered by the use of plasmids.

Infection with the plague bacillus can occur through two routes. Cutaneous infection is the classic bubonic plague. Flea bites were the traditional route of inoculation for cutaneous infection, but inoculation of cuts or abrasions from environmental contamination is possible. Invasive cutaneous infection results in lymphatic dissemination with the classic "buboe" developing in the regional lymph nodes. The lymphadenopathy measures up to 10 cm in size, and the infected lymph nodes may ulcerate and drain. Necrosis and ulceration are uncommon at the primary site of cutaneous infection. The progression of infection leads to dissemination via the lymphatics with systemic infection and death in 50% of cases. Cutaneous infection may be directly invasive into the circulation and bypass the classic lymphatic manifestation of infection. The rapid vascular dissemination of the infection leads to ischemic necrosis of digits (**Figure 23.2**), systemic evidence of severe infection, and death in nearly all who do not have lymphatic containment of the primary cutaneous infection.

Although naturally occurring cutaneous plague infection is quite uncommon, it does have a characteristic presentation. Recognition of the large buboes should be sufficient to raise the index of suspicion. Gram stains of drainage from ulcerated nodes, or aspirated specimens from the enlarged lymph nodes, may identify the Gram-negative rod. Cultures by standard methods from Gram-negative bacteria will confirm the pathogen. Other diagnostic methods with antigen detection or polymerase chain reaction (PCR) assays might be useful in early detection among patients suspected of exposure, but are unlikely to be of value in those in whom clinical infection is identified.

Pulmonary infection is the second and most important route of infection when considering this bacterium as a biological weapon. Pulmonary infection begins 2–4 days after exposure, and has a characteristic pattern of symptoms that are similar to other community-acquired pneumonias. Cough, fever, dyspnea, and leukocytosis are present. Chest radiographs will identify bronchopneumonia. Without appropriate treatment, pulmonary infection results in dissemination

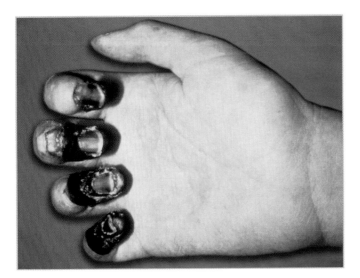

Figure 23.2 Digital necrosis due to plague infection. (From http://phil.cdc. gov/phil/details.asp, courtesy of CDC. ID no. 1957.)

and death in 24–48 h from onset of symptoms. Pulmonary aspirates will demonstrate Gram-negative rods on Gram stain. Sputum and blood cultures will identify the pathogen.

Recommended antibiotic therapy for both cutaneous and pulmonary infection is streptomycin, tetracycline, or doxycycline. Streptomycin is generally not available and other aminoglycoside choices are substituted. Quinolones have been used in experimental infections, but do not have a record of use in human infection. Tetracycline or doxycycline is recommended for postexposure prophylaxis. Ventilator support will be necessary for the pulmonary infections.

Infection control for pulmonary infections is important because of human transmission from expectorated, airborne organisms. This requires isolation of patients and full use of respiratory isolation procedures. With appropriate antibiotic therapy, the patients are generally thought to no longer be infectious by 48 h of treatment. Full and complete disinfection is necessary for rooms and all equipment used in the management of these patients.

■ Tularemia

Tularemia is caused by *Francisella tularensis*, which is an aerobic, Gram-negative coccobacillus. There are multiple subspecies variants of *F. tularensis*. It has been proposed as a biological weapon because the organism can be easily aerosolized and only a small inoculum of bacteria (<100) is necessary to cause human infection (Dennis et al. 2001). This clinical infection has a relatively low mortality rate among proposed bioweapons, but rather is an incapacitating infection that would pose an enormous logistical issue for management. It has been the focus of efforts to "weaponize" this pathogen by engineering resistant strains.

It is a naturally occurring infection in rabbits, squirrels, and other small mammals. It is transmitted to humans by mosquitoes and ticks, or from environmental inoculation of cutaneous wounds. *F. tularensis* is an intracellular parasite that infects macrophage cells, where it resides as an intracellular parasite. It retards intracellular killing by the host phagocytic cells due to a cellular capsule. It has recently been identified to infect erythrocytes (Horzempa et al. 2011). Intracellular replication leads to lysis of the host cell. The full scope of the virulence of this bacterium is not fully elucidated.

Tularemia infection occurs in different patterns. Local cutaneous infection follows skin inoculation and results in ulceration within 3–5 days. Lymphadenitis follows and regional lymph nodes become enlarged and tender. The infection from lymph nodes may ulcerate locally, or no ulceration may occur. Systemic access of bacteria proceeds from the lymph nodes. Oculoglandular infection may follow eye inoculation which results in a severe conjunctivitis syndrome with head- and neck-associated lymphadenopathy. Oropharngeal infection follows ingested of infected food or water and has been associated with ulceration, non-specific mucositis, and usually with regional lymphadenopathy. A typhoidal variant of tularemia occurs after cutaneous exposure where infection may have limited or no local manifestations or no lymphadenitis, and proceeds to a systemic infection with SIRS.

Inhalational tularemia is of greatest concern as a bioweapon. Infection follows 3–5 days after exposure, and follows either a pattern of severe fulminant pneumonia or a more protracted form of pulmonary infection. The infection pattern may demonstrate acute hemorrhagic edema with necrosis of lung parenchyma, or may have the indolent pattern of a caseating, granulomatous infection. Both patterns of pulmonary infection are associated with hilar adenopathy. In all forms of tularemia the infection has a variable rapidity of progression, and for many patients pursues a slow and indolent pattern. Human-to-human transmission has not been documented. Overall mortality rates are reported at 7%, but timely and effective treatment has reduced this rate to <2%.

Infections have a non-specific clinical presentation and make culture identification of the pathogen essential. The organism can be seen on Gram stains. Cultures of cutaneous exudates, sputum, and tissue samples from ulcerated lesions will recover the organism. Chocolate agar has been recommended. The organisms grow slowly in vitro and identification may take up to 5 days. Other diagnostic methods include fluorescent antibody stains, immunohistochemistry methods, and PCR identification from reference laboratories.

Naturally occurring pathogens are sensitive to aminoglycosides, and gentamicin is the recommended treatment. Therapy is recommended for a full 10 days. Doxycycline and quinolone antibiotics have also been used successfully for treatment. Relapse of infection has been a concern with the use of bacteriostatic drugs, and intravenous treatment has generally been recommended with a bactericidal agent (e.g., aminoglycoside). Tularemia infection responds promptly to antibiotic therapy and clinical failures must lead to an evaluation of the engineered resistant microbe. Standard infection control practices should be employed in managing patients. Oral doxycycline or ciprofloxacin has been recommended for postexposure prophylaxis for 14 days of administration. Effective disinfection practices are adequate for medical facilities and equipment after the treatment of tularemia.

Brucellosis

Brucellosis is a naturally occurring infection in sheep, goats, and cattle (Franco et al. 2007). Transmission to humans occurs from contract with infected animals or consumption of infected animal products (e.g., milk or cheese). Brucellosis is a suspected agent of bioterrorism because only small inocula are required for clinical infection, incubation time after exposure can be prolonged, diagnosis can be difficult, and the disease has a protracted course.

Human infection occurs from four different strains with *Brucella melitensis* as the most virulent strain. These bacteria are aerobic Gram-negative rods. A unique lipopolysaccharide with only modest pyrogenic effects is a major component of virulence. *Brucella* spp. are intracellular pathogens within macrophages and neutrophils.

Like other suspected bacterial bioweapons, brucellosis infection occurs in a cutaneous, gastrointestinal, or inhalational form. Cutaneous infection follows contact in a pre-existing open wound with infected animals, animal carcasses, or infected food products. Naturally occurring brucellosis infection commonly follows ingestion of the organisms. Inhalational disease occurs very uncommonly. Gastrointestinal and inhalational infections share the common pathophysiology of the pathogen being ingested but not killed, and then being transported to regional lymph nodes. Thus, the infection arises from the regional lymph nodes and is not primary to the gastrointestinal or pulmonary portal of entry. Clinical infection may not occur until 8 weeks after exposure.

Clinical brucellosis persists initially as a flu-like syndrome. Mild fever, myalgia, arthralgia, and malaise give the appearance of viral disease. The infection pursues a protracted course and dissemination is associated with visceral abscesses, meningitis, endocarditis, and other remote infections. Chronic infection is associated with substantial weight loss.

The diagnosis requires culture identification of the pathogen. Blood, bone marrow aspirates, or cultures of tissue/exudates from remote sites of infection are necessary for recovery of the organism.

Brucellosis is not a pulmonary infection and sputum cultures are not of value. The organism grows slowly in vitro, and positive cultures may require several weeks. Antibody detection methods and PCR studies are useful in earlier detection by reference laboratories. Chest radiographs are not helpful. Echocardiography may be necessary to evaluate possible endocarditis.

Long courses (≥6 weeks) of antibiotic therapy are required for management both to reduce the duration of the illness and to avoid metastatic infection. Combination doxycycline (100 mg twice daily) and rifampin (600–900 mg daily) have been recommended. Tetracyclines and aminoglycosides have also been used. Gentamicin (1 mg every 8 h) has replaced streptomycin because of availability, and is used only in the acute phase of treatment when intravenous administration is necessary. Quinolone antibiotics have in vitro activity but limited clinical experience. The long course of antibiotic therapy including even triple agents (doxycycline, rifampin, gentamicin) is recommended because of the risk of bacterial endocarditis. Postexposure prophylaxis remains of uncertain value, but suspected exposure events will likely lead to doxycycline utilization. The duration of postexposure prophylaxis is by physician choice.

Standard infection control practices are recommended. Human-to-human transmission is very unlikely, because the organisms are not expectorated and only cutaneous infection is a potential source of infection to others. Standard disinfection practices are appropriate after management of the cases.

Cholera

Cholera is a well-known infection to those areas of the world where a safe water supply is problematic. It continues to be a major source of epidemic infection. This enteric infection is caused by *Vibrio cholerae*. It is an aerobic Gram-negative rod which produces a potent enterotoxin. Malicious contamination of food or water becomes the mechanism for this organism to be an agent of bioterrorism.

Although not a spore-forming bacterium, it has both a metabolically active and a dormant state. Adverse environmental conditions result in the dormant state. Favorable environmental conditions result in active replication. Ingestion of a critical inoculum of *V. cholerae* results in binding of the organism to the enterocyte and production of the enterotoxin (Raufman 1998). The result is a severe secretory diarrhea. Death from cholera occurs not from invasive infection, but due to loss of extracellular volume and circulatory collapse.

The onset of profuse diarrhea is the major clinical sign for this diagnosis. Abdominal cramping is uncommon but tachycardia, tachypnea, and hypotension follow the onset of the diarrhea. The motile organisms can be recognized with phase microscopy of diarrheal stools. Cultures on specific media will identify the organism, but the severity of the diarrhea will require therapy before culture results.

Volume resuscitation of the patient is the critical component of treatment. Ringer's lactate or isotonic NaCl solution (0.9%) is used. Bicarbonate may be necessary to manage metabolic acidosis. Intravenous fluid support must be continued until the diarrhea has subsided and normal oral intake has resumed.

Antibiotic therapy is used. Tetracycline (500 mg, every 6 h x 3 days) or doxycycline (100 mg every 12 h x 3 days) is the preferred choice. A large single dose (1 g) of azithromycin has been successfully used for treatment (Saha et al. 2006). Other antibiotic choices (quinolones, erythromycin, trimethoprim–sulfamethoxazole) have been used. Antibiotics appear to reduce the duration and severity of the infectious event, but intravenous fluid support is the key to successful management. Postexposure antibiotic prophylaxis has not been well studied but would likely be employed in circumstances of a recognized exposure event. Standard infection control processes with appropriate handling of diarrheal stools should avoid human-to-human transmission. Standard disinfection practices are used for patient rooms and equipment.

Q fever

Coxielia burnetii is the pathogen of Q fever as a proposed agent of bioterrorism (Parker et al. 2006). It is a bacterium that has pathological and clinical characteristics similar to *Rickettsia* spp. It is an intracellular parasite but maintains viability and infectivity outside host cells. It is an endemic infection to goats, cattle, sheep, and birds. It has been labeled as a potential bioweapon because infection may occur after exposure to only a single organism and because of the airborne route of transmission. Infection may occur after ingestion or inhalation of the pathogen. The organism adheres to the plasma membrane of the target cell population, and is internalized into a phagosome. The organism may survive for years within the host as an intracellular parasite.

The hallmark of Q fever is a persistent low-grade fever. The patients characteristically have a flu-like syndrome with myalgias and malaise. A viral-like pneumonia is present on chest radiographs in about half of patients, and 20% will have a maculopapular rash. It is associated with endocarditis and a hepatitis syndrome. The infection may be of limited duration and severity in younger patients, but can be quite severe in elderly people. The acuity and severity of the infection depend on the inoculum size, route of exposure, and patient host factors. Plasmid-mediated variability may make specific strains quite virulent. The major pathological consequences of the disease are from chronic infection that persists over years.

Culture identification of the organism has proven to very difficult for the routine laboratory. The diagnosis is best established through the use of serological methods of antibody detection. PCR has also been more recently proposed for diagnosis.

The treatment for acute infections is doxycycline (100 mg twice daily) for 14 days. The treatment of chronic infection is prolonged antibiotic therapy because the agents that are used are bacteriostatic, and the organisms are intracellular in location. Doxycycline and hydrochloroquine for 18 months are the current recommendation. The hydrochloroquine is thought to adversely increase the pH within the phagosome that contains *C. burnetii*. Quinolones in combination with doxycycline have been used, but this therapy may be required for ≥3 years. Vaccine development is being pursued for areas with high rates of infection. Transmission from human to human has been reported but is rare. Standard infection control processes are used for infected patients, and standard decontamination of rooms and equipment is appropriate.

Glanders

Infection with *Burkholderia mallei* is referred to as glanders. This pathogen is an aerobic Gram-negative rod that is a human bacterial infection contracted from horses, mules, and donkeys. It is contracted by cutaneous exposure of non-intact skin, ingestion, or inhalation of the microbe. Cutaneous infection results in ulcerated lesions with regional adenopathy. Ingestion is associated with ulcerated lesions of the oropharynx. Pulmonary infection is an acute pneumonia or miliary disease. Fever, leukocytosis, and splenomegaly occur with acute glanders. The acute disease is usually fatal. A chronic and highly variable form of the infection occurs about 14 days after exposure of the host. The chronic form of the infection may proceed to resolution or relapse into an acute exacerbation with death of the host. As a small

inoculum of bacteria is necessary to cause the infection and high mortality rate of the acute infection, this organism has been actively pursued as a possible bioweapon.

Cultures of infected cutaneous lesions or of sputum will recover the pathogen with specific media (e.g., meat nutrient agar). Blood cultures are usually negative. Complement fixation tests, agglutination tests, immunoflorescence assays, and PCR are used by reference laboratories.

As the number of cases that have been managed with each drug regimen is small, uncertainty exists for antibiotic treatment and is based on in vitro sensitivities (Dow et al. 2010). For localized infection trimethoprim–sulfamethoxazole, doxycycline, amoxicillin/clavulanate, and quinolones have been used for 2–5 months in duration. Combinations of drugs are used for severe cases with systemic manifestations. No evidence supports postexposure prophylaxis with antibiotics. Human-to-human transmission is considered a low risk, so standard isolation precautions and standard disinfection of the healthcare environment are recommended.

A disease commonly associated with glanders is melioidosis (Cheng 2010). This infection is caused by *Burkholderia pseudomallei*. It is genetically similar to *B. mallei* and has many similar clinical and management features to glanders. Worldwide, it appears to be a more common infection in humans because of the presence of the organism in the soil. Treatment includes a broader array of antibiotics, including ceftazidime and the carbapenems, in addition to those drugs used in glanders. This bacterial pathogen has also been explored as a bioweapon.

VIRUSES

Smallpox

Without question smallpox is the one infection that is viewed with greatest concern as a bioweapon to be used against civilian populations (Henderson et al. 1999). Smallpox epidemics have been associated with large numbers of deaths and human misery in the past. The eradication of smallpox with a vigorous international immunization program has been one of the most remarkable success stories of public health efforts. The last identified infection was in 1977. By the mid-1980s, public immunization programs were discontinued. Only two repositories of the virus are known to exist at the Centers for Disease Control in Atlanta in the USA and the Institute for Viral Preparation in Moscow. As public immunization has been discontinued, it means that an entire generation under age 30 is unvaccinated and at risk. It is likely that remote immunization of the older population still affords significant protection. As the infection has airborne transmission and is readily passed from human to human, there has been real fear about viral cultures of the smallpox virus being in the possession of political dissidents.

This infection is caused by variola virus. Variola is a member of the Orthopox genera which includes cowpox, monkeypox, vaccinia, and other viruses that share a common antigenic character. It was successful vaccination of large populations of people with vaccinia that has provided immunological protection against smallpox infection.

Smallpox has a well-defined pathogenesis and humans are the natural host. Expectorated droplets containing virus are inhaled by the susceptible host. A small inoculum of inhaled virus is necessary to cause infection. The virus adheres to the oropharynx or respiratory mucosa. By 3–4 days after exposure, the virus has migrated to regional lymph nodes where proliferation occurs. An asymptomatic viremia occurs with dissemination to the spleen, bone marrow, and the regional lymph nodes of the infected host. A second viremia occurs about 8 days after the original exposure and the patients then experience fever and systemic symptoms. By 14 days, the patients experience a generalized viral syndrome of fever, headaches, myalgias, and even abdominal pain. A maculopapular rash occurs at this point which progresses to vesiculation and then pustule formation. The rash evolves into the classic crusting, umbilicated lesion (**Figure 23.3**). The patients remain infectious to others until the rash has resolved. Smallpox has a historically defined 30% mortality rate.

The characteristic cutaneous lesions of smallpox have traditionally made it a clinical diagnosis. The crusted, umbilicated lesions are most densely identified on the face and extremities, as opposed to the predominantly truncal crusted lesions that are typical of chickenpox. Scrapings from the skin lesions will show Guarnieri bodies on light microscopy, the virus can be visualized on electron microscopy, and it can be cultured. PCR techniques can be used to identify the viral DNA.

Early efforts in antiviral chemotherapy included treatment of smallpox with cytosine arabinoside and adenine arabinoside, but validation of effectiveness was not established before eradication of the infection. Animal studies supported cidofovir as another potential treatment. The care of the smallpox patient is supportive management. Smallpox patients were isolated in negative pressure rooms until resolution of cutaneous lesions was complete. All personnel obviously required immunization themselves. Strict barrier precautions were used. Disposable supplies were incinerated. Reusable linens were autoclaved before being laundered.

Concerns about the re-emergence of smallpox as a bioweapon has led to discussions about the resumption of immunization programs. However, vaccination is not without significant complications, detailed in **Table 23.2**. These complications can lead to major disability and even death. As these complication statistics come from clinical studies of ≥40 years ago (Lane et al. 1970), the prevalence of immunosuppressed patients in current society may make the frequency of immunization-associated complications greater than previously observed. The Advisory Committee on Immunization Practice has recommended to the Centers for Disease Control and Prevention (CDC) that immunization of the general population is not warranted. They have recommended immunization of emergency response teams and personnel in hospitals where identified cases would be managed

(Wharton et al. 2003). There remains no evidence that smallpox viral cultures have fallen into undesirable ownership and the world remains free of this infection for nearly 35 years. Nevertheless, a continued understanding of smallpox is necessary for prompt recognition should it re-emerge for any reason.

■ Equine encephalitis virus

The three equine encephalitis viruses (EEVs) are endemic infections for equine species (horses, mules, donkeys). They are transmitted by mosquitoes to humans. Exposure of humans from mosquito contact results in hematogenous transport of the virus to the central nervous system (CNS) to initiate the encephalitis process.

The three types of EEV include the Venezuelan EEV, Eastern EEV, and Western EEV. Each virus has unique virulence characteristics. Venezuelan EEV has been primarily identified in Central and South America and is a severely incapacitating disease, but has only a 1% mortality rate. Eastern EEV has a distribution of natural infection that is similar to Venezuelan EEV but also includes the eastern USA. Mortality rates with Eastern EEV are 50–70%. Western EEV occurs with multiple serotypes, in both North and South America, and has a 10% mortality rate.

Each of the three EEVs has been proposed as a bioweapon (Smith et al. 1997). They are easily grown in culture, easily stored, and quite infectious to humans, and the multiple types and subtypes will make the development of vaccines very difficult. As opposed to naturally occurring infection EEV as a bioweapon would be delivered as an aerosol, binds to respiratory epithelium, and is then transported to the CNS. It does not cause a viral pneumonia, and human-to-human transmission is thought to be a minimal risk. Some evidence suggests transmission of aerosol infection may be directly through olfactory nerves and then direct entry into the CNS.

Clinical disease begins 1–10 days after exposure. The disease begins as fever, myalgia, and malaise. It transitions into headaches and encephalitis. Leukopenia is observed. The diagnosis is made by cultures of the virus, and IgM antibody detection is useful but not positive until a week into the infection. Only supportive care is used, without any recommendations for antiviral chemotherapy. Standard infection control and disinfection are recommended.

■ Viral hemorrhagic fever

An array of different viruses are viral hemorrhagic fever (VHR) pathogens (**Table 23.3**). The number of different viruses and subspecies of recognized groups continue to expand. They share the common characteristics of fulminate febrile illnesses which are associated with clinical bleeding, shock, and death. These viruses can be cultured in large quantities, have the potential for airborne transmission, and have potential for human-to-human transmission. For these reasons, these agents have been evaluated by governments as bioweapons and represent a risk for use in bioterrorism (Marty et al. 2006).

The VHR viruses are single-stranded RNA viruses and have a lipid envelope (see Chapter 1). They commonly have rodent reservoirs and are transmitted by mosquitoes or ticks. Human-to-human transmission is by contact with infected blood or infected body fluids, or by inhalation of a fine aerosol. The endothelial cell is the host target. The incubation time for clinical infection after exposure may vary from only 2–3 days, to several weeks for the specific virus. Mortality rates approach 90% for selected infections (e.g., Marburg, Ebola).

The clinical presentations of these infections are highly variable, but have the hallmarks of the generic viral syndrome. Fever, myalgia,

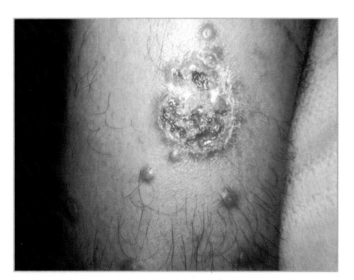

Figure 23.3 The pustules and crusting cutaneous lesions of smallpox.
(From http://phil.cdc.gov/phil/details.asp, courtesy of CDC/Dr John Noble Jr. ID no.: 10480, 1968.)

Table 23.2 Complications following primary and revaccination for smallpox.

Complication	Primary vaccination		Revaccination rate/million*
	Rate/million	Death rate of event	
Generalized vaccinia	241.5	0%	9.0
Progressive vaccinia	1.5	75%	3.0
Post-vaccinal encephalitis	12.3	25%	2.0
Eczema vaccinatum	38.5	10%	3.0

*Deaths are rare.

Table 23.3 Currently identified viruses of viral hemorrhagic fever.

Disease	Natural Locale
Arenaviruses	
Argentine hemorrhagic fever	South America
Bolivian hemorrhagic fever	South America
Brazilian hemorrhagic fever	South America
Lassa fever	Africa
Venezuelan hemorrhagic fever	South America
Flavivirus	
Dengue fever	Africa, Americas, Asia
Kyasanur forest disease	Africa, South America
Omsk hemorrhagic fever	Eastern Europe
Yellow fever	Africa, South America
Others	
Ebola/Marburg hemorrhagic fever (filovirus)	Africa
Hantavirus infection (hantavirus)	Asia, Europe, south-western USA
Crimean–Congo hemorrhagic fever (nairovirus)	Africa, Asia, Europe
Rift Valley fever (phlebovirus)	Africa

malaise, headaches, nausea/vomiting, diarrhea, and abdominal pain are commonly seen. Leukopenia and thrombocytopenia are common. Hemoconcentration may be an early finding due to plasma volume loss, until clinical bleeding becomes significant. Shock and the evolution of pulmonary, hepatic, and renal failure follow the rapid evolution of the clinical infection.

Although the clinical syndrome is readily recognized, documentation of the specific viral agent is challenging. The responsible virus can be cultured, but may require 3–10 days before identification is established. Detection of specific antibodies by enzyme-linked immunosorbent assay (ELISA) methods, and identification of the viral RNA through reverse transcriptase PCR via reference laboratories are usual methods for prompt diagnosis.

The treatment of VHF is supportive care. Maintenance of systemic perfusion and oxygenation are necessary for survival. Ribavirin therapy has been considered a potential treatment for these infections, but very little evidence supports use of this drug. Rigid infection control is important for personnel treating the patients and for laboratory workers handling the specimens for diagnosis. Disposables should be incinerated and linens autoclaved before laundry. Disinfection after patient care should be rigorous. International travel makes exposure events in remote areas of the world a risk for infection occurring at any location.

BIOLOGICAL TOXINS

Botulinum toxin

Botulinum toxin is an exotoxin product of *Clostridium botulinum*. It is considered one of the most potent toxins known. It can be readily produced and stored. There is an extensive military history concerning potential use as a bioweapon, and it represents a real threat for civilian populations (Arnon et al. 2001).

This toxin produces paralysis and has lethal effects from respiratory arrest. The toxin can be inhaled or ingested. By either route, the toxin gains systemic distribution and binds to the membrane of the presynaptic motor neurons. The toxin is internalized within the motor nerve cells and results in inhibition of acetylcholine release. The result disrupts the propagation of neurotransmission.

Rapid onset of paralysis is the characteristic finding of botulinum toxin paralysis within a few hours to several days after exposure. Dysarthria, dysphonia, and diplopia are early findings because the cranial nerves tend to be the first affected by this toxin. Paralysis proceeds in a descending fashion with the most severe motor nerve compromise being in the head and neck area. The paralysis is symmetric and there are no sensory changes. There are no changes in sensorium before hypoxemia. There is no febrile or other acute inflammatory response.

The diagnosis of botulinum poisoning is a clinical one. It should be clinically separated from Guillain–Barré syndrome or myasthenia gravis. Serum, gastric aspirate, stool specimen, and suspected food sources are sampled and submitted for the mouse bioassay. The mouse bioassay exposes the animals to the clinical specimen with and without the presence of the anti-toxin. The mouse bioassay is available only in special reference laboratories. Direct measures of the toxin are not available.

The management of botulism is prompt administration of the equine-derived antitoxin and supportive care for the associated failure of ventilation (Sobel 2005). Treatment cannot be delayed until the laboratory mouse bioassay results are available. Patients should not receive the antitoxin before the clinical specimens for the bioassay are recovered. As the antitoxin is effective only against extracellular toxin, the earliest possible administration is necessary to hopefully avoid the full impact on motor neurons. Toxin already internalized within cells in not affected by the antitoxin. As the antitoxin is of equine origin, a test dose is given before the full treatment is administered. Up to 10% of patients may have hypersensitivity reactions, and 2% may have anaphylaxis. The full treatment is the 10 ml vial in 100 ml of 0.9% saline and infused slowly over 30–60 min. For infant cases, human botulism immunoglobulin is used instead of the equine antitoxin (Chalk et al. 2011).

The supportive care of these patients may extend for weeks or even months. As the affected motor neurons have to regenerate new axonal twigs to restore muscle function, prolonged ventilator support is necessary. Tracheostomy may be necessary. The prolonged ventilator support puts these patients at risk for ventilator-associated pneumonia. Nutritional support is also necessary because of paralysis of the muscles of deglutition. It must be emphasized that botulism is a poisoning and not an infection. Antibiotics should not be employed unless a documented focus of infection is identified. The prolonged course of hospitalization requires that selection pressures for resistant organisms be avoided. If antibiotics become necessary, drugs associated with neuromuscular blockade (e.g., aminoglycosides) should be avoided.

In the event of a proven or suspected exposure event to botulinum toxin, patients should be decontaminated with removal of clothing, cleansing of skin, and washing or removal of hair. Decontaminated patients are not a risk for healthcare personnel. Standard infection control practices and disinfection of medical equipment are employed.

Ricin

Ricin is a protein that is extracted from the castor bean (Audi et al. 2005). It is extraordinarily toxic in humans with only 2 mg identified as a lethal dose in adults. It has been investigated by several governments as a bioweapon because of its ease of production and small doses necessary for a lethal effect. Ricin has actually been used in a political assassination.

Ricin can be delivered by injection, ingestion, or inhalation. Ingested ricin may be digested, with symptoms being gastrointestinal but with limited systemic uptake. Toxin gastrointestinal effects are vomiting and diarrhea, with extracellular fluid loss and hypovolemic shock being the major source of morbidity for the patient. Injected or inhaled ricin is distributed systemically and results in the inhibition of protein synthesis. Ricin accesses all cell populations. Symptoms begin within 6–8 h of exposure.

With inhalation, a necrotizing pneumonitis is seen due to local toxic events of the compound. Severe pulmonary failure may supervene the systemic effects of ricin as a cause of death in inhalation cases. Considerable discussion has focused on the weaponization of ricin for inhalational delivery. The powder product has to be finely processed to yield a size ≤5 μm to reach the alveolar region. The processing necessary to create the fine particle size has been a factor in discrediting ricin as a legitimate bioweapon by airborne exposure (Schap et al. 2009).

The diagnosis of ricin poisoning is suspected when a group of patients present with common symptoms after a suspicious public exposure. Gastrointestinal symptoms will be similar to food poisoning. Acute ventilator distress will herald inhalational injury. Clinical studies to detect ricin in serum specimens are not available in clinical laboratories, but detection of ricin or by antibody responses may be available through sophisticated reference laboratories.

The treatment for ricin poisoning is supportive care. There is no antidote available. Gastrointestinal exposure will require volume and hemodynamic support. Cases suspected of acute ricin ingestion may benefit from either gastric lavage or activated charcoal administration before the onset of symptoms. Inhalational cases will require ventilator and hemodynamic support. Decontamination of potentially exposed patients is necessary to avoid additional ricin exposure for patients and healthcare personnel. Secondary contamination from ricin-exposed patients is not a risk after effective decontamination. Standard environmental disinfection is employed within the hospital.

Other microbial toxins

The number of potential toxins to be derived from microbes and plants are numerous. Many may not have been appreciated as potential weapons of terror. An array of mycotoxins cause contact, gastrointestinal, and inhalational risks. Staphylococcal enterotoxins have been appreciated as potential ingestion or inhalation risks from naturally occurring clinical infections or from laboratory accidents. The exposures to the various toxins are quite similar, with patients having a food poisoning clinical picture. Inhalation causes the non-specific respiratory distress syndrome requiring ventilatory support. Clinical specimens are obtained for analysis by reference laboratories. Treatment is supportive care.

RECOGNITION OF BIOTERRORISM

A reality of life in the twenty-first century is that microbes or microbial products may be used as bioweapons against civilian populations. It means that surgeons and other healthcare professionals engaged in the care of acutely injured and acutely ill patients need to be sensitized to this possibility. The character of such an assault is totally unpredictable. It may vary from a crop duster scattering particles across an urban area, or contaminants placed into a ventilation system of an auditorium. Contamination with spores or powders on a pedestrian thoroughfare might result in multiple people being exposed unknowingly over time. A public exposure event may not be appreciated until infected or poisoned patients actually arrive at the emergency facility. Of course conventional explosions may have biological contaminants that will expose injured casualties, but also rescue personnel. For surgeons and emergency personnel, it means that all malicious clinical events with the intention of hurting civilian or political targets may represent more than immediately meets the eye. It means that reporting mechanisms must be in place for the identification of unusual infections or unknown sicknesses, so that public health officials can identify a cluster of unusual clinical events occurring within a community and among patients within a common geographical locale. With the vast number of bacteria, viruses, and microbial cell products in a world with widely disseminated technology for the production of these agents, it is not a matter of whether a biological event will occur among civilian populations, but when it will happen.

REFERENCES

Arnon SS, Schechter R, Inglesby TV, et al. Botulism toxin as a biological weapon: medical and public health management. *JAMA* 2001;**285**:1059–70.

Audi J, Belson M, Patel M, Schier J, Osterloh J. Ricin poisoning: a comprehensive review. *JAMA* 2005;**294**:2342–51.

Centers for Disease Control and Prevention. Bioterroism agents/diseases. Available at: www.bt.cdc.gov/agent/agentlist-category.asp (accessed January 10, 2012).

Chalk C, Benstead TJ, Keezer M. Medical treatment for botulism. *Cochrane Database Syst Rev* 2011;(**3**):CD008123.

Cheng AC. Melioidosis: advances in diagnosis and treatment. *Curr Opin Infect Dis* 2010;**23**:554–9.

Dennis DT, Inglesby TV, Henderson DA, et al. Tularemia as a biological weapon: medical and public health management. *JAMA* 2001;**285**:2763–73.

Dow SW, Estes DM, Schweizer HP, Torres AG. Present and future therapeutic strategies for melioidosis and glanders. *Exp Rev Anti Infect Ther* 2010;**8**:325–38.

Franco MP, Mulder M, Gilman RH, Smits HL. Human brucellosis. *Lancet Infect Dis* 2007;**7**:775–86.

Fry DE. Disaster planning for unconventional acts of civilian terror. *Curr Probl Surg* 2006;**43**:253–315.

Fry DE, Schecter WP, Parker JS, Quebbeman EJ, and the Governors' Committee on Blood Borne Infection and Environmental Risk of the American College of Surgeons. The surgeon and acts of civilian terrorism: biological agents. *J Am Coll Surg* 2005;**200**:291–302.

Inglesby TV, Henderson DA, Bartlett JG, et al. Anthrax as a biological weapon. *JAMA* 1999;**281**:1735–45.

Inglesby TV, Dennis DT, Henderson DA, et al. Plague as a biological weapon: medical and public health management. Working Group on Civilian Biodefense. *JAMA* 2000;**283**:2281–90.

Henderson DA, Inglesby TV, Bartlett JG, et al. Smallpox as a biological weapon: medical and public health management. Working Group on Civilian Biodefense. *JAMA* 1999;**81**:2127–37.

Horzempa J, O'Dee, Stolz DB, et al. Invasion of erythrocytes by *Francisella tularensis*. *J Infect Dis* 2011;**204**:51–59.

Lane JM, Ruben FL, Neff JM, Miller JD. Complications of smallpox vaccination, 1968;results of ten statewide surveys. *J Infect Dis* 1970;**122**:303–9.

Marty AM, Jahrling PB, Geisbert TW. Viral hemorrhagic fever. *Clin Lab Med* 2006;**26**:345–86.

Parker NR, Barralet JH, Bell AM. Q Fever. *Lancet* 2006;**367**:679–688.

Raufman J-P. Cholera. *Am J Med* 1998;**104**:386–94.

Saha D, Karim MM, Khan WA, Ahmed S, Salam MA, Bennish ML. Single-dose azithromycin for the treatment of cholera in adults. *N Engl J Med* 2006;**354**:2452–62.

Schap LJ, Temple WA, Butt GA, Beasley MD. Ricin as a weapon of mass terror-separating fact from fiction. *Environ Int* 2009;**35**:1267–71.

Smith JF, Davis K, Hart MK, et al. Viral encephalitides. In: Zajtchuk R, Bellamy RF (eds), *Medical Aspects of Chemical and Biological Warfare*. Washington DC: US Department of the Army, 1997: 561–89.

Sobel J. Botulism. *Clin Infect Dis* 2005;**41**:1167–73.

Sweeney DA, Hicks CW, Cui X, Li Y, Eichacker PQ. Anthrax infection. *Am J Respir Crit Care Med* 2011;**184**:1333–41.

Wharton M, Strikas RA, Harpaz R, et al. Recommenation for using smallpox vaccination in a pre-event vaccination program. Supplemental recommendations of the Advisory Committee of the Immunization Practices and the Healthcare Infection Control Practices Advisory Committee. *MMWR* 2003;**52**:1–16.

Chapter 24

Microbial translocation, gut origin sepsis, probiotics, prebiotics, selective gut decontamination

Edwin A. Deitch, Jordan E. Fishman, Gal Levy

■ INTRODUCTION

Since the late twentieth century, the role of the gut in the pathogenesis of infection, sepsis and organ failure in surgical and intensive care unit (ICU) patients has evolved considerably. Until this time, evaluation of intestinal function had been limited largely to monitoring gastric pH and intestinal motility. This approach has led clinicians to equate normal intestinal motility with normal intestinal function and to assume that, if stress-induced gastric bleeding can be prevented, all will be well. However, over the last three decades it has become increasingly clear that the gastrointestinal (GI) tract is not a passive organ and that intestinal dysfunction is not limited to ileus and upper GI bleeding. Instead, today we recognize that the GI tract and its microbial contents may influence the patient's clinical outcome and that the gut has important endocrine, immunological, metabolic and barrier functions in addition to its traditional role in nutrient absorption, e.g., it is the intestinal barrier that prevents the spread of intraluminal bacteria and endotoxins to systemic organs and tissues. Failure of intestinal bacteria function, leading to the escape of bacteria or their products (endotoxin), has been termed "bacterial translocation" (Berg and Garlington 1979). When one considers the enormous concentrations of bacteria and endotoxins present in the distal small bowel and colon (10^{10} anaerobes and 10^5–10^8 each of Gram-positive and Gram-negative aerobic and facultative organisms), the fact that sepsis originating in the gut and endotoxemia do not occur in normal, healthy individuals is in many respects a testimony to the effectiveness of the intestinal mucosal barrier.

Nevertheless, under certain pathophysiological conditions, intestinal barrier function can be impaired or overwhelmed to such an extent that bacterial (endotoxin) translocation does occur (Deitch 1990). The three basic mechanisms documented experimentally to promote bacterial translocation (Deitch 1990) are as follows:
1. Disruption of the ecological balance of indigenous intestinal flora, resulting in the overgrowth of Gram-negative enteric bacilli
2. Impairment of host immune and antibacterial defenses
3. Physical disruption of the intestinal mucosal barrier.

These same conditions that experimentally are associated with loss of intestinal barrier function are commonly observed in the critically ill or injured patient at risk for enteric bacteremia or the multiple-organ dysfunction syndrome (MODS), e.g., these at-risk patients are frequently immunocompromised and the antibiotic, anti-ulcer, and dietary regimens that they receive may disrupt the normal ecology of the intestinal flora, resulting in intestinal overgrowth with Gram-negative enteric bacilli and other potentially pathogenic microorganisms. Likewise, several clinical and laboratory studies indicate that impairment of upper intestinal antibacterial defenses is important in the development of nosocomial pneumonias (Driks et al. 1987, Tryba 1987), whereas life-threatening infection with bowel-associated bacteria, in which no infective focus can be found even at autopsy, is a major clinical problem in several groups of patients including burns patients (Jarrett et al. 1978, Chitkara and Feierabend 1981), victims of trauma (Garrison et al. 1982, Border et al. 1987), and patients with MODS (Goris et al. 1985, Carrico et al. 1986). Thus, although still controversial, the phenomenon of bacterial translocation has assumed clinical importance with the recognition that intestinal barrier failure may play a role in the development of systemic infection, sepsis originating in the gut, and MODS in the critically ill or injured individual.

However, to fully understand the implications of bacterial translocation and gut-derived sepsis, it is important to fully understand and define these key terms, because these terms mean different things to different people. Therefore, before we explore each of these topics, we will establish a common vocabulary (**Box 24.1**) and clarify the important point that bacterial translocation and gut-derived sepsis may occur independently of each other, i.e., bacterial translocation

---

Box 24.1 Bacterial translocation and gut-derived sepsis: a common vocabulary.

Bacterial translocation is best defined as the process by which intestinal bacteria or *Candida* spp. cross the intestinal mucosal barrier to reach the mesenteric lymph nodes, from which they may or may not spread systemically and cause infection.
The diagnosis of bacterial translocation requires the identification of intestinal bacteria in the intestinal lymph nodes.
Gut-derived sepsis is best defined as the process whereby gut-derived, proinflammatory, tissue-injurious, microbial and non-microbial factors induce or contribute to the development of systemic inflammatory response syndrome (SIRS), acute respiratory distress syndrome (ARDS), or multiple-organ dysfunction syndrome (MODS). This process may or may not occur in the presence or absence of systemic infection originating in the gut or bacterial translocation.
The diagnosis of gut-derived sepsis is based on measurements of gut barrier function (permeability) together with the clinical response of the patient.

may occur in the absence of gut-derived sepsis or the patient may have gut-derived sepsis in the absence of documented bacterial translocation. Therefore, when applying these two terms to clinical practice, the two terms should not be linked together but looked at separately. In fact, as discussed later in this chapter, the phenomenon and clinical relevance of bacterial translocation have been largely studied in patients undergoing abdominal surgery as well as animal models. In contrast, the incidence and clinical importance of gut-derived sepsis and its consequences, such as organ failure, have been largely studied in the critically ill or injured ICU patient populations, where the diagnosis is based on measurements of gut permeability and not bacterial translocation. Thus, the abdominal surgery population in which bacterial translocation can be directly measured are not generally critically ill and have a low likelihood of developing MODS. In contrast, bacterial translocation cannot be directly measured in the critically ill patient population, who are at the highest risk of developing gut-derived sepsis and MODS.

BACTERIAL TRANSLOCATION AND GUT-ORIGIN SEPSIS: A HISTORICAL PERSPECTIVE

This notion that the gut can be the reservoir for bacteria or fungi causing systemic infections is not new, e.g., beginning in the late 1800s, it was postulated that peritonitis could result from virulent bacteria migrating across an intact intestinal wall (Balzan et al. 2007), and this concept was experimentally validated in the 1940s when enteric-origin bacteria were recovered from the peritoneal washings

of uremic dogs (Schweinburg and Frank 1949). In the 1960s, Fine et al. published some of the earliest clinical studies establishing that intestinal bacteria and endotoxin originating in the gut are capable of gaining entry into the systemic circulation during shock states (Ravin and Fine 1962, Caridis et al. 1972, Woodruff et al. 1973). These authors proposed that a relationship existed for shock, intestinal ischemia, and systemic endotoxemia. However, over the next 20 years, the concept of an "intestinal factor" in shock-induced sepsis fell out of favor. This was largely due to experiments in germ-free animals indicating that these germ-free animals were only modestly more resistant to certain shock states than animals with a normal gut microflora.

The concept of sepsis originating in the gut lay dormant for almost 20 years. However, experimental animal studies performed in the late 1970s and early 1980s by Wolochow et al. (1966), Berg and Garlington (1979), and Deitch et al. (1985), and subsequently in the mid-1980s by Wells et al. (1986) and Inoue et al. (1988), established that bacteria can translocate from the gut to systemic organs and tissues. It was at this time that the term "bacterial translocation" was coined. This concept of bacterial translocation provided a biological explanation for how bacteria could breach the intestinal mucosal barrier and lead to systemic infections (**Figure 24.1**). Shortly thereafter, it was proposed that gut barrier failure leading to the translocation of bacteria and endotoxin could lead to septic states originating in the gut and that the gut was the "motor of multiple organ failure" (Carrico et al. 1986, Border et al. 1987, Deitch et al. 1987, Deitch 1992). Thus, by the mid- to late 1980s, the gut hypothesis of MODS had appeared. During the decade from 1985 to 1995, bacterial and endotoxin translocation across the compromised gut became viewed as a major contributor to systemic infection and MODS after shock, mechanical trauma, and

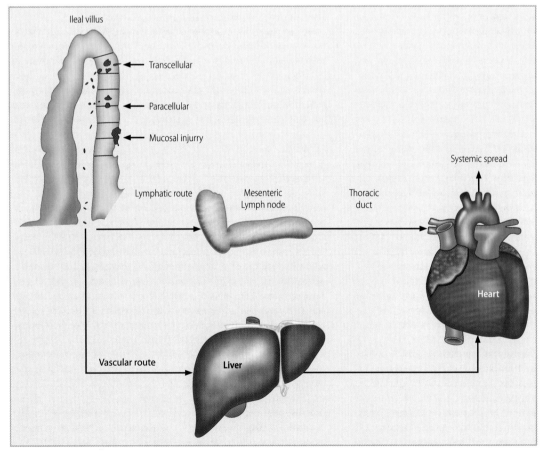

Figure 24.1 Potential route of bacterial translocation from intestine to systemic organs and tissues, which include lymphatic and blood-borne (portal vein) routes.

Ileal villus

Transcellular

Paracellular

Mucosal injurry

Systemic spread

Lymphatic route

Mesenteric Lymph node

Thoracic duct

Heart

Vascular route

Liver

burns, and in ICU patients as well as in patients undergoing major surgery (Deitch 1992).

Early clinical studies attempting to validate the bacterial translocation model in patients used the strategy of culturing the mesenteric lymph nodes of patients undergoing surgery, because translocation to the mesenteric lymph node was viewed as the initial and key step in the bacterial translocation process. These initial proof-of-principle clinical studies documented that bacterial translocation to the mesenteric lymph nodes occurred in patients undergoing abdominal surgery for inflammatory bowel disease (Ambrose et al. 1984), simple small bowel obstruction (Deitch 1989), or trauma (Moore et al. 1992). However, no such studies were carried out in patients with systemic inflammatory response syndrome (SIRS), sepsis, acute respiratory distress syndrome (ARDS), or MODS. These positive studies prompted additional clinical studies examining the peripheral blood, abdominal fluid, and portal blood of organ donors. In one such study, translocation of bacteria and endotoxin was observed in over half of all organ donors despite normal light and electron microscope examination of the bowel wall (Van Goor et al. 1994). Of more import, however, the bacteria cultured from the mesenteric lymph nodes (MLNs) were found to be identical to the GI flora, thus strengthening the hypothesis that the bacterial source was the GI tract. This finding was further strengthened by studies demonstrating that, in patients with both a documented postoperative septic source and bacterial translocation, as evidenced by a positive MLN culture, the bacteria isolated from the MLN culture was identical to the bacteria isolated from the septic source about half the time (Sedman et al. 1994, O'Boyle et al. 1998, MacFie et al. 1999, 2005, Woodcock et al. 2000, Chin et al. 2007).

In addition, bacterial genomic studies comparing the bacteria collected from MLN cultures with the indigenous colonic bacteria of patients undergoing colon resection found that the cultured bacteria were identical to those in the colon, thus serving to further strengthen the notion that the gut served as a bacterial reservoir for infection (Reddy et al. 2007). The transition from phenomenology to clinical relevance followed with the publication of six additional clinical series, totaling 2125 patients undergoing abdominal surgery. In these studies, the incidence of bacterial translocation to the MLN ranged between 5% and 21%, and the rate of infectious complications was two- to threefold higher in patients with bacterial translocation (Sedman et al. 1994, O'Boyle et al. 1998, MacFie et al. 1999, 2005, Woodcock et al. 2000, Chin et al. 2007). Thus, studies in surgical patients undergoing major operations appeared to validate the concept of bacterial translocation and found a significant association between the occurrence of bacterial translocation and an increased risk of postoperative infections.

However, although bacterial translocation had been documented to occur in patients undergoing major operations and in organ donors, the studies linking bacterial and endotoxin translocation to MODS in critically ill or injured patients in the ICU was indirect, and used increased intestinal permeability as a marker for patients at increased risk for developing gut-derived sepsis or MODS. These studies showed that gut permeability was increased in thermally injured, trauma, and ICU patients, but only about a third of these studies found a clear association between the magnitude of the increase in gut permeability and infectious complications, although the evidence linking increased gut permeability to the development of MODS was stronger (Pisarenko and Deitch 2010). Further support for the concept of gut injury contributing to MODS came from studies in ICU and trauma patients, indicating that gut ischemia, as reflected by gastric tonometry, was a better predictor of the development of ARDS and MODS than global indices of oxygen delivery (Ivatury et al. 1995). On the other hand, studies trying to correlate increased plasma endotoxin levels

with the development of ARDS and MODS in these high-risk patients were unsuccessful. In an attempt to directly correlate bacterial and endotoxin translocation with the subsequent development of ARDS and MODS, Moore et al. (1991) carried out a prospective study where portal vein catheters were placed in severely injured trauma patients shortly after their arrival at hospital. Serial portal blood samples were then tested for bacteria or the presence of endotoxin. Although 30% of the enrolled patients subsequently developed MODS, only 2% of all the portal vein cultures collected were positive for bacterial growth and endotoxin was not present in any of the portal blood samples. Given the compelling results of this study, doubt was cast on the clinical relevance of bacterial translocation to the development of MODS. Although bacterial translocation did appear to predispose to infectious complications in postoperative surgical patients, this study and others caused a reassessment of the role of bacterial translocation in the pathogenesis of MODS.

One potential explanation for the failure of Moore et al. to find bacteria or endotoxins in the portal system is that MODS-inducing factors were exiting the gut via the intestinal lymphatics rather than the portal blood. This observation would be consistent with preclinical studies showing that the primary route of translocating bacteria exiting the gut is via the lymphatics (Mainous et al. 1991). It would also help explain why increased gut permeability and gut ischemia are better predictors of the development of MODS than the presence of gut-derived bacteremia or endotoxemia. Based on an extensive series of studies, it was shown that gut-derived factors, carried in the intestinal lymphatics rather than the portal vein, are responsible for the early development of ARDS and MODS in stress conditions (Magnotti et al. 1998, 1999, Deitch et al. 2004a, Senthil et al. 2006). The synthesis of these observations into a coherent, experimentally testable hypothesis occurred over the last decade and has been termed the "gut lymph hypothesis" of SIRS, ARDS, and MODS (Deitch and Xu 2006). This theory postulates that the early onset of SIRS and organ failure after trauma or shock is due to non-bacterial, tissue injury-related, proinflammatory factors liberated from the stressed gut which reach the systemic circulation via the mesenteric lymphatics (Deitch and Xu 2006). This hypothesis is based on several major experimental observations. First, ligation of the major intestinal lymph duct, which prevents intestinal lymph from reaching the systemic circulation, prevents the development of early ARDS and MODS. Specifically, it prevents acute lung injury, cardiac dysfunction, neutrophil activation, increased endothelial permeability, bone marrow suppression, and red blood cell dysfunction in multiple preclinical models of trauma, shock, burn injury, or gut ischemia. Second, in vitro studies of mesenteric lymph from shocked animals, but not sham-shocked animals, leads to neutrophil activation, and cardiomyocyte and endothelial cell injury, as well as red blood cell dysfunction. Last, injection of shock lymph into healthy mice and rats recreates a systemic sepsis state and causes ARDS and MODS. Thus, the gut lymph hypothesis fulfills a modified set of Koch postulates (**Box 24.2**). Although no human clinical studies directly testing this hypothesis have been performed to date, this hypothesis has been verified in multiple rodent, porcine, and non-human primate studies. The strength of this working hypothesis is that it helps resolve the paradox of how gut-derived sepsis and MODS can occur, and yet neither bacteria nor endotoxins are found in portal vein blood samples. It also explains the relationship between increased gut permeability and MODS. Thus, currently, the original bacterial translocation paradigm has been expanded to include the gut lymph hypothesis (**Figure 24.2**).

Although it seems important to maintain normal intestinal barrier function in the critically ill or injured patient, maintenance of barrier function is exceedingly difficult. As previously mentioned, these patients are frequently immunocompromised and their bowel flora is often disrupted. In addition, they may have had major blood loss or hypotension and may be receiving vasoactive drugs. All can result in splanchnic vasoconstriction and intestinal mucosal injury. Thus,

the need to optimize intestinal barrier function in high-risk patients presents a clinical challenge. To develop strategies to maintain normal intestinal barrier function as well as limit bacterial translocation, it is necessary to understand each of the components that contribute to the intestinal barrier.

■ THE INTESTINAL BARRIER: DEFENSES AND MECHANISMS

The initial step in the translocation of bacteria from the intestinal tract is the adherence of bacteria to the epithelial cell surface or to ulcerated areas of the intestinal mucosal surface. Once adherence occurs, the bacteria then cross the mucosal barrier and reach the lamina propria in a viable state, at which point bacterial translocation has technically occurred. However, unless the bacteria or their products (endotoxins) are able to invade the lymphatics or bloodstream and then spread systemically, the process is unlikely to be of significance. In fact, there is increasing evidence that a limited amount of bacterial translocation may be a physiologically normal process that is important in the development and maintenance of intestinal and systemic immunity.

The host has a complex series of defense mechanisms to prevent or limit potentially pathogenic bacteria from adhering to the intestinal mucosa. These defense mechanisms of barrier function consist of three basic elements: The stabilizing influence of the normal intestinal microflora, and mechanical and immunological defenses (**Box 24.3**). One major component of the barrier worthy of special mention is the indigenous (normal) microflora. The protective role of the normal intestinal microflora was initially described by van der Waaij et al. (1971), who showed that intestinal colonization or overgrowth with potentially pathogenic microorganisms was

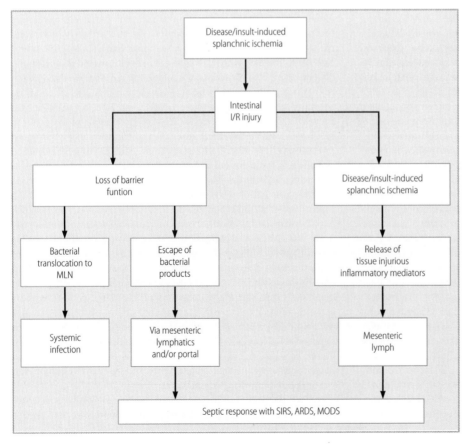

Figure 24.2 Schematic overview showing the different potential pathways and mechanisms by which a systemic insult can lead to bacterial translocation and/or gut-derived sepsis. In this paradigm, shunting of blood away from the splanchnic circulation leads to a gut ischemia–reperfusion injury, which in turn results in gut injury (loss of barrier function) and inflammation. In addition to the process of bacterial translocation, the stressed and inflamed gut appears to be the source of non-microbial sepsis and multiple-organ dysfunction syndrome-inducing factors that reach the systemic circulation via the intestinal lymphatics.

promoted by the disruption of the normal intestinal flora. They coined the term "colonization resistance" to describe this protective role of the normal intestinal flora. It is now clear that the obligate anaerobic bacteria are one major element responsible for colonization resistance, because the anaerobes outnumber the enteric Gram-negative and aerobic Gram-positive bacteria by 1000- to 10 000-fold. By associating closely with the intestinal epithelium, they form a physical barrier limiting the direct binding of potential pathogens with the mucosa. Due to increased sensitivity of the obligate anaerobes, this anaerobic barrier is lost when broad-spectrum antibiotics are administered (Berg 1981) as well as during periods of physiological or nutritional stress (Deitch 1990). Consequently, loss of this anaerobic "barrier" facilitates the association of potential pathogenic bacteria with the intestinal epithelium. As discussed later, these physiological observations were the rationale behind the development and the clinical use of anaerobic-sparing oral antibiotics to selectively decontaminate the intestinal tract as well as the use of prebiotics and probiotics.

A second line of defense against bacterial translocation or the absorption of endotoxins is provided by the mechanical defenses of the bowel, which include the intestinal mucous layer (Kim and Ho 2010), intestinal peristalsis, and the intestinal epithelium. The intestinal epithelium is coated by a mucous gel layer 30–50 μm thick. This gel layer prevents the adherence of bacteria to epithelial cell surface receptors and also provides a favorable environment for anaerobic bacteria. The presence of a normal continuous, mucous layer prevents tissue colonization by potential pathogens (Kim and Ho 2010). Elimination of this mucous layer has been shown to result in bacterial overgrowth with Gram-negative enteric bacteria and to increase the numbers of these bacteria adhering directly to the intestinal epithelium. Most recently, loss of the mucus layer has been shown to allow digestive enzymes and other toxic factors within the gut lumen to reach the underlying intestinal epithelial layer, leading to autodigestion and increased gut permeability (Sharpe et al. 2008). In the small intestine, normal peristalsis prevents the prolonged stasis of bacteria in close proximity to the intestinal mucosa, and thereby reduces the chances that bacteria will have adequate time to penetrate the mucous layer. When peristalsis is impaired, as occurs with intestinal obstruction or ileus, bacterial stasis and overgrowth result (Savage et al. 1968). This combination of events promotes bacterial penetration through the mucus and facilitates bacterial translocation.

The intestinal immune system, known as the gut-associated lymphoid tissue (GALT), regulates the local immune response to soluble and particulate antigens within the bowel. The exact role of the GALT in preventing bacterial adherence and translocation is unclear; however, it appears that secretory IgA produced by antigen-primed B lymphocytes lining the mucosal surface prevents mucosal invasion by binding to bacteria and blocking their attachment to epithelial cells, without activating other arms of the immune system (Tomasi et al. 1983). However, the importance of the GALT as opposed to the systemic immunoinflammatory system in the prevention of bacterial translocation or sepsis originating in the gut is unclear.

Although both an intact epithelial barrier and a normal functioning immune system are important for adequate gut barrier function, it appears that an intact mucosa will prevent bacterial translocation in rats with selectively impaired cell-mediated immunity (Suzuki et al. 2010). Thus, the physical barrier of the mucosa may be of primary importance in preventing or limiting bacterial translocation, especially in a host with a normal gut flora, whereas the immune system may serve a secondary or supportive role to the intestinal mucosal barrier. This is a similar role played by other mechanical barriers, such as the skin. The importance of loss of mucosal barrier function in the pathogenesis of bacterial translocation after thermal injury (Ma et al. 1989), limited periods of hemorrhagic shock (Deitch et al. 1988), or endotoxin challenge (Deitch et al. 1988) was highlighted by the results of early studies documenting that bacterial translocation can be largely prevented by limiting mucosal injury. In fact, one of the factors that most of the stress and injury models of bacterial translocation have in common is reduced splanchnic blood flow and histological evidence of mucosal edema or injury. Mucosal injury in these models, as well as in stressed patients, appears to be due to a gut ischemia–reperfusion injury. This ischemia–reperfusion-induced mucosal injury is mediated in part by xanthine oxidase-generated oxygen free radicals, as well as by the tissue destructive products generated by increased nitric oxide synthase (NOS) activity. Consequently, a major concept from these studies is that splanchnic circulation is very sensitive to alterations in intravascular volume, and injury- or stress-induced splanchnic vasoconstriction, which may ultimately lead to an ischemia–reperfusion (I/R) injury of the intestinal mucosa, impaired intestinal barrier function, and intestinal inflammation.

The mechanisms by which gut I/R leads to gut injury has also evolved over the last decade, with the recognition that injury-induced loss of gut barrier function and the generation of non-microbial factors carried in the lymphatics appears to be more important in the pathogenesis of gut-induced MODS than translocating bacteria. Based on this recent work, it appears that gut injury during low flow states is not just due to systemic factors but also involves processes occurring on the luminal side of the gut wall (**Figure 24.3**), i.e., although previous studies investigating the mechanisms of gut I/R-induced injury have focused on the systemic factors associated with the gut I/R response, they have largely ignored the non-microbial intraluminal contents of the gut, especially the mucous gel layer. However, if the mucous gel hydrophobic barrier is lost, this would allow luminal digestive enzymes, especially the pancreatic proteases, to come into direct contact with the underlying epithelial layer of the intestinal villi. In this circumstance, the host's intestinal lining would be enzymatically digested in a fashion similar to that of ingested proteins and other foodstuffs. Thus, if the mucous gel barrier were damaged and/or gut barrier failure occurred, the host would be in danger of being not only significantly injured by its own gut bacteria but also digested by its own intraluminal digestive enzymes.

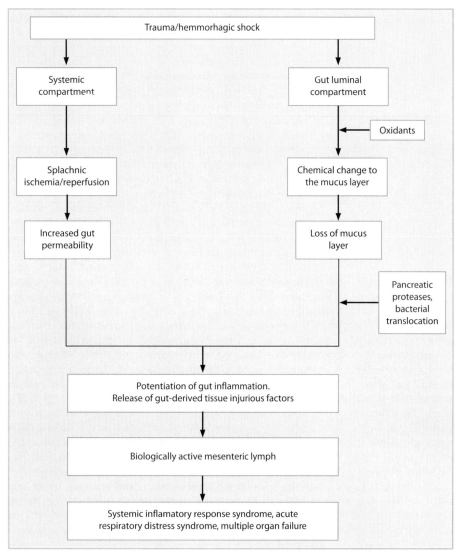

Figure 24.3 Schematic overview of the multifactorial processes leading to the development of increased gut permeability and biologically active mesenteric lymph that includes both systemic events (ischemia–reperfusion) and luminal factors within the gut lumen. The luminal components include loss of the protective mucus barrier, the deleterious effects of digestive enzymes, as well as bacteria and their products.

Although the concept of the mucous layer being an important protective barrier is well established in the stomach, where stress- or ischemia-induced loss of the gastric mucous layer contributes to gastric mucosal injury by intraluminal acid, few studies have investigated the consequences of loss of the mucous layer in other parts of the intestine. One potential reason for the limited attention being focused on the mucous layer under conditions of gut ischemia or stress is that the mucous layer is dissolved and lost during ordinary histological fixation procedures. Thus, what is not seen is not studied. In this light, recently published studies evaluating the mucous layer in gut I/R and trauma/hemorrhagic shock (T/HS) models document that T/HS leads to a significant loss of the unstirred mucous layer as well as increased villous injury, enterocyte apoptosis, and gut permeability (Rupani et al. 2007, Qin et al. 2008, 2011). In addition, gut permeability was greatest at the time of maximal mucus loss. The importance of maintaining the gut mucous gel layer is highlighted by a recent study showing that the enteral administration of high-molecular-weight polyethylene glycol (a mucus surrogate) prevented lethal sepsis originating from the gut (Wu et al. 2004). In addition, pharmacological studies have documented that the decisive barrier to the transport of a compound across the gut wall was related to the mucous layer and not the lipid membrane of the underlying enterocytes. Thus the mucous layer of

the gut is more of a barrier to the egress of compounds within the gut lumen than the enterocyte layer (Nimmerfall and Rosenthaler 1980). This concept of the major protective role of the gut mucous layer was convincingly shown in a recent proof-of-principle study of the normal intestine, where removal of the mucous layer was associated with increased gut permeability and pancreatic protease-induced gut necrosis (Sharpe et al. 2008).

Although the role of the pancreas as a factor in the pathogenesis of shock has a long history (Glenn and Lefer 1971, Lefer and Glenn 1971), this area was neglected for almost 30 years, until experiments showed that pancreatic enzymes are critical factors in intestinal I/R-induced shock and neutrophil activation in 2000 (Kistler et al. 2000, Mitsuoka et al. 2000). The studies investigating the effects of pancreatic proteases in gut I/R and T/HS models have generated the following four conclusions about the role that pancreatic proteases play in gut injury and the development of SIRS, ARDS, and MODS (Sharpe et al. 2008):

1. Pancreatic proteases contribute to gut injury in gut I/R models and this may be potentiated by the augmented destruction of the mucous layer.
2. The interaction of pancreatic proteases with the ischemic gut contributes to T/HS- and gut I/R-induced SIRS, ARDS, and MODS

through the generation of non-microbial proinflammatory and tissue injurious factors.

3. After T/HS, pancreatic proteases are necessary for the production of biologically active factors in mesenteric lymph, which transforms gut ischemia into a systemic toxic and inflammatory response.

4. Although T/HS decreases splanchnic blood flow resulting in a gut I/R injury, in the absence of pancreatic proteases, this systemic hemodynamic insult is not sufficient to produce toxic mesenteric lymph, neutrophil activation, or lung injury.

Thus, pancreatic proteases appear to be a necessary component in the pathogenesis of T/HS-induced MODS originating from the gut (Schmid-Schönbein et al. 2001, Mitsuoka et al. 2002, Deitch et al. 2003, Kramp et al. 2003, Waldo et al. 2003, Cohen et al. 2004, Caputo et al. 2007).

An additional component of the intraluminal compartment that has become important in understanding the pathogenesis of gut injury and gut-origin sepsis is the intestinal bacteria. Experimental studies in germ-free animals subjected to hemorrhagic shock (Ferraro et al. 1995) or superior mesenteric artery occlusion (Souza et al. 2004) indicate that these germ-free animals have better survival and less intestinal injury than their wild-type litter mates with normal gut flora. Studies in animals with intestinal bacterial overgrowth also indicate that the gut flora can amplify the magnitude of gut-related distant organ injury in non-lethal gut I/R models (Magnotti et al. 1999). Recent studies of normal animals document that bacterial overgrowth can induce the production of biologically active, proinflammatory, mesenteric lymph (Deitch et al. 2004b). Thus, it appears clear that the normal gut flora, as the conditions within the gut change, has the capacity to potentiate organ injury and contribute to the systemic septic response under conditions of stress or injury, even in the absence of bacterial translocation. Consequently, although the normal intestinal bacterial flora does not appear to play a direct role in the initial pathogenesis of shock-induced mucosal injury (Deitch et al. 1990), once the mucosal barrier has been breached, translocating bacteria do contribute to the problem. Thus, the gut flora and their products, although not initiating gut injury or adverse systemic effects, act as secondary insults to the damaged or stressed gut, thereby potentially exacerbating the local and systemic consequences of the initial insult. Of note, this ability of the gut flora to potentiate gut injury and MODS can occur even in the absence of measurable signs of systemic bacterial translocation or endotoxemia.

THERAPEUTIC OPTIONS AND APPROACHES

As a general principle, therapies directed at preventing or limiting bacterial translocation and/or gut injury are based on an understanding of the host's physiological defenses which maintain normal intestinal barrier function, limit stress-induced gut injury, and help maintain a stable gut flora. Therapies also include management of pathophysiology changes associated with bacterial translocation and gut barrier failure. Conceptually, these therapeutic approaches can be divided into four basic groups:

1. Preventive therapies
2. Therapies directed at maintaining a stable gut flora, thereby limiting the risk of bacterial translocation and the development of systemic infections
3. Therapies focused on limiting the development of gut injury and dysfunction, thereby supporting gut barrier function and hence reducing the incidence of gut-origin sepsis and MODS

4. Non-gut based therapies directed at limiting the systemic consequences of gut-origin sepsis (**Box 24.4**).

Box 24.4 Therapeutic options to maintain gut barrier.

1. **Support commensal gut flora and maintain microbial homeostasis**
   a. Probiotics/prebiotics/synbiotics
   b. SDD/SOD
   c. Limiting therapies that disrupt gut flora (antacids, broad-spectrum antibiotics)
2. **Support gut barrier function**
   a. Probiotics
   b. Early enteral feeding (Including tropic feeding regimens)
   c. Antioxidants (especially selenium)
   d. Specific nutrients (glutamine, omega-3 fatty acids)
3. **Prevent additional injury by adhering to basic critical care practices**

Although some therapies have overlapping effects, this conceptual approach has the advantage of providing a rationale therapeutic framework. Consequently, the remainder of this section discusses each of these four basic therapeutic goals separately.

■ Prevention

The best management of intestinal barrier failure and bacterial translocation unquestionably lies in its prevention. The two most important preventive goals are to maintain intestinal perfusion and avoid or limit therapies that disrupt the normal ecology of the gut flora. As inadequate tissue (intestinal) perfusion, a persistent inflammatory state, infection, and inadequate nutritional support appear to be the most common clinical factors predisposing to intestinal barrier failure and MODS, it seems logical that therapeutic efforts should be directed at their early treatment or prevention. Prevention takes different forms in different patients, e.g., in patients with pancreatitis, it has been shown that early and aggressive volume resuscitation is the most effective current therapy to limit the progression of pancreatitis and hence its systemic consequences, including gut barrier failure (Fritz et al. 2010, Talukdar and Swaroop Vege 2011). Likewise, an early definitive surgery approach, including prompt repair of injuries, avoiding abdominal compartment syndrome, debridement of necrotic tissues, control of bacterial contamination, and early fixation of fractures is associated with a significant reduction in the incidence of gut-derived sepsis and MODS (Diaz et al. 2010, Cotton et al. 2011). The basic concept behind this approach is that immediate treatment of all treatable injuries is the best way to limit the inflammatory response and thereby restore a more normal physiological state for maintenance of splanchnic perfusion. Similar principles apply to the non-trauma patient, for whom early definitive primary or reoperative surgery to remove necrotic tissue and control infection is of major benefit in preventing the secondary failure of other organs including the bowel. In considering prevention, it is wise to remember that systemic inflammation and/or infection can result in shunting of blood away from the gut and, thereby, increase the risk of gut injury and dysfunction. Therefore prompt resolution of inflammatory states and control of infections will reduce the likelihood of secondary changes in gut function including ileus, disruption of the normal gut flora, and increased intestinal permeability.

■ Therapies directed at maintaining a stable gut flora

Probiotics, prebiotics, and synbiotics

Probiotics are food supplements containing viable bacteria, and prebiotics are food supplements consisting of non-digestible fibers, whereas synbiotics are the combination of probiotics and prebiotics. Both probiotics and prebiotics are distinguished by their ability to exert beneficial effects on the host (**Table 24.5**). Over the last decade, the use of these agents as adjuncts to more traditional therapies has emerged and there is a growing body of data to suggest their usefulness in the treatment of both acute and chronic illnesses.

The rationale for the development and use of probiotics was based on the following four major lines of evidence: 1) that many postoperative infections are caused by the patient's own gut flora, 2) basic and clinical therapeutic strategies directed at maintaining a normal gut flora reduces bacterial translocation and systemic infections, 3) studies demonstrating that enteral nutrition and selective gut decontamination are associated with a decreased incidence of infection and 4) experimental studies indicating that certain members of the normal gut flora, such as probiotic lactobacilli, limit experimentally-induced bacterial translocation and are gut-protective (Ruan et al. 2007). This ability of probiotics to limit bacterial translocation is due to influences upon all three pathogenic mechanisms associated with bacterial translocation; which include preventing/limiting intestinal bacterial growth with potentially pathogenic bacteria, loss of gut barrier function and impaired immunity (**Box 24.5**), e.g., probiotics stabilize the gut flora by preventing intestinal overgrowth with potential pathogenic bacteria through their direct antimicrobial effects (i.e., lactic acid production) as well as by competitive growth (Servin 2004). Although probiotics

have been shown experimentally to decrease intestinal hyperpermeability and modulate immunity, the mechanisms by which this occurs are less clear (Walker 2008).

Similar to probiotics, prebiotics can also have gut-beneficial effects, especially in the presence of probiotics. Intraluminal intestinal fermentation of prebiotics by probiotics serves both to support probiotic growth and to provide colonocyte nutrient sources, such as omega-3 fatty acids (Bengmark 1999). Therefore most clinical studies have used synbiotic combinations of probiotics and prebiotics. Furthermore, as certain probiotic strains are able to act synergistically (Timmerman et al. 2004), most current clinical trials use a combination of probiotics and prebiotics to optimize the therapeutic potential.

The clinical use of probiotics and synbiotics is a relatively recent event with the first prospective randomized clinical trial (PRCT) testing the ability of synbiotics to decrease infections being published in 2002 (Rayes et al. 2002). In this German study of patients undergoing major abdominal surgery, the patients receiving synbiotics had a 10% versus a 30% postoperative infection rate in the control group. Since this pioneering clinical trial, PRCTs of probiotics/synbiotics have been carried out, largely in four major patient populations. These are patients undergoing major abdominal operations, patients with severe acute pancreatitis, patients undergoing liver transplantation, and mechanically ventilated patients in the ICU. The rationale for studying these four patient populations is their documented increased risk of bacterial translocation and sepsis originating from the gut. The largest number of studies were performed in patients undergoing elective major abdominal procedures and a meta-analysis of these studies was published in 2009 (Pitsouni et al. 2009). This meta-analysis of nine clinical studies documented that the perioperative administration of probiotics and/or synbiotics reduced the overall postoperative infection rate by more than 50% and significantly decreased length of stay, although there was no mortality advantage. This failure to show a mortality benefit is not surprising, because the mortality rate of these studies was low and averaged about 3% (Pitsouni et al. 2009). In spite of the overall benefits observed in this meta-analysis, two of the nine studies did not find a reduction in the incidence of postoperative infections due to the heterogeneity in the types of probiotics used as well as the exact probiotic/synbiotic treatment regimen employed. Consistent with this 2009 meta-analysis, an earlier review of 14 studies documented that, in most of the studies, perioperative probiotic/synbiotic therapy reduced the incidence of postoperative infections (van Santvoort et al. 2008). However, four of the five studies that failed to show clinical benefit were from the same group with unique regimens, further stressing the concept that not all probiotics/synbiotics are clinically equivalent. Thus further work needs to be done to better define optimal clinical probiotic, prebiotic, and synbiotic regimens. However, most of the studies carried out since 2005 used a synbiotic regimen consisting of four different lactic acid bacteria and four prebiotics (Symbiotic).

The second largest group of PRCT studies was carried out in mechanically ventilated ICU patients, with the first study being published in 2006. A meta-analysis of these PRCT trials was published in 2010 testing whether probiotics/synbiotics decreased the incidence of ventilator-associated pneumonia (VAP). This study found that the probiotic-treated patients had 40% less VAP than the control group (Siempos et al. 2010). This decreased incidence of VAP was associated with a decreased length of stay but not an improvement in mortality. In most of these studies, Synbiotic 2000 FORTE, consisting of five bacterial species and four prebiotics, was used. In the same year that this meta-analysis was published, a French group published a single-center PRCT trial designed to assess whether probiotic/

Box 24.5 Probiotics, prebiotics, and synbiotics.

1. **Definitions**
   - *Probiotics:* food supplements containing live bacteria that theoretically have beneficial effects on the host. These are commercially available viable microorganisms which, when administered in adequate amounts, either as individual strains or in various combinations have health benefits for the host.
   - *Prebiotics:* Non-digestable, non-absorbable, non-fermentable orally delivered fibers (sugars) that stimulate the growth or activity of certain bacteria of the gastrointestinal tract, to the benefit of the host.
   - *Synbiotics:* food supplements containing both probiotics and prebiotics.
2. **Biology**
   - Probiotics:
     - stabilize gut flora by maintaining non-pathogenic bacteria
     - stabilize intestinal barrier by blocking adhesion sites for pathogenic bacteria
   - enhances immune system
   - Prebiotics
     - act as "nutrient source" for probiotics and other beneficial intestinal bacteria
     - when fermented by probiotics provide a colonocyte food source
     - encourage growth of non-pathogenic bacteria while inhibiting growth of pathogenic bacteria

synbiotic therapy improved survival in mechanically ventilated ICU patients (Barraud et al. 2010). They used a commercial multi-bacterial product called 5 Ergyphilus. Although they found no difference in overall mortality between the groups, a subgroup analysis found that the administration of probiotics improved survival in patients with severe sepsis. However, of concern, this therapy increased the mortality rate of patients with non-severe sepsis. The explanation for the differential effects of synbiotic therapy on mortality between the severely septic patients versus patients with non-severe sepsis is unclear. It does, however, stress the need for more and larger studies in ICU patient populations.

Although the data are more limited, most of studies testing the ability of probiotics/synbiotics to reduce infections in patients with severe acute pancreatitis, as well as in patients undergoing liver transplantation, have shown efficacy (Oláh et al. 2002, Rayes et al. 2005). The important exception is a study by Basselink et al. (2008). In this study of severe acute pancreatitis, termed "PROPATRIA," patients treated with the probiotic Ecologic 641 had increased infectious complications and a higher mortality. The explanation for these conflicting results remains to be resolved. However, in a subsequent subgroup analysis of the patients enrolled in the PROPATRIA study, the adverse effects of the probiotic therapy were largely confined to the group of patients who had early organ failure (Besselink et al. 2009). From this observation, they (Besselink et al. 2009) and others (Soeters 2008) have proposed that probiotics may result in adverse consequences when administered into compromised GI tracts with increased permeability and compromised oxygen delivery.

Although the Basselink acute pancreatitis study (Besselink et al. 2008) raises concern, the meta-analyses and most of the PRCTs using probiotics show clinical benefit. However, it is difficult to directly compare the individual trials because both the probiotic agent and dosage used vary from trial to trial. Yet, based on findings from studies of the basic biology of the probiotics, differences in the exact probiotic bacteria administered between the different clinical trials may be of significant potential clinical importance, e.g., to have a beneficial effect, the probiotic administered must adhere to the intestinal epithelium via the same receptor as the target pathogenic bacteria. In this fashion, the probiotic bacteria can prevent pathogenic attachment or even displace attached pathogenic bacteria. This point is highlighted by the work of Collado et al. (2005), who demonstrated that the ability of different probiotic bacteria to prevent pathogenic intestinal bacterial binding as well as displace previously bound pathogenic bacteria to human intestinal epithelium varied based on the potentially pathogenic bacteria. Thus, if the specific pathogenic bacterium is known, the most appropriate probiotic can be selected that optimally inhibits future adherence and displaces adhered pathogens. Consequently, as different probiotics may differentially occupy specific intestinal epithelial cell receptors, the inhibition of pathogen adhesion is highly variable and strain dependent.

Which probiotic/synbiotic formulation is best for which clinical situation is currently the most important clinical question to be answered. Not only must the question of which species or combinations of species to use in specific clinical scenarios be addressed, but also it would be important to better define the optimal doses of these agents as well as the best methods and vehicles for their delivery. Current commercial prebiotic, probiotic, and synbiotic products are attempting to address this notion that different prebiotic fibers and probiotic bacteria may exert different effects and/or interact synergistically by producing products that contain multiple different probiotics and prebiotics (**Box 24.6**). Nevertheless, based on the high safety profile of these products and evidence from most studies that they are effective

Box 24.6 List of commercial probiotics/synbiotics.

1. **Single strains**
   - *Lactobacillus plantarum* 299V (Rayes et al. 2002, van Santvoort et al. 2008, Pitsouni et al. 2009, Siempos et al. 2010)
   - *Lactobacillus casei rhamnosus* (Siempos et al. 2010)
2. **Commercial prebiotic/synbiotic formulations**
   - Symbiotic 2000 Forte (Rayes et al. 2005, van Santvoort et al. 2008, Pitsouni et al. 2009, Siempos et al. 2010)
   - Symbiotic 2000 (van Santvoort et al. 2008, Pitsouni et al. 2009)
   - Trevis (van Santvoort et al. 2008, Pitsouni et al. 2009)
   - Yakult BL Seichoyaku (van Santvoort et al. 2008, Pitsouni et al. 2009)
   - Yakult 400 (van Santvoort et al. 2008, Pitsouni et al. 2009)
   - Bifies (van Santvoort et al. 2008)
   - 5-Ergyphilus (Barraud et al. 2010)
   - Ecologic 641 (Besselink et al. 2008)
3. **Commercial prebiotic formulations**
   - Oligomate 55 (van Santvoort et al. 2008, Pitsouni et al. 2009)
   - Raftilose (van Santvoort et al. 2008)

A recent Google search of the term probiotic has revealed that there are upwards of 1000 probiotic formulas that are commercially available. Commercial probiotic formulations are not regulated by the US Food and Drug Administration, and, as such, not all may be equally effective. Above is a list of the probiotic formulations/strains used in prospective randomized clinical trials mentioned in this chapter.

in reducing infections and shortening length of hospital stay, they appear to be a worthwhile clinical tool. Lastly, in thinking about the use of probiotics, prebiotics, and synbiotics, we believe that the timing of their administration may be critical, e.g., the prophylactic administration of these agents electively before major operations seems to have been a uniformly beneficial strategy. This may be because gut barrier function is intact and the patient's gut flora has been at most modestly perturbed. In contrast, administering probiotic bacteria at high doses to patients with established gut injury and increased permeability may result in these low virulence bacteria translocating across the injured mucosa, thereby contributing to increased systemic inflammation and altered immune defenses. Hopefully, as more information becomes available, these types of questions can be answered.

■ Selective digestive tract decontamination

The use of oral non-absorbable prophylactic antibiotic administration is another therapeutic approach employed to prevent intestinal colonization or overgrowth with potentially pathological bacteria. The first clinical study of selective decontamination of the digestive tract (SDD) was published by Stoutenbeck et al. in 1984, where this technique was found to reduce the infection rate in a cohort of trauma patients. Since then, the clinical efficacy of SDD has been tested in multiple different patient populations. The current technique of SDD has three parts and was designed primarily to selectively suppress and eradicate potentially pathogenic Gram-negative aerobic bacteria and fungi in the oropharynx and upper and lower intestines (**Box 24.7**). The three basic concepts on which SDD is based are that (1) nosocomial infections are a common problem in the ICU, (2) these infections directly

Box 24.7 Prophylactic antibiotic decontamination regimens. Three different regimens have been used, from most to least aggressive: selective digestive tract decontamination, selective gut decontamination, and selective oral decontamination.

1. **Selective digestive tract decontamination (SDD)**
   - Targets oral pathogens, intestinal pathogens, and respiratory tract flora
   - **Goal of therapy**: non-absorbable antimicrobial oral/intestinal therapies targeting Gram-negative organisms, *Staphylococcus aureus*, and yeasts to prevent infection after gut barrier failure plus systemic antimicrobial therapy targeting respiratory flora-mediated pneumonias
   - **Regimen**: 4 days of intravenous cefotaxime (1000 mg every 6 h); application of topical paste to the oral cavity and pharynx (polymyxin E, tobramycin, and amphotericin B, each at a concentration of 2%), and gastric lavage every 6 h with an antibiotic solution (10 ml of a suspension of 100 mg polymyxin E, 80 mg tobramycin, and 500 mg amphotericin B)
   - **Benefits**: 40–50% reduction in the rate of nosocomial infection and a lesser reduction (3.5%) in mortality
   - **Perceived detriments** (to date unproven): Increased risk of development of resistant organism pneumonia. Increased threat of *Clostridium difficile* colitis.
2. **Selective gut decontamination (SGD)**
   - Provides total decontamination of oral cavity and gastrointestinal tract without systemic antibiotic therapy
   - **Goal of therapy**: Non-absorbable antimicrobial oral/intestinal therapies targeting Gram-negative organisms, *S. aureus*, and yeasts to prevent infection after gut barrier failure. Maintenance of normal gut flora through avoidance of anti-aerobic antibiotics
   - **Regimen**: Application of topical paste to the oral cavity and pharynx (polymyxin E, tobramycin, and amphotericin B, each at a concentration of 2%), and gastric lavage every 6 h with an antibiotic solution (10 ml of a suspension of 100 mg polymyxin E, 80 mg tobramycin, and 500 mg amphotericin B)
   - **Benefits**: Reduction in the rate of hospital-acquired infection and a decrease in mortality greater than that of SOD but less than that of SDD (3%). Risk of development of resistant organism pneumonias is theoretically decreased
   - **Perceived detriments** (to date unproven): Increased threat of *C. difficile* colitis.
3. **Selective oral decontamination (SOD)**
   - Provides decontamination of the oral cavity only. Thought to prevent contamination of endotracheal tube colonization-mediated pneumonia and aspiration pneumonia.
   - **Goal of therapy**: Non-absorbable antimicrobial oral therapy targeting Gram-negative organisms, *S. aureus*, and yeasts to prevent secondary infections
   - **Regimen**: (1) Application of topical paste to the oral cavity and pharynx (polymyxin E, tobramycin, and amphotericin B, each at a concentration of 2%) or (2) chlorhexidine gluconate (0.12% oral rinse, 0.2% oral rinse, or 2% oral gel) applied every 8 h
   - **Benefits**: Reduction in the rate of systemic infection from ventilator-associated pneumonia and aspiration pneumonia. No risk of *C. difficile* colitis; no risk of generating a multidrug-resistant pneumonia from prophylaxis
   - **Detriments**: Reduction in mortality less than that of regimens in which systemic or gastrointestinal tract decontamination occurs

contribute to mortality, and (3) most of these infections are caused by bacteria and fungi that have colonized the oropharynx, stomach, and intestine. Consequently, the goals of SDD are to decrease the colonization rate of these high-risk patients, thereby reducing the incidence of infection and improving survival. As documented by multiple PRCTs and summarized in meta-analyses (van Nieuwenhoven et al. 2001, Chan et al. 2007), SDD has been repeatedly shown to decrease the absolute rate of infections in multiple ICU patient populations ranging from trauma patients to postoperative patients. Although the absolute reduction in infection rates has varied from series to series, on average the incidence of pneumonias, urinary tract infections, and primary bacteremias has been reduced by 50% or more. Although most of the early studies were not able to consistently document a survival advantage with SDD, selected single-center prospective trials, as well as new, recent meta-analyses, have documented that SDD significantly reduces mortality in medical, surgical, and trauma ICU patients (D'Amico et al. 1998, Nathens and Marshall 1999, van Nieuwenhoven et al. 2001, Krueger et al. 2002, de Jonge et al. 2003, Stoutenbeek et al. 2006, Dellinger et al. 2008, de Smet et al. 2009). Although the reduction in mortality observed with SDD has varied between studies, most studies have shown an absolute reduction in mortality rate of >3–4%, which translates into an overall reduction in mortality of approximately 11%.

As a result of the risk of antibiotic resistance, several studies have used a selective oral decontamination (SOD) approach rather than SDD as an alternative to the prevention of VAP (Pugin et al. 1991, Bergmans et al. 2001). The advantage of SOD is that no systemic antibiotics are given and the need for oral antibiotics is reduced (Box 24.7). This approach is based on the key role of oropharyngeal colonization in the pathogenesis of VAP and evidence that SOD is effective in preventing VAP (Bonten et al. 2004, Chan et al. 2007). The efficacy of SOD versus SDD in preventing VAP and improving mortality was recently tested in a multicenter clinical trial enrolling 5939 patients (de Smet et al. 2009). The results of this study showed that the two therapeutic approaches were comparable with SDD reducing 28-day mortality by 3.5% and SOD reducing mortality by 2.9%. Thus, the use of SDD or SOD to control oropharyngeal and intestinal colonization with potentially pathogenic bacteria appears a viable therapeutic option.

■ Therapies direct at supporting gut barrier function

As previously discussed, gut barrier failure and increased intestinal permeability have been found to be relatively common in critically ill patients, major injury and major surgery, in several clinical studies, have been found to be associated with increased morbidity and mortality (Pape et al. 1994, Reintam et al. 2006). Consequently, significant investigative effort has been directed toward understanding the mechanisms leading to gut injury, to develop effective therapies to prevent and/or limit gut barrier failure and restore the failed gut barrier. To date, the most effective therapies involve various nutritional and gut-barrier-enhancing strategies; one of the most important concepts is that the gut has specific nutritional needs distinct from the rest of the body. Importantly, the lack of enteral feeding itself can result in impaired gut barrier function (Gatt and MacFie 2010). This concept is based on both clinical and preclinical studies documenting that lack of enteral feeding (starvation), as well as standard total parenteral nutrition (TPN), leads to gut atrophy as well as major changes in gut function (**Figure 24.4**). The direct benefits of enteral as opposed to parenteral nutrition in reducing infection was first reported by Moore et al. (1989), who demonstrated that abdominal trauma patients randomized to the total enteral nutrition group had a reduced rate of

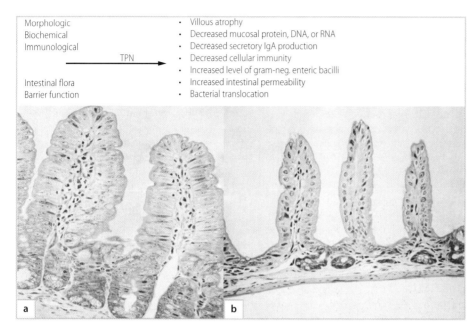

Morphologic	• Villous atrophy
Biochemical	• Decreased mucosal protein, DNA, or RNA
Immunological	• Decreased secretory IgA production
	• Decreased cellular immunity
	• Increased level of gram-neg. enteric bacilli
Intestinal flora	• Increased intestinal permeability
Barrier function	• Bacterial translocation

Figure 24.4 Schematic illustration of the effects of total parenteral nutrition on the gut and the gut flora as well as representative illustrations of the profound atrophy of the gut which occurs after even 5 days of starvation. (a) Normal gut. (b) Following TPN administration

infection (37% vs 17%) and septic morbidity (3% vs 20%), compared with patients receiving TPN. Since then, many studies, in multiple patient populations, have validated the clinical benefits of early enteral feeding, e.g., one recent meta-analysis of 30 PRCTs comparing enteral with parenteral nutrition in hospitalized patients found that enteral nutrition was associated with a significantly lower rate of infectious complications and a reduced length of hospital stay (Peter et al. 2005).

Furthermore, a meta-analysis of five PRCTs of enteral versus parenteral nutrition in patients with acute pancreatitis found that the mortality rate of the enterally fed patients was significantly reduced compared with parenterally fed patients (4% vs 16%) (Petrov et al. 2008). Support for enteral nutrition in patients undergoing major abdominal surgery was documented in a Cochrane review of patients undergoing colon surgery, in which enteral feeds were found to significantly reduce mortality (Andersen et al. 2006). This reduction in overall mortality was later confirmed in a meta-analysis (Lewis et al. 2008). As a result of these and other such studies, early enteral nutrition has been included in the enhanced recovery after surgery group recommendations for colorectal surgery (Lassen et al. 2009).

The exact reasons why enteral nutrition is superior to parenteral nutrition in maintaining intestinal barrier function, reducing sepsis originating from the gut and decreasing the incidence and/or severity of MODS in high-risk ICU patients has been extensively investigated. One hypothesis is that gut barrier failure and sepsis originating from the gut may be more severe in ICU patients receiving TPN due to the fact that current parenteral nutrition formulations lack bowel-specific nutrients and tropic factors (Wilmore et al. 1988). For this reason, these intravenous nutrition solutions will not fully support intestinal structure and function. Advances in nutrient pharmacology and physiology have shown that specific nutrients, such as glutamine and short-chain fatty acids, as well as trace minerals and even certain non-digestible fibers (prebiotics), exert beneficial tropic effects on the gut. Most of the work in this area has been directed at studying glutamine, because, in addition to being an enterocyte-specific nutrient and having important antioxidant activities, plasma glutamine levels rapidly drop during stress states (Avenell 2009). Although the results of clinical trials testing the efficacy of glutamine are confusing, due to a number of confounding factors, two recent meta-analyses

indicate that either parenteral or enteral glutamine supplementation is clinically beneficial (Avenell 2006, 2009). Similar to the studies with glutamine, recent work has shown that the administration of enteral diets high in omega-3 fatty acids (fish and borage oils) rather than omega-6 fatty acids (vegetable oil and main component in intralipid) reduces mortality in patients with severe sepsis (Pontes-Arruda et al. 2006). In fact, intravenous omega-3 fatty acids also show a survival benefit in ICU patients (Heller et al. 2006). Although extensive preclinical and limited clinical studies have implicated numerous other nutrients, vitamins, and minerals as well as prebiotic fibers as having potential gut protective effects, too little is known to accurately assess their therapeutic benefits. Nevertheless, it is clear that early enteral feeding and the enteral and/or parenteral administration of glutamine and omega-3 fatty acids are gut protective and clinically beneficial in high-risk surgical as well as ICU patients.

A second hypothesis of why enteral nutrition appears superior to parenteral is based on the concept that enteral feeding induces a number of gut-supportive mechanisms, e.g., enteral feeding stimulates the production and release of gut-derived intestinal hormones and growth factors, several of which have been shown to have gut tropic properties. In addition, as exemplified by prebiotics, the intraluminal digestion of fibers by the host microflora releases various nutrients, such as omega-3 fatty acids which are preferred enterocyte fuels. This hypothesis has been validated in animal studies, where limited amounts of enteral feeding have been documented to preserve or improve gut function and morphology (Omura et al. 2000, Ohta et al. 2003, Ikezawa et al. 2008). As it is not always possible to successfully administer full enteral support in critically ill patients, several studies have investigated whether limited enteral feeding would be comparable to full enteral feeding in these high-risk patients. One such PRCT study by Rice et al. (2011) found that mechanically ventilated patients randomized to a 6-day course of tropic levels of enteral feeding (10 ml/h) versus full enteral feeding had similar rates of organ failure and no difference in mortality was found between the groups. This and other studies support the concept that even limited amounts of early enteral feeding can have gut-protective effects which can translate into clinical benefits.

In trying to put this nutritional information into clinical perspective it is important to consider the patient population being treated as well as the therapeutic goal, e.g., preoperative as well as early postoperative nutrition can be administered to patients undergoing elective surgery, a strategy that has been shown to reduce postoperative infectious complications (Okamoto et al. 2009). However, this prophylactic perioperative approach is not possible in trauma, emergency surgery, or other high-risk patient groups, such as those with severe acute pancreatitis. In these patient groups, therapies are initiated after the disease process has become established, and thus the prevention of gut-barrier dysfunction and sepsis originating from the gut may not be fully possible. Instead, the goal is to limit the magnitude of gut dysfunction and to restore gut function to normal as quickly as possible.

Intestinal barrier failure and subsequent sepsis originating from the gut may be exacerbated by non-intestinal as well as intestinal factors, such as hypotension, hemodynamic instability, or vasoactive agents that decrease intestinal perfusion (i.e., I/R injury) and thereby increase intestinal permeability. All these systemic insults, as well as severe septic states, are associated with oxidant-mediated intestinal injury and experimental antioxidant therapies have been shown to successfully reduce bacterial translocation as well as gut injury in preclinical animal studies (Deitch 1990). Consequently, antioxidant therapies directed at preventing or limiting oxidant-mediated intestinal injury during stress states are a promising area of research. A limited number of clinical studies have examined whether antioxidants added to resuscitation fluids reduce infections and organ failure; the results are inconclusive. In contrast, a large number of PRCTs have studied antioxidants in ICU patients. As most of these studies focused more on the role of antioxidants as a group rather than individual antioxidants, there are few prospective trials evaluating the effect of individual agents. However, a meta-analysis has suggested that parenteral antioxidant supplementation is associated with a significant decrease in mortality, with this benefit being largely associated with parenteral selenium administration (Heyland et al. 2005). A subsequent PRCT of parenteral selenium supplementation in patients with septic shock, sepsis, and SIRS documented a reduction in the 28-day mortality rate from 50% in the control group to 40% in the selenium group (Angstwurm et al. 2007). Although additional studies are necessary to determine the effect of enteral selenium supplementation, the Society of Critical Care Medicine and the American Society for Parenteral and Enteral Nutrition recommend that selenium be specifically included as part of an antioxidant supplementation (Martindale et al. 2009). Thus, the role of antioxidants other than selenium remains unclear.

■ CONCLUSION

Much has changed since the original view of the gut as a digestive organ. Today, it is well recognized that gut failure has important physiological and clinical implications for many groups of surgical and ICU patients. Thus, beginning with studies showing that early enteral feeding can be clinically beneficial, efforts have been made to bolster gut function. Several of these strategies have focused on maintaining a normal gut flora and limiting gut overgrowth with potential pathogens. In the case of probiotics and prebiotics, most early studies are encouraging. Yet, more work is needed to better define the optimal patient groups for this therapy as well as the optimal probiotic/prebiotic/synbiotic formulae to be used in these specific patient populations. These gut-directed therapies are further supported by emerging evidence that the intestinal microflora are capable of up-regulating and downregulating mammalian gene products through receptor-based cross-talk (Kinross et al. 2009, Tsujimoto et al. 2009). This work highlights the potential benefits to the host of a normal gut flora as well as the fact that changes in the gut microflora may initiate corresponding changes in the host's own tissues which can modify the host's responses to various stresses and insults.

■ REFERENCES

Ambrose NS, Johnson M, Burdon DW, Keighley MR. Incidence of pathogenic bacteria from mesenteric lymph nodes and ileal serosa during Crohn's disease surgery. Br J Surg 1984;**71**:623–5.

Andersen HK, Lewis SJ, Thomas S. Cochrane Database of Syst Rev 2006;(**4**):CD004080.

Angstwurm MWA, Engelmann L, Zimmermann T, et al. Selenium in Intensive Care (SIC): results of a prospective randomized, placebo-controlled, multiple-center study in patients with severe systemic inflammatory response syndrome, sepsis, and septic shock. Crit Care Med 2007;**35**:118–26.

Avenell A. Glutamine in critical care: current evidence from systematic reviews. Proc Nutr Soc 2006;**65**:236–41.

Avenell A. Symposium 4: Hot topics in parenteral nutrition Current evidence and ongoing trials on the use of glutamine in critically-ill patients and patients undergoing surgery. Proc Nutr Soc 2009;**68**:261.

Balzan S, de Almeida Quadros C, de Cleva R, Zilberstein B, Cecconello I. Bacterial translocation: Overview of mechanisms and clinical impact. J Gastroenterol Hepatol 2007;**22**:464–71.

Barraud D, Blard C, Hein F, et al. Probiotics in the critically ill patient: a double blind, randomized, placebo-controlled trial. Intensive Care Med 2010;**36**:1540–7.

Bengmark S. Gut microenvironment and immune function. Curr Opin Clin Nutr Metab Care 1999;**2**:83–5.

Berg RD. Promotion of the translocation of enteric bacteria from the gastrointestinal tracts of mice by oral treatment with penicillin, clindamycin, or metronidazole. Infect Immun 1981;**33**:854–61.

Berg RD, Garlington AW. Translocation of certain indigenous bacteria from the gastrointestinal tract to the mesenteric lymph nodes and other organs in a gnotobiotic mouse model. Infect Immun 1979;**23**:403–11.

Bergmans DC, Bonten MJ, Gaillard CA, et al. Prevention of ventilator-associated pneumonia by oral decontamination: a prospective, randomized, double-blind, placebo-controlled study. Am J Respir Crit Care Med 2001;**164**:382–8.

Besselink MGH, van Santvoort HC, Buskens E. Probiotic prophylaxis in predicted severe acute pancreatitis: a randomised, double-blind, placebo-controlled trial. Lancet 2008;**371**:651–9.

Besselink MG, van Santvoort HC, Renooij W, et al. Intestinal barrier dysfunction in a randomized trial of a specific probiotic composition in acute pancreatitis. Ann Surg 2009;**250**:712–19.

Bonten MJM, Kollef MH, Hall JB. Risk factors for ventilator-associated pneumonia: from epidemiology to patient management. Clin Infect Dis 2004;**38**:1141–9.

Border JR, Hassett J, LaDuca J, et al. The gut origin septic states in blunt multiple trauma (ISS = 40) in the ICU. Ann Surg 1987;**206**:427–48.

Caputo FJ, Rupani B, Watkins AC, et al. Pancreatic duct ligation abrogates the trauma hemorrhage-induced gut barrier failure and the subsequent production of biologically active intestinal lymph. Shock 2007;**28**:441–6.

Caridis DT, Reinhold RB, Woodruff PW, Fine J. Endotoxaemia in man. Lancet 1972;**i**:1381–5.

Carrico CJ, Meakins JL, Marshall JC, Fry D, Maier RV. Multiple-organ-failure syndrome. Arch Surg 1986;**121**:196–208.

Chan EY, Ruest A, Meade MO, Cook DJ. Oral decontamination for prevention of pneumonia in mechanically ventilated adults: systematic review and meta-analysis. BMJ 2007;**334**:889.

Chin KF, Kallam R, O'Boyle C, MacFie J. Bacterial translocation may influence the long-term survival in colorectal cancer patients. Dis Colon Rectum 2007;**50**:323–30.

Chitkara YK, Feierabend TC. Endogenous and exogenous infection with *Pseudomonas aeruginosa* in a burns unit. *Int Surg* 1981;**66**:237–40.

Cohen DB, Magnotti LJ, Lu Q, et al. Pancreatic duct ligation reduces lung injury following trauma and hemorrhagic shock. *Ann Surg* 2004;**240**:885–91.

Collado MC, Gueimonde M, Hernández M, et al. Adhesion of selected *Bifidobacterium* strains to human intestinal mucus and the role of adhesion in enteropathogen exclusion. *J Food Prot* 2005;**68**:2672–8.

Cotton BA, Reddy N, Hatch QM, et al. Damage control resuscitation is associated with a reduction in resuscitation volumes and improvement in survival in 390 damage control laparotomy patients. *Ann Surg* 2011;**254**:598–605.

D'Amico R, Pifferi S, Leonetti C, et al. Effectiveness of antibiotic prophylaxis in critically ill adult patients: systematic review of randomised controlled trials. *BMJ* 1998;**316**:1275–85.

de Jonge E, Schultz MJ, Spanjaard L, et al. Effects of selective decontamination of digestive tract on mortality and acquisition of resistant bacteria in intensive care: a randomised controlled trial. *Lancet* 2003;**362**:1011–16.

de Smet AMGA, Kluytmans JAJW, Cooper BS, et al. Decontamination of the digestive tract and oropharynx in ICU patients. *N Engl J Med* 2009;**360**:20–31.

Deitch EA. Simple intestinal obstruction causes bacterial translocation in man. *Arch Surg* 1989;**124**:699–701.

Deitch EA. Bacterial translocation of the gut flora. *J Trauma* 1990;**30**:S184–9.

Deitch EA. Multiple organ failure. Pathophysiology and potential future therapy. *Ann Surg* 1992;**216**:117–34.

Deitch E, Xu D. Gut lymph hypothesis of early shock and trauma-induced multiple organ dysfunction syndrome: a new look at gut origin sepsis. *J Organ Dysfunct* 2006;**2**:70–9.

Deitch EA, Maejima K, Berg R. Effect of oral antibiotics and bacterial overgrowth on the translocation of the GI tract microflora in burned rats. *J Trauma* 1985;**25**:385–92.

Deitch EA, Berg R, Specian R. Endotoxin promotes the translocation of bacteria from the gut. *Arch Surg* 1987;**122**:185–90.

Deitch E, Bridges W, Baker J, et al. Hemorrhagic shock-induced bacterial translocation is reduced by xanthine oxidase inhibition or inactivation. *Surgery* 1988;**104**:191–8.

Deitch EA, Morrison J, Berg R, Specian RD. Effect of hemorrhagic shock on bacterial translocation, intestinal morphology, and intestinal permeability in conventional and antibiotic decontaminated rats. *Crit Care Med* 1990;**18**:529–36.

Deitch EA, Shi HP, Lu Q, Feketeova E, Xu DZ. Serine proteases are involved in the pathogenesis of trauma-hemorrhagic shock-induced gut and lung injury. *Shock* 2003;**19**:452–6.

Deitch EA, Forsythe R, Anjaria D, et al. The role of lymph factors in lung injury, bone marrow suppression, and endothelial cell dysfunction in a primate model of trauma-hemorrhagic shock. *Shock* 2004a;**22**:221–8.

Deitch EA, Lu Q, Feketeova E, et al. Intestinal bacterial overgrowth induces the production of biologically active intestinal lymph. *J Trauma* 2004b;**56**:105–10.

Dellinger RP, Levy MM, Carlet JM, et al. Surviving Sepsis Campaign: international guidelines for management of severe sepsis and septic shock: 2008. *Crit Care Med* 2008;**36**:296–327.

Diaz JJ, Cullinane DC, Dutton WD, et al. The management of the open abdomen in trauma and emergency general surgery: part 1-damage control. *J Trauma* 2010;**68**:1425–38.

Driks MR, Craven DE, Celli, BR, et al. Nosocomial pneumonia in intubated patients given sucralfate as compared with antacids or histamine type 2 blockers. The role of gastric colonization. *N Engl J Med* 1987;**317**:1376–82.

Ferraro FJ, Rush BF, Simonian GT, et al. A comparison of survival at different degrees of hemorrhagic shock in germ-free and germ-bearing rats. *Shock* 1995;**4**:117–20.

Fritz S, Hackert T, Hartwig W, et al. Bacterial translocation and infected pancreatic necrosis in acute necrotizing pancreatitis derives from small bowel rather than from colon. *Am J Surg* 2010;**200**:111–7.

Garrison RN, Fry DE, Berberich S, Polk HC. Enterococcal bacteremia: clinical implications and determinants of death. *Ann Surg* 1982;**196**:43–7.

Gatt M, MacFie J. Randomized clinical trial of gut-specific nutrients in critically ill surgical patients. *Br J Surg* 2010;**97**:1629–36.

Glenn TM, Lefer AM. Significance of splanchnic proteases in the production of a toxic factor in hemorrhagic shock. *Circ Res* 1971;**29**:338–49.

Goris RJ, te Boekhorst TP, Nuytinck JK, Gimbrère JS. Multiple-organ failure. Generalized autodestructive inflammation? *Arch Surg* 1985;**120**:1109–15.

Heller AR, Rössler S, Litz RJ, et al. Omega-3 fatty acids improve the diagnosis-related clinical outcome. *Crit Care Med* 2006;**34**:972–9.

Heyland DK, Dhaliwal R, Suchner U, Berger MM. Antioxidant nutrients: a systematic review of trace elements and vitamins in the critically ill patient. *Intensive Care Med* 2005;**31**:327–37.

Ikezawa F, Fukatsu K, Moriya T, et al. Reversal of parenteral nutrition-induced gut mucosal immunity impairment with small amounts of a complex enteral diet. *J Trauma* 2008;**65**:360–5.

Inoue S, Wirman JA, Alexander JW, Trocki O, Cardell RR. *Candida albicans* translocation across the gut mucosa following burn injury. *J Surg Res* 1988;**44**:479–92.

Ivatury R, Simon R, Havriliak, et al. Gastric mucosal pH and oxygen delivery and oxygen consumption indices in the assessment of adequacy of resuscitation after trauma: A prospective, randomized study. *J Trauma* 1995;**39**:128.

Jarrett F, Balish E, Moylan J. Clinical experience with prophylactic antibiotic bowel suppression in burn patients. *Surgery* 1978;**83**:523–7.

Kim YS, Ho SB. Intestinal goblet cells and mucins in health and disease: recent highlights and progress. *Curr Gastroenterol Rep* 2010;**12**:319–30.

Kinross J, Roon von A, Penney N. The gut microbiota as a target for improved surgical outcome and improved patient care. *Curr Pharm Des* 2009;**15**:1537–45.

Kistler EB, Hugli TE, Schmid-Schönbein GW. The pancreas as a source of cardiovascular cell activating factors. *Microcirculation* 2000;**7**:183–92.

Kramp WJ, Waldo S, Schmid-Schönbein GW, et al. Characterization of two classes of pancreatic shock factors: functional differences exhibited by hydrophilic and hydrophobic shock factors. *Shock* 2003;**20**:356–62.

Krueger WA, Lenhart FP, Neeser G, et al. Influence of combined intravenous and topical antibiotic prophylaxis on the incidence of infections, organ dysfunctions, and mortality in critically ill surgical patients: a prospective, stratified, randomized, double-blind, placebo-controlled clinical trial. *Am J Respir Crit Care Med* 2002;**166**:1029–37.

Lassen K, Soop M, Nygren J, et al. Consensus review of optimal perioperative care in colorectal surgery: Enhanced Recovery After Surgery (ERAS) Group recommendations. *Arch Surg* 2009;**144**(10:961–9.

Lefer AM, Glenn TM. Role of the pancreas in the pathogenesis of circulatory shock. *Adv Exp Medicine Biol* 1971;**23**, 311–35.

Lewis SJ, Andersen HK, Thomas S. Early enteral nutrition within 24h of intestinal surgery versus later commencement of feeding: a systematic review and meta-analysis. *J Gastrointest Surg* 2008;**13**:569–75.

Ma L, Ma J, Deitch E. Genetic susceptibility to mucosal damage leads to bacterial translocation in a murine burn model. *J Trauma* 1989;**29**:1245–51.

MacFie J, O'Boyle C, Mitchell CJ, et al. Gut origin of sepsis: a prospective study investigating associations between bacterial translocation, gastric microflora, and septic morbidity. *Gut* 1999;**45**:223–8.

MacFie J, Reddy BS, Gatt M, et al. Bacterial translocation studied in 927 patients over 13 years. *Br J Surg* 2005;**93**:87–93.

Magnotti LJ, Upperman JS, Xu DZ, Lu Q, Deitch EA. Gut-derived mesenteric lymph but not portal blood increases endothelial cell permeability and promotes lung injury after hemorrhagic shock. *Ann Surg* 1998;**228**:518–27.

Magnotti LJ, Xu DZ, Lu Q, Deitch EA. Gut-derived mesenteric lymph: a link between burn and lung injury. *Arch Surg* 1999;**134**:1333–40.

Mainous MR, Tso P, Berg RD, Deitch, EA. Studies of the route, magnitude, and time course of bacterial translocation in a model of systemic inflammation. *Arch Surg* 1991;**126**:33–37.

Martindale RG, McClave SA, Vanek VW, et al. Guidelines for the provision and assessment of nutrition support therapy in the adult critically ill patient: Society of Critical Care Medicine and American Society for Parenteral and Enteral Nutrition: Executive Summary. *Crit Care Med* 2009;**37**:1757–61.

Mitsuoka H, Kistler EB, Schmid-Schönbein GW. Generation of in vivo activating factors in the ischemic intestine by pancreatic enzymes. *Proc Natl Acad Sci U S A* 2000;**97**:1772–7.

Mitsuoka H, Kistler EB, Schmid-Schönbein GW. Protease inhibition in the intestinal lumen: attenuation of systemic inflammation and early indicators of multiple organ failure in shock. *Shock* 2002;**17**:205–9.

Moore FA, Moore EE, Jones TN, et al. TEN versus TPN following major abdominal trauma--reduced septic morbidity. *J Trauma* 1989;**29**:916–22.

Moore FA, Moore EE, Poggetti R, et al. Gut bacterial translocation via the portal vein: a clinical perspective with major torso trauma. *J Trauma* 1991;**31**:629–36.

Moore FA, Moore EE, Poggetti RS, Read RA. Postinjury shock and early bacteremia. A lethal combination. *Arch Surg* 1992;**127**:893–7.

Nathens AB, Marshall JC. Selective decontamination of the digestive tract in surgical patients: a systematic review of the evidence. *Arch Surg* 1999;**134**:170–6.

Nimmerfall F, Rosenthaler J. Significance of the goblet-cell mucin layer, the outermost luminal barrier to passage through the gut wall. *Biochem Biophys Res Commun* 1980;**94**:960–6.

O'Boyle CJ, MacFie J, Mitchell CJ, et al. Microbiology of bacterial translocation in humans. *Gut* 1998;**42**:29–35.

Ohta K, Omura K, Hirano K, et al. The effects of an additive small amount of a low residual diet against total parenteral nutrition-induced gut mucosal barrier. *Am J Surg* 2003;**185**:79–85.

Okamoto Y, Okano K, Izuishi K, et al. Attenuation of the systemic inflammatory response and infectious complications after gastrectomy with preoperative oral arginine and omega-3 fatty acids supplemented immunonutrition. *World J Surg* 2009;**33**:1815–21.

Oláh A, Belágyi T, Issekutz A, et al. Randomized clinical trial of specific lactobacillus and fibre supplement to early enteral nutrition in patients with acute pancreatitis. *Br J Surg* 2002;**89**:1103–7.

Omura K, Hirano K, Kanehira E, et al. Small amount of low-residue diet parenteral nutrition can prevent decreases in intestinal mucosal integrity. *Ann Surg* 2000;**231**:112–18.

Pape HC, Dwenger A, Regel G, et al. Increased gut permeability after multiple trauma. *Br J Surg* 1994;**81**:850–2.

Peter JV, Moran JL, Phillips-Hughes J. A metaanalysis of treatment outcomes of early enteral versus early parenteral nutrition in hospitalized patients. *Crit Care Med* 2005;**33**:213–20.

Petrov MS, van Santvoort HC, Besselink MGH, et al. Enteral nutrition and the risk of mortality and infectious complications in patients with severe acute pancreatitis: a meta-analysis of randomized trials. *Arch Surg* 2008;**143**:1111–7.

Pisarenko, V., Deitch, E. Bacterial translocation and gut derived sepsis: Do they exist? In: Deutschman CS, Neligan PJ (eds), *Evidence-based Practice of Critical Care*. Philadelphia, PA: Saunders, 2010: 172–7.

Pitsouni E, Alexiou V, Saridakis V, et al. Does the use of probiotics/synbiotics prevent postoperative infections in patients undergoing abdominal surgery? A meta-analysis of randomized controlled trials. *Eur J Clin Pharmacol* 2009;**65**:561–70.

Pontes-Arruda A, Aragão AMA, Albuquerque JD. Effects of enteral feeding with eicosapentaenoic acid, gamma-linolenic acid, and antioxidants in mechanically ventilated patients with severe sepsis and septic shock. *Crit Care Med* 2006;**34**:2325–33.

Pugin J, Auckenthaler R, Lew DP, Suter PM. Oropharyngeal decontamination decreases incidence of ventilator-associated pneumonia. A randomized, placebo-controlled, double-blind clinical trial. *JAMA* 1991;**265**:2704–10.

Qin X, Caputo FJ, Xu DZ, Deitch EA. Hydrophobicity of mucosal surface and its relationship to gut barrier function. *Shock* 2008;**29**:372–6.

Qin X, Sheth SU, Sharpe SM, et al. The mucus layer is critical in protecting against ischemia-reperfusion-mediated gut injury and in the restitution of gut barrier function. *Shock* 2011;**35**:275–81.

Ravin HA, Fine J. Biological implications of intestinal endotoxins. *Fed Proc* 1962;**21**, 65–8.

Rayes N, Hansen S, Seehofer D, et al. Early enteral supply of fiber and Lactobacilli versus conventional nutrition: a controlled trial in patients with major abdominal surgery. *Nutrition* 2002;**18**–8:609–15.

Rayes N, Seehofer D, Theruvath T, et al. Supply of pre- and probiotics reduces bacterial infection rates after liver transplantation--a randomized, double-blind trial. *Am J Transplant* 2005;**5**:125–30.

Reddy BS, MacFie J, Gatt M, et al. Commensal bacteria do translocate across the intestinal barrier in surgical patients. *Clin Nutr* 2007;**26**:208–15.

Reintam A, Parm P, Redlich U, et al. Gastrointestinal failure in intensive care: a retrospective clinical study in three different intensive care units in Germany and Estonia. *BMC Gastroenterol* 2006;**6**:19–26.

Rice TW, Mogan S, Hays MA, et al. Randomized trial of initial trophic versus full-energy enteral nutrition in mechanically ventilated patients with acute respiratory failure. *Crit Care Med* 2011;**39**:967–74.

Ruan X, Shi H, Xia G, et al. Encapsulated Bifidobacteria reduced bacterial translocation in rats following hemorrhagic shock and resuscitation. *Nutrition* 2007;**23**:754–61.

Rupani B, Caputo FJ, Watkins AC, et al. Relationship between disruption of the unstirred mucus layer and intestinal restitution in loss of gut barrier function after trauma hemorrhagic shock. *Surgery* 2007;**141**:481–9.

Savage DC, Dubos R, Schaedler RW. The gastrointestinal epithelium and its autochthonous bacterial flora. *J Exp Med* 1968;**127**:67–76.

Schmid-Schönbein GW, Kistler EB, Hugli TE. Mechanisms for cell activation and its consequences for biorheology and microcirculation: Multi-organ failure in shock. *Biorheology* 2001;**38**:185–201.

Schweinburg FB, Frank HA. Transmural migration of intestinal bacteria during peritoneal irrigation in uremic dogs. *Proc Soc Exp Biol Med* 1949;**71**:150–3.

Sedman PC, MacFie J, Sagar P, et al. The prevalence of gut translocation in humans. *Gastroenterology* 1994;**107**:643–9.

Senthil M, Brown M, Xu D-Z, et al. Gut-lymph hypothesis of systemic inflammatory response syndrome/multiple-organ dysfunction syndrome: validating studies in a porcine model. *J Trauma* 2006;**60**:958–65.

Servin AL. Antagonistic activities of lactobacilli and bifidobacteria against microbial pathogens. *FEMS Microbiol Rev* 2004;**28**:405–40.

Sharpe S, Doucet D, Qin X. Role of intestinal mucus and pancreatic proteases in the pathogenesis of trauma–hemorrhagic shock-induced gut barrier failure and multiple organ dysfunction syndrome. *J Organ Dysfunct* 2008;**4**:168–76.

Siempos II, Ntaidou TK, Falagas ME. Impact of the administration of probiotics on the incidence of ventilator-associated pneumonia: A meta-analysis of randomized controlled trials. *Crit Care Med* 2010;**38**:954–62.

Soeters PB. Probiotics: did we go wrong, and if so, where? *Clin Nutr* 2008;**27**:173–8.

Souza DG, Vieira AT, Soares AC, et al. The essential role of the intestinal microbiota in facilitating acute inflammatory responses. *J Immunol* 2004;**173**:4137–46.

Stoutenbeek CP, van Saene HK, Miranda DR, Zandstra DF. The effect of selective decontamination of the digestive tract on colonisation and infection rate in multiple trauma patients. *Intensive Care Med* 1984;**10**:185–92.

Stoutenbeek CP, Saene HKF, Little RA, et al. The effect of selective decontamination of the digestive tract on mortality in multiple trauma patients: a multicenter randomized controlled trial. *Intensive Care Med* 2006;**33**:261–70.

Suzuki K, Kawamoto S, Fagarasan S. GALT: organization and dynamics leading to IgA synthesis. *Adv Immunol* 2010;**107**:153–85.

Talukdar R, Swaroop Vege S. Early management of severe acute pancreatitis. *Curr Gastroenterol Rep* 2011;**13**:123–30.

Timmerman H, Koning C, Mulder L. Monostrain, multistrain and multispecies probiotics--A comparison of functionality and efficacy 1. *Int J Food Microbiol* 2004;**96**:219–33.

Tomasi TB. Mechanisms of immune regulation at mucosal surfaces. *Rev Infect Dis* 1983;**5**(suppl 4):S784–92.

Tryba, M. Risk of acute stress bleeding and nosocomial pneumonia in ventilated intensive care unit patients: Sucralfate versus antacids. *JAMA* 1987;**83**(suppl 2):117–24.

Tsujimoto H, Ono S, Mochizuki H. Role of Translocation of Pathogen-Associated Molecular Patterns in Sepsis. *Dig Surg* 2009;**26**:100–9.

van der Waaij D, Berghuis-de Vries JM, Lekkerkerk Lekkerkerk-v. Colonization resistance of the digestive tract in conventional and antibiotic-treated mice. *J Hyg* 1971;**69**:405–11.

van Goor H, Rosman C, Grond J, et al. Translocation of bacteria and endotoxin in organ donors. *Arch Surg* 1994;**129**:1063–6.

van Nieuwenhoven CA, Buskens E, van Tiel FH, Bonten MJ. Relationship between methodological trial quality and the effects of selective digestive decontamination on pneumonia and mortality in critically ill patients. *JAMA* 2001;**286**:335–40.

van Santvoort HC, Besselink MG, Timmerman HM, et al. Probiotics in surgery. *Surgery* 2008;**143**:1–7.

Waldo SW, Rosario HS, Penn AH, Schmid-Schönbein GW. Pancreatic digestive enzymes are potent generators of mediators for leukocyte activation and mortality. *Shock* 2003;**20**:138–43.

Walker W. Mechanisms of action of probiotics. *Clin Infect Dis* 2008;**46**:S87–91.

Wells CL, Rotstein OD, Pruett TL, Simmons RL. Intestinal bacteria translocate into experimental intra-abdominal abscesses. *Arch Surg* 1986;**121**:102–7.

Wilmore D, Smith R, O'dwyer S, Jacobs D. The gut: a central organ after surgical stress. *Surgery* 1988;**104**:917–32.

Wolochow H, Hildebrand GJ, Lamanna C. Translocation of microorganisms across the intestinal wall of the rat: effect of microbial size and concentration. *J Infect Dis* 1966;**116**:523–8.

Woodcock NP, Sudheer V, El-Barghouti N, Perry EP, MacFie J. Bacterial translocation in patients undergoing abdominal aortic aneurysm repair. *Br J Surg* 2000;**87**:439–42.

Woodruff PW, O'Carroll DI, Koizumi S, Fine J. Role of the intestinal flora in major trauma. *J Infect Dis* 1973;**128**:S290–4.

Wu L, Zaborina O, Zaborin A, et al. High-molecular-weight polyethylene glycol prevents lethal sepsis due to intestinal Pseudomonas aeruginosa. *Gastroenterology* 2004;**126**:488–98.

Chapter 25 Sepsis: systemic inflammation and organ dysfunction

John C. Marshall

Sepsis is one of the most common and potentially treatable causes of morbidity and mortality for surgical patients. Sepsis claims more than 200 000 North American victims a year – exceeding the annual toll of acute myocardial infarction (Angus et al. 2001) – and its prevalence has been increasing (Martin et al. 2003). Its diagnosis and optimal management remain incompletely understood by clinicians, and significant advances in its treatment have proven elusive. Yet a robust understanding of the optimal management of the septic patient is emerging in recent years, and strategies for improving survival are becoming increasingly well established.

■ SEPSIS: THE EVOLUTION OF A CONCEPT

Microorganisms are the most prevalent and diverse forms of life. Not only were primitive bacteria the first living species on the planet, but viable bacteria have been found in environments that would usually be considered inimical to life – in deep sea thermal jets, in Antarctic ice, and in rock from deep below the earth's surface. Microbes play a beneficial role in processes such as the breakdown of dying vegetable matter to form soil or the fermentation of plants and fruits to yield alcohol. But they are also agents of diseases that have, on occasion, wreaked havoc on human populations. The impact of this threat is apparent in our genome. The most highly polymorphic genes are those involved in antibacterial defenses. A single organism – *Plasmodium* sp., the cause of malaria – has been credited with the emergence of many polymorphisms in the hemoglobin gene, including the mutations responsible for sickle cell diseases and thalassemia. An understanding of the complex interactions between the microbial and human worlds is important to the understanding of the derangements that occur during sepsis.

■ Host–microbial interactions in evolution

Multicellular organisms have an evolutionarily ancient and biologically complex relationship with the microbial world. Bacteria and viruses are not simply a ubiquitous feature of our environment, they are also a fundamental part of whom we are. More than a billion years ago, simple unicellular organisms were parasitized by primitive protobacteria and, as a result, acquired the ability to generate energy. This development enabled cellular specialization and the emergence of multicellular species. These protobacteria became the mitochondria of cells of the animal world and the chloroplasts of the plant world. Over time, genetic material has been transferred between the mitochondrion and the host cell nucleus, and only 13 protein-coding genes remain in human mitochondrial DNA, whereas 22% of nuclear genes share a bacterial origin. Thus the

human genome and the cellular building blocks of life are partially microbial in origin.

As multicellular organisms evolved, they acquired microbial populations that established residence on epithelial surfaces such as the oropharynx, gut, vagina, and skin. The gastrointestinal tract of the healthy human is colonized by as many as 5000 distinct species of bacteria, and the total number of bacterial cells is 10 times greater than the number of human cells (Ley et al. 2006). Patterns of colonization are complex, but stable over time, and strikingly similar from one person to the next (Lee 1985). Epithelial colonization by microorganisms plays a critical role in the normal function of that surface. The normal flora of the gut plays a critical role in gut development and homeostasis, promoting the expression of epithelial cell enzymes involved in digestion, and even the development of the microvasculature of the intestinal villi (Xu and Gordon 2003). In the absence of a normal gut flora, host resistance to external infectious threats is significantly impaired (Dubos and Schaedler 1960). Moreover bacterial products such as lipopolysaccharide or endotoxin exert hormone-like effects, activating innate immune cells such as neutrophils and macrophages for increased antimicrobial activity (Marshall 2005). Our health and vitality are fundamentally dependent on our normal interactions with the microbial world.

At the same time, bacteria and viruses represent one of the most significant threats to our individual and collective survival. During the Middle Ages, the bubonic plague killed a quarter of the population of Europe, and endemic infections such as tuberculosis, malaria, and dengue, or epidemic infections such as severe acute respiratory syndrome (SARS) and influenza continue to exact a substantial toll. Infection is both an important cause of the diseases that surgeons treat, and a feared complication of the procedures that we use for treatment.

As effective methods of eradicating microorganisms using antimicrobial agents, or of eliminating foci of invasive infection using source control measures, have evolved, it has become apparent that the morbidity of sepsis arises from more than simply the cytopathic consequences of sustained uncontrolled microbial proliferation. At the same time, advances in our understanding of the biology of host–microbial interactions have shown that the response of the host against infection is also the vector of the illness that we have come to call sepsis.

■ Evolving concepts of sepsis

The word "sepsis" is attributed to Hippocrates (460–370 BCE) who believed that living tissues broke down through one of two distinct processes (Majno 1991). "Sepsis" was the term used to describe tissue breakdown in a manner that was unpleasant, foul smelling, and inducing of disease; examples of the Hippocratic concept of sepsis included the festering of wounds, the rotting of plants, and the vapors arising from the bad air of swamps which gave rise to the word "malaria."

In contrast, "pepsis" was tissue breakdown in a manner that supported life and health, and was exemplified by the digestion of food (hence the origins of the word "peptic") or the fermentation of grapes to produce wine. His ideas were articulated more than two millennia before the identification of microorganisms, yet are remarkably prescient in their recognition that these processes could be both beneficial and harmful to the host.

Bacteria were first visualized in the seventeenth century by Antony van Leeuwenhoek, the inventor of the microscope; however, it was not until the work of Louis Pasteur in the nineteenth century that the role of bacteria in the pathogenesis of infection was established, and the germ theory of disease born. With this evolving model of infection as a product of bacterial invasion, the word "sepsis" was seconded to denote the process, and the words sepsis and infection were used interchangeably, although sepsis generally denoted a more severe form of infection. Indeed as recently as 40 years ago, a major medical dictionary defined sepsis as "the presence of pus-forming organisms within the bloodstream" (Sweet and Williams 1972). By implication, the equation of infection with the clinical syndrome suggested that sepsis was a direct consequence of the proliferation of microorganisms or the release of their toxins within the host.

This model, however, proved inadequate. Although bacteria or bacterial products such as endotoxin can trigger clinical manifestations characteristic of sepsis in both humans and experimental animals, multiple lines of evidence over the past half century have shown that the syndrome arises indirectly – through the release of inflammatory mediators by the host – rather than through any direct toxic effects of the microorganism. One of the more compelling experiments that established this concept involved studies in which endotoxin from Gram-negative bacteria was administered to inbred mice (Michalek et al. 1980). Two otherwise genetically identical strains of mice – the C3h HeN and C3h HeJ strains – differ by a point mutation in a single gene. That mutation, which developed spontaneously decades ago, resulted in differential susceptibility to bacterial endotoxin: Although mice of the C3h HeN parent strain became ill after endotoxin injection, mice of the C3h HeJ strain could tolerate otherwise lethal doses with no apparent ill effects. When investigators created chimeric mice by irradiating mice of each strain to eliminate their own bone marrow, and repopulating the irradiated mice with bone marrow of the opposite strain, it was found that susceptibility to endotoxin could be transferred. In other words, the effects of endotoxin did not result from a direct toxic effect of the bacterial product on the host, but rather occurred indirectly, through products released from bone marrow cells in response to endotoxin exposure.

This subtle shift in concept – from sepsis as a direct consequence of bacteria to sepsis as an indirect consequence of the response of the host – has profound clinical implications which are discussed in greater detail throughout this chapter. One of the most important is that the host response itself is a legitimate target for intervention in the treatment of sepsis.

Terminology has changed with this shift in scientific concept, although contemporary conventions still fail to fully embody the nuances of a complex biological process (**Box 25.1**). *Infection* denotes a microbial phenomenon – the presence of viable microorganisms invading normally sterile host tissues – whereas *sepsis* describes the response of the host to that process of microbial invasion. As a host response is appropriate and essential for survival, the maladaptive consequences of the septic response are called *severe sepsis* when the response results in organ dysfunction and *septic shock* when it leads to cardiovascular instability. Moreover, as the response of the host is not specific to an infectious etiology, but can occur also in response to sterile tissue injury or ischemia, or other processes that result in inflammatory mediator release, the term "systemic inflammatory response syndrome" (SIRS) was coined to describe the response, independent of its cause. The interrelationship of infection, sepsis, and SIRS is represented graphically in **Figure 25.1**. It is important to recognize that SIRS is a concept, not a disease. The SIRS criteria have been widely criticized as being too non-specific to inform management decisions (Vincent 1997), yet the concept that a clinical syndrome of systemic inflammation, independent of cause, can be recognized marks an important advance in an evolving understanding of a complex biological process.

> **Box 25.1 Definitions of infection, sepsis, SIRS and septic shock.**
>
> *Infection:* The invasion of normally sterile tissues by viable microorganisms
> *Sepsis:* The maladaptive host response to infection
> *Systemic inflammatory response syndrome (SIRS):* The characteristic maladaptive host response, independent of cause
> *Severe sepsis:* Sepsis in association with organ dysfunction
> *Septic shock:* Sepsis in association with an inability to provide adequate oxygen delivery to tissues

More recently, recognition that patients with sepsis represent a highly heterogeneous population has stimulated interest in the concept that more sophisticated descriptive staging systems are needed. Adjuvant therapy in oncology is guided by the use of staging systems that stratify cancers, not only on the basis of their site of origin and histological type, but also on the degree of local and regional spread, and, increasingly, on the basis of expression of specific tumor markers. By analogy to oncology, the PIRO model (**p**redisposition, **i**nsult, **re**sponse, **o**rgan dysfunction – **Table 25.1**) has been proposed as a model that may be applicable to patients with acute illness (Levy et al. 2003). The PIRO model is still a concept, and an evolving work in progress, but may provide a means of resolving the enormous heterogeneity

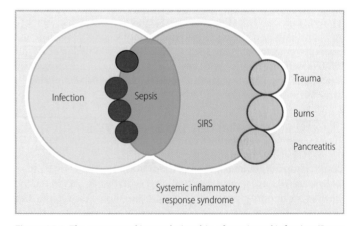

Figure 25.1 The conceptual interrelationship of sepsis and infection (Bone et al. 1992). Infection is a microbial process – the invasion of normally sterile host tissues – that evokes a response in the host that can be both protective and injurious. The response is not specific to infection, but can be elicited by sterile inflammatory stimuli such as burns, trauma, and acute pancreatitis; it has been termed the systemic inflammatory response syndrome (SIRS). Thus sepsis is present when infection elicits SIRS (and, perhaps more accurately, an injurious response characterized by organ dysfunction). It is apparent as well that infection may occur in the absence of a systemic response.

Table 25.1 The PIRO (predisposition, insult, response, organ dysfunction) model (from Levy et al 2003).

Domain	Present	Future
Predisposition	Premorbid illness with reduced probability of short term servival. Cultural or relisious beliefs, age, sex	Genetic polymorphisms in components of inflammatory response (e.g., TIR, TNF, IL-1, CD14); enhanced understanding of specific interactions between pathogens and host diseases
Insult infection	Culture and sensitivity of infecting pathogens; detection of disease amenable to source control	Assay of microbial products (LPS, mannan, bacterial DNA); gene transcript profiles
Response	SIRS, other signs of sepsis, shock, CRP	Nonspecific markers of activated inflammation (e.g., PCT or IL-6) or impaired host responsiveness (e.g., HLA-DR); specific detection of target of therapy (e.g., protein C, TNF, PAF)
Organ dysfuntion	Organ dysfunction as number of failing organs or composite score (e.g., MODS, SOFA, LODS, PEMOD, PELOD)	Dynamic measures of cellular response to insult – apoptosis, cytopathic hypoxia, cell stress

CRP, C-reactive protein; IL, interleukin; LODS, Logistic Organ Dysfunction; LPS, lipopolysaccharide; MODS, multiple-organ dysfunction syndrome; PAF, platelet-activating factor; PCT, procalcitonin; PELOD, Pediatric Logistic Organ Dysfunction; PFMOD, PEdiatric Multiple Organ Dysfunction; SIRS, systemic inflammatory response syndrome; SOFA, Sequential Organ Failure Assessment; TIR, toll/interleukin-1 receptor; TNF, tumor necrosis factor.

of patients with acute inflammatory disorders so that more focused studies of appropriate therapy can be undertaken.

From sepsis to organ dysfunction

The development of clinically important physiological organ system insufficiency is the hallmark of the entity of severe sepsis; conversely, organ dysfunction in the acutely ill patient invariably follows a clinical insult characterized by inflammation and tissue injury. The cardinal signs of local inflammation described by Galen and Celsus two millennia in the past have their counterpart in the systemic inflammatory disorder that is so common in the contemporary intensive care unit (ICU): Organ dysfunction – *functio laesa* – is one of the core elements. The process has come to be one of the defining syndromes, and has been given many names – multiple organ failure, remote organ dysfunction, or, addressing specific affected systems, acute respiratory distress syndrome (ARDS), acute kidney injury (AKI), or disseminated intravascular coagulation (DIC). Most prefer the designation the multiple organ dysfunction syndrome (MODS), to underline the fact that the process is a systemic one, of variable severity, and potentially reversible (Bone et al. 1992). Unlike the local impairment of function that accompanies local inflammation (impaired mobility of an acutely arthritic joint, for example), the MODS is largely an iatrogenic byproduct of the successes of intensive care (Marshall 2010). The early evolution of ARDS, for example, reflects the leakage of resuscitation fluids into the lung parenchyma because of increased capillary permeability, and becomes clinically manifest only because patients are kept alive through the intervention of intubation and mechanical ventilation. Its further evolution is at least in part shaped by further injury to the inflamed lung resulting from the effects of positive pressure mechanical ventilation.

An inability to maintain oxygenation of the blood, perfusion of the tissues, or removal of by products of metabolism is rapidly lethal. As a consequence, organ dysfunction is both the final pathway to death during sepsis and systemic inflammation, and the raison d'être of the contemporary ICU.

EPIDEMIOLOGY OF SEPSIS, SIRS, AND MODS

Unlike cancer, sepsis lacks a defined pathological phenotype and, unlike heart disease or stroke, there is no single characteristic anatomic abnormality. These vagaries of description render estimates of the

prevalence of sepsis difficult. Nevertheless, it is evident that sepsis is a leading cause of global mortality and disability, and a common complication of a disparate group of common diseases including cancer, trauma, and cardiovascular disease.

Four of the top ten causes of death on the World Health Organization's list are infectious diseases – lower respiratory tract infections, diarrheal diseases, tuberculosis, and HIV/AIDS – and infection is a common morbid complication of others including trauma, prematurity, and stroke. Thus it is reasonable to conclude that sepsis is one of the leading, if not the leading, causes of death.

Estimates of its incidence derive from large population-based studies using administrative data. Martin and colleagues estimated the incidence of sepsis in the USA to be 240 cases per 100 000, a threefold increase over two decades (**Figure 25.2**). Rates were significantly higher in men than women, and in non-white than in white individuals (Martin et al. 2003). Using a different methodological approach, Angus and co-workers came up with the surprisingly similar estimate that there are approximately 750 000 cases of severe sepsis annually in the USA, and that more than 200 000 deaths a year are attributable to sepsis (Angus et al. 2001). Similar estimates have been derived from studies from Europe (Brun-Buisson et al. 2004) and Australia (Finfer et al. 2004a).

Although the incidence of sepsis is increasing, its mortality appears to be on the decline. Data from the Surviving Sepsis Campaign based on more than 15 000 patients around the world reveal an overall in-hospital mortality rate of 31% (Levy et al. 2010), and data from recent randomized controlled trials of novel therapies suggest a contemporary 28-day mortality rate of approximately 25%, compared with a mortality rate of [3]40% in the 1990s. The extent to which these changes reflect improvements in care or differences in case ascertainment is not known.

From a surgical perspective, sepsis and MODS arise in two discrete contexts. First they may be a manifestation of a community-acquired illness such as peritonitis secondary to perforated diverticulitis or an acute necrotizing soft-tissue infection. Second, they may develop as a complication of an elective or emergency surgical procedure; in the latter case, new-onset organ dysfunction is often the initial harbinger of a clinically occult complication.

THE BIOLOGY OF THE INFLAMMATORY RESPONSE

The biological response to infection of injury is enormously complex, having evolved over the course of half a billion years as multicellular

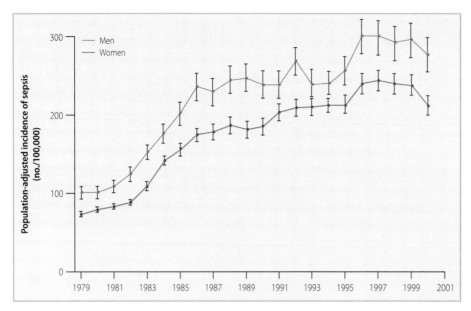

Figure 25.2 The epidemiology of sepsis in the USA (Martin et al. 2003). Rates of sepsis tripled over the last two decades of the twentieth century; men were consistently more likely to be affected than women.

organisms emerged. The immune system is conveniently, though imperfectly, stratified into the innate immune system and the adaptive immune system. Innate mechanisms are those that are encoded in the germline and can be rapidly mobilized in response to a threat. The innate immune system is potent but non-specific, and so bystander injury is a consequence of its activation. Its cellular elements include neutrophils, monocytes, and macrophages. The adaptive immune system develops in response to exposure to a specific antigen; its responses are highly specific, but dependent on prior exposure. Its cellular elements include lymphocytes and dendritic cells. The two arms of the immune system interact at multiple levels, and so the distinction is somewhat arbitrary. Our primary focus here will be the innate immune system, both because it provides an immediate and potent response to an acute threat and because its activation contributes to the organ injury of MODS.

Recognition of danger

The primary role of the innate immune system is the recognition of danger, and the expression of an immediate response to that danger. The recognition of danger in the environment of the cell is accomplished through the activation of cell surface proteins that are collectively known as pattern recognition receptors (PRRs). At least four classes of such receptors exist – the toll-like receptors (TLRs), the NOD (nucleotide oligomerization domain)-like receptors (NLRs), the retinoic acid-inducible gene I (RIG) receptors, and the C-type lectin receptors. Each recognizes conserved patterns that communicate potential danger, and are collectively known as danger-associated molecular patterns, or DAMPs. DAMPs include viruses, bacterial products such as endotoxins, and bacterial proteins such as flagellin, but also include an array of substances normally found within the cell, the presence of which in the extracellular environment indicates local cell damage; these include oxidized phospholipids, heat shock proteins (HSPs), uric acid, and elastase. The binding of a DAMP results in the association of an array of signaling proteins to the receptor, leading to the expression of inflammatory gene products. We focus here on the biology of the best characterized of these, the TLRs.

TLRs in humans comprise a family of 11 structurally similar proteins that are expressed as transmembrane receptors. Their name derives from their similarity to *toll* – a fruit fly gene that was originally identified as necessary for dorsoventral patterning during embryonic development (this role was considered to be very cool by the German scientists who found the gene, so they called it *toll* – the German word for 'neat' or 'cool'). Individual TLRs bind specific DAMPs (**Box 25.2**), providing a measure of specificity to the response, although the subsequent signaling cascades evoke similar gene expression patterns. TLR4 is the receptor for endotoxin, but also for a variety of host-derived DAMPs, whereas TLR2 binds products of Gram-positive bacteria, and TLR3, -7, and -8 recognize molecular patterns characteristic of viruses.

Box 25.2 Toll-like receptors (TLRs) and their ligands.

TLR1: Triacyl lipopeptides
TLR2: Lipoteichoic acid, bacterial lipoprotein, heat-specific protein HSP70
TLR3: Double-stranded RNA
TLR4: Endotoxin, elastase, heparan, HSP60, oxidized phospholipids
TLR5: Flagellin
TLR6: Mycoplasma lipopeptide
TLR7: Imiquod, single-stranded RNA
TLR8: Viral DNA, single-stranded RNA
TLR9: Bacterial DNA CpG motifs

Modulation of gene expression after receptor engagement

The engagement of a TLR results in receptor clustering, and attracts a series of adapter molecules to the intracellular tail of the receptor (**Figure 25.3**). These protein–protein interactions are facilitated by enzymes that add a phosphate group (kinases) or remove a phosphate group (phosphatases) to the amino acids tyrosine, serine, and threonine in the adapter proteins. This process of protein–protein

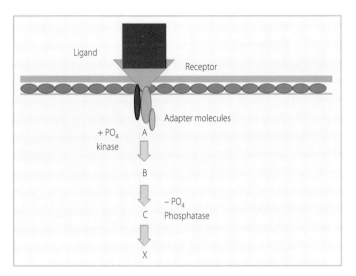

Figure 25.3 Signal transduction after engagement of a receptor. Gene transcription in response to a stimulus from the extracellular environment occurs through a process called signal transduction. The engagement of a cell surface receptor by its ligand results in receptor clustering, and in the recruitment of adapter proteins to the intracellular tail of the receptor. This process, in turn, results in recruitment of additional intracellular proteins, and the activation of transcription factors – proteins that pass into the nucleus of the cell and regulate gene expression. These protein–protein interactions depend on transient changes in protein structure, one of the most common being phosphorylation of an amino acid (typically tyrosine, serine, or threonine) using a phosphate group derived from ATP. An enzyme that adds a phosphate group to its target protein is called a kinase, whereas one that removes a phosphate group is known as a phosphatase.

interaction enables a signal to be transferred from the cell membrane to the interior of the cell, ultimately activating transcription factors such as NF-kB which, on activation, are able to translocate from the cytoplasm into the nucleus. Within the nucleus they bind the promoter region of target genes, stimulating or suppressing the transcription of genes, the expression of which is altered during inflammation. Studies in healthy volunteers given a single bolus of endotoxin have revealed that the transcription of >3700 genes is influenced by this single signal (Calvano et al. 2005).

Apoptosis in sepsis and systemic inflammation

Apoptosis, or programmed cell death, is a physiological mode of cell death that enables the body to remove cells without evoking an inflammatory response. It plays a fundamental role in normal growth and development, facilitating, for example, the deletion of cells in the web space of the palm to create fingers, or enabling the turnover of cells such as blood or epithelial cells. Apoptosis plays a role as well in the controlled removal of transformed or virally infected cells. Both excessive and inadequate apoptosis can play a role in the pathogenesis of disease. AIDS and *Clostridium difficile* colitis are examples of illnesses caused by excessive apoptosis of CD4+ lymphocytes and colonic epithelial cells, respectively. Impaired apoptosis contributes to the pathogenesis of cancer and to keloid formation.

Apoptosis is a complex and tightly regulated process. It can be initiated in response to both extracellular stimuli that result in ligation of cell death receptors of the Fas or CD95 family, and stimuli such as ionizing radiation that produce increased mitochondrial permeability.

Apoptosis occurs through the activity of a family of enzymes called caspases which cleave target proteins at specific peptide sequences adjacent to an aspartic acid residue. The result is the degradation of an intact cell into membrane-bound vesicles that are phagocytosed by macrophages, and so fail to evoke an inflammatory response.

Depending on the cell population evaluated, apoptosis can be shown to be both excessive and impaired in sepsis. Increased apoptosis of lymphocytes contributes to the characteristic lymphopenia, and prevention of this in animal models results in improved survival. Intestinal epithelial cell apoptosis is also increased after multiple trauma and sepsis. On the other hand, neutrophils are constitutively apoptotic cells that normally survive only hours in the circulation. In trauma and sepsis, inflammatory stimuli activate survival pathways within the neutrophil which enables longer survival in an activated state.

Early mediators of inflammation

Prominent among the genes whose expression is initially induced after activation of PPR are interleukin-1 IL-1) and tumor necrosis factor (TNF), two key proinflammatory cytokines. Each exerts varied and sometimes overlapping effects, but the importance of both is underlined by the fact that their manipulation in a variety of animal models has striking effects on subsequent mortality.

IL-1 is produced by a variety of cells, particularly monocytes and macrophages. Signaling through PRR leads to activation of an intracellular signaling complex called the inflammasome, which is necessary for the activation of IL-1. Once released from the cell, IL-1 exerts a variety of activities, acting on the hypothalamus to increase core temperature, on lymphocytes to promote their activation, and on neutrophils to prolong their survival by inhibition of apoptosis. IL-1 is actually a member of a family of related proteins, including IL-1 variants, IL-18, and IL-33. One of these – the IL-1 receptor antagonist (IL-1Ra) – is also synthesized in response to the same stimuli that trigger IL-1 release. IL-1Ra binds to the IL-1 receptor on target cells, but this binding does not result in intracellular signaling, so IL-1Ra serves as a competitive antagonist of IL-1 activity. Intriguingly, the IL-1 receptor is a member of the TLR family, although IL-1 activation from its precursor form requires the activity of caspase-1, an enzyme initially identified in apoptosis. Increased understanding has made it clear that apparently disparate processes such as inflammation, anti-inflammation, coagulation, and cell death are intimately interrelated.

TNF is synthesized as a protein that is expressed on the cell membrane, and released into the cellular environment when it is cleaved by TNF-converting enzyme. TNF interacts with cells through the CD95 family of death receptors, the engagement of which can result in apoptosis. Binding of TNF to its receptor can paradoxically cause either cell activation and new gene expression or apoptosis, depending on other associated cell signals. With inflammation, the role of TNF in activating gene transcription predominates; however, it was first identified as a protein that could kill tumor cells. The TNF receptor can also be cleaved from the cell surface and binds circulating TNF.

The list of inflammatory mediators that are activated and released after engagement of a pattern recognition receptor is long, and includes a variety of protein cytokines (e.g., IL-6, IL-8, IL-10, and macrophage migration inhibitory factor [MIF]) as well as lipid mediators such as prostaglandins, leukotrienes, and platelet-activating factor (PAF). How these interact to create the phenotype of systemic inflammation is poorly understood, but several important features are well recognized.

Late mediators of inflammation

The initial activation of innate immune cells results in the release of a number of early mediators that act on target cells to enhance or modify the resulting response. A coherent grand scheme of this process has yet to be articulated; however, it is instructive to consider a few key processes.

Inducible nitric oxide synthase (iNOS) is a gene expressed in a variety of cells, in particular endothelial cells; the enzyme NOS catalyzes the conversion of the amino acid citrulline to the amino acid arginine, and in the process releases nitric oxide (NO). NO is a short-lived but potent inhibitor of vascular smooth muscle contraction. Its release results in vasodilation, a property that underlies the therapeutic use of NO donors such as nitroglycerin, nitrates, and sodium nitroprusside. Local release of NO results in locally increased blood flow – the *rubor* of a local inflammatory response. A disseminated increase in NO release secondary to upregulation of the activity of iNOS produces the systemic vasodilatory state characteristic of sepsis.

Inflammatory stimuli can also trigger the expression of tissue factor on the surface of innate immune cells or endothelium; tissue factor interacts with factor VIIa, resulting in the activation of factor X and leading to local coagulation. Local induction of coagulation is responsible for the formation of the fibrin capsule that encloses an abscess, or for the adhesions that follow peritoneal injury. Intravascular activation of coagulation results in DIC.

A variety of early inflammatory mediators, including both IL-1 and TNF, acting on neutrophils can activate survival pathways, avoid apoptosis, and permit survival in an activated state – a process that prolongs neutrophil antibacterial activity, but also contributes to the bystander injury that accompanies neutrophil activation; it is an important factor in the early pathogenesis of the ARDS.

Other late-acting mediators of inflammation include IL-10, which exerts anti-inflammatory activity, and transforming growth factor β (TGF-β), which plays an important role in fibrosis and tissue repair. High mobility group box 1 (HMGB1) is another late-released proinflammatory mediator that exerts its activities, in part, by binding and activating TLR4, thus prolonging the expression of an inflammatory response.

THE CLINICAL PHENOTYPE OF THE INFLAMMATORY RESPONSE

Activation of the cellular and biochemical processes above as part of a systemic inflammatory response results in characteristic abnormalities of cardiovascular, metabolic, and immunological homeostasis which create a characteristic clinical syndrome.

Cardiovascular alterations

Abnormalities of cardiovascular homeostasis are particularly prominent during a septic response (Dellinger 2003). They define the most severe form of the syndrome – septic shock – and contribute significantly to its morbidity and mortality by impairing oxygen delivery to the tissues.

Two key early alterations shape the vascular response – vasodilation and increased capillary permeability (**Figure 25.4**). As discussed above, vasodilation results from increased local generation of NO. A single cause of increased capillary permeability has not been identified (Goldenberg et al. 2011). Multiple inflammatory mediators can reproduce the phenomenon by impeding intracellular barrier

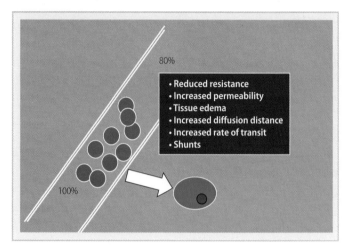

Figure 25.4 Vascular alterations in sepsis. Resuscitated sepsis is typically characterized by mixed venous oxygen saturation levels that are higher than the normal value of 70%. Multiple factors contribute to this. Reduced resistance results in higher rates of flow, providing less time for oxygen to diffuse from red cells in the microvasculature. Increased capillary permeability results in tissue edema, increasing the distance that oxygen must diffuse, and so reducing the gradient. Moreover shunting through the microvasculature leads to stasis in some capillaries and very rapid flow in others.

function, and even by increasing transcellular fluid flow. The combination of reduced small vessel resistance and increased permeability results in an extracellular redistribution of the normal intravascular fluids, and a relative reduction in the functional intravascular volume. This reduction results in a fall in blood pressure, a reflex increase in heart rate, and hypoperfusion or shock. As fluid resuscitation proceeds, these two physiological derangements create the characteristic features of resuscitated sepsis, in particular the elevated mixed venous oxygen saturation seen in septic shock.

The diffusion of oxygen from the red blood cell to cells in the microenvironment of the capillary bed is a passive process, driven by the concentration difference between oxygen in the red cell and oxygen in the tissues. In health, the saturation of oxygen in the red cells leaving the lung is 100%. As the cells traverse through the microcirculation, approximately 25–30% of that oxygen diffuses from the red cell into the adjacent tissues, so that the oxygen saturation of venous blood returning to the heart (denoted SVO_2) is about 70%. In hypovolemic shock, or early during unresuscitated septic shock, the SVO_2 is lower, reflecting the fact that tissue hypoxia has created a greater oxygen gradient. In resuscitated distributive or septic shock, however, the SVO_2 is increased, often up to 80% or more. Multiple factors contribute to this. First, fluid resuscitation in the face of increased capillary permeability creates a greater distance between the red cell and the tissues, rendering the diffusion gradient less steep. Second, alterations in flow at the microvascular level result in the creation of functional shunts, with some capillaries occluded, and others wide open. Finally, reduced tone at the postcapillary venule results in reduced resistance to flow through the microvasculature, with the result that the time available for unloading of oxygen is reduced.

Increased and patchy microvascular thrombosis, secondary to the activation of coagulation, is another cardiovascular manifestation of systemic inflammation. Moreover studies of red cells and leukocytes have demonstrated reduced cellular deformability of both cell types, with the result that capillaries become occluded with these more rigid cells and microthrombi secondary to the activation of coagulation.

Depression of myocardial contractility has also been described in sepsis, and attributed to a still poorly characterized myocardial depressant factor. Right heart dysfunction is particularly prominent. On the other hand, the cardiac output is usually elevated. Cardiac output (denoted Q) is the product of the heart rate and the stroke volume. The heart rate is elevated for a variety of reasons, including reduced peripheral vascular resistance, fever, and increased sympathetic activity. The stroke volume is also increased because of the reduced peripheral vascular resistance.

◼ Metabolic alterations

Metabolic processes are dramatically altered in association with the activation of a systemic inflammatory response. Patterns of protein synthesis by the liver are altered as part of the acute phase response (Gabay and Kushner 1999). Acute phase reactants such as C-reactive protein (CRP), a_1-antitrypsin, complement proteins, and serum amyloid A protein are increased, whereas other proteins – notably albumin – are suppressed. Hepatic synthesis of the anticoagulant, protein C, is also inhibited, contributing to a net procoagulant state. The net consequence of this change in patterns of protein synthesis is enhanced antimicrobial activity and augmentation of host defense capacity. CRP binds to phosphocholine, a DAMP associated with bacterial cells and injured tissue. Lipopolysaccharide-binding protein binds endotoxin, and a_1-antitrypsin provides local protection against proteases such as elastase released during inflammation. Reduced synthesis of iron-binding proteins such as transferring reduces the availability of iron – an essential cofactor for bacteria.

Multiple endocrine disorders have been described (Vanhorebeek et al. 2006); in general, anabolism is reduced while catabolism is increased. Insulin resistance is characteristic, and results in elevated serum glucose levels (Andersen et al. 2004), and a worse clinical prognosis. It is unclear whether increased morbidity results from reduced insulin availability or responsiveness, or from the direct effects of hyperglycemia. It is, however, apparent that judicious control of hyperglycemia using exogenous insulin can improve clinical outcomes (Van den Berghe et al. 2001), although strict glycemic control to maintain normoglycemia is associated with a poorer outcome, perhaps because of the adverse effects of hypoglycemia (Brunkhorst et al. 2008, Finfer et al. 2009).

Impaired adrenocortical function and reduced vasopressin release have been implicated in the pathogenesis of the cardiovascular alterations of systemic inflammation. Varying degrees of acute adrenal insufficiency have been documented in critical illness in both adults (Annane et al. 2000) and children (Menon et al. 2010), and the provision of exogenous glucocorticoids improves hemodynamic function, although the impact on mortality is less clear (Annane 2002, Sprung et al. 2008). Reduced pituitary synthesis of adrenocorticotropic hormone (ACTH) has been observed, and may account for the changes in adrenocortical function (Polito et al. 2011). Vasopressin levels are reduced in sepsis, and treatment of septic shock with exogenous vasopressin results in improved outcomes, particularly for patients with lesser degrees of shock (Russell et al. 2008).

Muscle atrophy – a result of increased proteolysis and reduced myofibrillar synthesis – is common in acute illness (Derde et al. 2012), and plays a significant role in delayed weaning from mechanical ventilation and in return to normal activities after ICU and hospital discharge (Herridge et al. 2011).

◼ Immunological alterations

Immunological homeostasis is equally altered in the patient with sepsis and the patient with organ dysfunction (Marshall et al. 2008).

Although efforts have been made to describe this process as either an excessive or an inadequate response, or to suggest that an initial state of enhanced inflammation is followed by a state of immune suppression (the so-called compensatory anti-inflammatory response syndrome or CARS), the reality is that evidence of both augmented and impaired immune responsiveness coexists.

Cells of the innate immune system – neutrophils, monocytes, and macrophages – typically show evidence of basal activation, accompanied by an impaired ability to respond further after exposure to inflammatory stimuli, e.g., basal production of reactive oxygen intermediates by the neutrophil and release of TNF by circulating monocytes are enhanced, but only a modest enhancement of these processes occurs when cells are exposed to inflammatory stimuli ex vivo, and activity is ultimately less than that seen in healthy cells exposed to the same stimuli. Expression of TLRs is increased. The phagocytosis and killing of bacteria are altered only minimally or not at all. Neutrophil survival is markedly increased as a consequence of the activation of an endogenous survival program (Jimenez et al. 1997).

On the other hand, the adaptive immune system shows extensive evidence of downregulation. Delayed-type hypersensitivity responsiveness is reduced, resulting in a state of anergy (Christou et al. 1995), and lymphocyte proliferation in response to mitogenic stimuli is decreased. Antibody responses are variably affected: Production of antibody to a protein antigen such as tetanus toxoid is reduced, whereas antibody production in response to pneumococcal capsular polysaccharide, a polysaccharide antigen, is normal or increased. Lymphocyte apoptosis is also increased (Hotchkiss and Karl 2003).

The hallmark of immune dysfunction in systemic inflammation is an increased susceptibility to nosocomial infection with a characteristic group of largely endogenous pathogens. These are not the typical infecting organisms of classic immunodeficiency disorders, and susceptibility to them reflects the spectrum of derangements in host defense mechanisms that occur in the critically ill patient. The upper gastrointestinal tract becomes colonized with organisms such as staphylococci, enterococci, *Escherichia coli*, and *Pseudomonas* and *Candida* spp. – the same spectrum of organisms that predominate in ICU-acquired infections (Marshall et al. 1993). These organisms share a number of features that favor their emergence and infectivity. They form biofilms, and so can grow on surfaces such as vascular and urinary catheters or endotracheal or nasogastric tubes. They also tend to be relatively resistant to first-line antibiotics, and so are selected out under antibiotic pressure. They are also able to translocate across an intact gut mucosa, likely accounting for the development of occult bacteremia with organisms such as enterococci, and for the development of infected peripancreatic necrosis. Finally organisms such as *Pseudomonas* spp. can increase their virulence in response to stress in the host. Although alteration in innate and adaptive immune function may predispose to nosocomial infection, the disruption of physical barriers such as the skin by vascular lines, of anatomic defenses such as the upper airway by endotracheal tubes, of chemical barriers such as gastric acidity, and of the microbial barriers created by the indigenous flora are likely to play a much more important role in the pathogenesis of these infections.

◼ THE MULTIPLE ORGAN DYSFUNCTION SYNDROME

Organ dysfunction of varying degrees of severity is a common manifestation of a systemic inflammatory response. The process has been called MODS, although the concept is sufficiently complex and of such importance to the optimal management of the critically ill patient that its origins and implications merit further consideration. MODS is at once a cardinal manifestation of an activated inflammatory response, a reflection of the successes of ICU care, and a consequence of the sequelae of that care.

MODS evolves only because patients who otherwise would have died of lethal physiological organ insufficiency can be kept alive using a spectrum of organ support technologies. The development of dialysis, positive pressure mechanical ventilation, and techniques for central monitoring of cardiovascular function after the Second World War created the preconditions for the first ICUs in the late 1950s. The development of ICUs created a spectrum of disorders that developed only because the patient could be kept alive on life support – ARDS, AKI, septic shock, DIC, and acute stress ulceration of the stomach. The late Arthur Baue (1975) suggested that these were not separate processes, but rather the specific organ system manifestations of a common process that he termed "multiple or progressive systems failure." Other terms such as multiple organ failure or remote organ dysfunction have been used, but the current preferred terminology is the MODS, emphasizing that the process can involve any organ, is variable in its severity, and is potentially reversible. Baue further emphasized that the challenge is not the failure of any single system, but rather the interactions between systems, and perhaps, most importantly, emphasized that MODS is a process to be prevented, rather than a disease to be treated.

For the surgeon, the prevention of MODS encompasses the entire spectrum of judgment and management decisions that comprise the optimal care of a vulnerable critically ill patient. Our focus below, therefore, is on the ICU management strategies that are associated with the lowest risk of additional iatrogenic injury, and so with the best clinical outcomes.

◼ Respiratory dysfunction

Impaired gas exchange in the lung, with reduced levels of oxygen in the blood, is the functional manifestation of the respiratory dysfunction of MODS. Following early descriptions of acute respiratory failure developing in association with peritonitis, Ashbaugh et al. (1967) proposed

the term the "acute respiratory distress syndrome," and defined it as arterial hypoxemia, in association with diffuse bilateral pulmonary infiltrates on chest radiograph in the absence of pulmonary edema. This somewhat arbitrary definition has been refined several times, and its vagaries underline the fact that variable degrees of measurable physiological alterations and lung injury are a common feature of systemic inflammation.

Increased capillary permeability with interstitial edema is the earliest abnormality in ARDS. Widening of the alveolar wall results in reduced diffusion of oxygen from the alveolus into the adjacent capillary, whereas diffusion of carbon dioxide is unaffected. As a result, an early manifestation is arterial hypoxemia with a normal or even reduced carbon dioxide tension. The influx of activated neutrophils into the lung causes a further increase in local capillary permeability, increasing the resultant hypoxemia (**Figure 25.5a**).

However, these initial physiological responses to an activated systemic inflammatory response represent only a part of the phenotype of ARDS. Hypoxemia leads the treating clinician to intubate the patient and initiate positive pressure ventilation. This intervention can attenuate hypoxemia, but the exogenous distending pressure results in further injury to the lung from inflammation (**Figure 25.5b**). Ultimately the pathophysiology of acute lung injury reflects a combination of processes – increased capillary permeability and enhanced neutrophil influx as early events, further injury from positive pressure ventilation and over-distension of alveolar units, and subsequently reparative processes including vascular thrombosis and activation of local fibrosis.

Lung injury can be minimized by prophylactic measures to prevent ventilator-associated pneumonia (VAP), including elevation of the head of the bed, and the use of the orotracheal route for intubation, closed endotracheal suction systems (Dodek et al. 2004), and lung protective methods of ventilatory support. These last include the use of non-invasive ventilation where feasible (Ferrer et al. 2009) and pressure-limited ventilatory approaches during mechanical ventilation (Brower et al. 2000, Meade et al. 2008). Limiting the amount of fluids administered after ICU admission (National Heart, Lung, and Blood Institute Acute Respiratory Distress Syndrome [ARDS] Clinical

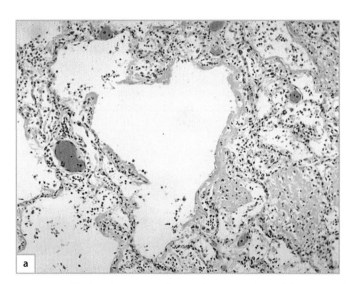
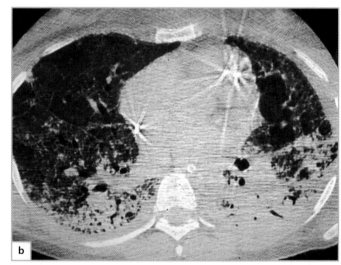

Figure 25.5 The lung in acute respiratory distress syndrome (ARDS). (a) A photomicrograph of the lung of a patient who died of ARDS reveals massive pulmonary infiltration by neutrophils, edema of the alveolar walls, intravascular thrombosis, and fibrin deposition in the alveoli; all of these contribute to impaired gas exchange. (b) A CT scan of a patient with ARDS reveals the further iatrogenic nature of the lung injury, showing consolidation in the dependent posterior lung zones, and cystic changes in the anterior anti-dependent areas resulting from over-distension of the lung.

Trials Network 2006), or active diuresis with diuretics and albumin (Martin et al. 2005), can shorten the duration of ventilator dependency.

Cardiovascular dysfunction

The cardiovascular derangements of systemic inflammation have been described earlier, and consist primarily of reduced peripheral vascular resistance and increased capillary permeability. Once again, the process of resuscitation and support can result in further injury. Intravenous fluids increase preload, but, in the setting of altered capillary permeability, they increase tissue edema, resulting in impaired pulmonary gas exchange, reduced myocardial contractility, reduced abdominal wall compliance and the abdominal compartment syndrome, and impairment of gut, brain, and renal function (Prowle et al. 2010). Moreover vasopressors such as norepinephrine, dopamine, and epinephrine can compromise blood flow, increasing the risk of complications such as anastomotic leaks (Zakrison et al. 2007), and the use of large doses of inotropes to augment cardiac output has been found to increase mortality (Hayes et al. 1994). For reasons that are not at all clear, and despite the increase in myocardial work associated with the response to critical illness, myocardial infarction is a relatively uncommon complication; atrial dysrhythmias, on the other hand, occur relatively frequently (Goodman et al. 2008).

Support of the cardiovascular system after ICU admission hinges on supporting preload through the administration of fluids, afterload through the judicious use of vasopressor agents, and myocardial contractility through the use of inotropic agents. Optimal strategies are not well defined. There is no convincing evidence that goal-directed strategies targeting either mixed venous oxygen saturation or cardiac index improve survival (Gattinoni et al. 1995). Both albumin and saline are equally efficacious as replacement fluids (Finfer et al. 2004b), and the tolerance of moderate degrees of anemia is preferable to more liberal transfusion strategies (Hebert et al. 1999).

Renal dysfunction

The renal dysfunction of MODS is characterized primarily by an inability to clear creatinine and other solutes from the blood. The term AKI has become the preferred term to describe the process, and, recognizing that graded degrees of dysfunction occur, the RIFLE criteria have been developed to describe these, reflecting **r**isk, **i**njury, **f**ailure, **l**oss, and **e**nd-stage disease (**Box 25.3**) (Bellomo et al. 2004).

Box 25.3 The RIFLE criteria for acute kidney injury.

Risk: Glomerular filtration rate (GFR) decreased >25%, serum creatinine increased 1.5 times or urine production of <0.5 ml/kg per h for 6 h

Injury: GFR decreased >50%, doubling of creatinine or urine production <0.5 ml/kg per h for 12 h

Failure: GFR decreased >75%, tripling of creatinine or creatinine >355 µmol/l (with a rise of >44) (>4 mg/dl) OR urine output <0.3 ml/kg per h for 24 h

Loss: Persistent acute kidney infection or complete loss of kidney function for >4 weeks

End-stage renal disease: Complete loss of kidney function for >3 months

---

The pathological findings in sepsis-induced AKI are minimal, and the pathogenesis of injury is incompletely understood (Bougle and Duranteau 2011). Reduced renal blood flow – either global or regional – with resulting cellular hypoxia likely contributes to injury and kidney dysfunction. However, the classic concept of acute tubular necrosis does not reliably reflect the histological findings, and mounting evidence suggests that renal epithelial cell apoptosis plays an important role (Havasi and Borkan 2011). Remote tissue injury, such as occurs during ventilator-induced lung injury, has been shown to induce renal apoptosis (Imai et al. 2003).

Support of the dysfunctional kidney is accomplished through renal replacement therapy. In contrast to chronic renal failure, the indication for institution of dialysis therapy for AKI is less frequently hyperkalemia or acidosis, and more frequently for regulation of volume status. Continuous dialysis techniques such as continuous venovenous hemofiltration (CVVH) or slow low-efficiency dialysis (SLED) that enables fluid removal without resulting hemodynamic instability are widely used.

Gastrointestinal dysfunction

Multiple abnormalities of gastrointestinal function are apparent in the patient with MODS; however, these are often clinically occult and difficult to quantify. Striking changes occur in patterns of microbial colonization of the small bowel and colon, with overgrowth of the small bowel by organisms commonly isolated from ICU-acquired infections (Marshall et al. 1993), and a reduction in the complexity of the colonic flora with a particular reduction in the density of anaerobic bacteria (Shimizu et al. 2006). These changes, together with alterations in gut epithelial barrier function, predispose to translocation of viable bacteria and bacterial products such as endotoxin into the host, although the mechanisms through which these changes lead to systemic disease are complex and poorly understood (Alverdy et al. 2003). Ileus and intolerance of enteral feeding are a common manifestation of gut dysfunction. Acute upper gastrointestinal tract bleeding as a result of so-called "stress ulceration" was common in the early years of intensive care, but has become uncommon today (Cook et al. 1998).

Hyperbilirubinemia is the classic manifestation of liver dysfunction in sepsis, although, similar to stress ulceration, its prevalence appears to be decreasing. Although patterns of protein synthesis are altered as part of the acute phase response described earlier, clinically significant derangements of hepatic synthetic or secretory function are extremely rare in the absence of primary liver pathology.

Enteral feeding is a key intervention in minimizing gastrointestinal dysfunction in the septic patient. Feeding stimulates gastrointestinal peristalsis, attenuating stasis and bacterial overgrowth, stimulates the release of gastrointestinal hormones, and maintains the integrity of the gut mucosa. Conversely, total parenteral nutrition is associated with an increased risk of cholestasis, particularly when administered early during the ICU stay (Casaer et al. 2011).

Neuromuscular dysfunction

Altered levels of consciousness manifested as delirium or somnolence and profound acquired neuromuscular weakness are common manifestations of the neuromuscular derangements of sepsis and critical illness. Multiple factors are implicated including disruption of day–night sleeping cycles, tissue edema, and circulating mediators of inflammation; however, the iatrogenic effects of commonly used

ICU medications and prolonged bed rest play a particularly important role (Vasilevskis et al. 2010). Corticosteroids, for example, have been shown to be a risk factor for prolonged weakness in survivors of ARDS (Herridge et al. 2003), whereas benzodiazepines are associated with an increased risk of delirium when compared with dexmedetomidine (Riker et al. 2009).

Sedation vacations, accomplished by daily interruption of sedation (Kress et al. 2000) and more active programs of physiotherapy (Schweickert et al. 2009), can enhance neuromuscular recovery and accelerate weaning from mechanical ventilation.

Hematological dysfunction

Although mild anemia is a common feature of systemic inflammation, the most striking abnormalities are those involving the coagulation system (Marshall 2001). Thrombocytopenia either present on admission or developing over the ICU stay occurs in up to 40% patients, and is associated with an increased risk of death (Hui et al. 2011). Thrombocytopenia often signals the presence of intravascular activation of coagulation, or DIC, characterized by consumption of coagulant proteins resulting in an increased prothromin time and increased levels of fibrin degradation products. Enhanced expression of tissue factor on endothelial cells contributes to activation of intravascular coagulation, whereas the synthesis and activation of anticoagulant proteins such as protein C, tissue factor pathway inhibitor, and antithrombin are impaired (van der Poll et al. 2011).

Although coagulopathy is associated with adverse outcome in sepsis, and plausibly plays a pathogenic role in the evolution of MODS, effective treatment strategies are not available. Recombinant activated protein C (drotrecogin alpha activated or Xigris) was reported to improve survival in severe sepsis, particularly in those patients with septic shock or DIC (Bernard et al. 2001). However, a recent randomized trial of 1696 patients failed to replicate the beneficial results of the original study, and the drug has been withdrawn from the market. Similar promising early results with antithrombin or tissue factor pathway inhibitor have likewise not withstood the rigors of subsequent trials.

Measuring the severity of organ dysfunction

A number of scoring systems have been developed to measure the severity of MODS, including the Multiple Organ Dysfunction (MOD) Score (**Table 25.2**) (Marshall et al. 1995), the Sequential Organ Failure Assessment (SOFA) score (Vincent et al. 1996), and the Logistic Organ Dysfunction (LOD) score (Le Gall et al. 1996). All are similar in the systems that they incorporate, and in the equal weighting given to each system; they differ in relatively minor ways in the variables used to define dysfunction.

The MOD score uses a single physiological variable to characterize dysfunction in each system, selected on the basis of specific criteria as being the optimal indicator of dysfunction in the specific system (Marshall 1993). By analogy to the PO_2/FiO_2 ratio used to quantify pulmonary dysfunction, which corrects the oxygen tension by consideration of the concentration of inspired oxygen needed to achieve that value, the MOD score uses a variable called the pressure-adjusted rate (PAR) to describe cardiovascular failure. The PAR is calculated as the product of the heart rate (HR) and central venous pressure (CVP), divided by the mean arterial pressure (MAP):

$$PAR = HR \times CVP/MAP.$$

Increasing abnormality is reflected in increasing values, and the PAR reflects the impact of fluid challenge on pressure; in the absence of a CVP measurement, a normal value of 8 is imputed for the CVP. Variables in the MOD score are calibrated so that, within any system, a score of 0 reflects normal function, whereas a score of 4 reflects markedly abnormal function and a risk of death of at least 50%.

Organ dysfunction scores can serve several purposes. Calculated on the day of admission, the *admission score* serves as a severity measure. Measured on a daily basis, the *daily score* can reflect net improvement or deterioration in an individual patient. Calculated over a period of time (e.g., the ICU stay) by recording the worst value in each system, independent of the day it occurred, the *aggregate score* measures the overall severity of organ dysfunction. By subtracting the admission score from the aggregate score, it is possible to calculate a *delta score* that quantifies new, and potentially preventable, organ dysfunction

Table 25.2 The Multiple Organ Dysfunction (MOD) score (from Marshall et al. 1995).

Organ system	0	1	2	3	4
Respiratory[a] (PO_2/FiO_2 ratio)	>300	226–300	151–225	76–150	<75
Renal[b] (serum creatinine)	<100	101–200	201–350	351–500	>500
Hepatic[c] (serum bilirubin)	<20	21–60	61–120	121–240	>240
Cardiovascular[d] (PAR)	<10.0	10.1–15.0	15.1–20.0	20.1–30.0	>30.0
Hematological[e] (platelet count)	>120	81–120	51–80	21–50	≤20
Neurological[f] (Glasgow Coma Scale)	15	13–14	10–12	7–9	≤6

[a]The PO_2/FiO_2 ratio is calculated without reference to the use or mode of mechanical ventilation, and without reference to the use or level of positive end-expiratory pressure.

[b]The serum creatinine level is measured in μmol/l, without reference to the use of dialysis.

[c]The serum bilirubin level is measured in μmol/l.

[d]The pressure-adjusted heart rate (PAR) is calculated as the product of the heart rate and right atrial (central venous) pressure (RAP), divided by the mean arterial pressure (MAP):

PAR = Heart rate × RAP/MAP.

[e]The platelet count is measured in platelets ´ 10^3/ml.

[f]The Glasgow Coma Scale score is preferably calculated by the patient's nurse, and is scored conservatively (for the patient receiving sedation or muscle relaxants, normal function is assumed unless there is evidence of intrinsically altered mental status).

that has arisen over the ICU stay. Finally, a combined mortality and morbidity measure can be created by recording the aggregate score for survivors and the aggregate score plus 1 for non-survivors.

Organ dysfunction scores have been most frequently used in research to compare baseline severity, and describe clinical course; their use as tools in the ICU management of critically ill patients has not been extensively evaluated.

The iatrogenic roots of MODS

Early descriptions of MODS emphasized its association with infection (Fry et al. 1980, Bell et al. 1983), even suggesting that new onset of organ dysfunction can be a valid sign of occult infection and an indication for exploratory laparotomy (Polk and Shields 1977). In the early postoperative period, the development of organ dysfunction – particularly respiratory insufficiency, renal dysfunction, atrial arrhythmias, or confusion – is not uncommonly a harbinger of a major surgical complication. However, improvements in diagnostic imaging have essentially obviated the need for blind surgical exploration, and, for the patient in the ICU, the etiology of new organ dysfunction more frequently reflects the iatrogenic consequences of ICU support than a missed diagnosis of infection. Indeed MODS is by definition an iatrogenic process, because it arises only in survivors of otherwise lethal illness, and ongoing ICU supportive care contributes to its evolution.

If the conceptual importance of MODS in the twentieth century was as sign of occult infection, its importance in the twenty-first century is as a reminder of the inadvertent consequences of ICU support (Marshall 2010): The clinical challenge is to support physiological function while minimizing the harm associated with that support.

MANAGEMENT OF SEPSIS

The core principles in the management of the septic patient include the following:
- Resuscitate the patient to ensure adequate tissue perfusion
- Identify and treat a focus of infection with appropriate antibiotics and source control measures
- Provide the necessary support for failing organ systems while minimizing further iatrogenic injury.

These have recently been synthesized into evidence-based management guidelines developed by the Surviving Sepsis Campaign (Dellinger et al. 2008). Although the focus is the patient with sepsis (i.e., new-onset organ dysfunction as a consequence of infection), it is often unclear in the early stages of patient management whether infection is the trigger for physiological instability, and the principles apply equally to patients whose illness arises from an acute sterile inflammatory process such as pancreatitis.

Resuscitation of the septic patient

A relative or absolute intravascular volume deficit is common in unresuscitated septic shock, occurring because of ongoing losses, reduced intake, peripheral vasodilation, and increased capillary permeability. Reduced oxygen delivery to the tissues results in anaerobic metabolism; measurement of serum lactate can provide information on the severity of the energy deficit, and so lactate assay is recommended as a diagnostic tool in the early resuscitation of the septic patient.

The initial step in resuscitation is the administration of intravenous fluids to optimize circulatory function. The optimal resuscitative fluid remains controversial; however, in the absence of compelling evidence for the superiority of any particular fluid, resuscitation should be initiated using a crystalloid such as 0.9% saline or Ringer lactate, with an initial rapid infusion of 30 ml/kg. Subgroup analyses of the 7000 patient Australia/New Zealand SAFE Trial that showed no overall mortality difference when patients received either saline or albumin, because the resuscitative fluid suggested the possibility that albumin might be superior to saline in the management of sepsis, but harmful in the setting of head injury (Finfer et al. 2004b). On the other hand, the use of synthetic colloids has been associated with increased rates of AKI (Brunkhorst et al. 2008). Several large international trials currently under way should help to clarify the role of synthetic colloids as acute resuscitative fluids.

Fluid resuscitation should be administered to target specific physiological endpoints, although which is the best measure of the adequacy of resuscitation is also a matter of debate. A reduction in heart rate and an increase in blood pressure suggest a therapeutic response to fluids, although they are relatively insensitive markers of resuscitation adequacy, and impacted by other factors such as pain and anxiety. Urine output can be an effective and dynamic marker of the adequacy of intravascular fluid volumes, and has the added advantage of reflecting both renal flow and renal function. Either acute or chronic renal impairment may render urine output unreliable. Measures of cardiac preload such as CVP, or of oxygen extraction such as central venous O_2 saturation ($ScvO_2$) also provide useful information on the adequacy of fluid resuscitation.

If perfusion remains compromised despite apparently adequate filling pressures (e.g., if blood pressure or urine output remains low despite a normal or elevated CVP), then vasopressor agents are used to increase blood pressure. Norepinephrine, epinephrine, and dopamine all exert vasopressor activity; norepinephrine is the most commonly used agent in North America and Europe, a practice supported by a meta-analysis suggesting improved survival when norepinephrine is used rather than dopamine (De et al. 2012).

Finally, if tissue perfusion remains compromised despite adequate filling volumes and vasoactive drug therapy, augmentation of cardiac output with an inotropic agent such as dobutamine, or of oxygen-carrying capacity through blood transfusion, may provide additional benefit.

A defined protocol for initial resuscitation has been popularized by Rivers et al. (2001) who proposed the concept of multimodal, early, goal-directed therapy in the management of severe sepsis. The Rivers protocol calls for the placement of a central venous catheter for monitoring, and the rapid administration of crystalloids targeting a CVP of 8 mmHg. If the mean arterial pressure remains low despite this initial fluid challenge, norepinephrine is added, targeting a MAP of 65 mmHg. A $ScvO_2$ is measured, and if the value is <70%, dobutamine and/or transfusion is administered (**Figure 25.6**). Using such a protocol in the emergency department of a single urban hospital, Rivers et al. demonstrated a mortality reduction from 46% to 30% for patients presenting with septic shock. Several large studies are currently in progress to validate the concept and to assess the relative importance of the differing elements of the protocol.

Diagnosis and treatment of infection

Although a distributive shock state may result from a variety of non-infectious causes, infection is both a common and a readily treatable cause of the physiological derangement, and so its early detection and management are critical to a favorable outcome.

The specific site of an inciting infection is often readily apparent based on the pattern of signs and symptoms at clinical presentation.

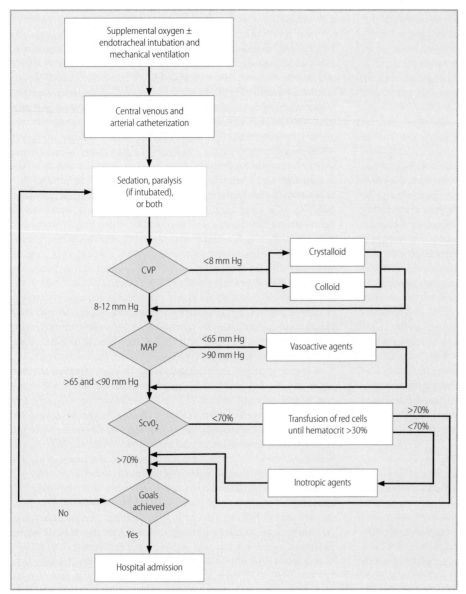

Figure 25.6 Early goal-directed therapy for sepsis and septic shock (Rivers et al. 2001). The strategy popularized by Rivers and colleagues begins in the emergency department with measurement of central venous pressure (CVP), and infusion of fluids to raise the CVP to ≥8 mmHg Vasopressors are added if this fails to increase the mean arterial pressure to at least 65 mmHg, and transfusion and inotropes administered as needed to increase the central venous oxygen saturation to at least 70%.

Documentation of the site of infection is based on the history and physical findings combined with appropriate imaging of chest radiograph, ultrasonography, and computed tomography (CT). Additional investigations such as lumbar puncture are dictated based on clinical presentation. A microbiological diagnosis should also be sought before anti-infective therapy is started, by obtaining two sets of blood cultures, along with cultures guided by the presumptive anatomic diagnosis.

Broad-spectrum empirical antibiotic therapy, based on the assumed anatomic focus and presumptive spectrum of pathogens, should be started as soon as cultures have been obtained, and ideally within an hour of initial presentation. Observational studies show that mortality increases strikingly with every hour of delay in initiating appropriate antibiotic therapy (Kumar et al. 2006). Antibiotic selection is discussed in Chapter 2.

Early source control is a key element of initial management for many infections. Source control measures are those that use physical interventions such as drainage (for infected fluids such as those found in an abscess), debridement (for infected or necrotic solid tissue), or device removal (for colonized foreign bodies and medical devices) to eradicate a focus of infection. In general, source control removes foci of microbial growth, and drainage converts a closed space infection to a controlled sinus or fistula. In selecting a method of achieving source control, the optimal approach accomplishes the anatomic objective with the least degree of physiological and anatomic disruption; thus percutaneous and minimally invasive approaches have emerged as the preferred initial intervention in feasible circumstances. (Marshall et al. 2004b).

Support of the septic patient

Beyond the initial resuscitation and treatment of infection, supportive care of impaired organ function while minimizing the adverse sequelae of the support-related interventions is paramount. For the intubated patient, a ventilatory mode that minimizes further ventilator-induced lung injury should be used. The best-studied approach is that popularized by ARDSNet in the USA (Brower et al. 2000), which limits tidal volumes to 6 ml/kg, using sedation and paralysis as needed. Newer strategies such as high-frequency oscillation may well play an increasingly important role in the future (Sud et al. 2010).

Although aggressive fluid resuscitation contributes to survival when used early during the course of sepsis, there is some evidence that a persistently positive fluid balance is harmful in the period after ICU admission (Boyd et al. 2011), and that conservative fluid management strategies result in improved clinical outcomes. Similarly, there is no evidence that normalization of hemoglobin levels through transfusion improves outcome, but rather a suggestion that indiscriminate transfusion may be harmful (Hebert et al. 1999).

Although broad-spectrum empirical therapy is appropriate in the initial management of the septic patient, once the results of culture and sensitivity testing become available, the antibiotic spectrum should be narrowed and, if cultures are negative, antibiotics should be stopped altogether.

Evidence-based strategies should be implemented to prevent nosocomial complications, including pharmacological prophylaxis against deep venous thrombosis, and interventions to prevent VAP and central venous catheter infections. Data from randomized controlled trials and systematic reviews indicate that the risk of nosocomial ICU-acquired infection and even mortality can be reduced through the use of selective decontamination of the digestive tract (SDD), particularly in surgical patients (Nathens and Marshall 1999). SDD is an antibiotic-based prophylactic regimen that uses topical agents active against Gram-negative bacteria (tobramycin and polymyxin B) and fungi (amphotericin B), leaving the Gram-positive and anaerobic flora intact. For reasons that are unclear, SDD has not been widely adopted outside Europe. Finally maintenance of blood glucose levels in the near normal range appears to improve outcome, although targeting strict normoglycemia has been found to increase mortality (Finfer et al. 2009).

TARGETING THE MEDIATORS OF SYSTEMIC INFLAMMATION

Contemporary understanding of the biological mechanisms that result in organ injury has raised the prospect that therapies targeting host-derived mediators of inflammation might improve outcomes in sepsis. Unfortunately this promise has been agonizingly difficult to realize. Upwards of 100 phase 2 and 3 clinical trials have been conducted, evaluating a spectrum of interventions (**Figure 25.7**). Despite some inconsistent evidence of clinical benefit, the net result of this enormous body of work is that there are currently no novel mediator-directed treatments available. Lack of convincing evidence of efficacy, however, does not equate to convincing evidence of lack of efficacy, and a strategy aimed at a variety of targets may yet find a clinical role.

Endotoxin

Endotoxin is the prototypical microbial trigger of innate immunity, and evokes the clinical manifestations of sepsis and lethality in both animals and humans. Endotoxemia is also common in critically ill patients, although importantly its presence does not necessarily signal the presence of Gram-negative infection, and levels may be elevated even without infection, suggesting the gut as a source of circulating endotoxins (Marshall et al. 2004a). A variety of strategies to neutralize endotoxin have been evaluated, including monoclonal antibodies, endogenous neutralizing proteins such as bactericidal permeability increasing protein, high-density lipoprotein, soluble CD14, and intestinal alkaline phosphatase, and synthetic antagonists including a non-toxic lipid that binds TLR4 without inducing activation, a lipid emulsion, and the antibiotic polymyxin B. Recent studies, using an extracorporeal polymyxin B column, have shown improved survival in severe peritonitis. Its utility is the focus of an ongoing North American clinical trial.

Tumor necrosis factor

The neutralization of TNF using either specific neutralizing antibodies or soluble receptor constructs has been evaluated in a dozen clinical trials. In aggregate, data derived from more than 7000 patients enrolled in these studies reveal a statistically significant, albeit small, benefit in 28-day survival (see Figure 25.7). None of these studies was individually compelling enough to lead to regulatory approval of anti-TNF therapies, although they have emerged as mainstays in the management of other inflammatory disorders, notably arthritis and inflammatory bowel disease.

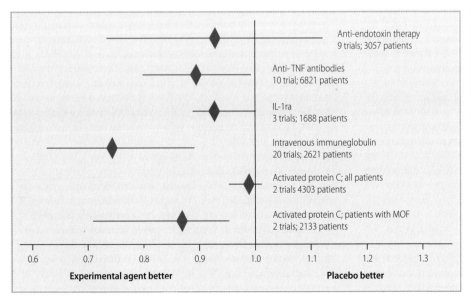

Figure 25.7 **Mediator-targeted therapy in sepsis (Marshall 2008).** Pooled data from studies of agents that neutralize endotoxin, tumor necrosis factor, or interleukin-1, provide exogenous immunoglobulin, or administer the endogenous anticoagulant, activated protein C, show a small but consistent signal for benefit, although for none of these has the effect been sufficiently robust that a commercial therapy is available for use.

Interleukin-1

The activity of interleukin-1 is regulated through the release of a natural occurring inhibitor, the IL-1Ra, a protein that shares homology with IL-1, and binds to the IL-1 receptor without inducing its activation. Recombinant IL-1Ra has been evaluated in three clinical trials which, in aggregate, show a 5% improvement in survival. As in the case of anti-TNF therapies, the signal was insufficient to support therapeutic approval as a therapy for sepsis, although recombinant IL-1Ra has found a role in other inflammatory disorders.

Activated protein C

Protein C is a naturally occurring anticoagulant protein synthesized by the liver, activated through its interactions with endothelial cell thrombomodulin. Once activated it functions as an anticoagulant by binding the endothelial cell protein C receptor, and exerting anti-inflammatory activity. Recombinant activated protein C (drotrecogin alpha activated) was licensed for use in severe sepsis and septic shock in 2001 on the basis of findings from the PROWESS trial which showed a significant 6.1% mortality reduction in septic patients (Bernard et al. 2001). Observational studies supported the conclusions of the PROW-ESS trial; however randomized trials in children and less ill adults failed to replicate the earlier evidence of benefit. As a result, European regulatory authorities mandated a further placebo-controlled trial of drotrecogin alpha activated in septic shock. The trial – PROWESS Shock – showed no benefit to patients receiving the agent, and the drug has been withdrawn from the market.

Corticosteroids

As pharmacological agents with broad anti-inflammatory activity, corticosteroids have a long history of use in the management of sepsis, but an inconsistent evidentiary base. The first contemporary sepsis studies evaluated high-dose methylprednisolone in sepsis, and failed to show benefit. However, observational studies suggesting that relative adrenal insufficiency was common in critically ill patients prompted evaluation of low-dose hydrocortisone, and an influential French study suggested that the use of pharmacological doses of hydrocortisone together with fludrocortisone improved survival. A subsequent trial reported that steroid use could hasten the resolution of shock without altering survival, and the role of corticosteroids remains controversial. Systematic reviews of the available data do show benefit, and our approach is to consider the use of hydrocortisone in the treatment of vasopressor-dependent hypotension, continuing treatment if the shock resolves, but terminating it if there is no apparent effect.

Intravenous immunoglobulin

A number of small clinical trials of intravenous immunoglobulin have suggested efficacy in treating sepsis and, when these are aggregated in a meta-analysis, the signal for benefit is strong. The quality of these studies is variable, and the evaluation of intravenous immunoglobulin in large and well-designed trials is needed.

Other approaches and the failure of sepsis trials

A variety of other strategies has been evaluated including: Recombinant anticoagulant proteins such as antithrombin, tissue factor pathway inhibitor, and soluble thrombomodulin; agents that block the interaction of PAF with its receptor or accelerate its degradation; recombinant lactoferrin; inhibitors of NOS; and ibuprofen. Each has shown promise in pre-clinical models, but failed in sepsis trials. The reasons for this ongoing lack of connection are many (Marshall 2008).

The entry criteria for sepsis trials have been the so-called sepsis syndrome or a variant, first developed almost 30 years ago for the first large trial of methylprednisolone in sepsis. The criteria are non-specific, and identify a highly heterogeneous population of patients who do not share common sites, bacteriology, or patterns of circulating endogenous mediators. The same criteria are used despite the fact that the targets are biologically diverse; studies are conducted without confirming that the target of intervention is present, or that intervention alters target levels or improves physiological parameters. The dose and duration of therapy are typically established in an arbitrary manner, rather than titrated to a response, and some of the agents tested have ultimately proven to be biologically inactive. A fundamental rethink of the approach to sepsis research is needed, and this may lead to a re-evaluation of strategies that have previously failed.

CONCLUSIONS

Sepsis is an enormously complex process both biologically and conceptually. The inflammatory response is effected though the coordinated interaction of literally hundreds of distinct host-derived molecules. These are expressed at low levels, and exert their most potent activities locally in the microenvironment of a contained insult. Moreover their activities are redundant. Remarkably, manipulation of any of more than three dozen of these before challenge will protect a mouse against a lethal endotoxin challenge (**Box 25.4**) (Marshall 2003); conversely, it would seem implausible that neutralization of any single mediator after challenge might alter outcome. Moreover it is unclear when these mediator responses are a host adaptation and therefore when they are beneficial and not an independent threat.

The conceptual challenges of sepsis rival the biological challenges. Microorganisms normally colonize the multicellular host, and contribute symbiotically to health. Although the endogenous flora can cause

---

Box 25.4 Mediators, the manipulation of which improves survival in murine endotoxemia (adapted from Marshall 2003).

Cytokines
- **Neutralization of:** IL-1, IL-12, IL-18, IL-31, IL-33, TNF, IFNα, TGFβ, LIF, MIF, G-CSF, HMGB-1, MIP-1α, MFP-14, LBP, PTH-RP
- **Administration of:** IL-1Ra, IL-4, IL-10, IL-13, IFNα, HGF, LIF, CRP, MCP-1, BPI, CAP18, TSG-14, VLDL, VIP, C3, C4, melatonin

Receptors
- **Inhibition of:** TNF receptor, p55, IL-1R, PAF receptor, LECAM-1, TREM-1, LDL receptor, CD11a, CD14
- **Activation of:** VIP receptor, adenosine A3 receptor

Non-proteins
- **Neutralization of:** PAF, PLA2
- **Administration of:** Vitamin B12, vitamin D3

Signal transduction
- **Inhibition of:** hck, COX-2, p38, jnk, NF-kB, iNOS, caspase-3
- **Activation of:** Stat4, Stat6, IκB, HSP70, hemoxygenase

Coagulation factors
- **Inhibition of:** PAI-1, tissue factor
- **Administration of:** TFPI, APC

infection, indiscriminate eradication of this flora can predispose to bacterial translocation, superinfection, and antimicrobial resistance. Endotoxin may be better considered an endogenous hormone than an exogenous toxin (Marshall 2005). Moreover endotoxin is commonly present in patients who do not meet conventional criteria for sepsis, and absent in those who do. Finally, the clinical syndrome is driven not only by host–microbial interactions, but also by the consequences of clinical intervention. Normalization of physiology does not neces-sarily result in improved clinical outcomes. Clearly, advanced staging systems of sepsis and MODS are necessary.

These challenges notwithstanding, however, results from the Surviving Sepsis Campaign have shown that adequate resuscitation, early treatment with antibiotics, appropriate source control, and optimal ICU support can improve survival by up to 6% (Levy et al. 2010). Attention to basic principles of surgery and infection control remains the mainstay of management.

■ REFERENCES

Alverdy JC, Laughlin RS, Wu L. Influence of the critically ill state on host-pathogen interactions within the intestine: gut-derived sepsis redefined. *Crit Care Med* 2003;**31**:598–607.

Andersen SK, Gjedsted J, Christiansen C, Tønnesen E. The roles of insulin and hyperglycemia in sepsis pathogenesis. *J Leukoc Biol* 2004;**75**:413–21.

Annane D, Sebille V, Troche G, et al. A 3-level prognostic classification in septic shock based on cortisol levels and cortisol response to corticotropin. *JAMA* 2000;**2834**:1038–45.

Annane D, Sebille V, Charpentier C, et al. Effect of treatment with low doses of hydrocortisone and fludrocortisone on mortality in patients with septic shock. *JAMA* 2002;**288**:862–71.

Angus DC, Linde-Zwirble WT, Lidicker J, et al. Epidemiology of severe sepsis in the United States: Analysis of incidence, outcome, and associated costs of care. *Crit Care Med* 2001;**29**:1303–10.

Ashbaugh DG, Bigelow DB, Petty TL, Levine BE. Acute respiratory distress in adults. *Lancet* 1967;**ii**:319–23.

Baue AE. Multiple, progressive, or sequential systems failure. A syndrome of the 1970s. *Arch Surg* 1975, **110**:779–81.

Bell RC, Coalson JJ, Smith JD, Johanson WG. Multiple organ system failure and infection in adult respiratory distress syndrome. *Ann Intern Med* 1983;**99**:293–8.

Bellomo R, Ronco C, Kellum JA et al. Acute renal failure – definition, outcome measures, animal models, fluid therapy and information technology needs: the Second International Consensus Conference of the Acute Dialysis Quality Initiative (ADQI) Group. *Crit Care* 2004;**8**:R204-R212.

Bernard GR, Vincent J-L, Laterre PF, et al. Efficacy and safety of recombinant human activated protein C for severe sepsis. *N Engl J Med* 2001;**344**:699–709.

Bone RC, Balk RA, Cerra FB, et al. ACCP/SCCM CONSENSUS CONFERENCE. Definitions for sepsis and organ failure and guidelines for the use of innovative therapies in sepsis. *Chest* 1992;**101**:1644–55.

Bougle A, Duranteau J. Pathophysiology of sepsis-induced acute kidney injury: the role of global renal blood flow and renal vascular resistance. *Contrib Nephrol* 2011;**174**:89–97.

Boyd JH, Forbes J, Nakada TA, et al. Fluid resuscitation in septic shock: a positive fluid balance and elevated central venous pressure are associated with increased mortality. *Crit Care Med* 2011;**39**:259–265.

Brower RG, Matthay MA, Morris A, et al. Ventilation with lower tidal volumes as compared with traditional tidal volumes for acute lung injury and the acute respiratory distress syndrome. *N Engl J Med* 2000;**342**:1301–8.

Brun-Buisson C, Meshaka P, Pinton P, Vallet B. EPISEPSIS: a reappraisal of the epidemiology and outcome of severe sepsis in French intensive care units. *Intensive Care Med* 2004;**30**:580–8.

Brunkhorst FM, Engel C, Bloos F, et al. Intensive insulin therapy and pentastarch resuscitation in severe sepsis. *N Engl J Med* 2008;**358**:125–39.

Casaer MP, Mesotten D, Hermans G, et al. Early versus late parenteral nutrition in critically ill adults. *N Engl J Med* 2011;**365**:506–17.

Calvano SE, Xiao W, Richards DR, et al. A network-based analysis of systemic inflammation in humans. *Nature* 2005, **437**:1032–7.

Christou NV, Meakins JL, Gordon J, et al. The delayed hypersensitivity response and host resistance in surgical patients - 20 years later. *Ann Surg* 1995;**222**:534–48.

Cook DJ, Guyatt GH, Marshall JC, et al. A randomized trial of sucralfate versus ranitidine for stress ulcer prophylaxis in critically ill patients. *N Engl J Med* 1998;**338**:791–7.

De BD, Aldecoa C, Njimi H, Vincent JL. Dopamine versus norepinephrine in the treatment of septic shock: a meta-analysis. *Crit Care Med* 2012;**40**:725–30.

Dellinger RP. Cardiovascular management of septic shock. *Crit Care Med* 2003;**31**:946–55.

Dellinger RP, Levy MM, Carlet JM, et al. Surviving Sepsis Campaign: international guidelines for management of severe sepsis and septic shock: 2008. *Crit Care Med* 2008;**36**:296–327.

Derde S, Hermans G, Derese I, et al. Muscle atrophy and preferential loss of myosin in prolonged critically ill patients. *Crit Care Med* 2012;**40**:79–89.

Dodek P, Keenan S, Cook D, et al. Evidence-based clinical practice guideline for the prevention of ventilator-associated pneumonia. *Ann Intern Med* 2004;**141**:305–13.

Dubos RJ, Schaedler RW. The effect of the intestinal flora on the growth rate of mice, and their susceptibility to experimental infections. *J Exp Med* 1960;**111**:407–17.

Ferrer M, Sellares J, Valencia M, et al. Non-invasive ventilation after extubation in hypercapnic patients with chronic respiratory disorders: randomised controlled trial. *Lancet* 2009;**374**:1082–8.

Finfer S, Bellomo R, Lipman J, et al. Adult-population incidence of severe sepsis in Australian and New Zealand intensive care units. *Intensive Care Med* 2004a;**30**:589–96.

Finfer S, Bellomo R, Boyce N, et al. A comparison of albumin and saline for fluid resuscitation in the intensive care unit. *N Engl J Med* 2004b;**350**:2247–56.

Finfer S, Chittock DR, Su SY, et al. Intensive versus conventional glucose control in critically ill patients. *N Engl J Med* 2009;**360**:1283–97.

Fry DE, Pearlstein L, Fulton RL, Polk HC. Multiple system organ failure. The role of uncontrolled infection. *Arch Surg* 1980;**115**:136–40.

Gabay C, Kushner I. Acute-phase proteins and other systemic responses to inflammation. *N Engl J Med* 1999;**340**:448–54.

Gattinoni L, Brazzi L, Pelosi P, et al. A trial of goal-oriented hemodynamic therapy in critically ill patients. *N Engl J Med* 1995;**333**:1025–32.

Goldenberg NM, Steinberg BE, Slutsky AS, Lee WL. Broken barriers: a new take on sepsis pathogenesis. *Sci Transl Med* 2011;**3**:88ps25.

Goodman S, Weiss Y, Weissman C. Update on cardiac arrhythmias in the ICU. *Curr Opin Crit Care* 2008;**14**:549–54.

Havasi A, Borkan SC. Apoptosis and acute kidney injury. *Kidney Int* 2011;**80**:29–40.

Hayes MA, Timmins AC, Yau EHS, et al. Elevation of systemic oxygen delivery in the treatment of critically ill patients. *N Engl J Med* 1994;**330**:1717–22.

Hebert PC, Wells G, Blajchman MA, et al. A multicentre randomized controlled clinical trial of transfusion requirements in critical care. *N Engl J Med* 1999;**340**:409–17.

Herridge MS, Cheung AM, Tansey CM, et al. One-year outcomes in survivors of the acute respiratory distress syndrome. *N Engl J Med* 2003;**348**:683–93.

Herridge MS, Tansey CM, Matte A, et al. Functional disability 5 years after acute respiratory distress syndrome. *N Engl J Med* 2011;**364**:1293–304.

Hotchkiss RS, Karl IE. The pathophysiology and treatment of sepsis. *N Engl J Med* 2003;**348**:238–50.

Hui P, Cook DJ, Lim W, et al. The frequency and clinical significance of thrombocytopenia complicating critical illness: a systematic review. *Chest* 2011;**139**:271–8.

Imai Y, Parodo J, Kajikawa O, et al. Injurious mechanical ventilation and end-organ epithelial cell apoptosis and organ dysfunction in an experimental model of acute respiratory distress syndrome. *JAMA* 2003;**289**:2104–12.

Jimenez MF, Watson RWG, Parodo J, et al. Dysregulated expression of neutrophil apoptosis in the systemic inflammatory response syndrome (SIRS). *Arch Surg* 1997;**132**:1263–70.

Kress JP, Pohlman AS, O'Connor MF, Hall JB. Daily interruption of sedative infusions in critically ill patients undergoing mechanical ventilation. *N Engl J Med* 2000;**342**:1471–7.

Kumar A, Roberts D, Wood KE, et al. Duration of hypotension before initiation of effective antimicrobial therapy is the critical determinant of survival in human septic shock. *Crit Care Med* 2006;**34**:1589–96.

Lee A. Neglected niches. The microbial ecology of the gastrointestinal tract. *Adv Microbial Ecol* 1985;**8**:115–62.

Le Gall JR, Klar J, Lemeshow S, et al. The logistic organ dysfunction system – A new way to assess organ dysfunction in the intensive care unit. *JAMA* 1996;**276**:802–10.

Levy MM, Fink M, Marshall JC, et al. 2001 SCCM/ESICM/ACCP/ATS/SIS international sepsis definitions conference. *Crit Care Med* 2003;**34**:1250–6.

Levy MM, Dellinger RP, Townsend SR, et al. The Surviving Sepsis Campaign: results of an international guideline-based performance improvement program targeting severe sepsis. *Crit Care Med* 2010;**38**:367–74.

Ley RE, Peterson DA, Gordon JI. Ecological and evolutionary forces shaping microbial diversity in the human intestine. *Cell* 2006;**124**:837–48.

Majno G. The ancient riddle of (Sepsis). *J Infect Dis* 1991;**163**:937–45.

Marshall JC. A scoring system for the multiple organ dysfunction syndrome (MODS). In: *Sepsis: Current perspectives in pathophysiology and therapy.* Berlin: Springer-Verlag, 1993: 38–49.

Marshall JC. Inflammation, coagulopathy, and the pathogenesis of the multiple organ dysfunction syndrome. *Crit Care Med* 2001;**29**(suppl):S106.

Marshall JC. Such stuff as dreams are made on: Mediator-targeted therapy in sepsis. *Nature Rev Drug Disc* 2003;**2**:391–405.

Marshall JC. Lipopolysaccharide: an endotoxin or an exogenous hormone? *Clin Infect Dis* 2005;**41**:S470–80.

Marshall JC. Sepsis: Rethinking the approach to clinical research. *J Leukoc Biol* 2008;**83**:471–82.

Marshall JC. Critical illness is an iatrogenic disorder. *Crit Care Med* 2010;**38**:S582–9.

Marshall JC, Christou NV, Meakins JL. The gastrointestinal tract. The "undrained abscess" of multiple organ failure. *Ann Surg* 1993;**218**:111–19.

Marshall JC, Cook DJ, Christou NV, et al. Multiple organ dysfunction score: A reliable descriptor of a complex clinical outcome. *Crit Care Med* 1995;**23**:1638–52.

Marshall JC, Foster D, Vincent J-L, et al. Diagnostic and prognostic implications of endotoxemia in critical illness: Results of the MEDIC study. *J Infect Dis* 2004a;**190**:527–34.

Marshall JC, Maier RV, Jimenez M, Dellinger EP. Source control in the management of severe sepsis and septic shock: an evidence-based review. *Crit Care Med* 2004b;**32**:S513–26.

Marshall JC, Charbonney E, Gonzalez PD. The immune system in critical illness. *Clin Chest Med* 2008;**29**:605–16, vii.

Martin GS, Mannino DM, Eaton S, Moss M. The epidemiology of sepsis in the United States from 1979 through 2000. *N Engl J Med* 2003;**348**:1546–54.

Martin GS, Moss M, Wheeler AP, et al. A randomized, controlled trial of furosemide with or without albumin in hypoproteinemic patients with acute lung injury. *Crit Care Med* 2005;**33**:1681–7.

Meade MO, Cook DJ, Guyatt GH, et al. Ventilation strategy using low tidal volumes, recruitment maneuvers, and high positive end-expiratory pressure for acute lung injury and acute respiratory distress syndrome: a randomized controlled trial. *JAMA* 2008;**299**:637–45.

Menon K, Ward RE, Lawson ML, et al. A prospective multicenter study of adrenal function in critically ill children. *Am J Respir Crit Care Med* 2010;**182**:246–51.

Michalek SM, Moore RN, McGhee JR, et al. The primary role of lymphoreticular cells in the mediation of host responses to bacterial endotoxin. *J Infect Dis* 1980;**141**:55–63.

Nathens AB, Marshall JC. Selective decontamination of the digestive tract in surgical patients. *Arch Surg* 1999;**134**:170–6.

National Heart, Lung, and Blood Institute Acute Respiratory Distress Syndrome (ARDS) Clinical Trials Network. Comparison of two fluid-management strategies in acute lung injury. *N Engl J Med* 2006;**354**:2564–75.

Polito A, Sonneville R, Guidoux C, et al. Changes in CRH and ACTH synthesis during experimental and human septic shock. *PLoS One* 2011;**6**:e25905.

Polk HC, Shields CL. Remote organ failure: a valid sign of occult intraabdominal infection. *Surgery* 1977;**81**:310–13.

Prowle JR, Echeverri JE, Ligabo EV, et al. Fluid balance and acute kidney injury. *Nat Rev Nephrol* 2010;**6**:107–15.

Riker RR, Shehabi Y, Bokesch PM, et al. Dexmedetomidine vs midazolam for sedation of critically ill patients: a randomized trial. *JAMA* 2009;**301**:489–99.

Rivers E, Nguyen B, Havstad S, et al. Early goal-directed therapy in the treatment of severe sepsis and septic shock. *N Engl J Med* 2001;**345**:1368–77.

Russell JA, Walley KR, Singer J, et al. Vasopressin versus norepinephrine infusion in patients with septic shock. *N Engl J Med* 2008;**358**:877–87.

Schweickert WD, Pohlman MC, Pohlman AS, et al. Early physical and occupational therapy in mechanically ventilated, critically ill patients: a randomised controlled trial. *Lancet* 2009;**373**:1874–82.

Shimizu K, Ogura H, Goto M, et al. Altered gut flora and environment in patients with severe SIRS. *J Trauma* 2006;**60**:126–33.

Sprung CL, Annane D, Keh D, et al. Hydrocortisone therapy for patients with septic shock. *N Engl J Med* 2008;**358**:111–24.

Sud S, Sud M, Friedrich JO. High frequency oscillation in patients with acute lung injury and acute respiratory distress syndrome (ARDS): systematic review and meta-analysis. *BMJ* 2010;**340**:2327.

Sweet FA, Williams MD. *Stedman's Medical Dictionary*, 22nd edn. Baltimore, MA: Williams & Wilkins, 1972.

Van den Berghe G, Wouters P, Weekers F, et al. Intensive insulin therapy in the surgical intensive care unit. *N Engl J Med* 2001;**345**:1359–67.

van der Poll T, de Boer JD, Levi M. The effect of inflammation on coagulation and vice versa. *Curr Opin Infect Dis* 2011;**24**:273–8.

Vanhorebeek I, Langouche L, Van den Berghe G. Endocrine aspects of acute and prolonged critical illness. *Nat Clin Pract Endocrinol Metab* 2006;**2**:20–31.

Vasilevskis EE, Ely EW, Speroff T, et al. Reducing iatrogenic risks: ICU-acquired delirium and weakness--crossing the quality chasm. *Chest* 2010;**138**:1224–33.

Vincent JL. Dear SIRS, I'm sorry to say that I don't like you. *Crit Care Med* 1997;**25**:372–4.

Vincent J-L, Moreno R, Takala J, et al. The SOFA (sepsis-related organ failure assessment) score to describe organ dysfunnction/failure. *Intensive Care Med* 1996;**22**:707–10.

Xu J, Gordon JI. Inaugural Article: Honor thy symbionts. *Proc Natl Acad Sci U S A* 2003;**100**:10452–9.

Zakrison T, Nascimento BAJr, Tremblay LN et al. Perioperative vasopressors are associated with an increased risk of gastrointestinal anastomotic leakage. *World J Surg* 2007;**31**:1627–34.

Index

Note: Page numbers in **bold** or *italic* refer to tables or figures respectively.